CRITICAL CARE SECRETS

Polly E. Parsons, M.D.
Assistant Professor of Medicine
University of Colorado School of Medicine
Staff, Division of Pulmonary Medicine
Denver General Hospital
Denver, Colorado

Jeanine P. Wiener-Kronish, M.D.
Associate Professor of Anesthesia and Medicine
Associate, Cardiovascular Research Institute
University of California, San Francisco,
   School of Medicine
San Francisco, California

HANLEY & BELFUS, INC./Philadelphia
MOSBY – YEAR BOOK, INC./St. Louis • Baltimore • Boston • Chicago • London
   Philadelphia • Sydney • Toronto

Publisher: HANLEY & BELFUS, INC.
                  210 S. 13th Street
                  Philadelphia, PA 19107
                  (215) 546-7293

North American and worldwide sales and distribution:

                  MOSBY–YEAR BOOK, INC.
                  11830 Westline Industrial Drive
                  St. Louis, MO 63146

In Canada: MOSBY–YEAR BOOK, INC.
                  5240 Finch Avenue East
                  Unit 1
                  Scarborough, Ontario M1S 5A2
                  Canada

CRITICAL CARE SECRETS

ISBN 1-56053-015-4

Library of Congress catalog card number 92-70041

Last digit is the print number: 9   8   7   6   5   4   3   2

CONTENTS

CONTRIBUTORS

Charles M. Abernathy, M.D.
Professor of Surgery, University of Colorado School of Medicine; Associate Director of Surgery, Denver General Hospital, Denver, Colorado

Olivia Vynn Adair, M.D.
Assistant Professor, Department of Medicine, Cardiology Division, University of Colorado School of Medicine; Director of Coronary Care Unit and of Non-Invasive Cardiology Unit, Denver General Hospital, Denver, Colorado

Elizabeth L. Aronsen, M.D.
Pulmonary Fellow, Department of Medicine, University of Colorado School of Medicine, Denver, Colorado

Suzanne Z. Barkin, M.D.
Assistant Professor, Department of Radiology, University of Colorado School of Medicine; Staff Radiologist, Denver General Hospital, Denver, Colorado

Tomas Berl, M.D.
Professor of Medicine, University of Colorado School of Medicine, Denver, Colorado

Daniel H. Bessesen, M.D.
Assistant Professor of Medicine, Division of Endocrinology, University of Colorado School of Medicine, Denver General Hospital, Denver, Colorado

Mary Bessesen, M.D.
Instructor of Internal Medicine, University of Colorado School of Medicine; Attending Physician, Denver General Hospital, Denver, Colorado

Robert A. Bethel, M.D.
Associate Professor of Medicine, University of Colorado School of Medicine; Associate Faculty Member, National Jewish Center for Immunology and Respiratory Medicine, Denver, Colorado

Raymond N. Blum, M.D.
Assistant Clinical Professor, Division of Infectious Disease, Department of Medicine, University of Colorado School of Medicine; Denver General Hospital, Denver, Colorado

Mark W. Bowyer, M.D.
Staff General Surgeon and Co-Director of Surgical Intensive Care Unit, Department of Surgery, David Grant USAF Medical Center, Travis Air Force Base, California

Charles B. Cairns, M.D.
Assistant Professor of Surgery, Division of Emergency Medicine, University of Colorado School of Medicine; Attending Physician, University of Colorado Health Sciences Center, Denver, Colorado

Anthony C. Campagna, M.D.
Senior Fellow, Pulmonary and Critical Care Medicine, University of California at San Francisco, School of Medicine, San Francisco, California

E. Michael Canham, M.D.
Assistant Clinical Professor of Medicine, University of Colorado School of Medicine, Denver; Chairman, Department of Medicine, Aurora Presbyterian Hospital, Aurora, Colorado

Stephen V. Cantrill, M.D.
Associate Director, Emergency Medical Service, Denver General Hospital, Denver, Colorado

Edmund Casper, M.D.
Associate Professor of Psychiatry, and Director, Alcohol, Drugs and Psychiatric Service, University of Colorado School of Medicine, Department of Health and Hospitals, and Denver General Hospital, Denver, Colorado

Arlene B. Chapman, M.D.
Assistant Professor of Medicine, University of Colorado School of Medicine, University Hospital and Denver General Hospital, Denver, Colorado

Robert Mitchell Claytor, III, R.N. B.S.N
Clinical Nurse III, University of California, San Francisco, Medical Center, San Francisco, California

Robert M. Cook, M.D.
Senior Pulmonary Fellow, Department of Medicine, University of Colorado School of Medicine, Denver, Colorado

Georgia H. Couderc, R.N., B.S.N.
Head Nurse, Intensive Care Unit, University of California, San Francisco, Medical Center, San Francisco, California

Jeffrey S. Cross, M.D.
Chief Resident, Department of Surgery, University of Colorado School of Medicine, Denver, Colorado

Ira M. Dauber, M.D.
Clinical Assistant Professor of Medicine, University of Colorado School of Medicine, Denver, Colorado

Julie Ann Dearwater, R.N., B.S.N.
Clinical Nurse III, Intensive Care Unit, University of California, San Francisco, Medical Center, San Francisco, California

Teresa A. DeLong, R.N., M.S.
Intensive Care Unit, University of California, San Francisco, Medical Center, San Francisco, California

Julia A. Drose, B.A., R.D.M.S., R.D.C.S.
Instructor, Department of Radiology, Division of Diagnostic Ultrasound, University of Colorado School of Medicine; Chief Sonographer, University of Colorado Health Sciences Center, Denver, Colorado

Richard T. Ellison, III, M.D.
Clinical Director of Infectious Diseases and Associate Professor of Medicine, University of Massachusetts Medical School, Worcester, Massachusetts

Enrique Fernandez, M.D.
Associate Professor, Division of Pulmonary Sciences, Department of Medicine, University of Colorado School of Medicine, and National Jewish Center for Immunology and Respiratory Medicine, Denver, Colorado

Christina Finlayson, M.D.
Resident in Surgery, University of Colorado School of Medicine, Denver, Colorado

Mark W. Geraci, M.D.
Fellow, Division of Pulmonary Sciences, Department of Medicine, University of Colorado School of Medicine, Denver, Colorado

Carlos E. Girod, M.D.
Fellow, Division of Pulmonary Sciences, Department of Medicine, University of Colorado School of Medicine, Denver, Colorado

Connie Glavis, M.S., R.N., CCRN
Assistant Clinical Professor, Department of Physiological Nursing, University of California, San Francisco, School of Medicine; Clinical Nurse Specialist, Adult Critical Care, University of California, San Francisco, Medical Center, San Francisco, California

David M. Guidot, M.D.
Instructor, Division of Pulmonary Sciences, Department of Medicine, University of Colorado School of Medicine, Denver, Colorado

James B. Haenel, R.R.T.
Clinical Instructor in Surgery and Director of Respiratory Therapy, University of Colorado School of Medicine and Denver General Hospital, Denver, Colorado

Michael E. Hanley, M.D.
Assistant Professor of Medicine, University of Colorado School of Medicine, Denver General Hospital, Denver, Colorado

Alan S. Hanson, M.D.
Renal Fellow, Department of Medicine, University of Colorado School of Medicine, Denver, Colorado

Diane M. Hartman, M.D.
Resident in Genitourologic Surgery, University of Colorado School of Medicine, Denver, Colorado

Kathryn L. Hassell, M.D.
Instructor, Division of Hematology, Department of Medicine, University of Colorado School of Medicine, Denver, Colorado

John E. Heffner, M.D.
Director of Medical Critical Care, Department of Medicine, St. Joseph's Hospital and Medical Center, Phoenix, Arizona

Marsha J. Heinig, M.D., Ph.D.
Assistant Professor of Radiology, University of Colorado School of Medicine; Staff Radiologist, Denver General Hospital, Denver, Colorado

Richard L. Hock, M.D.
Instructor and Staff Physician, Ambulatory Care/Internal Medicine, University of Colorado School of Medicine and Denver Veteran Affairs Medical Center, Denver, Colorado

Fred D. Hofeldt, M.D.
Professor of Medicine, University of Colorado School of Medicine; Director of Medicine, and Chief, Endocrine Division, Denver General Hospital, Denver, Colorado

James L. Jacobson, M.D.
Clinical Assistant Professor, Department of Psychiatry, University of Colorado School of Medicine, Denver, Colorado

Michael R. Johnston, M.D.
Head, Division of Thoracic Surgery, Mount Sinai Hospital, Toronto, Ontario, Canada

Susan L. Kelley, M.D.
Director of Clinical Cancer Research, Bristol-Myers Squibb Pharmaceutical Research Institute, Wallingford, Connecticut; Clinical Assistant Professor of Medicine, Yale University School of Medicine, New Haven, Connecticut

Brian J. Kelly, M.D.
Head, Neuroscience Intensive Care Unit, National Naval Medical Center, Bethesda; Assistant Professor of Neurology, Uniformed Services University of the Health Sciences, Bethesda; National Naval Medical Center, Bethesda, Maryland

Joyce S. Kobayashi, M.D.
Associate Professor, Department of Psychiatry, University of Colorado School of
Medicine; Director, Neuropsychiatric Clinic and Psychiatric Consultation Services,
Denver General Hospital, Denver, Colorado

Ken Kulig, M.D.
Assistant Professor of Surgery, Division of Emergency Medicine, University of Colorado
School of Medicine, Denver, Colorado

Susan M. Lehr, R.N., B.S.N, CCRN
Clinical Nurse III, University of California, San Francisco, Medical Center, San
Francisco, California

Stuart L. Linas, M.D.
Professor of Medicine, University of Colorado School of Medicine, Denver General
Hospital, Denver, Colorado

Steven R. Lowenstein, M.D., M.P.H.
Associate Professor of Medicine, Surgery, and Preventive Medicine and Biometrics,
Department of Surgery, Division of Emergency Medicine, University of Colorado School
of Medicine; Associate Director, Department of Emergency Medicine, University of
Colorado Health Sciences Center, Denver, Colorado

Vincent J. Markovchick, M.D., FACEP
Associate Professor of Surgery, Division of Emergency Medicine, University of Colorado
School of Medicine; Director of Emergency Medical Services, Denver General Hospital;
Program Director, Denver Affiliated Residency in Emergency Medicine, Denver,
Colorado

John A. Marx, M.D.
Chairman, Department of Emergency Medicine, Carolinas Medical Center, Charlotte;
Clinical Professor, Department of Emergency Medicine, University of North Carolina at
Chapel Hill, School of Medicine, Chapel Hill, North Carolina

Susan R. Mason, M.D.
Private Practice, Infectious Diseases; Active Staff, St. Anthony's Hospital, Lutheran
Medical Center, Humana Hospital Mountain View, Denver, Colorado

Michael T. McDermott, M.D.
Staff Internist/Endocrinologist, Fitzsimmons Army Medical Center, Aurora; Denver
General Hospital, University of Colorado Health Sciences Center, Denver, Colorado

Mari McQuitty, R.N.
Clinical Nurse III, Intensive Care Unit, University of California, San Francisco, Medical
Center, San Francisco, California

Philip S. Mehler, M.D.
Clinical Assistant Professor of Medicine, University of Colorado School of Medicine;
Director of Internal Medicine, Columbine Hospital, Denver, Colorado

York E. Miller, M.D.
Associate Professor of Medicine, University of Colorado School of Medicine, Denver,
Colorado

Ernest E. Moore, M.D.
Professor and Vice Chairman of Surgery, University of Colorado School of Medicine;
Chief of Surgery, Denver General Hospital, Denver, Colorado

Frederick A. Moore, M.D.
Assistant Professor of Surgery, University of Colorado School of Medicine; Chief,
Surgical Critical Care, Denver General Hospital, Colorado

Sue Anne Murahata, M.D.
Private Practice, Denver, Colorado

Thomas A. Neff, M.D.
Professor of Medicine, University of Colorado School of Medicine; Head, Pulmonary Service, Denver General Hospital, Denver, Colorado

Dorre K. Nicholau, M.D., Ph.D.
Department of Anesthesia, University of California, San Francisco, School of Medicine, San Francisco, California

Polly E. Parsons, M.D.
Assistant Professor, Division of Pulmonary Sciences, Department of Medicine, University of Colorado School of Medicine; Staff, Pulmonary Division, Denver General Hospital, Denver, Colorado

Richard A. Peters, M.D.
Director, Surgical Intensive Care Unit, and Chief of Thoracic Surgery, David Grant USAF Medical Center, Travis Air Force Base, California

Jean-François Pittet, M.D.
Cardiovascular Research Institute, University of California, San Francisco, School of Medicine, San Francisco, California

Peter T. Pons, M.D.
Assistant Professor of Emergency Medicine, Department of Surgery, University of Colorado School of Medicine; Associate Director, Emergency Department, Denver General Hospital, Denver, Colorado

Thomas Rehring, M.D.
Resident in Surgery, Denver General Hospital, Denver, Colorado

Randall R. Reves, M.D., M.Sc.
Associate Professor of Medicine, Division of Infectious Disease, University of Colorado School of Medicine; Staff Physician, and Chairman, Infection Control Committee, Denver General Hospital, Denver, Colorado

Jonathan Ritvo, M.D.
Advanced Physician Specialist, Alcohol, Drug and Psychiatric Service, Denver Health and Hospitals; Department of Psychiatry, University of Colorado School of Medicine, Denver, Colorado

John W. Schaefer, M.D.
Professor of Medicine, University of Colorado School of Medicine; Chief of Gastroenterology, Denver General Hospital, Denver, Colorado

Hildegarde M. Schell, R.N., B.S.N.
Clinical Nurse, University of California, San Francisco, Medical Center, San Francisco, California

Jeffrey R. Schelling, M.D.
Instructor, Department of Medicine, University of Colorado School of Medicine, Denver, Colorado

Lynn M. Schnapp, M.D.
Pulmonary and Critical Care Fellow, Cardiovascular Research Institute, University of California, San Francisco, School of Medicine, San Francisco, California

David E. Schwartz, M.D.
Assistant Clinical Professor of Anesthesia and Medicine, Departments of Anesthesia and Medicine, University of California, San Francisco, School of Medicine, San Francisco, California

Marvin I. Schwarz, M.D.
Professor of Medicine, and Head, Division of Pulmonary Sciences, University of Colorado School of Medicine; University Hospital, National Jewish Center for Immunology and Respiratory Medicine, Denver General Hospital, Denver, Colorado

Stuart I. Senkfor, M.D.
Renal Fellow, Department of Medicine, University of Colorado School of Medicine, Denver, Colorado

Joseph I. Shapiro, M.D.
Assistant Professor of Medicine and Radiology, University of Colorado School of Medicine, Denver, Colorado

Thomas J. Stelzner, M.D.
Assistant Professor of Medicine, Division of Pulmonary Sciences, University of Colorado School of Medicine, Denver, Colorado

Nancy L. Szaflarski, R.N., M.S., CCRN, FCCM
Doctoral Student in Critical Care, Department of Physiological Nursing, University of California, San Francisco, San Francisco, California

Marshall R. Thomas, M.D.
Assistant Clinical Professor, Department of Psychiatry, University of Colorado School of Medicine, Denver, Colorado

Christopher L. Tyler, M.D.
Fellow in Pulmonary Medicine, Cardiovascular Research Institute, University of California, San Francisco, School of Medicine, San Francisco, California

Carolyn H. Welsh, M.D.
Associate Professor of Medicine, Division of Pulmonary Sciences, University of Colorado School of Medicine, Denver, Colorado

Madeline J. White, M.D.
Staff Physician, Denver General Hospital, Denver, Colorado

Thomas A. Whitehill, M.D.
Lecturer in Surgery, Department of Vascular Surgery, University of Michigan School of Medicine, Ann Arbor, Michigan

Jeanine P. Wiener-Kronish, M.D.
Associate Professor of Anesthesia and Medicine, and Associate, Cardiovascular Research Institute, University of California, San Francisco, School of Medicine, San Francisco, California

Carter Willis, M.D.
Assistant Clinical Professor, Department of Anesthesia, University of California, San Francisco, School of Medicine, San Francisco, California

Eugene E. Wolfel, M.D.
Associate Professor of Medicine, Division of Cardiology, University of Colorado School of Medicine; Staff Cardiologist, University Hospital and Denver General Hospital, Denver, Colorado

Martin R. Zamora, M.D.
Assistant Professor of Medicine, Division of Pulmonary Sciences, University of Colorado School of Medicine, Denver, Colorado

PREFACE

Over the last few years, critical care medicine has emerged into an important subspecialty, encompassing major medical fields such as internal medicine, surgery, anesthesia, and emergency medicine. Although there are some aspects of critical care medicine that are unique to each branch of medicine, the fundamentals required to care for critically ill patients transcend the various subspecialties.

Critical Care Secrets is designed for house officers and medical students who are learning to care for the critically ill—whether the patients be in an intensive care unit (medical, surgical, neurosurgical), the operating room, the recovery room, or the emergency room.

Like the other books in the Secrets series, *Critical Care Secrets* is not intended to be a traditional textbook. Rather, its format consists of questions and answers designed both to provide factual information for the reader and to stimulate discussion. We hope you find the book enjoyable, readable, and useful.

Polly E. Parsons, M.D.
Jeanine Wiener-Kronish, M.D.

I: Basic Life Support

1. CARDIOPULMONARY RESUSCITATION

Charles B. Cairns, M.D., and Steven R. Lowenstein, M.D., M.P.H.

1. When is cardiopulmonary resuscitation (CPR) indicated?
A reasonable guide appeared in the first paper describing clinical experience with closed-chest CPR: "Not all dying patients should have cardiopulmonary resuscitation. . . . The cardiac arrest should be sudden and unexpected. The patient should not be in the terminal stages of a malignant or other chronic disease, and there should be some possibility of a return to a functional existence."[5]

2. What are the ABCs of resuscitation?
*A*irway, *B*reathing, and *C*irculation.

3. How should CPR be performed?
The ABCs should guide and steady the resuscitation of all critically ill patients.
1. Open the airway by performing a head tilt–chin lift or a head tilt–jaw thrust. These maneuvers cause anterior displacement of the mandible and lift the tongue and epiglottis away from the glottic opening. Tidal volumes are adequate with either maneuver. To improve airway patency, suction the mouth and oropharynx, and insert a plastic oropharyngeal airway.
2. Assist breathing by performing mouth-to-mouth, mouth-to-mask, or bag-valve-mask breathing. The recommended technique will depend on the clinical setting, the equipment available, and the rescuer's skill and training. These techniques can sustain ventilation and oxygenation indefinitely in ideal situations (e.g., the OR), but in the emergency setting they are suboptimal. Air leaks at the facemask result in inadequate lung ventilation. Furthermore, insufflation of the stomach, followed by emesis and aspiration, is an ever-present threat. To reduce these risks, deliver slow, even breaths, pausing for full deflation between breaths, and avoid excessive peak inspiratory pressures. Use the Sellick maneuver (apply digital pressure to the cricoid cartilage) to further reduce the hazard of vomiting and aspiration.
3. After opening the airway and initiating rescue breathing, check for spontaneous circulation by palpating for a carotid or femoral pulse. If the patient is pulseless, begin chest compressions. Place the heels of the hands, one atop the other, on the lower half of the sternum; avoid the ribs and the xiphoid process. Compress the chest smoothly and forcefully 80 to 100 times per minute. If there are two rescuers, interpose one artificial breath after every five chest compressions. If only one rescuer is available, the recommended sequence is 15 compressions followed by 2 breaths.

4. Are there any exceptions to the rule of the ABCs?
Yes. (1) When a patient in a monitored setting experiences sudden ventricular tachycardia or ventricular fibrillation, the first priority is electrical defibrillation. Never delay defibrillation to perform airway opening, endotrachial intubation, or CPR. (2) In traumatic cardiac arrest, closed-chest CPR is ineffective. In trauma, the etiology of the arrest may be a tension pneumothorax, cardiac tamponade, or exsanguinating hemorrhage from the thorax or abdomen. An immediate thoracotomy, not CPR, is indicated in trauma patients.

1

In significant craniofacial trauma or forceful deceleration, a fracture or dislocation of the cervical spine may be present. When an injury to the neck is suspected, a jaw thrust (and never a head tilt) should be used to open the airway.

5. What is the mechanism of blood flow during CPR?

Two basic models explain the mechanism of blood flow during CPR. In the **cardiac pump model,** the heart is squeezed between the sternum and spine. Chest compression results in systole, and the atrioventricular valves close normally, ensuring unidirectional, antegrade flow. During the relaxation phase (diastole), intracardiac pressures fall, the valves open, and blood is drawn into the heart from the lungs and vena cavae.

In the **thoracic pump model,** the heart is considered a passive conduit. Chest compression results in uniformly increased pressures throughout the heart and thorax. Forward blood flow is achieved selectively in the arterial system, because the stiff-walled arteries (for example, the carotid) resist collapse; also, retrograde flow is prevented in the great veins by one-way valves. Aspects of both models have been substantiated in animal models, and both pumps probably contribute to blood flow during CPR.

6. Is blood flow to the brain and heart adequate during CPR?

In both models, blood flow to the brain is a function of the aortic-to-jugular venous pressure difference during systole (the compression phase of CPR). The cerebral flow measured experimentally is approximately 30% of normal. Blood flow to the heart occurs during the relaxation phase of CPR and is a function of the aortic-to-right atrial pressure difference in diastole. Unfortunately, net myocardial flow is essentially nil during closed-chest CPR, and even retrograde coronary flow has been demonstrated.

7. What is the main determinant of successful resuscitation?

The quantity of myocardial blood flow. In experimental models, this myocardial blood flow correlates with the aortic-to-right atrial pressure gradient generated during the diastolic phase of CPR. The minimal pressure gradient necessary for restoration of spontaneous circulation and successful defibrillation is 20–25 mm Hg.

8. What is the role of pharmacologic therapy during CPR?

The immediate goal of pharmacologic therapy is to improve myocardial blood flow, the key physiologic parameter conducive to the return of spontaneous circulation. Alpha-adrenergic agonists, such as epinephrine, augment the aortic-to-right atrial diastolic gradient by increasing arterial vascular tone. Although pure alpha-adrenergic agents, such as methoxamine and norepinephrine, also increase arterial pressure and myocardial blood flow, none has been shown to be superior to epinephrine.

9. What are the most common causes of cardiopulmonary arrest?

Most cardiopulmonary arrests in the hospital setting are caused by **ventricular fibrillation** (VF) or **ventricular tachycardia** (VT), which usually occur with ischemic heart disease. Yet, drug toxicity, electrolyte disturbances (hypokalemia or hypomagnesemia), and prolonged hypoxemia are also important inciting factors. A surprisingly high proportion (30–50%) of in-hospital arrests are brady-asystolic at the onset. One common cause of this rhythm is unrecognized hypoxia or acidemia. Another cause of brady-asystole is heightened vagal tone, which may be precipitated by drugs, anesthetic agents, inferoposterior myocardial infarction (Bezold-Jarisch reflex), or invasive procedures. **Electromechanical dissociation** (EMD) is the third common arrest rhythm. The most common etiology of EMD is prolonged arrest itself; typically, after 8 minutes or more of VF, electrical defibrillation is futile and induces a slow, wide-complex EMD, which is terminal and known as pulseless idioventricular rhythm. EMD may also present as an inciting, rather than a terminal, rhythm. Examples are tension pneumothorax, cardiac tamponade, exsanguination, anaphylaxis, or pulmonary embolus. These are discussed in detail below.

10. What are the most common immediately reversible causes of cardiopulmonary arrest?

The alert clinician should recognize at the bedside the following treatable causes of cardiopulmonary arrest:

1. **Hyperkalemia** is encountered in patients with renal insufficiency, diabetes, and profound acidosis, and occurs especially frequently in patients receiving beta-blocking drugs. Hyperkalemia is heralded by slow conduction (wide, slurred QRS complexes) and the absence of P waves. Treatment includes calcium chloride, sodium bicarbonate, and an insulin-glucose infusion.

2. **Anaphylaxis** causes arrest by asphyxia or shock and should be suspected whenever cardiac arrest occurs after drug administration or in the radiology suite. Rapid tracheal intubation and administration of crystalloid and epinephrine are the cornerstones of resuscitation.

3. **Cardiac tamponade** presents with hypotension, a narrowed pulse pressure, elevated jugular venous pressure, distant and muffled heart sounds, and low-voltage QRS complexes on the EKG. Trauma victims and patients with malignancies are at greatest risk. Pericardiocentesis or subxiphoid pericardiorrhaphy may be lifesaving.

4. **Tension pneumothorax** must be recognized without delay. Most often it occurs in trauma patients or in patients receiving positive-pressure ventilation (especially after subclavian venipunctures). The signs of tension pneumothorax are rapid-onset hypotension, hypoxia, and high airflow resistance. Subcutaneous emphysema and reduced breath sounds on the affected side are commonly noted.

5. **Hypovolemia** must be recognized. "Absolute" hypovolemia occurs in such settings as gastrointestinal hemorrhage or rupture of an abdominal aneurysm; "relative" hypovolemia occurs in sepsis or anaphylaxis.

6. **Torsade de pointes** is an undulating form of ventricular tachycardia characterized by rapid reversals of the polarity ("twisting of the points") on the EKG. The predisposing cause is prolongation of the QT interval, which may be congenital or induced by drugs (e.g., phenothiazines or type IA antiarrhythmic agents). Treatment includes cardioversion, followed by magnesium, isoproterenol, and rapid ventricular pacing.

7. **Toxic cardiopulmonary arrest** must also be recognized. Carbon monoxide poisoning occurs after prolonged exposure to smoke or inhalation of the exhaust from incomplete combustion. High-flow and hyperbaric oxygen, along with management of acidosis, are the cornerstones of treatment. Cyanide poisoning occurs surprisingly often, especially during fires involving synthetic materials. The antidotes are intravenous sodium nitrite and sodium thiosulfate. Tricyclic antidepressant drugs act as type IA antiarrhythmic agents and cause slowing of cardiac conduction, ventricular arrhythmias, hypotension, and seizures. Vigorous alkalinization and seizure control are required.

8. **Primary asphyxial causes of cardiac arrest** are common. In addition to anaphylaxis, obstructive asphyxia may occur after foreign body aspiration, inflammatory conditions of the hypopharynx (epiglottitis or retropharyngeal abscess), or cervicofacial trauma. The latter results in edema or hematoma formation, subcutaneous emphysema, or laryngeal or tracheal disruption.

11. How common is iatrogenic cardiopulmonary arrest?

Errors of omission and commission contribute to the incidence and poor outcome of in-hospital cardiopulmonary arrests. In a recent study[2] of 562 in-hospital arrests, a major unsuspected diagnosis was present (and proved by autopsy) in 14% of cases. The most common missed diagnoses were pulmonary embolus and bowel infarction, which together accounted for 89% of all missed conditions. As many as 15% of in-hospital arrests are probably avoidable; retrospective reviews indicate that respiratory insufficiency and hemorrhage are often undetected, and that aberrations in vital signs and patients' complaints (especially dyspnea) are frequently ignored in the hours that precede arrest.

Direct iatrogenesis may also contribute to in-hospital cardiopulmonary arrests. Almost every procedure, including gastroscopy, bronchoscopy, barium enema, carotid sinus massage, and placement of Swan-Ganz catheters, has, on occasion, caused cardiac arrest. The injudicious use of lidocaine, aminophylline, digoxin, sedative-hypnotics, and anesthetic agents may be responsible for arrests throughout the hospital.

12. How should ventricular fibrillation be treated?
The essential ingredient is **speed;** the prognosis dims (and the defibrillation success rate decreases approximately 4%) with every minute of delay. An initial defibrillation dose of 200 joules is recommended to minimize myocardial damage and to prevent the development of post-countershock pulseless bradyarrhythmias.

13. What about incessant ventricular fibrillation?
(1) Perform endotracheal intubation and ensure adequate ventilation. (2) Administer magnesium sulfate, which may be an effective antifibrillatory agent. (3) Administer epinephrine to augment aortic diastolic blood pressure and improve myocardial perfusion. (4) Administer lidocaine or procainamide. Bretylium tosylate is an alternative antidysrhythmic agent. However, neither lidocaine nor any other drug (including magnesium) has been proved to be efficacious in improving defibrillation success rates or in restoring a perfusing rhythm in patients in ventricular fibrillation.

14. Is pulseless idioventricular rhythm treatable?
Delayed electrical countershock frequently results in asystole or a pulseless idioventricular rhythm, which is often untreatable and results in death. In animal experiments, high-dose epinephrine (0.1–0.2 mg/kg) has helped to restore cardiac contractility and pacemaker activity and may improve the outcome of post-countershock brady-asystole.

15. How should asystole be treated?
Asystole should be treated according to a three-step approach:

1. Confirm the absence of cardiac activity (a flat-line electrocardiogram may be recorded because of technical mistakes). Verify the absence of pulses at the carotid or femoral artery. Check for loose or disconnected battery cables and monitor leads. Rotate the monitoring leads 90° and increase the amplitude to detect occult, fine ventricular fibrillation.

2. Atropine should be administered to counter hypervagotonia, which may accompany inferoposterior myocardial infarction, acidosis, drug or anesthetic administration, or hypoxia. The third step is to give epinephrine.

3. High-dose epinephrine (0.1–0.2 mg/kg) is recommended to treat this ominous condition.

16. Is electrical fibrillation or pacemaker therapy used for asystole?
Electrical defibrillation should be reserved for instances in which the differentiation between asystole and fine ventricular fibrillation is difficult; in these ambiguous situations, defibrillation should be employed, after administration of high-dose epinephrine. Pacemaker therapy is often attempted for asystole, but it is seldom effective in restoring a pulsatile rhythm.

17. What are the appropriate routes of administration of drugs during resuscitation?
Intravenous administration is the preferred route. If a central venous catheter is in place, then the most distal port should be used. Otherwise, use of a peripheral vein catheter will result in a slightly delayed onset of action, although the peak drug effect is similar to that

of the central route. Intracardiac administration should be reserved for cases of open cardiac massage.

A number of drugs (epinephrine, atropine, lidocaine) are absorbed systemically after endotracheal administration, yet the effectiveness of this route during CPR is suspect. Pulmonary blood flow and hence systemic absorption are minimal during CPR. Recent animal studies suggest that comparable hemodynamic responses occur only with endotracheal doses of epinephrine ten times that of the intravenous doses.

Virtually every resuscitation drug can be administered in conventional doses via the intraosseous route. This method is preferred in pediatric patients, in whom an intravenous line cannot be established rapidly.

18. What is the usual outcome of in-hospital CPR?
Most patients who receive CPR in the hospital do not survive. In fact, only 5–20% of patients live to be discharged home. Furthermore, many patients who do survive have severe impairments of independence and mental fitness; many would choose not to undergo CPR again. It is not yet possible to predict confidently the outcome of in-hospital resuscitation. In one often-cited study, prearrest azotemia, cancer, pneumonia, sepsis, and a home-bound life-style were predictors of death. In most studies that control for comorbidity and illness severity, advanced age is not an independent predictor of outcome.

19. What is a DNR order?
The do-not-resuscitate (DNR) order is an accepted means to protect the right of hospitalized patients to refuse unwanted resuscitative care, even if it is lifesaving.

20. How is the DNR decision reached?
In a chronic, progressive, and irreversible illness, especially when death is imminent and expected, the physician should give careful consideration to the possible futility of CPR. Among the factors that the physician should weigh, in close communication with the patient and family, are: reversibility of the patient's disease; imminence of death; the patient's baseline physical and mental health; and information about the patient's wishes, gathered from the patient, advance directives, or close relatives. A DNR order does not mean that other treatments, such as antibiotics, intensive care, or comfort measures, must be withheld. Although alluring, it is not possible to state with certainty for a given patient the probability of successful CPR or to define "futility" for a given diagnosis (for example, cancer, congestive heart failure, or emphysema). Therefore, the DNR decision can seldom be reached by the physician alone. In almost every case, the appropriateness and desirability of CPR must be evaluated after an open and frank discussion with the patient or his or her surrogates, after a thorough assessment of the patient's diagnosis, condition, prognosis, and treatment options, and with primacy and respect given to the patient's expressed wishes if they are known.

CONTROVERSIES

21. Should epinephrine be given in "high" doses?
For: The conventional dose of epinephrine (0.5–1.0 mg IV every 5 minutes) was derived empirically from animal studies and then applied arbitrarily to humans. No dose-response studies were performed. The "standard" 1-mg dose of epinephrine actually reduces myocardial blood flow in experimental studies and has never been proved to be efficacious in human cardiac arrest. Recent animal experiments and human trials indicate that "high-dose" epinephrine (0.1–0.2 mg/kg) results in higher rates of restoration of spontaneous circulation compared with standard doses. These preliminary and limited clinical trials have not demonstrated any evidence of detrimental side effects.

Against: While recent human trials may have demonstrated a higher rate of return of spontaneous circulation with "high-dose" epinephrine, no trial has demonstrated improved neurologic recovery. Until a well-designed study is performed, current therapy should remain standard. This is especially true because the result of high-dose treatment may be an increased number of neurologically impaired survivors.

22. Is sodium bicarbonate indicated in routine management of cardiopulmonary arrest?

For: When cardiopulmonary arrest occurs, acidemia follows. Even if CPR is performed "correctly," tissue perfusion is suboptimal and metabolic acidosis occurs. In addition, and more importantly, alveolar hypoventilation (respiratory acidosis) occurs. Buffering is necessary to counter the pernicious effects of acidemia. A severe fall in pH interferes with the vascular and myocardial responses to adrenergic drugs and endogenous catecholamines and reduces cardiac chronotropy and inotropy. Also, acidosis leads to ventricular irritability and a lower threshold for ventricular fibrillation. Finally, below a pH of 7.2, myocardial contractile function may decline, resulting in refractory EMD. Although the primary treatment of the acidemia of cardiac arrest is adequate ventilation, metabolic acidosis often progresses inexorably. Sodium bicarbonate is the only buffer commonly available, and its use traditionally has been recommended when the pH falls to a life-threatening range, usually below 7.2. Sodium bicarbonate may be particularly useful in attenuating post-resuscitation myocardial dysfunction.

Against: The primary treatment of the acidemia of cardiac arrest is adequate ventilation, which, in clinical and animal studies, correlates with survival. The metabolic acidosis is usually unimportant in the first 15–18 minutes of resuscitation. If ventilation is maintained, the arterial pH usually remains above 7.2; moderate acidosis in this range does not interfere with defibrillation and may actually augment cardiac contractility and protect against, rather than precipitate, EMD.

Most important, sodium bicarbonate is a poor buffering agent for cardiac resuscitation. Sodium bicarbonate causes volume overload, hyperosmolarity, hypernatremia, and hyperkalemia, even when used as recommended. Iatrogenic alkalosis may cause arrhythmias, cerebral vasoconstriction, lactic acid production, and a left shift of the oxygen/hemoglobin saturation curve, further limiting tissue oxygen delivery. The bicarbonate ion, after combining with hydrogen ion, generates new carbon dioxide. Biologic membranes are highly permeable to carbon dioxide (but are much more slowly permeable to sodium bicarbonates). Therefore, administration of sodium bicarbonate causes a paradoxical intracellular acidosis. Intramyocardial hypercarbia causes a profound decline in cardiac contractile function and will lead to failure of resuscitation. Myocardial PCO_2 in human resuscitation may reach levels in excess of 250 mm Hg, further highlighting the risks of administering carbon dioxide–generating agents such as sodium bicarbonate. Within the myocardial cell, hypercapnia impairs contractility and results in refractory EMD.

Because no buffer therapy is needed in the first 15 minutes of arrest (so long as adequate lung ventilation is maintained), and since the optimal acid-base status for resuscitation has not been established, sodium bicarbonate is not recommended. Only restoration of the spontaneous circulation—not a buffering agent—can reverse the development of intramyocardial hypercarbia.

23. Is there a place for routine calcium administration during CPR?

For: Adequate levels of ionized calcium are necessary for effective cardiovascular function. In the setting of ionized hypocalcemia, administration of calcium chloride improves cardiovascular hemodynamics. Recent human and animal trials have confirmed that ionized calcium levels fall precipitously during prolonged (> 7.5 minutes) cardiac arrest. The only prospective, double-blinded study of calcium administration in cardiac arrest suggested that calcium (calcium chloride, 500–100 mg IV) may facilitate restoration of circulatory function, eespecially when the QRS complex is wide.

Against: Calcium overload is thought to play an important role in ischemic and reperfusion cell injury, and increases in intracellular calcium are associated with cell death. There is no evidence that calcium administration increases neurologic recovery or hospital discharge rates. Currently, calcium should be administered only to patients with hyperkalemia, calcium-channel blocker overdose, or hypocalcemia.

BIBLIOGRAPHY

1. American Heart Association: Standards and guidelines for cardiopulmonary resuscitation (CPR) and emergency cardiac care (ECC). JAMA 255:2905, 1986.
2. Bedell SE, Fulton EJ: Unexpected findings and complications at autopsy after cardiopulmonary resuscitation (CPR). Arch Intern Med 146:1725–1728, 1986.
3. Callaham ML: High dose epinephrine therapy and other advances in treating cardiac arrest. West J Med 152:697–703, 1990.
4. Charlop S, Kahlam S, Lichstein E, Frishman W: Electromechanical dissociation: Diagnosis, pathophysiology, and management. Am Heart J 118:355–360, 1989.
5. Jude JR, Kouwenhoven WB, Knickerbocker GG: Cardiac arrest: Report of application of external cardiac massage on 118 patients. JAMA 178:1063–1070, 1961.
6. Lowenstein SR: Cardiopulmonary resuscitation in non-injured patients. In Wilmore DW, Brennan MF, Harken AH, et al (eds): Care of the Surgical Patient. New York, Scientific American, 1990, pp 1–24.
7. Paradis NA, Koscove EM: Epinephrine in cardiac arrest: A critical review. Ann Emerg Med 19:1288–1301, 1990.
8. Paradis NA, Martin GB, Rivers EP, et al: Coronary perfusion pressure and the return of spontaneous circulation in human cardiopulmonary resuscitation. JAMA 263:1106–1113, 1990.
9. Paradis NA, Martin GB, Rosenberg J, et al: The effect of standard and high-dose epinephrine on coronary perfusion pressure during prolonged cardiopulmonary resuscitation. JAMA 265:1139–1144, 1991.
10. Stempien A, Katz AM, Messineo FC: Calcium and cardiac arrest. Ann Intern Med 105:603–606, 1986.
11. Urban P, Scheidegger D, Buchmann B, Barth D: Cardiac arrest and blood ionized calcium levels. Ann Intern Med 109:110–113, 1988.
12. Weil MH, Rackon EC, Trevino R, et al: Difference in acid-base state between venous and arterial blood during cardiopulmonary resuscitation. N Engl J Med 315:153–156, 1986.

2. PULMONARY AND TISSUE GAS EXCHANGE

Nancy L. Szaflarski, R.N., M.S.

PHYSIOLOGY AND PATHOPHYSIOLOGY OF GAS EXCHANGE

1. What is hypoxemia? Name six causes of hypoxemia in the critically ill adult.

Hypoxemia is commonly defined as an arterial partial pressure of oxygen (PaO_2) of less than 60 torr. It may be caused by one or more of the following:

1. The inspired partial pressure of oxygen may become inadequate owing to a significant decrease in barometric pressure (e.g., altitude ascent) or to an inadequate fraction of inspired oxygen (FiO_2). Hypoxemia can develop in critically ill patients during air transport in nonpressurized aircraft, especially when they are dependent on supplemental oxygen at ground level. Hypoxemia can also develop in patients dependent on oxygen therapy when the FiO_2 is inadvertently lowered by accidental disconnection of oxygen delivery systems.

2. Alveolar hypoventilation is a source of hypoxemia that is represented by an elevated alveolar partial pressure of carbon dioxide ($PACO_2$), which is reflected in an elevated arterial partial pressure of carbon dioxide ($PaCO_2$). Because the partial pressures of alveolar nitrogen and water vapor change minimally at a constant barometric pressure, an increase in $PACO_2$ results in a decrease in the partial pressure of alveolar oxygen (PAO_2). If minute ventilation is suppressed because of central nervous system impairment (e.g., disease, narcotics, sedatives), neuromuscular disease (e.g., Guillain-Barré syndrome, myasthenia gravis), or parenchymal lung disease, hypoxemia may result.

3. True diffusion barriers do not commonly exist in critically ill adults. Diffusion impairments can cause hypoxemia by decreasing the amount of functional alveolar-capillary surface area or by thickening the alveolar-capillary membrane. Examples include pulmonary fibrosis and sarcoidosis. The chance of developing hypoxemia from diffusion defects in critically ill adults is enhanced if pulmonary blood flow is greatly increased. Because blood spends less time in the pulmonary circuit when pulmonary flow is increased, hypoxemia may develop because the time for the transfer of oxygen is decreased. Thus a patient with pulmonary fibrosis and sepsis syndrome, for example, is at greater risk for hypoxemia than is a patient without sepsis.

4. Ventilation-perfusion ($\dot{V}/\dot{Q}$) mismatches that result in decreased ventilation in relation to perfusion (low $\dot{V}/\dot{Q}$ units) cause hypoxemia and are responsive to oxygen therapy. Diseases that cause alveoli to become partially filled with fluid (e.g., blood, pus, edema) or collapsed (e.g., pneumothorax, atelectasis, pleural effusion) predispose to hypoxemia.

5. The worst form of a low $\dot{V}/\dot{Q}$ unit, termed **intrapulmonary shunt**, represents continued pulmonary perfusion in the face of absent ventilation. Intrapulmonary shunt is nonresponsive to oxygen therapy but is responsive to positive end-expiratory pressure.

6. The sixth cause of hypoxemia involves two simultaneous processes. Given a significant degree of preexisting intrapulmonary shunt ($> 30\%$) from lung disease, a drop in cardiac output or an increase in oxygen consumption may worsen preexisting hypoxemia because a lower mixed venous partial pressure of oxygen ($P\bar{v}O_2$) results from either decreased cardiac flow and/or increased oxygen consumption. Venous blood returning to the pulmonary circuit will thus be further deoxygenated. Due to the existing lung disease causing the intrapulmonary shunt, the impaired lung will not be able to oxygenate the mixed venous blood well. A greater degree of hypoxemia will result than if just an intrapulmonary shunt existed. This sixth cause is succinctly referred to as "a low $P\bar{v}O_2$ in the face of a preexisting intrapulmonary shunt."

2. What is intrapulmonary shunt ($\dot{Q}s/\dot{Q}t$)? What data are required for its calculation?

Intrapulmonary shunt is the percentage of cardiac output that passes through the pulmonary capillary bed without exchanging with alveolar air because of fluid-filled or collapsed alveoli. Values of intrapulmonary shunt of up to 5% are found in normal individuals. This small degree of shunt is due to normal, anatomic drainage of deoxygenated blood from thebesian, bronchial, and pleural veins into the left atrium and ventricle.

Shunt values of up to 20% in critically ill adults are usually not life-threatening. Values of 20–30% can be life-threatening if cardiac function is impaired, and values of greater than 30% are life-threatening because they result in severe arterial hypoxemia.

The procurement of simultaneous arterial and mixed venous blood gases is needed to calculate an intrapulmonary shunt. Mixed venous blood is obtained from the distal port of a pulmonary artery flotation catheter. This mixed venous blood sample should be carefully withdrawn from the distal port at a rate of no greater than 3 ml/min in order to avoid obtaining arterialized blood from the pulmonary capillaries. Faster withdrawal may result in inaccurate values of $P\bar{v}O_2$ and mixed venous oxygen saturation. An accurate value of hemoglobin is also needed for shunt calculation. The oxygen content for arterial mixed venous and capillary blood is determined, and the following formula is used to determine intrapulmonary shunt:

$$\dot{Q}s/\dot{Q}t = \frac{CcO_2 - CaO_2}{CcO_2 - C\bar{v}O_2}$$

where CcO_2 equals capillary oxygen content, CaO_2 equals arterial oxygen content, and $C\bar{v}O_2$ equals mixed venous oxygen content.

3. What effect does acidemia have on tissue oxygenation?

A decrease in pH (increase in hydrogen ions) of arterial blood causes the oxyhemoglobin dissociation curve to shift to the right (see figure below) because of a change in hemoglobin affinity for oxygen related to a change in the protein structure of hemoglobin. The affinity of hemoglobin for oxygen becomes less in acidemia, whereby more oxygen is available to the tissues. This phenomenon is viewed as compensatory because it makes more oxygen available to compromised tissues. The effects of curve shifts are primarily appreciated when the PaO_2 falls within the steep portion of the curve. Thus more oxygen will be released to the tissues in acidemia when the PaO_2 is lower.

The parameter used to express any curve shift is known as "P_{50}," which symbolizes the partial pressure of oxygen when 50% of the hemoglobin is saturated. A normal P_{50} in adults is 27 torr. In acidosis, the P_{50} is increased.

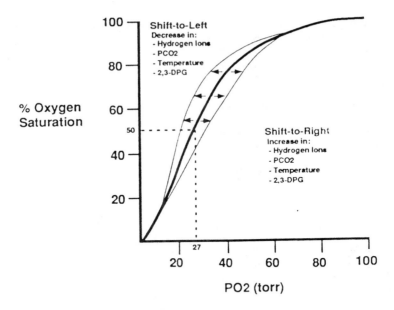

Oxyhemoglobin dissociation curve.

4. What is "oxygen supply"? Are the terms "oxygen transport" and "oxygen delivery" interchangeable with the term "oxygen supply"?

Oxygen supply is the total amount of oxygen delivered to the tissues per minute, and is commonly expressed in millimeters per minute (ml/min). The terms oxygen transport, oxygen delivery, and oxygen supply are interchangeable and represent the same concept. Factors determining oxygen supply ($\dot{S}O_2$) include cardiac output (CO), arterial oxygen saturation (SaO_2), hemoglobin level (Hgb), and arterial partial pressure of oxygen (PaO_2).

5. Can oxygen supply be easily determined at the patient's bedside?
Yes. In order to determine oxygen supply in a critically ill adult, one needs to obtain an accurate thermodilution cardiac output while simultaneously obtaining a specimen for arterial blood gas analysis. A recent hemoglobin value is also needed.

6. How is $\dot{S}O_2$ calculated?
$\dot{S}O_2$ = CO × arterial oxygen content × 10
      = CO × (oxygen-carrying capacity + dissolved oxygen in plasma) × 10
      = CO × [(Hb × SaO_2 × 1.36) + (PaO_2 × 0.003)] × 10

7. What is the derivation of the variables in these equations?
Because arterial oxygen content is usually calculated and expressed in milliliters per deciliter, a factor of 10 is multiplied to the product of CO and arterial oxygen content in order to convert the result to milliliters per minute. A constant factor of 1.36 ml is used in the calculation of oxygen-carrying capacity to account for the average quantity of oxygen that one gram of hemoglobin can bind when fully saturated. A constant factor of 0.003 ml is used in the calculation of dissolved oxygen to represent the amount of oxygen that is dissolved into plasma per torr of partial pressure.

8. What is the normal value for $\dot{S}O_2$ in adults?
1000 ml/min.

9. Do normal values of $\dot{S}O_2$ guarantee adequate tissue oxygenation in critically ill adults?
No, because hypermetabolic states often exist (e.g., sepsis). In such states, the $\dot{S}O_2$ may need to be doubled or tripled in order to provide adequate oxygen transport to tissues. Also, normal values of $\dot{S}O_2$ do not guarantee that specific organs are receiving equal and adequate amounts of oxygen. The adequacy of $\dot{S}O_2$ in critically ill adults must be interpreted in conjunction with other measures that reflect the adequacy of tissue oxygenation (e.g., oxygen consumption, serum lactate values, end-organ function).

10. What is the most important determinant of oxygen supply?
Cardiac output.

11. Is "tissue oxygen consumption" the same as "tissue oxygen demand"?
These terms are often used synonymously in the literature. Tissue oxygen consumption is the quantity of oxygen that tissues extract during the time course of one minute. Tissue oxygen demand is the total quantity of oxygen needed to maintain aerobic tissue metabolism. In healthy individuals, these two terms are equivalent, because tissues have the capability of extracting more oxygen from arterial blood even during times of increased metabolism (e.g., mild to strenuous exercise). Healthy tissues have the flexibility of extracting between 25% and 80% of the oxygen flowing by them. However, in disease states in which tissue oxygen extraction is impaired (e.g., sepsis, ARDS), maximal oxygen extraction can be severely limited to 30–40%. In these disease states, tissue oxygen demand is often not synonymous with oxygen consumption. Tissue oxygen demands exceed oxygen consumption rates, and evidence of anaerobic metabolism may appear in the form of increased serum lactate levels.

12. If a pathophysiologic defect limits the ability of tissues and organs to extract oxygen, what factor is primarily responsible for determining the rate of oxygen consumption?
Oxygen supply. "Pathologic oxygen supply dependence" is used to express this phenomenon, in which oxygen consumption becomes dependent on oxygen supply over large ranges of $\dot{S}O_2$ because of peripheral defects in oxygen extraction. Pathologic oxygen supply dependence has been documented to occur in sepsis and ARDS. Research efforts are currently focused on investigating the effect of increasing oxygen supply in these states.

13. What common direct and indirect measurements are used to determine the presence of anaerobic metabolism in critically ill adults?

The evaluation of end-organ function remains the most common method for inferring inadequacy of tissue oxygenation. The noninvasive assessment of mentation and optimal urine flow rates of 0.5–1.0 ml/kg/hr can be of great assistance in detecting organ dysfunction caused by hypoxia. From an invasive viewpoint, other laboratory tests (e.g., serum bilirubin, prothrombin time, serum creatinine) can infer hypoxic failure of organs. Serum lactate levels have also been used as indirect evidence of anaerobic metabolism in critically ill adults. Although such levels may be useful in indicating the quantitative extent of such metabolism, lactate levels represent systemic values and do not delineate which particular tissues or organs are hypoxic.

BIBLIOGRAPHY

1. Ahrens TS: Concepts in the assessment of oxygenation. Focus Crit Care 14:36–44, 1987.
2. Ahrens TS: Blood gas assessment of intrapulmonary shunting and deadspace. Crit Care Nurs Clin North Am 1:641–648, 1989.
3. Dantzker DR: Oxygen delivery and utilization in sepsis. Crit Care Clin 5:81–98, 1989.
4. Dantzker DR: Physiology and pathophysiology of pulmonary gas exchange. Hosp Pract 1:135–157, 1986.
5. Dorinsky PM, Gadek JE: Mechanisms of multiple nonpulmonary organ failure in ARDS. Chest 96(4):885–892, 1989.
6. Dorinsky PM, Gadek JE: Multiple organ failure. Clin Chest Med 11:581–591, 1990.
7. Edwards JD: Practical application of oxygen transport principles. Crit Care Med 18:S45–S48, 1991.
8. George RB: Alveolar ventilation, gas transfer, and oxygen delivery. In George RB, Light RW, Matthay MA, Matthay RA (eds): Chest Medicine: Essentials of Pulmonary and Critical Care Medicine. Baltimore, Williams & Wilkins, 1990.
9. Reischman RR: Review of ventilation and perfusion physiology. Crit Care Nurse 8:24–30, 1987.
10. Reischman RR: Impaired gas exchange related to intrapulmonary shunting. Crit Care Nurse 8:35–49, 1987.
11. Rutherford KA: Advances in the treatment of oxygenation disturbances. Crit Care Nurs Clin North Am 1:659–667, 1989.
12. Schumacker PT, Cain SM: The concept of a critical oxygen delivery. Intens Care Med 13:223–229, 1987.
13. Schumacker PT, Samsel RW: Oxygen delivery and uptake by peripheral tissues: Physiology and pathophysiology. Crit Care Clin 5:255–269, 1989.
14. Snyder JV, Pinsky MR: Oxygen Transport in the Critically Ill. Chicago, Year Book Medical Publishers, 1987.
15. Weg JG: Oxygen transport in adult respiratory distress syndrome and other circulatory problems: Relationship of oxygen delivery and oxygen consumption. Crit Care Med 19:650–657, 1991.

3. NONINVASIVE MONITORING

Nancy L. Szaflarski, R.N., M.S.

1. How does pulse oximetry work?

Pulse oximetry is based on the techniques of spectrophotometry and plethysmography. **Spectrophotometry** involves the use of a light-emitting diode (LED) that intermittently emits red and infrared light at consistent, specified wavelengths through a peripheral vascular bed. Given that human oxyhemoglobin and deoxyhemoglobin have fixed patterns of light absorbance for red and infrared light, oxygen saturation of hemoglobin is measured using the intensity of light transmitted to a photodetector assuming a constant hemoglobin concentration.

Plethysmography uses the signal of pulsatile flow to determine arterial oxygen saturation of hemoglobin by changes in light absorbance. When blood volume increases in the arterial vascular bed with systole, light absorption increases and the amount of light received by the photodetector is diminished. This change in light absorption with pulsations makes the determination of arterial oxygen saturation more accurate because a ratio of transmitted to absorbed red and infrared light can then be obtained.

Transmission spectrophotometry is most commonly used in adults and involves sending red and infrared light signals through tissue. The placement of a sensor (containing the LED and photodetector) is usually on a digit. The reading that is obtained from a pulse oximeter is the arterial oxygen saturation of hemoglobin and should be abbreviated SpO_2, because the sources of inaccuracy of its determination differ from that of calculated oxygen saturations and those obtained from a multiwavelength oximeter.

2. Why is pulse oximetry inaccurate in the presence of dyshemoglobinemias?

Pulse oximeters measure only "functional" oxygen saturation. This term refers to the ratio of oxyhemoglobin (oxyHb) to all hemoglobin that is capable of transporting oxygen. The formula for functional oxygen saturation is:

$$\text{Functional oxygen saturation} = \frac{\text{oxyHb}}{\text{oxyHb} + \text{deoxyhemoglobin}}$$

If another type of hemoglobin becomes present in the blood (e.g., carboxyhemoglobin, methemoglobin), the pulse oximeter will not read it because the dyshemoglobin (dysHb) cannot bind with oxygen and become part of the "functional" hemoglobin pool. The readings of SpO_2 will be falsely high and not accurately reflect true arterial oxygen saturation (SaO_2). The degree of error will be proportionate to the degree of dyshemoglobinemia.

3. How is SaO_2 determined in a patient with dyshemoglobinemia?

The use of a pulse oximeter in a patient with suspected or known dyshemoglobinemia is contraindicated. A multiwavelength oximeter is needed to determine SaO_2 accurately in dyshemoglobinemia. Since it measures multiple wavelengths, a multiwavelength oximeter can measure all hemoglobin present in the blood regardless of whether it can transport oxygen. Multiwavelength oximeters measure "fractional" oxygen saturation based on the following formula:

$$\text{Fractional oxygen saturation} = \frac{\text{oxyHb}}{\text{oxyHb} + \text{deoxyhemoglobin} + \text{dysHb}}$$

4. When should dyshemoglobinemia be suspected?

(1) When the SpO_2 is inappropriately high for an arterial partial pressure of oxygen (PaO_2), (2) when the SpO_2 is appreciably greater than a measured value (via a multiwavelength oximeter) of SaO_2, or (3) when a measured SaO_2 level (via a multiwavelength oximeter) is inappropriately low for the PaO_2 level. To confirm suspicion, oxygen saturation is determined by a multiwavelength oximeter.

5. What are common limitations of pulse oximeters?

Nonmodifiable limitations are important to recognize because their effects are long lasting and often noncorrectable. Dyshemoglobinemia may cause falsely high SpO_2 readings. Intravenously administered dyes have been reported to cause falsely low SpO_2 readings. Hyperbilirubinemia has been reported to cause falsely low and high values. Severe anemia or induced hemodilutional states may limit the use of pulse oximetry because of inadequate hemoglobin concentration.

Modifiable limitations include optical inference caused by environmental light sources (e.g., surgical lamps, fluorescent lights, direct sunlight, fiber-optic light sources) and optical shunting. Optical shunting results when a portion of the light from the LED reaches the photodetector without passing through the pulsating vascular bed. A common cause of optical shunting is inappropriate sensor application or a sensor that has become loose from wear. Other modifiable limitations include: low perfusion signals that result from hypothermia, elevated systemic vascular resistance, or obliterative vascular disease; motion artifact limitations (e.g., from shivering, agitation, seizures, or tremors); and multiple pulsatile states such as severe right-sided heart failure, severe tricuspid insufficiency, high levels of positive end-expiratory pressure, intraaortic balloon pulsation, dependent extremities (location of sensor), and arteriovenous malformations.

6. If the SpO$_2$ is 90%, what is the predicted PaO$_2$?

Based on the normal oxyhemoglobin dissociation curve, the PaO$_2$ should be approximately 60 torr. However, curve shifts caused by acid-base disturbances, changes in ventilation and/or temperature, and levels of organic phosphates (e.g., 2,3-diphosphoglycerate) could increase or decrease PaO$_2$. The presence of such abnormalities as well as limitations affecting the accuracy of the SpO$_2$ reading must be considered before predicting the PaO$_2$.

7. How does capnography work?

Infrared absorption spectrophotometry is usually employed when capnography is used in adults in critical care units today. Infrared spectrophotometry is based on the fact that carbon dioxide (CO$_2$) absorbs infrared light. If a known spectrum of infrared light is beamed through a sample of end-tidal gas, the amount of infrared light that is absorbed will be proportional to the amount of CO$_2$ in the sampled gas. Sampling of end-tidal gas can occur by the use of mainstream or sidestream capnographs. Mainstream capnographs analyze end-tidal CO$_2$ by using a transducer that is placed directly in-line of the patient's breathing circuit. The transducer contains a light source and a photodetector. The response time for analysis using the mainstream method is very brief. Sidestream capnographs actively divert gas away from the patient's breathing circuit with a narrow sampling tube. Gas analysis occurs in the capnograph, which contains the light source and photodetector. Because gas samples are actively transported to the sidestream capnograph, transit times are unavoidable and result in slow response times.

8. What is a normal difference between the arterial partial pressure of carbon dioxide (PaCO$_2$) and the partial pressure of end-tidal carbon dioxide (PETCO$_2$)? What can increase this difference?

This difference, commonly referred to as the P(a-ET)CO$_2$ gradient, has been consistently reported as less than 6 torr in healthy subjects. This gradient can increase primarily owing to a decrease in PETCO$_2$. Pathophysiologic causes for a decrease in PETCO$_2$ include the development of high ventilation–perfusion ($\dot{V}/\dot{Q}$) units (> 0.8). High $\dot{V}/\dot{Q}$ units are frequently created when a decrease in pulmonary perfusion occurs due to obstruction or obliteration of the pulmonary vascular bed. If pulmonary perfusion decreases (e.g., COPD, pulmonary hypoperfusion, pulmonary emboli), the PETCO$_2$ will also decrease because less CO$_2$ is delivered to the alveolar-capillary interface, resulting in an increased P(a-ET)CO$_2$. The gradient may also increase owing to technologic failures. Endotracheal tube cuff leaks and accidental extubation cause a decrease in PETCO$_2$.

9. When a patient is placed on a capnograph, what is the most important *ventilatory* parameter to monitor serially?

Awareness of the PaCO$_2$ is critical in order to ensure that adequate ventilation is being provided. Because PETCO$_2$ and P(a-ET)CO$_2$ gradient can change with disease progression, disease improvement, or technologic failures, intermittent analysis of arterial blood gases is paramount to ensure safety. A $P(a-ET)CO_2$ gradient that appears to be normalizing (approaching 6 torr or less) may indeed reflect a normal gradient but may also suggest that the patient is becoming hypercarbic (e.g., $PETCO_2$ 42 torr; $PaCO_2$ 47 torr). A golden rule to remember is that the $PaCO_2$ will *always* be higher than the $PETCO_2$.

10. What is the "alveolar plateau" on a capnogram? What does it represent? What does absence of an "alveolar plateau" mean?
In a healthy individual, the alveolar plateau of the capnogram is represented by a nearly constant partial pressure of CO_2 during the expiratory phase (segment A-B in figure below). The alveolar plateau is "flat" primarily because the expired gas from all alveoli have similar ventilation–perfusion ($\dot{V}/\dot{Q}$) relationships. The actual value of $PETCO_2$ is determined at the very end of the plateau phase (point B in figure below). True alveolar gas is being analyzed when a distinct alveolar plateau is present.

Absence of alveolar plateau represents a pathophysiologic state, because $\dot{V}/\dot{Q}$ relationships vary throughout the lung. Exhaled gas will have varying concentrations of CO_2 because some alveoli will have low and high concentrations of CO_2. The defining characteristics of this situation are a slow, rising expiratory upstroke and, hence, loss of a defined alveolar plateau (segment a-B in figure below).

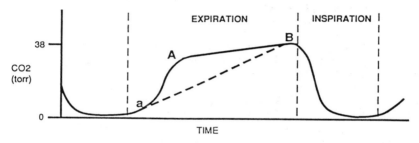

Capnogram demonstrating a normal alveolar plateau (segment A-B) and an abnormal loss of the alveolar plateau (segment a-B).

11. Has capnography been shown to assist in cardiopulmonary resuscitation efforts?
Yes. If cardiopulmonary resuscitation results in forward flow of blood, pulmonary perfusion will be regained and transport of carbon dioxide across the alveolar-capillary membrane will resume. Thus, with successful resuscitative efforts, the capnograph will show a progressive rise in $PETCO_2$, and a capnogram tracing will be restored. The evaluation of the efficacy of resuscitative efforts for critically ill patients who arrest while being monitored on capnography can thus be enhanced.

12. What potential factors can lead to decreased mixed venous oxygen saturation ($S\bar{v}O_2$) in a critically ill adult?
Four factors individually or in combination may cause a decline in $S\bar{v}O_2$ due to increased oxygen extraction at the tissue level: (1) low hemoglobin levels (can seriously impair the body's oxygen-carrying capacity); (2) low arterial oxygen saturation of hemoglobin; (3) decreases in systemic cardiac output; (4) increases in oxygen consumption ($\dot{V}O_2$) (cause venous blood to be more desaturated).

13. What is the significance of a decrease in $S\bar{v}O_2$?
It is a compensatory mechanism of the body. If not enough oxygen reaches the tissues or if oxygen demand is increased, normal tissues will extract a greater percentage of oxygen,

resulting in further desaturation of mixed venous blood. Hence, tissue oxygen extraction normally is inversely proportional to mixed venous oxygen saturation.

14. Which disease states that are prevalent among critically ill adults alter the tissue's ability to extract oxygen and often result in normal or high $S\bar{v}O_2$?
Sepsis and adult respiratory distress syndrome (ARDS).

15. What is the mechanism for this phenomenon in these disease states?
Two mechanisms have been proposed. (1) Altered blood flow to organs and tissues caused by a redistribution of cardiac output may occur due to anatomic, arteriovenous shunts or to a reduction in recruitable capillary reserves. This altered vascular pattern may preclude tissues and organs from extracting oxygen from blood because of reduced blood flow. (2) Endothelial injury may occur in these states due to the release of systemic mediators, causing edema formation in tissues and organs. Because edema can impair oxygen diffusion to tissues and organs, oxygen extraction would be impaired.

BIBLIOGRAPHY

 1. Ahrens T: $S\bar{v}O_2$ monitoring: Is it being used appropriately? Crit Care Nurs 10:70–72, 1990.
 2. Baker SA, Young DJ: Methemoglobinemia: The hidden diagnosis. Crit Care Nurs 10:50–53, 1990.
 3. Carlon GC, Ray C, Miodownik S, Kopec I, Groeger JS: Capnography in mechanically ventilated patients. Crit Care Med 16:550–556, 1988.
 4. Morley TF: Capnography in the intensive care unit. J Intens Care Med 5:209–223, 1990.
 5. Sanders AB, Kern KB, Otto CW, et al: End-tidal carbon dioxide monitoring during cardiopulmonary resuscitation: A prognostic indicator for survival. JAMA 262:1347–1351, 1989.
 6. Schnapp LM, Cohen NH: Pulse oximetry: Uses and abuses. Chest 98:1244–1250, 1990.
 7. St. John RE: Exhaled gas analysis: Technical and clinical aspects of capnography and oxygen consumption. Crit Care Nurs Clin North Am 1:669–679, 1989.
 8. Szaflarski NL, Cohen NH: The use of pulse oximetry in critically ill adults. Heart Lung 18:444–453, 1989.
 9. Szaflarski NL, Cohen NH: The use of capnography in critically ill adults. Heart Lung 20:363–372, 1991.
10. Von Rueden KT: Noninvasive assessment of gas exchange in the critically ill patient. AACN Clinical Issues in Critical Care Nursing 1:239–247, 1990.
11. Watson CB: Continuous measurement of mixed venous oxygen saturation: Shall we worship the golden calf? J Clin Monit 1:252–258, 1985.
12. Weil MH, Bisera J, Trevino RP, Rackow EC: Cardiac output and end-tidal carbon dioxide. Crit Care Med 13:907–909, 1985.
13. White KM: Completing the hemodynamic picture: $S\bar{v}O_2$. Heart Lung 14:272–280, 1985.
14. Wiedemann HP, McCarthy K: Noninvasive monitoring of oxygen and carbon dioxide. Clin Chest Med 19:239–254, 1989.

4. INVASIVE HEMODYNAMIC MONITORING

Mark W. Bowyer, M.D.

1. What tools are available for invasively monitoring the hemodynamic status of critically ill patients?
Arterial catheters, central venous pressure monitors, and pulmonary artery or Swan-Ganz catheters.

2. What data can be obtained with an arterial catheter?

Arterial catheters are used for moment-to-moment recording of blood pressure and to derive the mean arterial pressure (MAP), which is frequently used in the calculation of several derived hemodynamic variables. The MAP is calculated by adding the value for the diastolic pressure to the value obtained by subtracting the diastolic pressure from the systolic pressure, and dividing this sum by 3. Arterial lines also allow easy access for frequent withdrawal of blood and for measurement of arterial blood gases, which help tremendously in the care of critically ill patients.

3. Where and how are arterial catheters inserted?

The radial artery is the most commonly used because of its superficial location and collateral anastomoses with the ulnar artery. Other sites in order of decreasing frequency are the dorsalis pedis, femoral, brachial, and axillary arteries. After evaluation of the adequacy of the collateral circulation, the radial artery is cannulated percutaneously with an angiocath or much less frequently by cutdown.

4. What are the complications of radial arterial catheter monitoring?

Thrombosis is the most common complication, the risk of which increases with increased size of the catheter and duration of catheterization. Recanalization of the thrombosed artery usually occurs in 2–3 weeks. Other complications that occur much less frequently are embolization, infection, median nerve neuropathy, and pseudoaneurysm of the artery.

5. What is obtained with central venous pressure (CVP) monitoring?

CVP is a numerical value that represents the right atrial pressure or right ventricular filling pressure. In simplistic terms, CVP is an indication of fluid status and right cardiac function. In normal individuals, changes in CVP correlate with changes in left ventricular filling pressure. In patients with preexisting pulmonary or cardiac disease, and in patients with multisystem trauma, this correlation may no longer exist. As such, CVP can be a misleading index of volume status and should be interpreted with caution in critically ill patients.

6. How are CVP monitors placed?

A catheter is placed into the central venous system (superior vena cava or, less commonly, inferior vena cava or right atrium) usually via the subclavian or internal jugular vein. The patient is placed in a head-down (Trendelenburg) position and the catheter inserted using the Seldinger technique, which involves placing a soft, flexible wire through the needle that has been placed in the vein, removing the needle, inserting the catheter over the wire, and removing the wire. The catheter is secured with suture, and its position is confirmed with a chest x-ray.

7. What is a normal CVP? What factors may affect it?

In healthy persons, the CVP is 0–4 mm Hg, providing adequate filling of the right ventricle. Ten to 12 mm Hg is commonly considered the upper limit of normal for acutely ill patients. Several factors affect this value, including cardiac performance, blood volume, vascular tone, increased intraabdominal or intrathoracic pressures, and vasopressor therapy.

8. What is a Swan-Ganz catheter?

The Swan-Ganz or pulmonary artery catheter was introduced in 1970 by Harold James C. Swan, M.D., and William Ganz, M.D., both cardiologists. It is a multilumen catheter with a balloon on the tip that allows it to be flow directed through central venous access into the right side of the heart and then into the pulmonary artery.

9. What values can be measured with the Swan-Ganz catheter?
Direct measurement of pulmonary artery (systolic, diastolic, and mean) pressures, pulmonary artery wedge pressure, cardiac output, and mixed venous blood parameters.

10. What are the indications for use of the Swan-Ganz catheter?
This is an emotionally charged, highly controversial topic. In general, the greatest uses of data obtained with the catheter are in patients with complicated myocardial infarction, during complex general and cardiac surgery, in patients with severe cardiopulmonary disease, in critically ill patients with extensive multisystem failure, shock states, or major trauma, or in other situations in which hemodynamic status is difficult to assess adequately. The risks must be weighed against the benefits in each case. Use of this catheter should imply that the information derived will affect decisions regarding therapy.

11. What is the pulmonary artery wedge pressure (PAWP)? How is it measured?
The PAWP is a reasonably accurate measurement of the mean left atrial pressure, which closely parallels the left ventricular end-diastolic pressure (provided that left ventricular compliance and the mitral valve are normal). The PAWP is therefore considered to accurately reflect left ventricular diastolic dynamics and thus left ventricular function. The PAWP is obtained by inflating the balloon at the tip of the Swan-Ganz catheter, which has been inserted into the pulmonary artery. When the balloon fills the lumen of the vessel, the transducer measures the pressure transmitted across the pulmonary vasculature from the left atrium. The measurement is obtained at end expiration, when the value is least affected by transmitted pleural pressure.

12. How can you tell if the PAWP value is accurate?
1. The mean pulmonary capillary wedge pressure should be equal to or lower than the pulmonary artery diastolic (PAD) pressure and lower than the mean pulmonary artery pressure. If the PAWP is greater than the PAD pressure, the catheter tip may be in west zone 1 of the lung, where the alveolar pressure is greater than the arterial or venous pressure, and thus the PAWP will reflect airway pressure and not left atrial pressure. The catheter tip will enter zone 3, where venous and arterial pressures exceed alveolar pressure more than 95% of the time. In a supine patient, the catheter tip is likely to be in zone 3 if it is posteriorly positioned beneath the level of the left atrium. This can be confirmed with a lateral chest film. Zone 3 positioning can also be tested by addition of an incremental level of positive end-expiratory pressure (PEEP). If the wedge pressure increases by greater than half the increment of PEEP, zone 3 positioning is unlikely. When vascular pressure decreases or if increasing the PEEP raises the alveolar pressure, zone 3 may be converted to zone 2 or 1 and the catheter may need to be refloated in order to get accurate readings in a zone 3 region.
2. A characteristic waveform of left atrial pressure should be seen, with the wedge waveform disappearing promptly with balloon deflation and rapidly returning after balloon inflation. If less than a full balloon inflation (1.5 cc) produces a wedge trace, the catheter should be pulled back until such is the case.
3. The presence of mitral valve disease or impaired left ventricular function (decreased compliance) will lead to artificial elevation of measured PAWP values. When ventilated patients are placed on PEEP, pleural pressure will increase and therefore artificially increase the measured wedge value. In a normally compliant lung, about half of the administered PEEP is transmitted to the wedge. In stiff (noncompliant) lungs, about one-fourth to one-third is transmitted.

13. How is cardiac output measured?
Cardiac output is measured with the Swan-Ganz catheter using a thermodilution technique. The thermodilution technique involves injecting a solution that is colder than blood through

the right atrial port of the catheter and measuring the temperature change distally with a thermometer located 4 cm from the catheter tip. The area under the thermodilution curve (by computer) and the volume and temperature of the indicator injection allow calculation of the thermodilution cardiac output. Cardiac output varies depending at what point during the respiratory cycle the solution is injected; therefore, by convention, it is measured at end expiration. Cardiac output may also be measured by dye techniques or by the Fick principle, in which the cardiac output is said to equal the oxygen consumption divided by arteriovenous oxygen content difference times a factor of 10.

14. What is a mixed venous blood sample? How is it helpful?
Mixed venous blood is pulmonary artery blood that is drawn from the end of the Swan-Ganz catheter and represents blood from all organs of the body. The oxygen content of mixed venous blood is a sensitive indicator of the adequacy of oxygen delivery to the tissues. Oxygen delivery to the tissues can be improved by increasing cardiac output and hemoglobin content and maximizing oxygenation of the arterial blood. The mixed venous oxygen will be artificially elevated if blood is withdrawn too forcefully from the pulmonary artery catheter. This causes the pulmonary artery to collapse, and the blood obtained is pulled back from the pulmonary veins or left atrium and thus has an increased oxygen content and decreased CO_2 content. If the PCO_2 of the mixed venous sample is less than that obtained from the arterial blood sample, the mixed venous sample has been improperly drawn.

15. Which hemodynamic values can be derived from Swan-Ganz measurements? How are they calculated?
    1. **Cardiac index (CI)** = cardiac output ÷ body surface area
This measurement allows standardization of the cardiac output number to account for differences in body size when comparing patients.
    2. **Vascular resistance** represents the afterload against which the left and right ventricles must work. Pressure is a function of flow times resistance; therefore, resistance equals pressure divided by flow.
        (a) The afterload to the left ventricle is the **systemic vascular resistance (SVR)**, which is calculated as follows:

$$SVR = \frac{\text{mean arterial pressure} - \text{central venous pressure}}{\text{cardiac output}} \times \text{factor (80)}$$

        (b) The afterload to the right ventricle is the **pulmonary vascular resistance (PVR)**, calculated by:

$$PVR = \frac{\text{mean pulmonary artery pressure (MPAP)} - \text{PAWP}}{\text{cardiac output}} \times \text{factor (80)}$$

    3. **Stroke volume** is a measure of the volume of blood ejected by the heart with each beat and is calculated by dividing the cardiac output by the heart rate.
    4. **Oxygen transport** is the amount of oxygen delivered by the heart to the tissues.
    5. **Oxygen return** is the amount of oxygen returning to the heart.
    6. **Oxygen consumption** reflects the overall ability of the peripheral tissues to extract oxygen.
    O_2 consumption = CI (O_2 content arterial blood – mixed venous O_2 content).
    7. **Oxygen delivery** reflects the ability of the body to supply oxygen to the tissues. It must increase as the tissue demand increases with injury or illness.
    Oxygen delivery = arterial O_2 content × cardiac output
where O_2 content $= PO_2 \times .0031 + [Hgb] \times SaO_2 \times 1.34$
              .0031 = the solubility coefficient of oxygen
              1.34 = the milliliters of oxygen bound to Hgb when it is fully saturated

16. How can oxygen delivery be improved?
The oxygen delivery is most sensitive to changes in cardiac output. Cardiac output can be improved by increasing the preload (wedge), decreasing the afterload (SVR), or improving the function (contractility) of the heart. These changes can be accomplished with fluid or with a variety of pharmacologic interventions. Oxygen delivery may also be improved by increasing the hemoglobin content in the blood to increase the carrying capacity of oxygen.

17. What are considered normal hemodynamic values?

Central venous pressure	=	0–6 mm Hg
Right atrial pressure	=	0–6 mm Hg
Right ventricular pressure	=	25/0–6 mm Hg
Pulmonary artery pressure	=	25/6–12 mm Hg
Pulmonary artery wedge pressure	=	6–12 mm Hg
Mean arterial pressure	=	85–95 mm Hg
Aortic pressure	=	130/80 mm Hg
Cardiac index	=	$\geq$ 2.8–3.6 (L/min/m^2)
Systemic vascular resistance	=	770–1500 (dynes/sec/cm^5)
Pulmonary vascular resistance	=	20–120 (dyne/cm/sec^{-5})
Mixed venous oxygen content	=	15 ml/dl
Mixed venous oxygen tension	=	35–45 torr
Mixed venous oxygen saturation	=	70–75%
Oxygen delivery	=	600 ml/min/m^2
Oxygen consumption	=	150 ml/min/m^2

18. Which hemodynamic derangements would you expect to see with cardiogenic shock?
Cardiogenic shock is that which arises from a primary cardiac cause and leads to ineffective pumping of blood. This status is reflected hemodynamically by a decreased cardiac index, increased pulmonary artery wedge pressure, increased systemic vascular resistance, and inadequate delivery of oxygen to the tissues.

19. Which hemodynamic derangements would you expect to see with hypovolemic or traumatic shock?
Hypovolemic or traumatic shock results in depletion of vascular volume with resultant decreased cardiac index, decreased pulmonary artery wedge pressure, increased systemic vascular resistance, and inadequate delivery of oxygen to the tissues.

20. Which hemodynamic derangements would you expect to see with septic shock?
Classic septic shock results in a profound state of vasomotor collapse, which includes vasodilatation with tissue hypoxemia and leakage of intravascular fluid into the tissues. Hemodynamically, this is manifested by an early increase in cardiac index (hyperdynamic state), a profound decrease in the systemic vascular resistance, and a decrease in the wedge pressure. Oxygen delivery is adequate, but the peripheral tissues are unable to use this oxygen and therefore oxygen consumption will be low. As the sepsis continues, toxic factors released from infected tissues lead to further hypovolemia and cardiac depression.

21. Which hemodynamic derangements would you expect to see with neurogenic shock?
Neurogenic shock may result from spinal cord injury, spinal anesthesia, or drug overdose. It is the result of the loss of venous adrenergic tone with pooling of blood in the periphery. This leads to inadequate ventricular filling with resultant decreased wedge pressure and decreased cardiac index. The loss of adrenergic tone also results in a profound decrease in systemic vascular resistance.

22. What are the complications of Swan-Ganz catheterization?

Insertion of the Swan-Ganz catheter shares many of the complications associated with central venous monitoring in general: pneumothorax, hemothorax, inadvertent arterial puncture, infection, air embolism, arrhythmias, and chylothorax. Complications unique to Swan-Ganz catheters include ventricular rupture, valvular damage, pulmonary artery rupture, aneurysm, thrombosis or infarction, bundle branch blocks, ventricular arrhythmias, and knotting of the catheter.

23. How should pulmonary artery rupture be treated?

Pulmonary artery rupture as a complication of pulmonary artery catheterization is an infrequent but life-threatening complication. Most of these patients do not die as a result of exsanguination, but rather from causes secondary to aspiration and asphyxia; therefore the initial management should focus on fluid replacement, airway protection, and control of bleeding. Endotracheal intubation using a double-lumen tube is recommended with positioning of the patient in a lateral decubitus position with the side of the injury down. Fluid resuscitation, reversal of anticoagulation, and lowering of pulmonary hypertension are all useful adjuncts for control of the bleeding. Thoracotomy and pulmonary resection are rarely required because of frequent spontaneous cessation but should be done promptly if all other measures fail.

BIBLIOGRAPHY

1. Clark CA, Harmon EM: Hemodynamic monitoring: Arterial catheters. In Civetta JM, Taylor RW, Kirby RR (eds): Critical Care. Philadelphia, J.B. Lippincott, 1988, pp 289–292.
2. Clark CA, Harmon EM: Hemodynamic monitoring: Pulmonary artery catheters. In Civetta JM, Taylor RW, Kirby RR (eds): Critical Care. Philadelphia, J.B. Lippincott, 1988, pp 293–302.
3. Feng WC, Singh AK, Drew T, Donat W: Swan-Ganz catheter induced massive hemoptysis and pulmonary artery false aneurysm. Ann Thorac Surg 50:644–646, 1990.
4. Fletcher EC, Mihalick MJ, Siegel CO: Pulmonary artery rupture during introduction of the Swan-Ganz catheter: Mechanism and prevention of injury. J Crit Care 3:116–121, 1988.
5. Friesinger GC, Williams SV: Clinical competence in hemodynamic monitoring: A statement of physicians from the ACP/ACC/AHA Task Force on Clinical Privileges in Cardiology. Circulation 81:2036–2040, 1990.
6. Matthay MA, Chatterjee K: Bedside catheterization of the pulmonary artery: Risks compared to benefits. Ann Intern Med 109:826–834, 1988.
7. Putterman C: The Swan-Ganz catheter: A decade of hemodynamic monitoring. J Crit Care 4:127–146, 1989.
8. Smart FW, Hasserl FE: Complications of flow-directed balloon-tipped catheters. Chest 97:227–228, 1990.
9. Swan HJC, Ganz W, Forrester J, et al: Catheterization of the heart in man with the use of a flow-directed balloon catheter. N Engl J Med 283:447–451, 1970.
10. Voyce SJ, Rippe JM: Pulmonary artery catheters: An update. J Intens Care Med 6:175–192, 1990.
11. Wiedemann HP, Matthay MA, Matthay RA: Cardiovascular-pulmonary monitoring in the intensive care unit (Part I). Chest 85:537–549, 1984.
12. Wiedemann HP, Matthay MA, Matthay RA: Cardiovascular-pulmonary monitoring in the intensive care unit (Part 2). Chest 85:656–668, 1984.

5. INTERPRETATION OF ARTERIAL BLOOD GASES

E. Michael Canham, M.D.

1. What do arterial blood gas (ABG) instruments measure?
The current ABG instruments measure pH, PCO_2, and PO_2 using three separate electrodes. The blood gas samples are placed through an inlet into a temperature-controlled chamber (usually $37°C$) where the blood is exposed to these three electrode tips.

2. When should ABGs be analyzed?
Analysis of ABGs is used extensively in the critical care setting to evaluate both acid-base status and oxygen and carbon dioxide gas exchange. Analysis of ABGs is indicated in virtually all cardiopulmonary conditions.

3. What are the problems associated in obtaining ABGs?
The arterial puncture may result in acute hyperventilation, which is often minimized by good technique, by use of a small needle, or by instillation of a local anesthetic. After the sample is obtained, all air bubbles should be expelled and the syringe capped. Air bubbles that are mixed or agitated into the sample will equilibrate with the blood, possibly altering the PO_2 toward room air and lowering the PCO_2. The sample should be placed on ice unless the analysis is performed within 15 minutes. Plastic syringes may allow greater diffusion of gases than glass syringes and so should also be run promptly. In the absence of extreme leukocytosis, an iced, glass ABG syringe will maintain the PO_2 value for up to 3 hours.

4. Does the heparin within the ABG syringe influence the results? If so, how?
Heparin is placed within the ABG syringe as an anticoagulant. Many commercial blood gas kits have a predetermined quantity of heparin instilled into the syringe for convenience and to reduce the effect of heparin on the sample. Heparin is acidic and theoretically could reduce the sample pH if too small a specimen is obtained; however, because blood is a good buffer, the error for pH is generally minimal. Heparin may also affect the PCO_2 and PO_2 measurements by dilution. For example, the liquid heparin that fills the dead space of a 10-ml syringe and needle may be around .25 ml, so that a 1-ml blood sample would be diluted and the PCO_2 and bicarbonate levels in the sample will be 25% less. The potential error in the PO_2 value can also be large.

5. What does extreme leukocytosis ("leukocyte larceny") do to the ABG analysis?
The presence of large numbers of leukocytes or platelets will reduce the PO_2 value, giving a false impression of hypoxemia. This drop in PO_2 is negligible if the sample is stored in ice and analyzed within 1 hour. Presumably the ongoing metabolism of the cellular elements of blood consume oxygen, reducing PO_2.

6. What is the effect of temperature on ABG analysis?
The normal pH rises as the patient cools, and it falls with warming. When blood flows from the warm central body to the cool periphery, the H+ concentration and PCO_2 fall and the pH rises. Consequently, oxygen saturation rises with cooling and the PO_2 decreases. Temperature will not appreciably change oxygen or CO_2 content. For simplicity, accuracy, and ease of interpretation, the vast majority of ABG samples should be reported at $37°C$ so that temperature correction is not necessary.

7. What else may alter ABG analysis?

Halothane anesthesia will falsely increase PO_2 values, because the PO_2 electrode in blood gas instruments also responds to halothane.

8. Why does the CO_2 content of venous blood measured in the chemistry lab occasionally differ from the CO_2 content calculated from the blood gas lab?

This observed difference in plasma CO_2 content is likely owing to the difference between free-flowing arterial blood and peripheral blood obtained from a temporarily occluded vein.

9. How long after starting or stopping supplemental oxygen should one wait before ABGs can be drawn and reflect baseline or plateau values?

In patients with severe obstructive lung disease and air trapping, 25 minutes may be required; however, in the absence of significant lung disease, 5–7 minutes would be adequate.

10. What is the alveolar gas equation?

The alveolar gas equation is a formula used to approximate the partial pressure of oxygen in the alveolus (PAO_2).

$$PAO_2 = (PB - PH_2O)\, FiO_2 - \frac{PaCO_2}{R}$$

where PB is the barometric pressure, PH_2O is the water vapor pressure (usually 47 mm Hg), FiO_2 is the fractional concentration of inspired oxygen, and R is the gas exchange ratio. (The rate of CO_2 production to O_2 utilization is usually around .8 at rest.) For example, at sea level:

$$PAO_2 = (760 - 47).21 - \frac{40}{.8} = 100 \text{ mm Hg}$$

11. What is the alveolar-arterial PO_2 difference, or "A-a gradient" (AaO_2 gradient)?

After calculation of the PAO_2 from the alveolar gas equation, the AaO_2 gradient can be obtained by subtracting the PaO_2 measured from the ABGs. For example, at sea level (with $PCO_2 - 40$, $PO_2 - 92$):

$$PAO_2 - PaO_2 = AaO_2 \text{ gradient}$$
$$100 \text{ mm Hg} - 92 \text{ mm Hg} = 8 \text{ mm Hg}$$

The normal AaO_2 gradient is dependent on age, body position, and nutritional status. The AaO_2 gradient is widened under normal conditions by age, obesity, fasting, supine position, and heavy exercise. One predictive equation for estimating PO_2 (at PB = 760 mm Hg) in relation to age is as follows: $PO_2 = 109 - .43 \times$ age (in years).

12. How is the AaO_2 gradient useful?

The AaO_2 gradient may be widened by any significant cardiopulmonary condition that results in hypoxemia and/or hypocarbia. Hypoxemia caused by simple alveolar hypoventilation will not widen the AaO_2 gradient. Most pulmonary emboli, on the other hand, will widen the AaO_2 gradient, because even if hypoxemia does not occur, hypocarbia is very common.

13. What is the difference between a calculated versus a measured oxygen saturation?

The calculated oxyhemoglobin saturation is calculated from the measured values of PaO_2 and pH by the Severinghaus slide rule, by a nomogram, or by the blood gas instrument microprocessor. The measured oxyhemoglobin saturation is obtained with a co-oximeter (a spectrophotometer), which measures reduced hemoglobin, oxyhemoglobin, carboxyhemoglobin, and methemoglobin. Errors in the calculation of oxygen saturation may occur if carboxyhemoglobin is present, which is commonly seen in cigarette smokers. Carbon monoxide does not affect oxygen tension (PAO_2) but does bind and displace oxygen from hemoglobin. Consequently, the calculated oxygen saturation is falsely elevated.

The calculated oxygen saturation may also be in error if the oxyhemoglobin dissociation curve is displaced by changes in 2,3-diphosphoglycerate (2,3-DPG). The binding of 2,3-DPG to hemoglobin reduces the affinity of hemoglobin for oxygen, facilitating the unloading of oxygen at the tissue level. The binding of 2,3-DPG to hemoglobin shifts the oxyhemoglobin dissociation curve to the right. A common example of 2,3-DPG depletion occurs in the storage of blood. Consequently, a patient receiving multiple units of stored blood, with a leftward shift of the oxyhemoglobin dissociation curve, will have a calculated oxygen saturation less than the measured oxygen saturation.

Hemoglobinopathies will also cause a discrepancy between the measured and calculated oxygen saturation, depending on which way they shift the oxyhemoglobin dissociation curve (see page 9).

14. Given that oximetry is so readily available, painless, and accurate, why is ABG analysis necessary?
Oximetry and the newer technology that made it more accessible, affordable, and accurate have decreased the need for ABG analysis in monitoring oxygen saturation. In fact, in many hospitals the number of ABGs done has decreased with the influx of oximeters into virtually every department within a hospital. However, relying on oximetry alone can lead to misdiagnosis, increased cost, and potentially fatal respiratory arrest. Consider the following examples of pitfalls of using oximetry alone that have been observed in practice.

1. A patient was noted to have oxygen desaturation via oximetry during a routine check after minor orthopedic surgery. The physicians evaluated this oximetric abnormality by ordering a chest x-ray, pulmonary function tests, and a ventilation-perfusion lung scan, all of which were normal. Finally, ABG analysis was done and revealed alveolar hypoventilation alone with a normal AaO_2 gradient. The oxygen desaturation was simply the result of an increased PCO_2 from hypoventilation in a patient receiving narcotics.

2. Following an episode of smoke inhalation, a patient came to the emergency room for headache and nausea. The oxygen saturation by oximetry was normal, and the patient was nearly dismissed after symptomatic treatment alone. Fortunately, recognizing the limitation of oximetry in differentiating oxygenated hemoglobin from carboxyhemoglobin, the physician drew an ABG sample, which revealed profound carbon monoxide poisoning. The patient was treated appropriately with 100% oxygen and close monitoring.

3. Another example involved a house officer who was asked to see a febrile, septic patient with a respiratory rate of 40 and a chest x-ray revealing early alveolar infiltrates bilaterally. Oxygen was initiated, and with the use of oximetry, the oxygen saturation was titrated to 90%. The patient required FiO_2 of 100% by non-rebreather mask to achieve the 90% oxygen saturation. Unfortunately, the house officer did not draw an ABG sample and failed to realize that with marked hyperventilation and respiratory alkalosis, the oxyhemoglobin dissociation curve is shifted to the left, thereby causing a much higher oxygen saturation for a given PaO_2. Had ABG analysis been done at that time, it would have revealed pH 7.58, $PACO_2$ 22, PAO_2 50, and O_2 sat 90%, all clearly indicating intubation and assisted ventilation with PEEP. Later that evening, the patient suffered a near-fatal respiratory arrest.

BIBLIOGRAPHY

1. Asmussen E, Nielsen M: Alveolo-arterial gas exchange at rest and during work at different O_2 tensions. Acta Physiol Scand 50:153–160, 1960.
2. Cissik JH, Salustro J, Patton OL, Louden JA: The effects of sodium heparin on arterial blood gas analysis. Cardiovasc Pulm 5:17–21, 1977.

3. Cugell DW: How long should you wait? (editorial). Chest 67:253, 1975.
4. Cvitanic O, Marino PL: Improved use of arterial blood gas analysis in suspected pulmonary emboli. Chest 95:48–51, 1989.
5. Hansen JE: Arterial blood gases. In Mahler DA (ed): Pulmonary Function Testing. Clin Chest Med 5:227–237, 1989.
6. Hansen JE, Simmons DH: A systematic error in the determination of blood PCO_2. Am Rev Respir Dis 115:1061–1063, 1977.
7. Hess CE, Nichols AB, Hunt WB, Suratt PM: Pseudohypoxemia secondary to leukemia and thrombocytosis. N Engl J Med 301:361–363, 1979.
8. Raffin TA: Indications for arterial blood gas analysis. In Sox HC Jr (ed): Common Diagnostic Tests, 2nd ed. Philadelphia, American College of Physicians, 1990, pp 100–119.
9. Severinghaus JW: Blood gas calculator. J Appl Physiol 21:1108–1116, 1966.
10. Sorbini CA, Grassi V, Solinas E, Muiesan G: Arterial oxygen tension in relation to age in healthy subjects. Respiration 25:3–13, 1968.

6. FLUID THERAPY

Mark W. Bowyer, M.D.

1. What percent of total body weight is composed of water?
Total body water makes up 60% of body weight in an average male and approximately 50% in an average female.

2. How is total body water distributed?
A 70-kg lean adult man has a total body water of about 42 liters (60% of total body weight). This water is distributed into an intracellular compartment containing 66% (28 liters) and an extracellular compartment containing 34% (14 liters). The extracellular compartment is further subdivided into an intravascular (approximately 25% or 3.5 liters) and an interstitial (approximately 75% or 10.5 liters) subcompartment.

3. What happens to free water that is infused into the intravascular space?
When dextrose in water (D5W) is infused, the dextrose is metabolized, leaving free water. When added to the intravascular space, free water will equilibrate with the extracellular and intracellular compartments in proportion to their relative values.

4. What governs the distribution of fluid in the body?
The membranes between the fluid compartments are semipermeable, allowing rapid equilibration of free water and low-molecular-weight solutes. Particles/solutes unable to cross the membrane create oncotic pressure. The relative difference in oncotic pressure between various compartments governs the distribution of fluid. The rate of equilibration can be measured using the modified Starling equation, which asserts that fluid movement across a semipermeable membrane is equal to barrier conductance multiplied by the driving pressure.

5. What is "third spacing" of fluids?
The third space refers to extracellular fluid that is "nonfunctional," i.e., does not participate in the transport of nutrients to, or waste products from, the body cells. With burns, crash injuries, severe soft-tissue infections, postoperative wounds, and hemorrhagic shock, significant amounts of extracellular fluid are sequestered, with a resultant significant decrease in interstitial fluid and plasma volume. Attempts to restore extracellular and

intracellular fluid compartments with intravenous fluids lead to further sequestration in the nonfunctional third space, as it is in equilibrium with the other two. This leads to weight gain that can be of massive proportions. In acute injury, resolution of third spacing begins 48–72 hours after the event, with resultant resorption, diuresis, and weight loss. This may result in cardiac failure in patients with preexisting significant cardiopulmonary disease.

6. What are crystalloids?
Crystalloid fluids are mixtures of sodium chloride and other physiologically active solutes. Sodium is the major component, and the distribution of sodium will determine the distribution of the infused crystalloid. Only 20% of infused sodium chloride will remain in the vascular space.

7. What are colloids?
Colloids are high-molecular-weight substances that do not pass rapidly across capillary walls. They stay in the vascular space and exert an osmotic force (colloid osmotic pressure) that keeps fluid in the blood vessels. The most commonly used colloids are albumin, hetastarch, and dextran. Blood products are also considered to be colloids.

8. What are the commonly used crystalloids? What are their compositions?
Normal saline solution and lactated Ringer's solution are the most commonly used crystalloids. Normal saline solution is composed of 154 mEq of sodium and 154 mEq of chloride, with an osmolality of 308. Lactated Ringer's solution contains 130 mEq of sodium, 4 mEq of potassium, 3 mEq of calcium, 109 mEq of chloride, and 128 mEq of bicarbonate, with an osmolality of 273. In comparison, extracellular fluid contains 142 mEq of sodium, 4 mEq of potassium, 5 mEq of calcium, 3 mEq of magnesium, 103 mEq of chloride, and 27 mEq of bicarbonate, with an osmolality of 280–310.

9. What are the characteristics of albumin?
Albumin is responsible for 80% of the colloid osmotic pressure of plasma. As such, it is ideally suited for use in volume expansion. Infusion of 100 ml of a 25% solution will expand plasma volume by 500 cc.

10. What are the characteristics of hetastarch?
Hetastarch is a synthetic starch used as a plasma expander. Hetastarch increases plasma volume in an amount slightly in excess of the infused volume. Hetastarch has a longer half-life than albumin. Allergic reactions can occur rarely with hetastarch, and the metabolism of it produces an increase in measured amylase.

11. What are the characteristics of dextran?
Dextran is a polysaccharide derived from sugar beets and is available as a high-molecular-weight (avg. of 70,000) and low-molecular-weight (avg. of 40,000) product. Infusion of Dextran 40 expands the plasma volume to about two times the infused volume. Use of dextran is associated with an incidence of approximately 1% of anaphylaxis, renal failure, and interference with subsequent cross-matching of blood. If more than 1.5 gm/kg/day is infused, problems with bleeding may occur secondary to its interaction with factor VIII.

12. Describe the goals of fluid therapy.
The goals of fluid therapy are to maintain an adequate state of hydration and tissue perfusion with electrolyte balance. The adequacy of fluid therapy can be followed clinically by observation of vital signs, physical examination, measurement of input, output, and weights, urine output, serum electrolytes, and, if necessary, invasive monitoring.

13. What factors must be considered when estimating fluid needs of critically ill patients?
There are three categories of fluid loss. (1) Fluid loss, both sensible and insensible, occurs with normal body maintenance. (2) Fluid loss may result from existing fluid deficits such as in patients with shock. (3) Fluid loss may result from ongoing volume losses secondary to an underlying disease process.

14. How are maintenance fluid requirements calculated?
For a 70-kg patient, obligatory fluid losses that must be replaced include insensible losses from skin and lungs (about 800 ml), fecal losses (200 ml), and sweat. Additionally, enough urine must be produced to excrete a solute load of 600 mOsm produced each day by the body. Healthy people can concentrate urine to a maximum of 1200 mOsm/L and therefore can excrete this solute load with only 500 ml of urine. Critically ill patients have diminished urine-concentrating abilities and therefore have a minimum obligatory urine output of about 900 ml. Thus sensible and insensible losses account for 2000–2500 ml per day, giving a 24-hour fluid requirement of 30–35 ml/kg to maintain fluid balance.

15. What are fluid maintenance requirements for children?
Twenty-four-hour fluid requirements for children have been formulated based on weight:
   0–10 kg = 100 ml/kg
   11–20 kg = 1000 ml + 50 ml/kg for every kg above 10 kg
   > 20 kg = 1500 ml + 20 ml/kg for every kg above 20 kg

16. What are some of the sources of ongoing volume loss that must be replaced?
   1. Loss of body fluids—loss of gastric fluid from nasogastric suctioning, loss of biliary or pancreatic fluid, or loss of colon fluid secondary to diarrhea.
   2. Third-space losses—these are difficult to quantitate, but a rough rule of thumb is that one liter of fluid is third-spaced for each abdominal quadrant that is traumatized.
   3. Fever—each degree above 37° C adds 2–2.5 ml/kg/day of insensible water loss.
   4. Burns—contribute significantly to evaporative water losses.

CONTROVERSY

17. Should crystalloids or colloids be used for fluid resuscitation?
The colloid-crystalloid controversy has raged for more than 25 years with no consensus regarding which is most appropriate for resuscitation. The facts available are that colloids are much more expensive than crystalloids; crystalloid infusion requires 2–4 times more volume to achieve the same hemodynamic effect; colloids *do not* cause more pulmonary edema than crystalloids when pulmonary capillaries are damaged; and the bottom line— there is no difference in survival based on fluid choice alone. If the goal is to expand the plasma volume, colloids are a logical choice. If the goal is to replenish the entire extracellular space, then crystalloids should be used.

BIBLIOGRAPHY

1. Bisonni RS, Holtgrave DR, Lawler F, Morley DS: Colloids versus crystalloids in fluid resuscitation: An analysis of randomized controlled trials. J Fam Pract 32:387–390, 1991.
2. Davies MJ: Crystalloid or colloid: Dose it matter? J Clin Anesth 1:464–471, 1989.
3. Karanko MS, Klossne JA, Laaksonen VO: Restoration of volume by crystalloid vs. colloid after coronary artery bypass: Hemodynamics, lung waters, oxygenation and outcome. Crit Care Med 15:559–566, 1987.
4. Kaufman BS, Rackow EC, Falk JL: Fluid resuscitation in circulatory shock. Curr Stud Hematol Blood Transf 53:186–198, 1986.
5. Moss GS, Gould SA: Plasma expanders. Am J Surg 155:425–434, 1988.
6. Shoemaker WC: Fluids and electrolytes in the acutely ill adult. In Shoemaker WC, et al (eds): Textbook of Critical Care, 2nd ed. Philadelphia, W.B. Saunders, 1989, pp 1128–1151.

7. ENTERAL NUTRITION IN THE CRITICALLY ILL PATIENT

Anthony C. Campagna, M.D.

1. What is enteral nutrition?

Enteral nutrition is the administration of supplemental or total nutrient sources via the existing gastrointestinal tract of a patient who is unable to fulfill daily protein, caloric, and hydration requirements. Supplemental enteral nutrition may be given along with ad libitum or special diets for patients unable to meet all of their nutritional needs by mouth. More commonly in the ICU setting, enteral nutrition is used to provide total protein and caloric requirements and some hydration requirements for the patient.

2. What are the indications for initiation of enteral nutrition?

Any patients who will be unable to fulfill their nutritional requirements within 3–4 days should be considered candidates for supplemental nutrition. It has been shown that patients with head or abdominal trauma, bone marrow transplant candidates (even those who are not malnourished), patients undergoing cytoreduction, some postoperative surgical patients, and possibly malnourished cancer patients undergoing chemotherapy or radiation therapy might benefit from supplemental nutrition. Also, patients with significant nutritional depletion (defined as an unintentional weight loss of 10% or greater of usual body weight), protein malnutrition (kwashiorkor), or protein-calorie malnutrition (marasmus) will require supplemental nutrition. A functional gastrointestinal tract is necessary for enteral nutrition, and total parenteral nutrition may be necessary if clinical conditions prohibit enteral feeding.

3. In addition to weight loss, are there other indicators of malnutrition in the critically ill?

Anthropometric measurements such as the body mass index (BMI), mid-arm circumference (MAC), and triceps skinfold (TSF) are other indicators. These measurements correlate actual body part measurements and standard values with metabolic stress. In assessment of the critically ill patient, these should be measured on admission to the ICU, at 2–3 weeks, and monthly thereafter.

The creatinine-height index (CHI): actual 24-hour urinary creatinine divided by the ideal urinary creatinine multiplied by 100. When compared to standard calculations, this index estimates a measure of lean body mass by measuring muscle mass as a function of creatinine excretion. Serum albumin, prealbumin, and transferrin or total iron binding capacity (the "visceral proteins") may correlate to recent metabolic stress.

Other tests include total lymphocyte count and delayed hypersensitivity reaction assessment with skin testing for mumps, PPD, coccidioidin, streptokinase/streptodornase (SK-SD), and Candida as an assessment of immune function. Patients who are not receiving steroids may be considered anergic if they do not show a positive reaction to at least two of four antigens.

4. What types of enteral nutrition are available?

Currently, there are over 30 enteral nutrition solutions commercially available. They all contain, in different concentrations, protein (8–24%), carbohydrates (28–90%), and fat (1–55%) along with varying osmolalities (300–810 mOsm/kg H_2O) and concentrations of trace elements, vitamins, and electrolytes. Liquid bases include caseinates from milk, egg, free amino acids, soy, and lactalbumin. Individual patient nutritional requirements are necessary to choose the correct formula.

5. What is the Harris-Benedict equation? What is it used for?

For males, the Harris-Benedict equation is:

kcal/24 hr = 66.47 + [13.75 × (weight in kg)] + [5.0 × (height in cm)] – [6.76 × (age in years)].

For females:

kcal/24 hr = 655.1 + [9.56 × (weight in kg)] + [1.85 × (height in cm)] – [4.68 × (age in years)].

The Harris-Benedict equation estimates the basal energy expenditure (BEE) in nonstressed patients. In the critically ill, sepsis, trauma, head injury, or burns all increase energy requirements 20–30%, depending on the severity of the insult. The BEE may be multiplied by a stress factor and multiplied by an activity factor (1.25 if the patient is ambulatory) to better predict the true daily energy expenditure. The mean value of the sum of the "actual" and the "ideal" weights should be used as the weight value for obese patients to avoid overfeeding or underfeeding, respectively. The "actual weight" should be used in patients with recent or significant weight loss.

Reference: Schlictig R, Ayres SM: Nutritional Support of the Critically Ill. Chicago, Year Book, 1988, ch 3.

6. Are there any components of enteral feedings not found in current standard parenteral nutrition formulations?

Yes. Both formulations can contain long-chain fatty acids, amino acids, simple sugars, trace elements, and vitamins. However, nutrients found in enteral feedings but not found in current standard parenteral formulations are nucleic acids, medium- and short-chain fatty acids, complex carbohydrates (fiber), glutamine (important for gastrointestinal tract maintenance), peptides, and intact proteins (thought to be a superior source of nitrogen over amino acids for critically ill patients).

7. When is it appropriate to stop enteral feeding?

In the critically ill patient, enteral feeding should be continued until malnutrition is reversed (measured by anthropometric measurements and laboratory testing), an acceptable nitrogen balance is achieved, the external metabolic stress that prompted the enteral feeding is removed (e.g., burn injury, sepsis, respiratory failure requiring intubation, trauma), and the patient has a functioning gastrointestinal tract along with adequate mental status enabling fulfillment of protein, caloric, and hydration requirements. In all cases, specific nutritional goals should be addressed prior to initiation of enteral feeding.

8. What other clinical conditions should be considered when determining nutrient or fluid requirements in the critically ill?

1. **Organ failure:** cardiac (fluid overload), hepatic (end-stage liver disease), respiratory (CO_2 retention), renal (nephrotic syndrome, dialysis), gastrointestinal (malabsorption syndromes), endocrine (diabetes, insulin resistance secondary to sepsis, adrenal failure).

2. **Fistulas:** (surgical or spontaneous) viscus to viscus or viscus to cutaneous, involving any part of the gastrointestinal, biliary, or genitourinary system.

3. **Coagulation defects:** prolonged PT, PTT. Acquired antithrombin III deficiency secondary to protein malabsorption or nephrotic syndrome (a value of less than 75% of normal increases the risk of arterial or venous thrombosis).

4. **Chemotherapy** (agent, total and most recent dose, complications) and **radiation therapy** (total dose, location, and complications).

5. **Other:** nasogastric tube suctioning (metabolic alkalosis), diarrhea, renal tubular acidosis, ureteral diversion (hypokalemia).

9. What is the respiratory quotient? How is it determined? When is it used?

The respiratory quotient (RQ) is the ratio of the patient's carbon dioxide production to oxygen consumption and is measured most commonly in the ICU by the closed-circuit, indirect calorimetry method (metabolic cart). Caloric requirements are then derived from this ratio. For optimal calculation of a patient's caloric need, an RQ determination should be performed within 48–72 hours of ICU admission, again 3–4 days after the initiation of feeding, then as clinically indicated. An acceptable RQ is between 0.8 and 0.9 (physiologic range, 0.7–1.2) and can be manipulated by the fat and glucose content of the nutrition prescribed. In patients with respiratory failure or in ventilated patients, CO_2 production should be closely monitored (see question 4 in the next chapter).

10. How may nitrogen balance be estimated in the critically ill?
If a patient's 24-hour protein intake is known, and if the urine urea nitrogen (UUN) concentration measured from a 24-hour urine collection is known, then the patient's nitrogen balance may be estimated from the following equation:

$$\text{Nitrogen balance (gm/day)} = \frac{\text{protein intake (gm/day)}}{6.25} - [\text{UUN (gm/day)} + 4]$$

A negative number for the nitrogen balance signifies the patient is losing nitrogen or body cell mass (1 gm nitrogen = 30 gm of lean tissue) secondary to increased protein catabolism. These losses may be lessened with nutritional therapy.

11. Name four potential complications of enteral feeding in the critically ill patient.
    1. **Aspiration of feedings.** Although more common in nonintubated patients with altered mental status, even in patients with endotracheal tubes or tracheostomies, enteral feeding solution can leak around the inflated cuff and be aspirated into the lungs. Patients at risk for aspiration should have nasoduodenal instead of nasogastric tube placement or jejunostomy instead of a gastrostomy tube placement.
    2. **Pulmonary injury.** Pulmonary injury during placement of the feeding tube may range from mild hemorrhage secondary to tube trauma to puncture of the pleura resulting in pneumothorax. A chest roentgenogram to document correct position of the feeding tube prior to its use is a necessity. There have been many reports of enteral feeding solution entering the lung through a misplaced feeding tube in the bronchial tree, and causing mild respiratory insufficiency to frank pneumonia and death.
    3. **Diarrhea** (incidence approximately 30–40%). In critically ill patients with hypoalbuminemia, bowel edema and decreased absorption can lead to an increase in stool volume. Intravenous salt-poor albumin or total parenteral nutrition, both aimed at rapidly increasing serum albumin, and a peptide-based enteral diet (instead of a standard enteral diet) have all been suggested to combat this problem. Also, a protein-losing enteropathy may be present in the hypoalbuminemic patient with diarrhea. Several investigators have found correlation between the measurement of fecal alpha-1-antitrypsin level and elevated protein losses in the stool. In addition, some drugs (digoxin, quinidine, alpha-methyldopa, magnesium from antacids), lactose intolerance, fat malabsorption, concurrent antibiotics leading to *Clostridium difficile* infection, and hyperosmolar solutions given through feeding tube contribute to diarrhea during enteral feeding.
    4. **Nausea and vomiting.** More common in critically ill ICU patients with paralytic ileus, delayed gastric emptying or gastrointestinal edema.

12. Are there any contraindications to enteral feeding?
Critically ill patients who do not have a functional gastrointestinal tract (postoperative abdominal surgery, liver transplant) should not receive enteral feeding. Patients malnourished from a terminal illness and within 3 months of the end of their lives should probably receive only hydration therapy and not receive any type of supplemental nutrition. Patients malnourished from a terminal illness in whom the prognosis may be greater than 3 months should decide along with their family and physicians whether or not to begin supplemental

feeding. Also, in well-nourished patients immediately after surgery, it has never been shown that the routine use of jejunal feedings improves outcome.

BIBLIOGRAPHY

1. Baker JP, LeMoyne M: Nutritional support in the critically ill patient: If, when, how, and what. Crit Care Clin 3:97–113, 1987.
2. Benotti P, Blackburn GL: Protein and caloric or macronutrient metabolic management of the critically ill patient. Crit Care Med 7:520–525, 1979.
3. Blackburn GL, Bistrian BR, Maini BS, et al: Nutritional and metabolic assessment of the hospitalized patient. J Parenter Enteral Nutr 1:11–22, 1977.
4. Bower RH, Talamini MA, Sax HC, et al: Postoperative enteral vs parenteral nutrition—a randomized controlled study. Arch Surg 121:1040–1045, 1986.
5. Brinson RR, Pitts WM: Enteral nutrition in the critically ill patient: Role of hypoalbuminemia. Crit Care Med 17:367–370, 1989.
6. Fletcher JP, Little JM: A comparison of parenteral nutrition and early postoperative enteral feeding on the nitrogen balance after major surgery. Surgery 100:21–24, 1986.
7. Koruda MJ, Guenter P, Rombeau JL: Enteral nutrition in the critically ill. Crit Care Clin 3:133–153, 1987.
8. Schlictig R, Ayres SM: Nutritional Support of the Critically Ill. Chicago, Year Book, 1988, ch 3.
9. Talbot JM: Guidelines for the scientific review of enteral food products for special medical purposes. J Parenter Enteral Nutr 15(3 Suppl):99S–174S, 1991.

8. PARENTERAL NUTRITION IN THE CRITICALLY ILL PATIENT

Anthony C. Campagna, M.D.

1. What is parenteral nutrition?

Parenteral nutrition is the administration of supplemental or total nutrient sources via the peripheral or central venous route in patients who are unable to fulfill daily protein, caloric, and hydration requirements. Most commonly in the ICU, patients appropriate for parenteral nutrition will require total nutritional support. Central catheters allow administration of a much higher concentration of dextrose in water (25–45%) than do peripheral catheters, which are usually limited to a 5–15% dextrose solution.

2. What are the indications for beginning parenteral nutrition in the critically ill patient?

It is best to feed patients through the enteral route whenever possible. Parenteral nutrition provides no advantage (and may increase morbidity and cost) compared with enteral feedings in patients with a functioning gastrointestinal tract. Patients with requirements unable to be met by enteral feeding may benefit from parenteral feeding. Parenteral nutrition may be indicated in patients with an exacerbation of inflammatory bowel disease or pancreatitis, in bone marrow transplant patients with mucositis or diarrhea who need bowel rest, in some postoperative patients (e.g., after liver transplant or bowel resection), and in malnourished patients.

3. What are the daily protein, carbohydrate, fat, and water requirements for adults?

Protein. 1.0–1.5 gm/kg of ideal body weight per day (some sources recommend an upper limit of 2–3 gm/kg ideal body weight per day in severely stressed critically ill patients). In parenteral nutrition, protein should be given as a standard amino acid solution (see question 7 for comments on branched-chain amino acids).

Glucose. 2–4 gm/kg of ideal body weight per day given as dextrose. Some sources recommend an upper limit of 5 gm/kg ideal body weight—an upper limit of approximately 350 gm/day for a 70-kg patient.

Fat. If the caloric requirements cannot be reasonably met by protein and carbohydrates alone, it may be reasonable to add fat, beginning at 0.5 gm/kg/day as lipid. Increases may be initiated by approximately 0.5 gm/kg every 1–2 days to a maximum of 1.5–2.5 gm/kg/day. Serum triglyceride levels should be in an acceptable range before any increases are made. Fat in parenteral nutrition is usually given as long-chain fatty acids particularly linolenic acid (50–60%) along with linoleic, oleic, palmitic and stearic acid.

Water. Maintenance fluid requirements per hour are approximately: 5 cc/kg for the first 10 kg of body weight; 2.5 cc/kg for the next 10 kg of body weight, then 0.75 to 1 cc/kg for each 10 kg of body weight thereafter; e.g., a 70-kg nonstressed, afebrile patient for 24 hours will require approximately 2500 cc/day as maintenance fluid or 1500 cc of maintenance fluid per square meter of body surface area.

All of these recommendations are generalizations and should be modified, daily if necessary, in response to laboratory studies, respiratory quotient, respiratory status, core temperature, stress, and activity.

4. What are the potential disadvantages of total parenteral feeding in the critically ill?

1. **Complications of central venous access.** Immediate complications include pneumothorax, air embolism, vascular injury of the subclavian or carotid arteries, cardiac arrhythmias, hemothorax, loss of catheter integrity with embolism of a fragment, and tissue perforation of the thoracic duct, peripheral nerves, superior vena cava, or trachea. Delayed complications include thrombosis, arteriovenous fistula formation, pulmonary embolism, and infection (sepsis, catheter contamination, endocarditis). There is evidence that continuous low-dose heparin added to the parenteral nutrition may decrease the incidence of central vein thrombosis. It has also been shown that single-lumen rather than triple-lumen parenteral nutrition catheters can minimize the risk of catheter-related sepsis (see question 11 for additional comments on infection).

2. **Excess carbon monoxide (CO_2) production.** The oxidation of fat produces one-third less CO_2 than oxidation of glucose. Patients with respiratory failure or patients requiring mechanical ventilation may benefit from a parenteral nutrition solution of approximately 50% carbohydrates and 50% fat as lipid emulsion to prevent excess CO_2 production. However, the exact mixture of carbohydrate to fat should be a function of the measured respiratory quotient, serum triglycerides, and serum glucose levels.

3. **Hyperglycemia.** Continuous 24-hour parenteral feeding will produce hyperglycemia. Insulin may be added directly to the daily solution along with a sliding scale for subcutaneous regular insulin to assist the body's own insulin production in achieving euglycemia. Also, a serum glucose greater than 200 mg/dl can cause an osmotic diuresis and inhibit white blood cell function.

4. **Cost.** Parenteral nutrition may cost 2 to 10 times more and requires more laboratory testing than enteral feeding.

5. Name eight "trace elements" (along with their functions) that should be included in parenteral nutrition solutions. How often should they be added?

1. Zinc: protein synthesis of multiple enzymes
2. Copper: hemoglobin synthesis, erythrocyte survival
3. Iron: hemoglobin, myoglobin
4. Selenium: may protect sulfhydryl group oxidation
5. Manganese: cofactor of pyruvate carboxylase and superoxide dismutase
6. Chromium: glucose metabolism

7. Cobalt: formation of vitamin B12 (cyanocobalamin)
8. Iodine: thyroid function

Zinc, copper, manganese, selenium, chromium, and iodine should be given daily. Iron, 2 mg, may be given daily. Cobalt need not be added. Vitamin B12 fulfills the cobalt requirement. Copper and manganese should be withheld from patients with abnormal liver function. Manganese deficiency has not been described in humans on total parenteral nutrition.

6. What is the debate between giving protein as a standard amino acid solution versus a "branched-chain-enriched" amino acid solution?

It has been suggested that branched-chain amino acids (BCAAs)—leucine, isoleucine, valine—when given parenterally to stressed patients, will decrease the amount of skeletal muscle breakdown (the body's primary source of BCAA) during a catabolic state. In theory, parenteral BCAA, especially leucine, may increase muscle protein synthesis and decrease protein breakdown when glucose and fats are not available as fuel. Although some investigators have found a significant trend toward positive nitrogen balance in patients administered BCAA, others have not. Differences in study design, control "standard" parenteral nutrition solutions, and level of stress in the patients studied all may account for the differing results. Further studies are needed to better define which subgroups of patients may benefit from BCAA-supplemented nutrition.

7. Which vitamins are necessary to include in parenteral nutrition solutions? How often should they be added? How are they used by the body? How are their deficient states manifested?

The first nine vitamins are water soluble:

Vitamin C (ascorbic acid): collagen synthesis. Deficiency: scurvy (muscle weakness and tenderness, gum swelling, petechial hemorrhages, and anemia) and altered wound healing.

B1 (thiamine): ATP synthesis; formation of reduced nicotinamide adenine dinucleotide phosphate (NADPH) and pentose. Deficiency: peripheral neuropathy, beriberi (polyneuritis, heart disease, edema), Wernicke's encephalopathy, and Korsakoff's syndrome.

B2 (riboflavin): converted to flavin adenine dinucleotide (FAD) and flavin mononucleotide (FMN). Deficiency: photophobia, glossitis, fissuring and scaling of the lips (cheilosis), and pruritus.

B6 (pyridoxine): amino acid and lipid metabolism; glycogenolysis; porphyrin and neurotransmitter synthesis. Deficiency: increased renal and bladder calcium oxalate stones.

B3 (niacin): supplies the coenzymes nicotinamide adenine dinucleotide (NAD) and nicotinamide adenine dinucleotide phosphate (NADP). Deficiency: pellagra (dermatitis, diarrhea, dementia, and inflammation of mucous membranes).

Pantothenic acid: a component of coenzyme A; oxidation of fatty acids and pyruvate; acetylation of amines. Deficiency: fatigue, abdominal cramping, pain, and paresthesias.

Biotin: cofactor of acetyl-CoA carboxylase (fatty acid synthesis), pyruvate carboxylase (gluconeogenesis), and propionyl-CoA carboxylase (amino acid catabolism). Deficiency: hair loss, myalgias, paresthesias, atrophy of the tongue, and dermatitis.

Folic acid: Purine and pyrimidine synthesis. Deficiency: macrocytic anemia.

B12 (cyanocobalamin): DNA synthesis; folic acid metabolism. Deficiency: macrocytic (pernicious) anemia.

The remaining four vitamins are fat soluble:

Vitamin A: vision, cell growth, and differentiation. Deficiency: night blindness and follicular hyperdermatosis.

Vitamin D: bone mineralization. Deficiency: rickets (children), osteomalacia (adults).

Vitamin E: antioxidant; controls hydroperoxide formation. Deficiency: hemolysis.

Vitamin K: synthesis of clotting factors II, VII, IX, and X. Deficiency: excessive bleeding.

Although it is generally agreed that vitamins should be given daily, doses for critically ill patients have not been rigorously studied. Most pharmacies add standard doses based on requirements for healthy subjects. Vitamin K is not routinely added to the daily preparation. Empirically, it may be given subcutaneously once weekly or in response to an elevated prothrombin value.

8. What considerations should be made for electrolytes in the parenteral nutrition solution?
Current recommended ranges of electrolyte requirements in total parenteral nutrition are as follows:

Sodium chloride: 60–150 mEq/day
Potassium chloride: 60–100 mEq/day
Acetate (converted to HCO_3^-): 10–40 mEq/day (combined with Na^+ or K^+)
Chloride: 40–100 mEq/day (given as NaCl or KCl)
Calcium: 5–20 mEq/day (given as calcium gluconate)
Magnesium: 8–15 mEq (some sources recommend up to 45 mEq) per day as magnesium sulfate.

9. Can anything else be added directly or "piggybacked" into the parenteral nutrition solution?
Yes, as long as the medication has "physical" and "chemical" compatibility. A partial list of those which may be added directly is: albumin, aminophylline, cyclophosphamide, cytarabine, dopamine, furosemide, heparin, hydrocortisone, insulin, isoproterenol, lidocaine, methotrexate, methyldopa hydrochloride, metoclopramide and the H2 blockers, cimetidine, and ranitidine. When given over a 24-hour period of parenteral feeding, the dose of cimetidine can be reduced (routinely to as low as 900 mg for 24 hours), and the same prophylactic protective effect can be achieved as with full-dose bolus administration. Experimentally in humans, vancomycin has also been added directly to the parenteral nutrition solution with adequate peripheral blood levels achieved.

Although it is best to minimize injections into a parenteral nutrition catheter, antibiotics are routinely piggybacked into these lines. Antibiotics known to be compatible are penicillins, cephalosporins, aminoglycosides, clindamycin, and tetracycline.

10. Which laboratory parameters should be monitored and how often should they be monitored during total parenteral nutrition?
Baseline values for Na, K, Cl, HCO_3, serum glucose, BUN, creatinine, PO_4, Mg, albumin, calcium, liver function tests, and CBC with differential should be drawn. Daily intake, output, and weight along with urine dipstick for acetone and glucose should be recorded. Electrolytes and glucose should then be monitored daily for 3–4 days until stable, then checked every other day. Calcium, magnesium, phosphate, BUN, and creatinine should be tested every other day until stable, then may be checked every 3 or 4 days. Liver function tests and albumin should be checked every 10–14 days. If lipid emulsion is being administered, a triglyceride level approximately 4–5 hours after the end of the first infusion should be checked. More frequent testing may be necessary depending on the clinical situation.

11. How should the patient with a central venous parenteral feeding catheter and a fever be managed?
Management of a fever in a patient with a total parenteral nutrition catheter should include removal of the catheter over a guidewire, semiquantitative culture of the catheter tip, and, if not contraindicated, placement of a new catheter over the guidewire at the same site. In addition to a physical exam (including the skin and peripheral access sites), a chest roentgenogram and peripheral blood and urine cultures should be obtained. Echenique et al. have described a protocol for interpretation of blood cultures through the catheter, catheter tip

culture, peripheral blood cultures, and management. Purulence at the insertion site or hypotension due to possible sepsis should prompt catheter removal and reinsertion at a new site.

BIBLIOGRAPHY

1. Armstrong CW, Mayhall CG, Miller KB, et al: Prospective study of catheter replacement and other risk factors for infection of hyperalimentation catheters. J Infect Dis 154:808–816, 1986.
2. Baptista RJ: Medications compatible with hyperalimentation solutions. Nutr Support Serv 3:18–22, 1983.
3. Cochran EB, Kamper CA, Phelps SJ, Brown RO: Parenteral nutrition in the critically ill patient. Clin Pharm 8:783–799, 1989.
4. Driscoll DF, Bistrian BR: Clinical issues in the therapeutic monitoring of total parenteral nutrition. Clin Lab Med 7:699–714, 1987.
5. Echenique MM, Bistrian BR, Blackburn GI: Theory and technique of nutritional support in the ICU. Crit Care Med 10:546–549, 1982.
6. Imperial J, Bistrian BR, Bothe A, et al: Limitation of central vein thrombosis in total parenteral nutrition by continuous infusion of low-dose heparin. J Am Coll Nutr 2:63–73, 1983.
7. LeMoyne M, Jeejeebhoy KN: Total parenteral nutrition in the critically ill patient. Chest 89:568–575, 1986.
8. Pemberton LB, Lyman B, Lander V, Covinsky J: Sepsis from triple- vs. single-lumen catheters during total parenteral nutrition in surgical or critically ill patients. Arch Surg 121:591–594, 1986.
9. Shizgal HM: Parenteral and enteral nutrition. Annu Rev Med 42:549–565, 1991.
10. Vander Woude PV, Morgan RE, Kosta JM, Davis AT, et al: Addition of branched-chain amino acid to parenteral nutrition of stressed critically ill patients. Crit Care Med 14:685–688, 1986.
11. Vanhuynegem L, Parmentier P, Potvliege C: In situ bacteriologic diagnosis of total parenteral nutrition catheter infection. Surgery 103:174–177, 1988.
12. Veterans Affairs Total Parenteral Nutrition Cooperative Study Group: Perioperative total parenteral nutrition in surgical patients. N Engl J Med 325:525–532, 1991.
13. Weissman C, Hyman AI: Nutritional care of the critically ill patient with respiratory failure. Crit Care Clin 3:185–203, 1987.

9. MECHANICAL VENTILATION

Carolyn H. Welsh, M.D.

1. What are the indications for mechanical ventilation?

The majority (75%) of patients requiring mechanical ventilation have **ventilatory failure** with the inability to exchange air and adequately expire carbon dioxide (CO_2). This results in a high blood PCO_2 and low pH. Causes of this type of respiratory failure include sedation, general anesthesia, drug overdose, neuromuscular disease, chest wall deformity, and airway diseases such as chronic obstructive lung disease and asthma.

In general, patients with **acute ventilatory failure** require intubation and ventilation if they hypoventilate to a PCO_2 greater than 50 mm Hg with a pH of less than 7.30. Patients with acute superimposed on chronic ventilatory failure may have a much higher PCO_2, up to 80 mm Hg, before requiring intubation, since they develop chronic CO_2 retention with metabolic compensation.

A smaller number of patients require ventilation for **hypoxemia**, as they fail to oxygenate their blood even with supplemental oxygen. These patients are frequently able to ventilate well, as demonstrated by a low arterial PCO_2. Causes of hypoxemic respiratory failure include pneumonia, aspiration, adult respiratory distress syndrome (ARDS), and pulmonary emboli. Hypoxemic patients usually require mechanical ventilation if they have a PO_2 less than 50 mm Hg on a 100% oxygen nonrebreather mask.

2. How are ventilator settings determined?

Ventilator settings are chosen to optimize both oxygen exchange and acid base status. Most patients start with a fraction of inspired oxygen (FiO_2) of 1.00 (100% oxygen). If the PO_2 is high on arterial blood gas analysis, the FiO_2 is decreased incrementally to give a PO_2 of 60–90 torr. When possible, a fraction of inspired oxygen of 0.4–0.5 is selected to avoid oxygen toxicity.

As a general estimate, a tidal volume of 10–12 ml/kg is chosen, which is approximately 800 ml for a 70-kg person. For a routine postoperative patient, a respiratory rate of 10–15 breaths per minute is selected to deliver a minute ventilation (tidal volume × respiratory rate) of 8–12 liters per minute. Although these supraphysiologic tidal volumes are recommended, a recent study compared 12 mg/kg with 6 ml/kg tidal volumes and found that the lower tidal volumes were associated with a decreased incidence of pulmonary infection, duration of intubation, and length of ICU stay. The optimal choice of tidal volumes is controversial, but low tidal volumes will be used more frequently in the future.

3. What parameters are followed to see if a patient is receiving adequate ventilation?

The simplest method to assess adequacy of ventilation is observation of the patient for comfort, synchrony of chest and abdominal movement with delivered ventilator breaths, absence of cyanosis, and symmetry of chest movement. Observation can detect major problems. For example, if the right mainstem bronchus rather than the trachea is intubated, the right chest will move but the left will be stationary, and breath sounds can be auscultated to confirm this. Twenty to thirty minutes after initiation of ventilation or after ventilator changes, an arterial blood gas is drawn to check for adequacy of oxygenation ($PO_2 \geq 60$ mm Hg) and ventilation ($PCO_2 = 25$–45 mm Hg, pH = 7.33–7.49).

Important parameters to follow also include the peak and static airway pressures, which are recorded on a pressure manometer dial or digital printout. **Peak pressures** are the highest pressures measured during end inspiration. High peak pressures may indicate bronchospasm, inappropriate selection of ventilator settings, or pneumothorax. **Static pressures** reflect underlying properties of lung tissue and are measured during the last second of expiration by kinking the exhalation line or adding an inspiratory pause. Static pressures will be increased with processes that stiffen the lung such as ARDS, pulmonary edema, pneumonia, and fibrosis. Static pressures may be decreased with emphysema.

4. How can static pressures be normalized for changes in ventilator tidal volume?

During mechanical ventilation, static pressures may rise because of increases in the tidal volume settings as well as increases in lung stiffness. Thus, a decreased pressure may reflect a lower tidal volume rather than a change in the lung itself. We calculate static compliance as follows:

$$\frac{\text{tidal volume}}{(\text{static pressure} - \text{PEEP})}$$

where PEEP = positive end-expiratory pressure, and normal static compliance is 60–100 ml/cm H_2O.

By calculating compliance, we can compare information on lung stiffness despite changes in the tidal volume settings. Compliance decreases with processes that stiffen the lung, such as ARDS, pulmonary edema, pneumonia, and fibrosis, and can be followed serially to assess patient improvement.

5. What is oxygen delivery?

$$\text{Oxygen delivery} = \text{cardiac output} \times \text{oxygen content}$$
$$\text{Oxygen content} = (1.38 \times \text{Hgb} \times SaO_2) + (PaO_2 \times 0.003)$$

where Hgb is hemoglobin concentration, SaO_2 = arterial oxygen saturation, 1.38 = affinity constant of oxygen for hemoglobin, and 0.003 reflects the solubility of oxygen in plasma.

Delivery of oxygen to tissues is a more sensitive measure of dysfunction than a single PO_2 reading, since oxygen delivery incorporates PO_2, cardiac output, and hemoglobin concentration, all of which affect the utilization of oxygen. Oxygen delivery may be impaired when PO_2 is in the normal range. It is frequently compromised in the settings of cardiogenic shock, anemia, ARDS, and sepsis.

6. Do mechanical ventilators affect the cardiovascular system?
Positive-pressure ventilation decreases cardiac output and may lead to hypotension. The most common mechanism is that positive pressure in the thorax diminishes venous return to the heart and creates a low cardiac output state. Decreased cardiac output may result in poor tissue delivery of oxygen. In patients with cardiogenic pulmonary edema, the lowering of venous return to the heart during mechanical ventilation may lessen edema and actually improve oxygenation by shortening muscle fiber length and increasing contractility of the heart muscle.

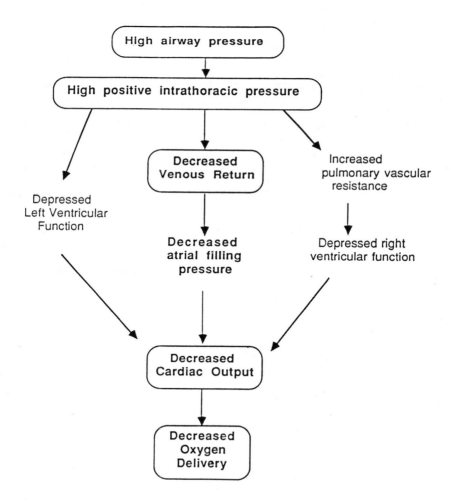

Three pathophysiologic mechanisms of decreased cardiac output and oxygen delivery during mechanical ventilation. Clinically, decreased venous return appears to be most important.

7. What is the most common complication of mechanical ventilation? Why? Other common complications?

Barotrauma. High airway pressures may induce rupture of the alveolar wall at its weakest point, leading to egress of air into the bronchovascular sheath. If air remains in the sheath, it tracks to the mediastinum and pleura, leading to pneumomediastinum, pneumothorax, pneumoperitoneum, and subcutaneous emphysema. If air enters the pulmonary vessels, the devastating air emboli syndrome characterized by livedo reticularis, cardiac arrhythmias, and unexplained altered mental status or stroke may ensue.

Other common complications of positive-pressure mechanical ventilation include increased intracranial pressure, fluid retention, renal failure, hyponatremia, local trauma to the nares and mouth, tracheal necrosis and hemorrhage from high endotracheal tube cuff pressures, and nosocomial infections such as sinusitis and pneumonia.

8. How important is nosocomial pneumonia in ventilated patients?

In ventilated patients, it is frequently difficult to distinguish clinical pneumonia from tracheal colonization with bacteria. Pneumonia is defined as fever, change in character of the sputum, rise in the white blood cell count, a Gram stain showing bacteria and more than 25 neutrophils per field in the absence of epithelial cells, and a positive bacterial culture. Colonization is characterized by a positive Gram stain or culture without the clinical changes of infection and white blood cell rise. Pneumonia clearly warrants treatment, whereas colonization does not.

Up to 30% of patients requiring mechanical ventilation for longer than 48 hours die from nosocomial pneumonia. Most of these pneumonias develop during the first 10 days of ventilation. Much of the increased risk is attributable to bacteremia from intravenous line contamination or to altered host immune function from immunocompromising diseases and treatments. In addition, mechanical disruption of mucociliary clearance by endotracheal tubes and suction catheters increases bacterial colonization and predisposes to infection. Although controversial, recent studies suggest that patients receiving antacids or H_2 receptor blockers to decrease gastric pH and prevent stress gastritis may have a slightly increased risk of nosocomial pneumonia.

9. How do assist control and intermittent mandatory ventilation (IMV) differ?

Assist control and IMV are commonly used ventilator modes of positive-pressure ventilation available on most commercial ventilators. Both modes share several common features and are standards of care. Both deliver a preset volume such that if set at a tidal volume of 800 ml and a rate of 10, both will deliver at least an 8-liter minute ventilation. To improve patient comfort and synchrony, both modes are designed to accommodate additional patient-initiated breaths.

These types of ventilation differ in that assist control delivers each initiated breath to the full preset tidal volume, whereas IMV delivers each initiated breath to only as much volume as pressure from the patient's muscles generates and also intermittently delivers the full preset tidal volume at the preset rate. Modern ventilators synchronize breath delivery to patient-initiated breathing, frequently referred to as **synchronized intermittent mandatory ventilation** (SIMV). (See figure on next page.)

10. When is assist control preferable to IMV?

To initiate an IMV breath on most ventilators, the patient must generate enough force to pop open both a demand valve for inspiration and a second valve for exhalation. Thus, IMV increases the work of breathing by the amount of work required to overcome the valve pressures. The effort required for this can be considerable, and has been measured as high as 6 cm H_2O pressure. Due to this increased work of breathing, IMV may hasten fatigue and compromise weaning in patients with neuromuscular weakness, severe COPD, or high minute ventilation needs. For these patients, the assist control mode may be preferable.

AIRWAY PRESSURE WAVEFORMS

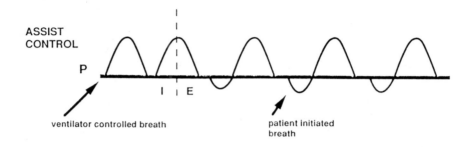

ASSIST
CONTROL

P

I E

ventilator controlled breath

patient initiated
breath

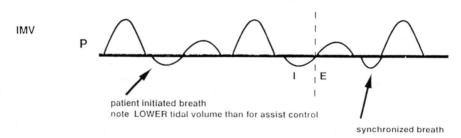

IMV

P

I E

patient initiated breath
note LOWER tidal volume than for assist control

synchronized breath

P = airway pressure during assist control and IMV modes of ventilation with upward deflections positive in pressure and downward negative. I = inspiration and E = expiration. In contrast to normal breathing, both phases of respiration are positive in pressure with ventilator-delivered breaths.

11. When is IMV preferable to assist control?

Patients with respiratory alkalemia (low PCO_2, high pH) may benefit from IMV, because the minute ventilation delivery with IMV is lower for a given respiratory rate due to delivery of a lower tidal volume for patient-initiated breaths. Two studies have directly compared IMV with assist control for the same patients. Both found a minimal decrease in pH for patients ventilated with IMV. Thus, with respiratory alkalemia, IMV may have a slight advantage over assist control.

12. How is respiratory alkalemia treated?

Respiratory alkalemia, particularly when the pH is greater than 7.60, may induce seizures or arrhythmias or may depress cardiac function. It may also decrease oxygen delivery by shifting the oxyhemoglobin dissociation curve to the left, preventing release of oxygen from hemoglobin to the tissues. To avoid these problems, several ventilator maneuvers and changes in patient management should be considered and implemented. Arterial blood gases should be checked to monitor for decreased oxygenation and to assess the efficacy of the changes.

    1. Decrease ventilator rate
    2. Decrease tidal volume
    3. Add dead space tubing to the ventilator circuit in 6-inch increments
    4. Switch from assist control to IMV mode
    5. Change the trigger valve sensitivity to less sensitive

6. Sedate the patient, and consider paralysis if medically indicated
7. Extubate

13. What do you do if a patient on the ventilator is agitated or the ventilator alarms?

Agitation should be used as a clue to machine malfunction or a change in the patient's medical status. It is important to remove the patient from the ventilator and ventilate with a resuscitation bag while evaluating the problem.

Common ventilator problems include (1) inadvertent disconnection of the patient from the ventilator, and (2) use of inappropriate ventilator settings such as low trigger sensitivity, low flow rates, or ventilator response delay. Always check the ventilator for problems with settings and connections, as these are easily correctable.

Changes in the patient's medical condition that may affect ventilation include both airway and neurologic problems: mucous plugs and copious secretions, bronchospasm, pneumothorax, pulmonary edema, sepsis, carbon dioxide retention, hypoxemia, lobar collapse, pulmonary emboli, pain, hallucinations, and awakening from sedation.

14. What is PEEP?

PEEP, positive end-expiratory pressure, is positive pressure applied to the expiration circuit. In effect, PEEP works by increasing the functional residual capacity of the lung, preventing collapse of some alveoli while overdistending others. This usually leads to improved ventilation-perfusion matching in the pulmonary circulation.

15. What are the indications for PEEP? How do you monitor its effects?

PEEP is used primarily to improve arterial oxygenation in severely hypoxemic patients or to decrease the fraction of inspired oxygen to avoid pulmonary oxygen toxicity. PEEP has also been advocated to decrease mediastinal bleeding immediately after open heart surgery, although this remains controversial. A large number of studies show no efficacy of PEEP in this regard, and recommend avoiding PEEP because of its potential for decreasing cardiac output. PEEP can be monitored with a "best PEEP" trial.

1. Use stepwise increments of 3–5 cm H_2O PEEP, starting at 0 cm.

2. Minimize the time interval between changes (20–30 minutes is ideal) to increase the likelihood that a response is due to PEEP itself rather than a change in the patient's condition.

3. Note and evaluate the response to each change with blood pressure measurements, an arterial blood gas sample, cardiac output, and oxygen delivery calculations. The best PEEP is that achieved when the inspired oxygen decreases to a minimal level without compromising oxygen delivery.

16. What is auto-PEEP?

Auto-PEEP, or intrinsic PEEP, is the inadvertent development of PEEP due to the ventilator delivery of a positive-pressure breath prior to complete exhalation of the previous breath. Thus, it is seen in patients with high minute ventilation, as in ARDS and in diseases of airflow limitation such as asthma and chronic obstructive lung disease. Since the ventilator manometer dial does not reflect auto-PEEP, detection involves occlusion of the expiratory port at end exhalation, allowing equilibration of airway and circuit pressure. The complications of auto-PEEP are similar to those of applied PEEP: diminished cardiac output and hypotension, barotrauma, and inaccurate pulmonary artery catheter measurements leading to inappropriate fluid and pressor administration or diuresis.

17. How can auto-PEEP be remedied?

Primary treatment for auto-PEEP is treatment of the underlying bronchospasm. Other treatment approaches include raising inspiratory flow rates to maximize expiratory time, increasing endotracheal tube size, and lowering minute ventilation by decreasing respiratory rate or tidal volume. If this dangerous problem persists, the patient should be sedated and perhaps paralyzed. Although some practitioners treat auto-PEEP by applying PEEP in centimeters equivalent to the original auto-PEEP, others think this enhances the risk of barotrauma and should be avoided.

18. Are there other options for positive-pressure mechanical ventilation in patients with respiratory failure?

Although mechanical ventilation saves lives, it has clear complications and limitations. For patients with acute bronchospasm in whom positive-pressure ventilation is risky, vigorous treatment of the underlying disease may abolish the need for mechanical ventilation. Frequent intermittent positive pressure breathing (IPPB) treatments may be used for patients with acute exacerbations of chronic obstructive lung disease to avoid long-term mechanical ventilation. Negative-pressure ventilators are used for pediatric patients and may be used for adults with normally compliant lungs as in neuromuscular disease. For patients with hypoxemic respiratory failure, continuous positive airway pressure (CPAP) masks may improve PO_2 and substitute for mechanical ventilation. Patients with ARDS who remain hypoxic despite 100% FiO_2 and PEEP are occasionally treated with extracorporeal membrane oxygenation (ECMO), bypassing the diseased lungs to better oxygenate blood and tissue.

BIBLIOGRAPHY

1. Ashbaugh DG, Petty TL: Positive end-expiratory pressure: Physiology, indications, and contraindications. J Thorac and Cardiovasc Surg 65:165–170, 1973.
2. Brown DG, Pierson DJ: Auto-PEEP is common in mechanically ventilated patients: A study of incidence, severity, and detection. Respir Care 31:1069–1074, 1986.
3. Culpepper JA, Rinaldo JE, Rogers RM: Effect of mechanical ventilator mode on tendency towards respiratory alkalosis. Am Rev Respir Dis 132:1075–1077, 1985.
4. Driks MR, Graven DE, Celli BR, et al: Nosocomial pneumonia in intubated patients given sucralfate compared with antacids or histamine type 2 blockers: The role of gastric colonization. N Engl J Med 317:1376–1382, 1987.
5. Fagon JY, Chastre J, Domart Y, et al: Nocosomial pneumonia in patients receiving continuous mechanical ventilation. Am Rev Respir Dis 139:877–884, 1988.
6. Hudson LD, Hurlow RS, Craig KC, Pierson DJ: Does intermittent mandatory ventilation correct respiratory alkalosis in patients receiving assisted mechanical ventilation? Am Rev Respir Dis 132:1071–1074, 1985.
7. Lee PC, Helsmoortel CM, Cohn SM, Fink MP: Are low tidal volumes safe? Chest 97:430–434, 1990.
8. Marini JJ, Culver BH: Systemic gas embolism complicating mechanical ventilation in the adult respiratory distress syndrome. Ann Intern Med 110:699–703, 1989.
9. Mathru M, Rao TLK, Venus B: Ventilator-induced barotrauma in controlled mechanical ventilation versus intermittent mandatory ventilation. Crit Care Med 11:359–361, 1983.
10. Pepe PE, Marini JJ: Occult positive end-expiratory pressure mechanically ventilated patients with airflow obstruction. Am Rev Respir Dis 126:166–170, 1982.
11. Tobin MJ, Dantzker DR: Mechanical ventilation and weaning. In Danzker D (ed): Cardiopulmonary Critical Care. Philadelphia, W.B. Saunders, 1991, pp 259–308.

10. WEANING FROM MECHANICAL VENTILATION

Enrique Fernandez, M.D.

1. What percentage of patients can be readily weaned from mechanical ventilation?
Most patients who require mechanical ventilation can be easily removed from ventilator support. At the University of Colorado, 77% of all surviving patients on ventilators were successfully removed from mechanical ventilators within 72 hours of the initiation of ventilatory support, 91% had ventilatory assistance withdrawn in less than 7 days, and approximately 9% of patients on ventilators required prolonged or lifelong ventilation.

2. When should weaning from mechanical ventilation be considered?
There are two "systems" to evaluate: the ventilatory pump and gas exchange.

Ventilatory Pump
Vital capacity of > 10–15 ml/kg body weight
Tidal volume > 4 ml/kg body weight
Minute ventilation < 10 L/min
Maximum minute ventilation > 2 times resting minute ventilation
Maximum negative inspiratory pressure (MIP) < -25 to -30 cm H_2O
Respiratory rate < 35 breaths/min (in adults)

Gas Exchange
PaO_2: > 80 torr with $FiO_2 < 0.6$
$PaCO_2$: < 45 torr (except in patients with chronic hypercapnia)
$P(A\text{-}a)O_2$: < 300–350 torr with $FiO_2 = 1.0$

3. Is there any single parameter or specific group of parameters that predicts weaning success?
No. The accuracy of various predictive measurements often depends on patient selection, duration of ventilatory support, level of physician aggressiveness, and other factors. Various predictive parameters have been evaluated, but in all cases there are patients successfully weaned despite poor predictive measurements and patients who fail weaning despite stellar numbers.

4. What additional factors should be considered when weaning patients from prolonged mechanical ventilation?
Patients who require prolonged mechanical ventilation typically may have chronic lung disease exacerbated by acute infection or another acute process, overwhelming acute pulmonary disease with previously normal lungs, respiratory failure associated with extrapulmonary organ system failure, or neuromuscular disease. In these patients, reported hospital discharge and 1-year survival rate range from 35–85%, respectively. Objective criteria for when to begin the weaning process in patients who require prolonged mechanical ventilation have not been established. It has been said that an MIP > 25 cm H_2O, a forced vital capacity (FVC) > 12–15 ml/kg, or a ratio of dead space to tidal volume (VD/Vt) < 0.6 may distinguish patients who will wean successfully from those who will not. The weaning approach should be gradual and consist of sessions of weaning of increasing duration interspersed between periods of mechanical ventilation. All factors related to failure to wean should be kept in mind and treated if present.

5. Describe several weaning methods that are available.
  1. **T-tube weaning.** One approach that has been used successfully in discontinuing mechanical ventilation following short-term ventilatory support is to allow the patient to

breathe on a T-piece circuit with an FiO_2 of approximately 0.4; if the patient remains comfortable, arterial blood gases are obtained after 30 minutes. Provided that oxygenation during spontaneous breathing has been maintained ($PaO_2 > 60$ mm Hg and similar to that on mechanical ventilator) and there is no significant CO_2 retention (< 5 mm Hg increase in $PaCO_2$) or acute fall in arterial pH, after suctioning and a brief rest period on the ventilator, the patient is extubated. If a T-tube system is used, the gas source flow to the inspiratory limb should be at least twice that of the patient's spontaneous minute ventilation in order to meet the patient's peak inspiratory flow rate. An extension piece, usually about 12 inches in length, should be added to the expiratory limb to prevent entrainment of room air.

2. **Intermittent mandatory ventilation (IMV) weaning.** The patient receiving IMV can breathe spontaneously but, in addition, receives periodic positive-pressure breaths from the ventilator at a preset volume and frequency. Machine-delivered cycles are usually provided initially at 10–12 breaths/min with a tidal volume (Vt) of 10–12 ml/kg. The IMV rate is then progressively decreased at intervals of 1–4 as long as spontaneous ventilation continues and arterial pH remains greater than 7.30. The patient's clinical status should be followed and adequacy of oxygenation assessed with oximetry or periodic measurement of arterial blood gases. The ventilator can be removed and extubation performed once the patient remains stable with adequate blood gas values on an IMV rate of zero for 1 hour. It has been suggested that IMV has several advantages. It may prevent the patient from "fighting" the ventilator, limit the need for sedation and muscle paralysis, reduce the likelihood of respiratory alkalemia, achieve a more normal matching of ventilation and perfusion, decrease oxygen consumption, reduce paradoxical breathing and respiratory muscle fatigue, and allow more rapid weaning from the ventilator. Data supporting these claims are minimal.

IMV and T-tube weaning techniques have been compared. No differences have been found in duration of the weaning time, in PaO_2, $PaCO_2$, cardiac index, shunt, oxygen consumption, or CO_2 production.

3. **Pressure-support ventilation (PSV).** PSV can be used for mechanical ventilation and/or weaning. This ventilatory mode augments a spontaneous breath with a fixed amount of positive pressure. The level of positive pressure is set by the physician, but the patient has control over the respiratory frequency, inspiratory time, and inspiratory flow rate. Tidal volume is determined by the level of PSV, patient effort, and pulmonary mechanics. Unlike IMV, PSV assists every breath initiated by the patient. A disadvantage of PSV is the need for each ventilatory cycle to be initiated by the patient. Consequently, patients with an unstable respiratory center output or rapidly changing lung mechanics may receive an inadequate level of ventilatory support. Low-level PSV (5–10 cm H_2O) can eliminate the pressure work required for spontaneous airflow through an endotracheal tube. Higher levels can be used to augment the patient's effort to produce tidal breaths equivalent to those supplied by conventional mechanical ventilation support. With this level of support, it appears that the patient's ventilatory muscle work is near zero. Weaning from PSV can be performed by gradually decreasing the pressure level in 3–6 cm of H_2O decrements as tolerated, and extubation can be performed at PSV of 5 cm H_2O.

4. **Continuous positive airway pressure (CPAP).** It has been suggested that CPAP be used in patients who benefit from PEEP while on the respirator but who are, in fact, able to support their respirations without ventilatory assistance.

6. How should the patient be monitored during a weaning trial?

To monitor a weaning trial, it is desirable to avoid respiratory arrest, improve comfort, assess daily progress, and predict the future course of the patient. Ideally there should be on-line monitoring of oxygenation, CO_2 production and elimination, efficiency of gas exchange, work of breathing, ventilatory drive center output, ventilatory muscle strength, fatigue, and efficiency of gas exchange. However, physical examination provides the most important integration of monitoring techniques currently available. Important physical findings that suggest that the patient may be failing weaning are:

- Recession of the suprasternal notch
- Retraction in the intercostal spaces
- Accessory muscle recruitment
- Abdominal paradoxical motion
- Rapid, shallow breathing
- Respiratory alternans

7. Name indications for the termination of weaning.

The decision to discontinue weaning and to reinstitute ventilatory support is usually based on careful clinical evaluation and assessment of the indices reflecting respiratory work, gas exchange, and cardiac function. Clinical signs of retraction of intercostal spaces, abdominal paradoxical motion, rapid shallow breathing, and respiratory alkalosis are all considered markers of intolerable load for the respiratory system. Other signs and/or laboratory values that should be considered as possible indications of failure of the weaning attempt include:

- Patient discomfort, anxiety, or progressive obtundation
- Diastolic pressure > 100 torr or rise or fall in systolic blood pressure of 20 torr (mean arterial pressure change > 15 torr)
- Pulse rate >110 beats/min or increased > 20 beats/min
- Respiratory rate > 30 breaths/min or increased > 10 breaths/min
- Tidal volume < 250–300 ml (in adults < 3–4 ml/kg of dry weight)
- Significant ECG changes (extrasystolic > 6/min; ST changes or ventricular conduction defects)
- $P(A-a)O_2$ > 400 torr (FiO_2 = 1.0)
- PaO_2 < 60 torr*
- $PaCO_2$ > 55 torr* or increased > 8 torr
- pH < 7.35*
- PCWP or LAP > 20 torr
- Cardiac index < 1.9 L/min/m².

* A lower PaO_2 and/or pH and a higher $PaCO_2$ are acceptable in patients with COPD.

8. What should you look for when a patient fails a weaning trial?

1. **Is the patient at optimal mechanical advantage for breathing?** It is important that patients being weaned from mechanical ventilation be upright during the procedure; most of the time, movement of the diaphragm is impeded by the abdominal contents in the recumbent or semirecumbent position.

2. **Does the size of the endotracheal tube impede breathing?** In patients already with airway obstruction, tubes may impose serious limitations on breathing, as shown below:

Tube Resistance (cm $H_2O/L/sec$)

	Flow Rate	Flow Rate
Tube size	(30 L/min)	(60 L/min)
6	11.5 (cm $H_2O/L/sec$)	20.2 (cm $H_2O/L/sec$)
7	5.9 (cm $H_2O/L/sec$)	9.9 (cm $H_2O/L/sec$)
8	3.7 (cm $H_2O/L/sec$)	6.1 (cm $H_2O/L/sec$)

Normal airway resistance: ± 2 cm $H_2O/L/sec$.

3. **Is reversible airway obstruction present?** Treatment with inhaled beta-agonist, atropine derivatives, or theophylline may be of benefit in some patients.

4. **Are secretions a problem?** Secretions might impede airflow. This impedance can be overcome by placing the patient in an upright position, suctioning the airway, and administering an inhaled bronchodilator.

5. **Is metabolic alkalemia impeding weaning?** The use of diuretics and nasogastric suction may lead to hypochloremic metabolic alkalemia; its correction as well as correction of any electrolyte imbalance might improve the chances for a successful weaning.

6. **Is breathing being depressed by drugs?** Sedative hypnotics and analgesic drugs might depress respiratory drive and produce alveolar hypoventilation and subsequent respiratory acidosis.

7. **Is hypophosphatemia or hypomagnesemia present?** Hypophosphatemia can lead to metabolic acidosis, osteomalacia, central nervous system dysfunction, red and white blood cell dysfunction, peripheral neuropathy, and respiratory failure—the latter, likely the result of skeletal muscle weakness and diaphragmatic dysfunction. Hypomagnesemia causes muscular weakness. Replacement therapy should be used to maintain normal serum levels.

8. **Is hypothyroidism present?** Hypothyroidism leads to decreased respiratory drive and muscular weakness, including the respiratory muscles.

9. **Is the patient's nutritional intake adequate?** Semistarvation depresses respiratory drive but also impedes wound healing, increases susceptibility to infection, decreases serum protein concentration, and interferes with the production of blood cells. Nutritional status should be maintained from the beginning of mechanical ventilation, and in patients in whom a prolonged course of respiratory care is anticipated, parenteral hyperalimentation should be started within 24 hours.

10. **Is the patient receiving excessive carbohydrate calories?** This may lead to hypercapnia and increased ventilatory requirements because the respiratory quotient (RQ) ($\dot{V}CO_2/\dot{V}O_2$) varies with the source of calories. The excess carbohydrates are converted to fat for storage. This process of lipogenesis has an RQ of 8.0 and, therefore, is associated with large increases in CO_2 production. A tip-off to such a circumstance is a high minute ventilation (> 25 L/min) in the face of a normal $PaCO_2$.

11. **What are the patient's normal arterial blood gas values?** This is very important in patients whose baseline arterial blood analysis, prior to the acute illness, showed a compensated respiratory acidosis with elevated $PaCO_2$ but normal pH. It is important that these values be maintained while the patient is being weaned from mechanical ventilation; otherwise, the patient who attempts to breathe spontaneously will have an increase in $PaCO_2$ and a decrease in pH, with the production of serious respiratory acidosis. This happens mainly in patients with COPD and compensated respiratory acidosis. In these patients the tidal volume of the respirator should first be decreased to approximately that which is normal for the patient.

12. **Is there a neuromuscular problem?** In patients with history of poliomyelitis, respiratory failure requiring intubation and mechanical ventilation may develop following surgery or minor respiratory illness. We should think of this diagnosis in patients with explained respiratory failure.

13. **Does the patient have normal diaphragmatic function?** This may be difficult to assess clinically. Unilateral or bilateral diaphragmatic paralysis may be diagnosed by fluoroscopic evaluation of the diaphragms with the patient off of ventilation.

14. **Are psychological factors being neglected?** Establishing an appropriate psychological environment and ensuring adequate sleep are very important. Psychological health also depends on body conditioning. Early ambulation is necessary for improving both muscle tone and psychological outlook.

9. Is respiratory muscle training feasible in patients who repeatedly fail weaning attempts?

If ventilatory dependence relates to the imbalance between ventilatory capability and demand, it would be important to improve the capability of muscles to perform work as well as to reduce the loads placed upon them. Muscle training is accomplished by sporadically imposing some degree of muscular overload. Performing small numbers of high-tension maneuvers augments mainly the maximum force that can be generated.

Moderate overloads for extended periods improve mainly endurance. Aldrich et al. examined the value of respiratory muscle training in 30 patients who had failed repeated attempts at weaning. Twelve patients undergoing training sessions were able to discontinue mechanical ventilation completely after 10–46 days, and another 5 patients were able to be weaned to nocturnal ventilation. Respiratory muscle training might be beneficial in patients who had failed weaning attempts repeatedly.

BIBLIOGRAPHY

1. Aldrich TK, Karpel JP, Uhrlass RM, et al: Weaning from mechanical ventilation: Adjunctive use of inspiratory muscle resistive training. Crit Care Med 17:143–147, 1989.
2. Grassino A, Macklem PT: Respiratory muscle fatigue and ventilatory failure. Ann Rev Med 34:625–647, 1984.
3. Lewis MJ, Belman MJ: Nutrition and the respiratory muscles. Clin Chest Med 9:337–348, 1980.
4. MacIntyre NR: New forms of mechanical ventilation in the adult. Clin Chest Med 9:47–54, 1988.
5. Mancebo J, Amaro P, et al: Effects of albuterol inhalation on the work of breathing during weaning from mechanical ventilation. Am Rev Respir Dis 144:95–100, 1991.
6. Marini JJ: Mechanical ventilation. In Simmons DH (ed): Current Pulmonology, Vol 9. Chicago Year Book Medical Publishers, 1988, pp 164–208.
7. Morganroth ML, Morganroth JL, Nett LM, Petty TL: Criteria for weaning from prolonged mechanical ventilation. Arch Intern Med 144:1012–1016, 1984.
8. Nett LM, Morganroth M, Petty TL: Weaning from mechanical ventilation: A perspective and review of techniques. In Bone RC (ed): Critical Care: A Comprehensive Approach. Park Ridge, IL, American College of Chest Physicians, 1984, pp 171–188.
9. Petty TL: IMV vs IMC. Chest 67:630–631, 1975.
10. Sahn SA, Laksminarayan S: Bedside criteria for discontinuation of mechanical ventilation. Chest 62:1002–1005, 1973.
11. Sharp JT: The respiratory muscles in chronic obstructive pulmonary disease. Am Rev Respir Dis 134:1089–1091, 1986.
12. Tobin MJ: State of the art: Respiratory monitoring in the intensive care unit. Am Rev Respir Dis 138:1625–1642, 1988.

11. TRACHEOTOMY

John E. Heffner, M.D.

1. Should all tracheotomies in critically ill patients be performed in the operating room?
Not necessarily. Tracheotomy in intubated patients undergoing mechanical ventilation can be done efficiently and safely in the intensive care unit, thereby avoiding patient transport and OR scheduling delays. The patient's critical care room must be transformed, however, to an OR environment, with adequate instrumentation, sterile fields, lighting, and suction.

2. Is emergency tracheotomy the surgical procedure of choice in apneic patients with acute upper airway obstruction?
No. Tracheotomy is acceptably safe when performed electively in an OR environment under controlled clinical conditions. Risks of surgical complications increase five-fold, however, when tracheotomy is applied in the emergency situation. An emergency cricothyroidotomy provides the greatest likelihood of successful airway placement with the lowest risks for complications in patients with acute upper airway obstruction who cannot undergo translaryngeal intubation.

3. Is cricothyroidotomy a suitable alternative to tracheotomy for long-term airway cannulation in patients undergoing mechanical ventilation?

Because of an increased risk for subglottic stenosis, most experts reserve cricothyroidotomy for emergency airway control with subsequent conversion to a standard tracheostomy as soon as possible. Exceptions include patients with anatomic variations that prevent tracheotomy, and terminally ill, ventilator-dependent patients who require an easily placed surgical airway to improve comfort.

4. How is a cricothyroidotomy performed?

The cricothyroid membrane is located approximately 2–3 cm below the thyroid notch. The membrane, which is typically 1 cm in height, lies below the vocal cords but within the subglottic larynx. A surgical scalpel is used to incise the overlying skin and stab the membrane. The resultant opening into the airway is enlarged with a spreader, allowing placement of a tracheostomy tube. Commercially available instruments designed for the emergency situation allow puncture of the membrane and introduction of an airway cannula in one maneuver.

5. Can mechanically ventilated patients with a tracheostomy speak?

Several techniques exist to promote speech in mechanically ventilated patients with a tracheostomy tube in place. Patients with low to moderate minute ventilation requirements can whisper intelligibly if the tracheostomy tube cuff is deflated to allow a small "cuff leak" during the ventilator inspiratory cycle. Addition of a small amount of positive end-expiratory pressure (PEEP) creates a leak throughout inspiration and expiration and promotes more spontaneous speech. A "speaking tracheostomy tube" provides an external cannula that directs compressed gas to exit the tube below the vocal cords, allowing some patients to communicate in whispered tones. An "electrolarynx" placed against the neck near the laryngeal cartilage generates a vibratory tone that can be articulated with practice into intelligible speech.

6. What precautions should be exercised in patients with a cuffed tracheostomy tube who undergo general anesthesia?

Some volatile anesthetics, such as nitrous oxide, diffuse more rapidly into a tracheostomy tube cuff than oxygen or nitrogen can diffuse out and thereby increase intracuff pressures. During a 2-hour operation, cuff pressures may increase from 15 mm Hg to over 80 mm Hg, which can cause ischemic injury to the tracheal mucosa. Appropriate precautions include frequent monitoring of cuff pressures in the OR or inflation of the tube cuff at the outset of the surgical procedure with the anesthetic gas mixture administered to the airway.

7. What is the ideal size of tracheostomy tube for a patient?

No one size is best for all patients because tracheal caliber and clinical situations vary. Small-caliber tubes may decrease the incidence of tracheal stenosis at the stoma site because of the smaller tracheal incision required. Unfortunately, small tubes present difficulties in airway suctioning, spontaneous ventilation, and fiber-optic bronchoscopy. Furthermore, small tubes have small cuffs that may damage the tracheal mucosa because they require high intracuff pressures to overdistend in order to seal the airway. Overly large tubes require wide stomas and prohibit adequate cuff inflation to cushion the rigid tube from the tracheal mucosa and to effectively prevent aspiration. The best approximation of ideal size requires the surgeon to select a tube with an outer diameter two-thirds the inner caliber of the patient's trachea at the point of insertion.

8. Should tracheostomy tube cuff pressures be checked periodically in patients undergoing mechanical ventilation?

Although not all experts agree, frequent monitoring of cuff pressure provides the best measure to prevent tracheal injury at the cuff site. Cuff pressures in excess of mucosal capillary perfusion pressures (usually less than 25 mm Hg) can rapidly cause mucosal ischemia and resultant tracheal stenosis. Reliance on minimal leak technique to inflate cuffs may prevent detection of patients with high cuff pressure requirements. These patients may often experience adequate seal with low cuff pressures after insertion of a tracheostomy tube of a different size or design.

9. What should the clinician consider in any patient with airway hemorrhage after the first 48 hours of insertion of a tracheostomy tube?
Bleeding within the first 48 hours of tracheotomy is usually a result of hemorrhage from the incisional wound. Any bleeding that develops longer than 48 hours after surgery, however, should suggest the possibility of a tracheoinnominate fistula. This life-threatening complication requires immediate evaluation by a thoracic surgeon capable of performing an emergency sternotomy for ligation of the innominate artery, because massive hemorrhage often develops after an initial "herald" episode of mild to moderate bleeding.

10. How should a patient be evaluated who continues to have cough and shortness of breath 2 months after removal of a tracheostomy tube?
Although these symptoms often accompany underlying lung disease, they also occasionally represent the only clinical manifestations of a tracheoesophageal fistula. If symptoms appear disproportionate to the patient's cardiopulmonary status, evaluation with a carefully performed esophagogram possibly enhanced by cine may identify a small fistula tract.

11. What are the indications for tracheotomy in critically ill patients?
Common indications include removal of airway secretions, relief of upper airway obstruction, provision of airway access for long-term mechanical ventilation, and prevention of aspiration.

12. What is a "mini-tracheotomy"?
Often patients require a tracheotomy solely for suctioning of airway secretions from the lower respiratory tract. Rather than persisting in long-term nasotracheal suctioning or proceeding to a standard tracheotomy, a mini-tracheotomy provides airway access with excellent patient tolerance. This procedure places a 7-French cannula through the tracheal rings by a needle and wire Seldinger technique. The mini-tracheotomy tube is just large enough to allow passage of a suction catheter for frequent removal of secretions.

13. What is the role of a fenestrated tracheostomy tube in the ICU?
Newer fenestrated tracheostomy tubes with multiple small holes in their greater curvature assist speech and weaning from tracheostomy in spontaneously breathing patients without stimulating growth of granulation tissue. After removal of an inner cannula (if present) and deflation of the cuff, patients can breathe around the cuff and through the fenestrations in addition to the stoma to decrease airway resistance. Placement of a one-way valve, such as the Passy-Muir valve, on the tracheostomy tube allows patients to inhale through the tube and exhale out their native upper airways, thereby promoting speech.

14. Why do patients aspirate after removal of a tracheostomy tube?
Scarring at the stoma site may interfere with the rostrocaudal excursion of the larynx during swallowing, which is necessary for glottic closure. Also, prolonged diversion of ventilation away from the glottis causes attenuation of the vocal cord adductor response that is important in aspiration prevention.

15. What is a tracheal button?
Tracheal buttons, such as the Olympic tracheal button, assist weaning from a tracheostomy tube. Designed as a straight, rigid plastic tube, tracheal buttons fit through the stoma to

maintain its patency in case patients need suctioning or reinsertion of a tracheostomy tube through the tract. The button is ideal for patients with borderline ventilatory status, because the distal end abuts the anterior tracheal wall and does not protrude into the airway to impede respiration or clearance of secretions by coughing.

CONTROVERSIES

16. What is the appropriate time to convert an intubated patient undergoing mechanical ventilation to a tracheotomy?

No study or accumulation of data from combined investigations has determined the ideal time to perform a tracheotomy in patients who require long-term mechanical ventilation. Recent consensus, however, is that the decision should be individualized, with a tracheotomy being performed when a patient appears likely to benefit from the procedure. The potential benefits of tracheotomy over prolonged translaryngeal intubation include improved comfort, enhanced ability to communicate, greater mobility, diminished risk for direct laryngeal injury, and possible acceleration of weaning from mechanical ventilation. Consensus further emphasizes that the decision for a tracheotomy in ventilator-dependent patients should be determined by a patient's anticipated likelihood of requiring prolonged mechanical ventilation rather than by the arbitrary duration of ventilator dependency that has already transpired. As an example, patients with respiratory failure should be evaluated within 7 days of treatment with a translaryngeal endotracheal tube for the probability of successful extubation within the first 10–14 days of intubation. Patients determined unlikely to improve rapidly on the basis of severity of disease should undergo tracheotomy at an early opportunity rather than waiting for an additional 1–2 weeks of respiratory failure.

17. Should tracheotomy be avoided whenever possible in critically ill patients because of the considerable risks of surgical complications?

Recent prospective studies indicate that tracheotomy in critically ill patients performed by experienced surgeons has an acceptably low rate of surgical complications. Mortality ranges from 0 to 1% and morbidity from pneumothorax, wound bleeding, subcutaneous emphysema, and airway obstruction should occur in less than 1 to 2.4%. Earlier reports of surgical complications resulting in 9 to 36% of tracheotomies derived from university hospitals where the procedure was performed by multiple surgical specialty trainees rather than a limited cadre of expert physicians.

BIBLIOGRAPHY

1. Bishop MJ: Physiology and Consequences of Tracheal Intubation. Problems in Anesthesia. Philadelphia, J.B. Lippincott, 1988.
2. Colice GL: Prolonged intubation versus tracheostomy in the adult. J Intern Med 2:85, 1987.
3. Finucane BT, Santora AH: Principles of Airway Management. Philadelphia, F.A. Davis, 1988.
4. Godwin JE: Special critical care considerations in tracheostomy management. Clin Chest Med 12:573–583, 1991.
5. Grillo HC, Mathisen DJ: Surgical management of tracheal strictures. J Cardiothorac Surg 68:511, 1988.
6. Heffner JE (ed): Airway Management in the Critically Ill Patient. Clin Chest Med 12(3):415–630, 1991.
7. Heffner JE: Management of the airway in mechanical ventilation. Clin Chest Med 9:23–35, 1988.
8. Heffner JE: Medical indications for tracheotomy. Chest 96:186–190, 1989.
9. Heffner JE, Miller KS, Sahn SA: Tracheostomy in the intensive care unit. Part I. Chest 90:269–274, 1986.

10. Heffner JE, Miller KS, Sahn SA: Tracheostomy in the intensive care unit. Part II. Chest 90:430–436, 1986.
11. Myers EN, Stool SE, Johnson JT: Tracheotomy. New York, Churchill Livingstone, 1985.
12. Plummer AL, Gracy DR: Symposium. Consensus conference on artificial airways in patients receiving mechanical ventilation. Chest 96:178, 1989.
13. Stock MC, Woodward CG, Shapiro BA, et al: Perioperative complications of elective tracheostomy in critically ill patients. Crit Care Med 14:861, 1986.
14. Whited RE: A prospective study of laryngotracheal sequelae in long-term intubation. Laryngoscope 94:367, 1984.
15. Wu WH, Suh C-W, Turndorf H: Use of the artificial larynx during airway intubation. Crit Care Med 2:152, 1974.

12. INTRAHOSPITAL TRANSPORT

James B. Haenel, R.R.T., and Frederick A. Moore, M.D.

1. Who are the primary members of the transport team?

The key member of the team is the patient. The escorts required to transport a patient safely to remote areas within the hospital will depend on the acuity of the individual patient as well as the type of hospital. Policies and procedures should be written that specify who accompanies the patient during transports and who stays with the patient at the destination site. For example, at our acute-care county hospital, which is staffed by M.D. residents in training, we follow these guidelines:

Guidelines for Transport

Type of Patient	Required Staff for Duration of Transport
Stable patient with IV line only	Staff to be determined by head nurse in consultation with MD or a designee
Stable patient with arterial line only	RN
Patient on ventilator	RN, ICU resident, RT
Patient with pulmonary artery catheter or any vasoactive drips	RN and ICU resident
Unstable patient	RN, ICU resident, RT
Patient with an artificial airway	RN, RT

There will always be situations in which personnel may not be available and the final decision regarding transport will be up to the attending physician. Attempts to stratify patients at high risk for an untoward event during transport by use of scoring systems such as the APACHE II or TRISS score have proved unsuccessful.

2. What is the reported incidence of complications during intrahospital transport of critically ill patients?

It is surprisingly high, ranging from 21% to 84% (average 40%), considering these rates are derived from patients who are aggressively monitored to determine the incidence of intrahospital transport complications. The incidence of adverse outcomes from transport-related complications is not well documented. One study noted that one death per month was caused by mishaps during intrahospital transport.

3. What are the most frequent complications encountered during intrahospital transport?

Complications During Intrahospital Transport

Cardiovascular	Pulmonary	Equipment
Hypotension	Hypoxemia	Power loss:
Hypertension	Respiratory acidosis	electrical
Hypertensive crisis	Respiratory alkalosis	battery
New cardiac arrhythmias	Airway obstruction	pneumatic
Cardiac arrest	Aspiration	Loss of: tubes, airways, IVs,
	Respiratory arrest	chest tubes, and drains

4. What is the primary cause of cardiopulmonary decompensation during transport?
Critically ill patients depend upon advanced supportive care technology to survive. Most critically ill patients need continuous mechanical ventilatory support during intrahospital transport. Most hospitals, especially smaller community hospitals, cannot justify the expense of a dedicated transport ventilator and therefore provide manual ventilation with a self-inflating bag during transit. While generally reliable for short-term use, these devices may not provide precise, prolonged ventilatory support. The accuracy of self-inflating bags is further hampered by the lack of feedback to the operator concerning delivered tidal volume and minute ventilation provided. Commonly, the manually ventilated patient experiences acute changes in acid-base balance as a result of either overzealous ventilation or unintentional hypoventilation. Arterial blood gas measurements made during transport have documented frequent changes from baseline alterations in both $PaCO_2$ ($>$ 10 torr) and pH ($>$ 0.05). The physiologic effects of acute alkalosis may predispose the already unstable myocardium to arrhythmias, with resultant hypotension. Hyperventilation may result in gas trapping due to insufficient exhalation time (auto-PEEP effect). The resulting hyperinflation can cause barotrauma as well as a rise in intrathoracic pressure, which in turn can decrease venous return or increase intracranial pressure. Alternatively, inadvertent hypoventilation causing acute hypercarbia may depress cardiac output, be arrhythmogenic, or increase cerebral blood flow.

5. What is a transport ventilator? How do its capabilities compare with those of a state-of-the-art ICU ventilator?
The latest ICU ventilators offer a sophisticated array of modes, flow patterns, alarms, trend capabilities, and microprocessor functions. With the development of highly responsive electromechanical valves acting in concert with microprocessors, the ICU ventilator becomes capable of altering and maintaining flow demands and inspiratory time in the face of a falling compliance or rising airway resistance, thus maintaining tidal volume delivery. In contrast to a state-of-the-art ICU ventilator, the transport ventilator usually consists of a small pole-mounted or even handheld device that offers one or two different modes of ventilation and is pneumatically powered. The ability to monitor tidal volume delivery continuously is critical to ensure that ventilation is being maintained. Other features of an ideal transport ventilator include simplicity of operation, light weight, versatility (pediatrics/adults), and capacity for delivering high levels of minute volume ($>$ 20 L/min). The transport ventilator should also have a responsive demand valve to minimize inspiratory work, PEEP/CPAP up to 25 cm H_2O, demand or continuous flow, variable FiO_2, and flow rates to 120 L/min; be pneumatically powered with minimal gas consumption; and have appropriate alarms.

6. What additional risk factors make transport hazardous?
A lack of appropriate monitors. Intuitively, it makes sense that when you take the sickest patient out of one of the most controlled environments within the hospital—the ICU—and

discontinue ongoing monitoring, complications during transit may go undetected until physiologic reserves have been exhausted. However, despite having what would appear to be adequate numbers of both monitors and personnel, many studies still report a significant number of complications.

7. What is the best transport monitor?

An experienced transport person who can clinically assess the patient's condition and is comfortable with the monitoring equipment is the best monitor. What equipment accompanies the patient is dependent upon the clinical scenario. For example, even the most experienced transport team member will not be able to detect a spontaneously wedged pulmonary artery catheter unless pulmonary artery pressure is continuously monitored. Likewise, when leaving the ICU to obtain a pulmonary ventilation/perfusion scan for the workup of an acute hypoxic event, one would be foolhardy not to continuously monitor the adequacy of oxygenation. Although end-tidal CO_2 monitoring is too cumbersome for routine transports, it can be invaluable in patients with difficult-to-control intracranial pressure.

8. What are the two sources of oxygen typically used in intrahospital transport? What are the advantages of each?

The most common appliances employed are gas cylinders and liquid oxygen reservoirs. The advantages of the gas cylinder are that it is portable, convenient, and lightweight (15 lbs). Unfortunately, the smaller cylinders (E size) cannot be used for prolonged transports, especially at high flow rates (e.g., at 20 L/min, with a full cylinder, oxygen can be supplied for only 30 minutes), and larger cylinders are bulky and weigh up to 150 lbs. The advantage of a liquid reservoir is that 1 cubic foot of liquid oxygen can be converted to 860 cubic feet of gaseous oxygen. The liquid oxygen reservoir, therefore, has high flow capabilities and can power portable ventilators even at high minute demands (< 30 L/min). These liquid oxygen reservoirs are quite heavy (80–150 lbs), require a separate cart or stand, and must always be in the upright position.

9. How long will a cylinder of oxygen last?

This depends on the cylinder size, cylinder pressure, and delivered flow rate in liters per minute. To calculate an approximate duration of time available, the following formula is used:

$$\text{Duration of flow in minutes} = \frac{\text{Gauge pressure in PSI} \times \text{Factor*}}{\text{Liter flow}}$$

* Factor = cylinder volume in cubic feet × 28.3 ÷ 2200 PSI

Factors to calculate duration of cylinder flow in minutes:

D	E	G	H & K
0.16	0.28	2.41	3.41

Example: How long will an E cylinder of oxygen last with a gauge pressure of 700 PSI, if the flow to the self-inflating bag is 15 L/min?

$$\frac{700 \times 0.28}{15} = 13 \text{ minutes}$$

You had better change out tanks before going!

10. If 100% oxygen is coming out of the cylinder, what FiO_2 is being delivered to the patient?

Delivered FiO_2 depends upon: (1) liter flow into the bag; (2) the volume of the reservoir attached to the bag; (3) the refill time during exhalation, i.e., the higher the bagging rate, the less time is available for the reservoir to refill with fresh oxygen gas, and therefore the FiO_2 will diminish. Most self-inflating manual resuscitators equipped with a reservoir and adequate flow (15 L/min) will deliver 90–100% oxygen.

11. Your patient requires a minute volume of 22 liters, an FiO_2 of 90%, and 10 cm H_2O PEEP. How do you provide these requirements during transport?

A standard portable oxygen regulator delivers a maximum flow of 15 L/min (on flush, slightly higher). Therefore, to deliver 22 L/min, two gas cylinders will need to be "T" connected to the self-inflating bag. With this setup, delivery of up to 90% FiO_2 is not a problem. The majority of manual resuscitators are capable of providing fairly accurate levels of PEEP up to 15 cm H_2O.

12. Is it necessary to apply suction to a chest tube during transit?

First, determine if the chest tube is functioning. Respiration-induced fluctuations in the water seal chamber's column level confirm that the tube is functioning and that all connections are secure. Patients receiving mechanical or hand-bag ventilation during transport will not require continuous suction (unless an unusually large air leak exists), because continuous positive intrathoracic pressure should result in evacuation of any pleural air through the water seal chamber. For spontaneously breathing patients who are not on CPAP, the lung may not be protected from collapse solely by the water seal chamber and may require continuous suction. During transport, the chest tube drainage system should be suspended below the level of the patient's chest to allow gravity to drain fluid.

BIBLIOGRAPHY

1. Braman SS, Dunn SM, Amic CA, Millman RP: Complications of intrahospital transport in critically ill patients. Ann Intern Med 107:469–473, 1987.
2. Crippen D: Critical care transportation medicine: New concepts in pretransport stabilization of the critically ill patient. Am J Emerg Med 8:551–554, 1990.
3. Ehrenwerth J, Sorbo S, Hackel A: Transport of critically ill adults. Crit Care Med 14:543–547, 1986.
4. Indeck M, Peterson S, Smith J, Brotman S: Risk, cost and benefit of transporting ICU patients for special studies. J Trauma 28:1020–1025, 1988.
5. Link J, Krause H, Wagner W, Papadopoulos G: Intrahospital transport of critically ill patients. Crit Care Med 18:1427–1429, 1990.
6. Smith I, Fleming S, Cernaiann A: Mishaps during transport from the intensive care unit. Crit Care Med 18:278–281, 1990.
7. Waddell G: Movement of critically ill patients within hospital. Br Med J 2:417–419, 1975.

II: Procedures

13. PULMONARY ARTERY CATHETERIZATION

Susan Lehr, R.N.

1. What is a pulmonary artery (PA) catheter?

The PA catheter, also known as a Swan-Ganz catheter, is a flow-directed, balloon-tipped catheter that is placed via the central venous circulation into the right atrium, through the right ventricle, and then out into the pulmonary artery. The catheter, with ports in the right atrium and pulmonary artery, can provide measurements of right- and left-sided heart function.

2. What are some critical conditions in which PA catheterization might be used?

Myocardial infarction, shock, pulmonary edema, or status post cardiac, vascular, or other major surgical procedures.

3. What is the significance of right arterial pressure measurements through a PA catheter?

The blue port of a Swan-Ganz line measures central venous pressure (CVP) in the right atrium, which indicates blood volume and adequacy of central venous return. CVP can be used to assess volume status and to differentiate between right- and left-sided cardiac failure. Normal CVP in a nonventilated patient is less than 2–6 mm Hg.

4. What is the waveform for right atrial pressure?

The CVP waveform has three positive waves. The first, or A wave, reflects atrial systole and corresponds to the PR interval on EKG. The second, the C wave, reflects the opening of the tricuspid valve, which is seen on the RS-T portion of the EKG. The third, or V wave, reflects ventricular systole against a closed tricuspid valve and corresponds to the period between the T wave and the next P wave.

5. When would right atrial pressure be elevated?

Elevated pressures may occur with right ventricular failure, constrictive pericarditis, cardiac tamponade, pulmonary hypertension, hypervolemia, tricuspid stenosis and/or regurgitation, or chronic left ventricular failure.

6. What is the waveform for the right ventricle?

As the catheter passes from the right atrium through the tricuspid valve, into the right ventricle, the waveform undergoes a marked change in appearance. The ventricle fills with blood while the pulmonary valve is closed, increasing in pressure until the pulmonary valve is opened, ejecting blood into the pulmonary artery. The systolic portion of the wave reaches pressures of 20–30 mm Hg. During diastole, the ventricle relaxes, the pulmonary valve closes and the tricuspid valve opens, causing passive filling of the ventricle when there is equilibrium between the right ventricle and right atrium. The diastolic measurement is less than 5 mm Hg, corresponding to the right atrial pressure. The waveform shows a high systolic pressure and low diastolic pressure, distinguishing it from other waveforms seen with pulmonary artery catheter.

7. What conditions may cause elevated right ventricular pressure?

Right ventricular failure, pulmonary hypertension, constrictive pericarditis, cardiac tamponade, chronic congestive heart failure, ventricular septal defect, and pulmonary valvular stenosis.

8. What is the appearance of a PA waveform?

The PA wave looks similar to the right ventricular (RV) waveform, except the dicrotic notch is present, reflecting the closure of the pulmonic valve. This pressure is measured through the yellow port of the PA catheter. During diastole, the wave reflects first an increase in pressure against closed valves and then a decrease as blood flows into pulmonary capillaries. PA systolic pressure reflects RV systolic pressure, and PA diastolic pressure reflects LA pressures and therefore LV end-diastolic pressures in the normal heart. Normal PA pressure is 20–30/10–12 mm Hg.

9. What causes elevation in PA pressure?

PA pressures are elevated in patients with increased pulmonary blood flow as seen in atrial or ventricular septal defects with left-to-right shunts, increased pulmonary vascular resistance (in patients with pulmonary hypertension or pulmonary disease), or in mitral stenosis or left ventricular failure (both of which cause increased LA pressure).

10. What is pulmonary artery wedge pressure (PAWP)?

PAWP is measured when the catheter is placed in the pulmonary artery, and the balloon at the end of the catheter is inflated to obstruct further blood flow in that artery. When the catheter is thus wedged, it reflects pressure in the pulmonary capillaries, left atrium, and in the left ventricle when the mitral valve is open during diastole. In this way, it reflects left ventricular end-diastolic pressure.

11. What is the appearance of the pulmonary capillary wedge pressure (PCWP) wave?

The PCWP wave is similar to the right atrial wave, consisting of three waves. The A wave reflects left atrial systole and is timed with the P wave of the EKG, although it is slightly delayed due to transmission through the pulmonary vasculature. The C wave represents closure of the mitral valve during initiation of ventricular systole. It is often not seen in the PCWP. The V wave reflects filling of the left atrium and the bulging of the mitral valve during ventricular systole. Between the A wave and the beginning of the V wave is the X descent, which reflects atrial relaxation. The Y descent, which occurs after the V wave, is due to rapid atrial emptying after the opening of the mitral valve.

12. What is the normal value for PCWP?

The normal range is approximately 12–15 mm Hg.

13. What conditions cause elevation of PCWP?

Left ventricular failure, mitral stenosis, mitral insufficiency, constrictive pericarditis, cardiac tamponade, and volume overload.

14. How are pulmonary artery pressures measured in a clinical situation?

Respiratory effort can markedly affect the accuracy of these measurements. During spontaneous inspiration in nonventilated patients, intrathoracic pressure is lowered, causing a decrease in catheter measurements. Just the opposite effect occurs in ventilated patients, with inspiration elevating the intrathoracic pressure. The optimal time for measurement is during end expiration, at which time the intrathoracic pressures are equilibrated and constant, giving a stable waveform. This measurement is especially imperative in patients on positive end-expiratory pressure (PEEP).

15. How are pulmonary artery pressures obtained in patients on PEEP?

It is not clinically acceptable to remove patients from PEEP to measure pulmonary artery pressures. The following formula provides an accurate measurement of PCWP on patients on PEEP greater than 10 cm H_2O:

$$PCWP \; (mm \; Hg) \; - \; \frac{[PEEP \; (cm \; H_2O) \times 0.75]}{3}$$

Another method of estimating pulmonary wedge pressure when PEEP is greater than 10 cm H_2O is to subtract half of the PEEP pressure from the measured PCWP.

16. How is the PA catheter inserted?

It is inserted at the bedside, often without the need for fluoroscopic guidance. A percutaneous insertion site is chosen, usually the subclavian, internal or external jugular veins, and less commonly the femoral or antecubital veins. Prior to insertion, it is imperative to test the proper function of the balloon to be sure that there is no leakage of air when the balloon is inflated, and that when inflated it covers the tip of the catheter. Once venous access is achieved, the catheter is inserted with transducer attached, and advanced into the vena cava, as evidenced by a sudden increase in pressure fluctuations due to respiratory effort. At this point, the waveforms on the monitor are closely observed to assist in guiding the tip of the catheter into the right atrium. Once in the right atrium, the balloon is fully inflated and the catheter is advanced through the right ventricle and quickly into the pulmonary artery (to avoid excess ventricular irritation). With the balloon fully inflated, the catheter is advanced until it is wedged in the pulmonary artery and typical pulmonary wedge pressure waves are observed.

17. How is distal migration of the catheter prevented?

It is quite common for the catheter, once inserted into the pulmonary artery, to migrate distally because the loop formed by insertion through the right ventricle shortens as the catheter is warmed to body temperature. Anticipation of this phenomenon is accomplished by inflating the balloon two to three times over several minutes, and recording how much air is needed to achieve proper wedging of the catheter tip. If less than 1.3–1.5 cc of air is required, the catheter needs to be retracted *with the balloon deflated*. Migration most frequently occurs during the first 24 hours. It is therefore important to record the volume needed to inflate the balloon to wedge position.

18. What is the proper technique for inflation and deflation of the balloon?

After inflation of the balloon and measurement of the wedge, the syringe should be removed from the catheter to allow passive flow of air out of the catheter. Never aspirate from the syringe, which may cause tearing of the balloon. Verify proper deflation of the balloon by observing the PA waveform on the monitor.

19. What are the criteria for true wedge pressure measurements?

1. A true wedge pressure reflects the pulmonary artery diastolic pressure in the normal heart. Therefore, the mean pulmonary artery wedge pressure should be lower than or equal to the pulmonary artery diastolic pressure, and lower than the mean pulmonary artery pressure.

2. The characteristic waveform (with A and V waveforms) should be observed. A dampened waveform, straight line, or variation in waveform owing to respiratory effort is not acceptable. The waveform should quickly disappear when the balloon is deflated and appear again when the balloon is reinflated.

3. With fast flushing of the catheter, the observable waveform is quickly elevated and then returns to baseline, indicating no catheter obstruction.

4. It is possible, although not always accurate, to analyze blood gas samples from the distal port with the balloon inflated. This sample should reflect alveolar-capillary gas levels that are highly saturated with oxygen.

5. As with all pressure readings, the transducer must be at the phlebostatic axis (level with the right atrium).

20. In which zone of the lung must the PA catheter be placed in order to obtain accurate data?

The catheter must be placed in zone 3 so that the PCWP approximates pulmonary venous pressure. In zone 3 pulmonary artery pressure is greater than pulmonary alveolar pressure, as is pulmonary venous pressure (pART > pALV < pVein). This allows flow of a continuous column of blood from the tip of the catheter to the pulmonary veins. If the catheter is placed in zone 2, then when the balloon is inflated pulmonary artery pressure will exceed pulmonary capillary pressure, causing the vessel distal to the balloon to collapse. A "wedge" pressure in this zone would reflect alveolar pressures, not venous pressures, which reflect left ventricular function. These are physiologic, not anatomic, zones, and they may vary according to clinical conditions. For example, large amounts of PEEP or hypovolemia may cause different pressure. The pressure recordings will appear to reflect zone 2 conditions. Fluid replacement or refloating of the Swan-Ganz catheter will ensure accuracy of the wedge readings. The clinician can be assured that the tip of the catheter is in zone 3 by obtaining a lateral chest x-ray. On this x-ray, the tip of the catheter should be located below the level of the left atrium. If the catheter is not in zone 3, the characteristic A and V waves will not be present. Instead, there will be variations caused by respiratory fluctuation. Furthermore, the wedge pressure may exceed the pulmonary artery diastolic pressure because it no longer reflects left atrial pressures.

21. When does pulmonary artery wedge pressure not equal pulmonary artery diastolic pressure?

If there is (1) inaccurate catheter position; (2) overwedging (overinflating the balloon; inflation should never exceed 1.5 cc of air); or (3) pulmonary disease such as COPD, ARDS, pulmonary embolus, or tachycardia greater than 130. Caution should be observed when mitral insufficiency is suspected because the V wave in the recorded capillary wedge pressure will elevate the pressure reading (reflecting elevated left atrial pressure). To obtain a better correlation between the pulmonary diastolic pressure and the pulmonary capillary wedge, use the A wave on the wedge pressure reading.

22. What conditions seen clinically preclude accurate measurements and do not allow accurate correlation between PCWP and left ventricular end-diastolic pressure (LVEDP)?

Conditions in which PCWP is greater than LVEDP:
- Mitral stenosis
- Left atrial prolapsing tumor (myxoma)
- Conditions of high intra-alveolar pressures (positive-pressure ventilation)

Conditions in which the PCWP is less than LVEDP:
- Stiff left ventricle
- High LVEDP (greater than 25 mm Hg)

23. What other useful data can be obtained with a PA catheter?

It is possible to measure cardiac output by two methods using a PA catheter. The thermodilution method is accomplished by injecting either normal saline or 5% dextrose solution into the proximal (blue) port of the catheter while hooking up the thermistor of the catheter to a specialized cardiac output analyzer. This analyzer is able to measure the change in temperature over time and thus reflects cardiac output. However, the use of cardiac index rather than cardiac output yields more individualized information. Cardiac index is obtained by dividing cardiac output by body surface area.

Another method, the arteriovenous oxygen difference (A-V DO_2), consists of withdrawing blood into a blood gas syringe simultaneously from the distal (yellow) port of the catheter and the arterial line. This blood must be withdrawn slowly, over approximately a minute, to obtain a true mixed venous blood gas sample. The A-V DO_2 is measured by subtracting the venous oxygen content (obtained from the distal catheter) from the arterial oxygen content. The normal value for an A-V DO_2 is 3–5.5 volumes %. Thus, a patient with an A-V differential of 2 volumes % might have a diagnosis of a high output state, such as sepsis, hyperthyroidism, or liver failure.

Systemic vascular resistance (SVR) can be measured from data taken from the pulmonary artery and the arterial line. The formula for measuring the SVR in dynes/sec/cm^{-5} is:

$$\frac{\text{Mean arterial pressure (MAP) – central venous pressure (CVP)} \times 80}{\text{Cardiac output (CO)}}$$

24. What are the clinical complications of PA catheterization?

Insertion may cause:

1. Pneumothorax

2. Ventricular irritability, especially serious in patients with acute myocardial infarction, is best avoided by securing the catheter at the insertion site so that it cannot migrate to the right ventricle. The usual precautions taken to correct electrolyte imbalance, hypothermia, and acidosis must be taken prior to insertion of a PA catheter.

3. Arterial puncture

4. Heart block, especially in patients with preexisting left bundle branch block

5. This may be avoided by quick insertion of the catheter and use of a temporary pacemaker.

6. Air embolus

7. Endocardial injury to chordae tendineae, papillary muscles, or valve cusps.

Infection

1. Local phlebitis at the insertion site. Prevention is enhanced by sterile insertion and by application of a sterile occlusive dressing. The catheter should not remain in the patient for longer than 72–96 hours.

2. Sepsis occurs in about 2% of patients. In addition to the above-mentioned precautions, the flush solution for maintaining catheter patency should be normal saline and not exceed 5% dextrose, sterile caps and stopcocks should be used, and the transducer should be changed frequently (every 48–72 hours). When readvancing the catheter, special caution is needed to ensure that the catheter has been maintained in its sterile sleeve.

Pulmonary artery rupture occurs only rarely, with the highest risk factor being pulmonary hypertension. However, there are special precautions to reduce this risk:

1. Be sure that the catheter is placed in the pulmonary artery so that full balloon inflation is required for wedging. This keeps the catheter tip from protruding past the balloon.

2. The balloon should be inflated slowly, and the stopcock at the balloon syringe should remain open at all times. When not actively wedging, the syringe should remain free of air.

3. Do not flush the catheter in the wedge position.

4. Do not overinflate the balloon. Never use more than 1.5 cc of air to inflate it.

Balloon rupture may be caused by overinflation, frequent inflation, or active deflation of the balloon with the syringe. With prolonged use, the exposure of the balloon to blood causes it to lose its elasticity.

BIBLIOGRAPHY

1. Carlson TA, Goldenberg IF, Murray PD, et al: Catheter-induced delayed recurrent pulmonary artery hemorrhage: Intervention with therapeutic embolism of the pulmonary. JAMA 261: 1843, 1989.

2. Chatterjee K, Matthay M: Right-heart catheterization is a diagnostic procedure, not a therapeutic intervention. J Intensive Care Med 6:101–104, 1991.
3. Gore JM, Goldberg RJ, Spodnick DH, et al: A community-wide assessment of the use of pulmonary artery catheters in patients with acute myocardial infarction. Chest 92:721, 1987.
4. Iberti TJ, Fischer EP, Leibowitz AB, et al: A multicenter study of physicians knowledge of the pulmonary artery catheter. JAMA 264:2928, 1990.
5. Matthay MA, Chatterjee K: Bedside catheterization of the pulmonary artery: Risks compared with benefits. Ann Intern Med 109:826, 1988.
6. Nadeau S, Noble WH: Misinterpretation of pressure measurements from the pulmonary catheter. Can Anaesth Soc J 33:352–363, 1986.
7. Pierson DJ, Hudson LD: Monitoring hemodynamics in the critically ill. Med Clin North Am 67:1343, 1983.
8. Sharkey SW: Beyond the wedge: Clinical physiology and the Swan-Ganz catheter. Am J Med 83:111–118, 1987.
9. Wiedemann HP, Matthay MA, Matthay RA: Cardiovascular-pulmonary monitoring in the intensive care unit (Part 1). Chest 85:537–549, 1984.
10. Wiedemann HP, Matthay MA, Matthay RA: Cardiovascular-pulmonary monitoring in the intensive care unit (Part 2). Chest 85:656–668, 1984.

14. THORACENTESIS

Christopher Tyler, M.D.

1. When is diagnostic thoracentesis indicated?

In a few clinical circumstances, such as an exacerbation of congestive heart failure, the clinician can observe a pleural effusion. Because asymptomatic pleural effusions often result from potentially lethal diseases such as tuberculosis and cancer, any nonresolving effusion should be investigated. Thoracentesis should be strongly considered in any circumstance in which the effusion is thought to be exudative. Fever, leukocytosis, weight loss, suspected malignancy, or pleural effusions that are nonresolving, unilateral, or recurrent demand further evaluation. Examination of the pleural fluid is the only way to differentiate empyema from uncomplicated parapneumonic effusions, and this differentiation is vital in deciding whether chest tube drainage is needed. If clinical evaluation suggests an exudative effusion, thoracentesis should be performed. If, after thoracentesis, there is still no diagnosis, one should consider pleural biopsy, pleuroscopy, or open pleural biopsy. Frequent causes of asymptomatic pleural effusion include recent childbirth or abdominal surgery, benign asbestos effusion, uremia, malignancy, and tuberculosis. Once malignant or granulomatous pleuritis has been excluded, observation may be prudent before proceeding to more invasive procedures.

2. What is the sensitivity of the chest x-ray in the ICU in the detection of pleural effusions?

Radiographic signs of a pleural effusion include increased homogeneous density super-imposed over the lung, loss of the hemodiaphragm silhouette, blunted costophrenic angle, apical capping, elevation of the hemodiaphragm, decreased visibility of lower-lobe vasculature, and accentuation of the minor fissure. The most frequent but least specific criterion for detecting pleural effusions is blunting of the costophrenic angle. Other helpful signs include loss of the hemodiaphragm and increased density of the hemothorax. A normal supine radiograph does not exclude a pleural effusion. Ruskin et al. studied the ability to detect pleural effusions by supine chest radiographs. Using the above criteria on supine radiographs, they found a sensitivity of 67% and a specificity of 70%.

3. What is the value of chest ultrasonographic guidance for thoracentesis?
Chest ultrasonography has been found to be significantly superior to decubitus roentgeno-grams alone for obtaining adequate fluid samples in small effusions. However, the technique has no such advantage in large effusions. Ultrasonography does not reduce the need for multiple attempts, nor does it decrease the incidence of complications.

4. What are Light's criteria?
Pleural fluid can be categorized as transudates or exudates. Light's criteria allow differentiation between a transudate and an exudate. An exudate is a fluid with a pleural serum protein ratio > 0.5, a ratio of pleural fluid to serum LDH > 0.6, and a pleural fluid LDH of greater than two-thirds the normal serum upper limit. A transudate meets none of these criteria.

5. What is the differential diagnosis of a transudate?
Congestive heart failure, pericardial disease, hepatic failure, nephrotic syndrome, peritoneal dialysis, postpartum pleural effusion, myxedema, sarcoidosis, and pulmonary embolism. Left ventricular failure accounts for the majority of cases. Pleural effusions are rarely associated with right-sided heart failure (cor pulmonale). The location of the effusion may be of some help in making the diagnosis: for example, effusions secondary to liver cirrhosis are usually right sided, whereas those secondary to nephrosis are usually bilateral.

6. What is the differential diagnosis of an exudative pleural effusion?
Pneumonia, empyema, viral pleurisy, tuberculosis, fungal diseases, amebiasis, pulmonary embolism, pancreatitis, esophageal perforation, abdominal abscess, rheumatologic diseases, asbestosis, and malignancy. Parapneumonic effusion complicates pneumonia in 40% of patients. The definition of empyema varies from author to author and can indicate frank pus in the pleural space or exudative effusions that have a positive Gram stain for bacteria. Bacteriologic evaluation reveals that roughly one-third of empyemas are anaerobic, one-third are mixed, and one-third are aerobic. Over one-third of patients with anaerobic pneumonia will have culture-positive pleural effusion, whereas only 5% of patients with aerobic pneumonias will have culture-positive pleural effusion. Anaerobic pleuropulmonary infections often present subacutely with significant weight loss.

7. What may the cellular composition of the pleural fluid suggest?
Bloody effusions with red cell counts of 100,000/mm suggest trauma, malignancy, or occasionally pulmonary embolism. Blood-"tinged" pleural fluid can occur with only 5000 cells/mm and is a common finding due to minor bleeding that occurs at the time of thora-centesis. White cell counts of greater than 1000/mm generally suggest exudative effusions, and the finding is nonspecific. However, a rapidly rising count may herald the development of empyema. If lymphocytes make up greater than 50% of the white cells, malignancy or tuberculosis is suggested and warrants further evaluation with pleural biopsy.

8. What are the indications for drainage of the pleural space?
Indications for tube thoracostomy and drainage include: (1) frank pus, (2) positive Gram stain or culture, (3) pleural fluid glucose less than 40 mg/dl, and (4) pleural fluid pH < 7.00. If the pleural fluid pH is greater than 7.20 and glucose level is more than 60 mg/ml, antibiotic therapy alone usually suffices. Parapneumonic effusions with a pH of 7.00 to 7.20 should be observed closely or drained, depending upon the clinical circumstances. Large pleural effusions should be drained when they cause respiratory compromise. Moderate or large pleural effusions often require drainage to afford an adequate evaluation of the underlying lung by chest x-ray or CT scan. After thoracic injury, tube thoracostomy is indicated for drainage of hemopneumothorax and allows assessment of ongoing bleeding.

9. What is the best approach to drainage of a loculated pleural effusion?

Chest tube or radiologically guided catheter drainage commonly fails if the catheter is not placed optimally within the loculation or if the fluid is hemorrhagic or fibrinous. Recent studies suggest that loculations that fail to respond to conventional drainage may respond to the instillation of lytic agents (such as urokinase) into the space. Serial instillations may be required. If this method fails, thoracotomy may be needed.

10. What is the effect of therapeutic thoracentesis on pulmonary function?

The improvement in vital capacity is small even when a large amount of pleural fluid is drained. In one series of patients who had an average of 1700 ml of fluid removed, the vital capacity increased an average of 400 ml.

11. What are the most common diagnoses made by analyses of pleural fluid and pleural biopsy specimens?

Aside from the diagnosis of nonspecific exudates and transudates and empyema, the most common definitive diagnoses made by pleural fluid and biopsy specimens are those of tuberculosis and cancer.

12. How is pleural biopsy performed?

The patient is typically seated upright slumped forward with his or her head on a pillow. After liberal local anesthesia, a small skin incision is made. The biopsy needle is inserted over the top of the rib to avoid the intercostal neurovascular bundle. Multiple specimens are obtained at 3, 6, and 9 o'clock positions.

13. What risks are encountered with pleural biopsy?

A small pneumothorax is common after biopsy and usually requires no specific intervention. Fortunately, major complications, including pulmonary injury with bronchopleural fistula, hemothorax, and infection, are rare. Seeding of the chest wall with malignant cells has been reported but is exceedingly rare and does not constitute a contraindication to the procedure. Pleural biopsy is a potent vagal stimulus, and premedication with atropine, 0.6–0.8 mg IM, is advised.

14. What are the indications for pleurodesis or pleural sclerosis?

Adhesion of the parietal and visceral pleura is useful in the management of persistent bronchopleural fistula, in recurrent malignant pleural effusions, and prophylactically in patients considered to be at high risk for recurrent pneumothoraces. The method employs instillation of a sclerosing agent or irritant into the pleural space after tube evacuation of the pleural effusion or pneumothorax and satisfactory opposition of the pleural surfaces has occurred. Common agents that sclerose the pleurae include doxycycline, bleomycin, and talc. Tetracycline for pleurodesis has recently been removed from the market. The procedure should never be considered if infection of the pleural space is suspected. Common causes of failure include large bronchopleural fistulas or rapid reaccumulation of pleural fluid (evidenced by continued significant chest tube output) that prevents adequate opposition of pleural surfaces.

15. What anesthesia is required during chemical pleurodesis?

Chemical pleurodesis is extremely painful for most patients. Sherman et al. suggest that 250 mg of lidocaine instilled into the pleural space should be considered the standard dose. In addition most patients should receive IM or IV morphine titrated to effect, with close hemodynamic monitoring. Some patients will require as much as 20–40 mg of morphine. Many authors advocate the use of benzodiazepines for amnesia.

16. What is the effect of patient positioning on the distribution of tetracycline in the pleural space during pleurodesis?

Patient rotation through various positions after instillation of tetracycline has been advocated empirically. However, scintigraphic imaging during pleurodesis using radiolabeled tetracycline has demonstrated neither tetracycline dispersed throughout the pleural space within seconds nor patient positioning had any effect on intrapleural distribution in four of five patients.

BIBLIOGRAPHY

1. Aelong Y, King R, Boutin C: Thoracoscopic talc poudrage pleurodesis for chronic recurrent pleural effusions. Ann Intern Med 15:778–782, 1991.
2. George R, Light R, Matthay MA, Matthay RA (eds): Chest Medicine, 2nd ed. Baltimore, Williams & Wilkins, 1990.
3. Irani DR, Underwood RD, Johnson EH, Greenberg SD: Malignant pleural effusions: A clinical cytopathologic study. Arch Intern Med 47:1133–1136, 1987.
4. Kohan JM, Poe RH, Israel RH, et al: Value of chest ultrasonography versus decubitus roentgenography for thoracentesis. Am Rev Respir Dis 133:1124–1126, 1986.
5. Landvater L, Hix WR, Mills M, et al: Malignant pleural effusion treated by tetracycline sclerotherapy: A comparison of single vs. repeated instillation. Chest 93:1196–1198, 1988.
6. Light RW, Stansbury DW, Brown SE: The relationship between pleural pressures and changes in pulmonary function after therapeutic thoracentesis. Am Rev Respir Dis 133:658–661, 1986.
6a. Lorch DG, Gordon L, Wooton S, et al: Effect of patient positioning on distribution of tetracycline in the pleural space during pleurodesis. Chest 93:527–529, 1988.
7. Moulton JS, Moore PT, Mencini RA: Treatment of loculated pleural effusions with transcatheter intracavitary urokinase. Am J Roentgenol 153:941–945, 1989.
8. Murray JF, Nadel JA (eds): Textbook of Respiratory Medicine. Philadelphia, W.B. Saunders, 1988.
9. O'Moore PV, Mueller PR, Simeone JF, et al: Sonographic guidance in diagnostic and therapeutic interventions in the pleural space. Am J Roentgenol 149:1–5, 1987.
10. Ruskin JA, Gurney JW, Thorsen MK, Goodman LR: Detection of pleural effusions on supine chest radiographs. Am J Roentgenol 148:681–683, 1987.
11. Sherman S, Ravikrishnan KP, Patel AS, Seidman JC: Optimum anesthesia with intrapleural lidocaine during chemical pleurodesis with tetracycline. Chest 93:533–536, 1988.
12. Siegel RD, Schiffman FJ: Systemic toxicity following intracavitary administration of bleomycin. Chest 98:507, 1990.
13. Smyrnios NA, Jederlinic PJ, Irwin RS: Pleural effusion in an asymptomatic patient: Spectrum and frequency of causes and management considerations. Chest 97:192–196, 1990.
14. Varkey B: Pleural effusions caused by infection. Postgrad Med 80:213–216, 219, 222–223, 1986.
15. Walsh FW, Alberts WM, Solomon DA, Goldman AL: Malignant pleural effusions: Pleurodesis using a small-bore percutaneous catheter. South Med J 82:963–965, 972, 1989.

15. CHEST TUBES

Richard A. Peters, M.D.

1. What is the purpose of a chest tube?

A chest tube is placed to evacuate fluid and air from the pleural space and reestablish a negative intrapleural pressure so that the lung may reexpand.

2. What is the normal intrapleural pressure?

Intrapleural pressure is normally -10 cm H_2O. The natural elastic forces of the chest wall cause the chest wall to move outward from a maximal expiration. The elastic fibers of the lung pull inward, making the lung tend to collapse. The net result is negative pressure in the closed pleural space. Because gravity tends to have a greater effect at the apex than at the base of the lung, the negative pressure is greater at the apex (–10 cm H_2O) than at the base (–2 cm H_2O). The pressure varies throughout the respiratory cycle, and at times during expiration the pressure may be positive.

3. How does a chest tube collection system work?
In the past, the chest tube went directly into a glass bottle, with the tip of the tube about 2 cm under the surface of the water. The patient had only to cough to generate positive pressure in the pleural space, and to push fluid or air out of the pleural space, past the water seal. When the patient inspired and generated a negative pressure in the pleural space, it was maintained by a narrow column of water in the bottle. The problem with this older system was twofold: (1) it required positive pressure generation in the pleural space, and (2) as fluid accumulated in the bottle, the patient had to generate ever increasing positive pressure to expel air and fluid. These deficiencies were overcome with a three-bottle system. The first bottle acts as the fluid collection bottle, the second as the water seal, and the third as a suction control apparatus. The modern, sealed plastic systems may look different from the old bottle systems; however, they still have only the same three compartments.

From Pleural Space

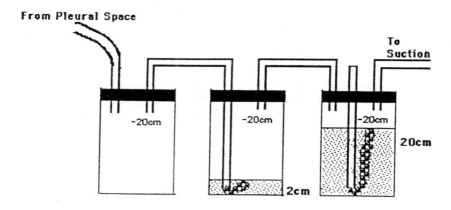

Three-bottle collection system.

4. How much suction is applied to the chest tube?
Under normal circumstances, about –20 cm H_2O is applied to the chest tube. The pressure is regulated by adjusting the depth of the tube or air vent in the last (suction) bottle. No matter how much wall suction is applied to the system, the appropriate pressure (–20 cm) is achieved when the air vent tube bubbles in the bottle system. A pressure of –20 cm H_2O is about the highest negative pressure in the pleural space in normal people, and consequently a –20 cm H_2O is usually adequate to keep the pleural space evacuated but not so high as to damage the lung. The highest pressure ever routinely used is –40 cm H_2O.

5. Where are chest tubes placed?
For a pneumothorax, the tube may be placed either in the second intercostal space in the midclavicular line or in the fourth or fifth space in the anterior or posterior axillary line. Tubes for hemothorax are routinely placed in the axillary position to promote dependent drainage. Chest tubes are rarely placed posteriorly, as they may be compressed and become nonfunctional and are quite uncomfortable in that position. In women, the tube leaves a more acceptable scar in the axillary position.

6. What size chest tube should be used?

The largest tubes, 36 French, should be used to drain a hemothorax. With their large diameter they are unlikely to be occluded with blood clots. On the other hand, most pneumothoraces can be drained with much smaller tubes; tubes as small as 10 French may be used; however, a 20–28 French tube is preferred in the critically ill, as the consequences of a failure of the tube to function due either to a large air leak or occlusion are poorly tolerated in the critically ill.

7. What are the complications of chest tube placement? How are they avoided?

Empyemas can complicate tube thoracostomy, but can be minimized by sterile technique. Placing a chest tube is an operation into a major body cavity and should be done in sterile fashion using a hat, mask, and gloves as a minimum, with as large an iodoform-prepared field as practical. The next most frequent complication is a recurrent pneumothorax after chest tube removal. This is avoided by meticulous attention to detail at the time of removal. Malfunction of a tube placed in the pleural space may be caused by a kink in the tube or by placement in a lung fissure so that the tube does not function. This problem should be recognized on the initial x-ray after tube placement and should be corrected. If the chest tube is not placed far enough into the chest, the distal hole may be pulled outside the pleural space as the skin sags around the sutures. This can be avoided by making sure that the last hole of the chest tube is at least 8 cm into the inner chest wall at the time of placement. Tubes can be placed totally outside of the chest, subcutaneously, or subdiaphragmatically with the obvious problems. The latter complication occurs when the physician does not properly count the interspaces and attempts placement below the fifth interspace. Laceration of the intercostal vessels can occur, usually infrequently.

8. How is a Heimlich valve used?

A Heimlich valve is a simple one-way flutter valve. It is held open at the proximal or patient end by a rigid ring. The distal end of soft rubber remains collapsed except when air is moving from the pleural space. It is frequently placed in line between the patient and the water seal during transport of the patient so that if the tubing becomes disconnected, pneumothorax will not occur. It may also be useful in lieu of a water seal system but is usually not used in critically ill patients.

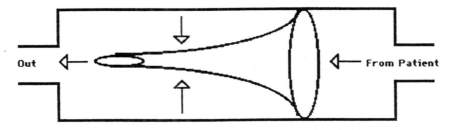

One-way air flow in the Heimlich valve.

9. What is barotrauma? What problems does it cause?

Pulmonary barotrauma is the dissection of air under pressure from the alveolus to the interstitium; the air can then further dissect to the mediastinum and out of the thoracic inlet to cause subcutaneous emphysema. The air can also dissect through the diaphragmatic hiatus to manifest as free or contained intraperitoneal air. These are alarming but relatively innocuous problems. The most disastrous event is the rupture of this air into the pleural space, resulting in a tension pneumothorax. The relationship of barotrauma to positive end-expiratory pressure (PEEP) is not clear but may be increased at levels of PEEP above 18 cm H_2O. The relationship of barotrauma to peak airway pressure is inconsistent and occurs only at very high peak pressure, usually greater than 60 cm. A sudden deterioration in status should prompt an immediate examination for presence of a tension pneumothorax.

10. When are chest tubes removed?

Chest tubes are pulled when the drainage falls below 100 ml/day, no air leak has been noted for 24 hours on water seal, and chest x-ray demonstrates complete expansion of the lung. Exceptions are (1) when a patient is on positive-pressure ventilation, it may be most appropriate not to remove a chest tube placed for a pneumothorax until the patient is off of the ventilator; (2) when tubes are placed for an empyema. In the case of an empyema, the pleural surfaces fuse and, in essence, an abscess cavity is being drained. In that case, when no fluctuation occurs in the water seal chamber with respiration, the tube may be cut off and converted to an open drain that is removed when the drainage has decreased. It is then immediately replaced with successively smaller tubes so that the tissue closes around a progressively smaller space and closes from the inside to the outside.

11. How do you know if an air leak is from the patient?

When a continued air leak is noted in the water seal chamber, the source of the leak must be found. The method of checking is simple. First, isolate the patient from the collection system. This is done by double clamping the chest tube before the first connection with a pair of large rubber-shod Kelly clamps. If an air leak is still present, the leak is from the system. Next, with the clamps still in place, double-check the connections. If they are secure and tightly sealed, the leak is in the collection system and it should be replaced. If, after clamping of the chest tube, the leak stops, then the leak is proximal. Recheck the x-ray to make sure the last hole is in the chest, then take down the chest tube dressing and make sure, with greased gauze around the tube at the chest, that air is not leaking around the tube and back into the chest.

12. How is a chest tube removed?

After taking down the dressing, place greased gauze on a 4 by 4 gauze dressing. Then, while holding this over the chest tube exit site and after cutting the suture holding the tube in place, have the patient take a large breath and perform a Valsalva maneuver. The tube is then rapidly pulled during an inspiratory Valsalva maneuver so that there is a positive pressure in the pleural space, preventing a pneumothorax. If great care is not taken during this maneuver, it may be necessary to reinsert the tube to take care of the resultant pneumothorax.

13. What is reexpansion pulmonary edema?

This is a rare condition in which a unilateral pulmonary edema develops on the side of the chest from which a pleural effusion or a pneumothorax was evacuated. Even though it is rare, it is serious and is associated with up to 20% mortality in recognized cases. The formation of edema is controlled by a balance between the intracapillary colloid osmotic and hydrostatic pressures, the pericapillary colloid osmotic and tissue pressures, and the capillary permeability. With reexpansion of the lung, there may be a change in permeability. There is a change in pleural pressure so that hydrostatic pressure is relatively unchanged at best. Most reported cases have occurred after drainage of large collections, i.e., greater than 2 liters that have existed for greater than 3 days. However, it has also been reported with effusions of short duration and smaller collections. Prophylaxis is predicated on these scant facts and consists of (1) clamping the chest tube for several hours after draining the initial 2 liters of a large chronic pleural effusion, and allowing the initial drainage to occur using water seal only; and (2) draining a large, chronic pneumothorax for the initial few hours using water seal only.

14. Should chest tubes be clamped when transporting patients?

No! There are very few times when chest tubes are ever clamped, and during transport is definitely not one of them. The risk of a pneumothorax or, worse, a tension pneumothorax, is very real. During transport when suction is usually unavailable, the patient is transported on water seal, and the water seal chamber must be kept at least 20 cm H_2O below the level of the patient to prevent reflux of fluid up the tube with any high negative intrathorax pressures that may occur. Lower is better. If the water seal chamber is above the level of the patient, the fluid can siphon back into the chest. It is frequently prudent to interpose a Heimlich valve between the chest tube and the rest of the system so that if anything happens to it while the patient is being moved, he or she still has a functioning one-way valve.

15. What is chest tube stripping?

Stripping is the practice of compressing the chest tube or drainage tubing coming from it—with either the thumb or forefinger on a greased tube or with a mechanical stripper with rollers on it on an ungreased tube—and pulling away from the chest wall while continuing to compress the tube. This generates tremendous negative pressures, up to -340 cm H_2O in the tube, and, presumably, in the pleural space as well. The reason for doing this is to dislodge any clots that may have formed in the tube and thus promote pleural drainage. However, there is no evidence that stripping the tube actually accomplishes this goal, and there is the theoretical possibility of damaging the pulmonary parenchyma as well. This is a procedure whose routine use should probably be abandoned.

16. What is the role of prophylactic antibiotics in tube thoracostomy?

Although the data are conflicting, there seems to be a decrease in the infectious complications of pneumonia and empyema with the use of prophylactic antibiotics when chest tubes are placed for traumatic hemo-pneumothoraces, and they are probably indicated in that setting. There is no evidence that they are helpful for chest tubes placed for simple spontaneous pneumothoraces.

17. How much blood draining from a hemothorax should prompt operative intervention?

About 1500 ml of blood draining from a hemothorax acutely represents approximately 40% of the circulating blood volume and should raise serious concerns that the hemorrhage may require operative intervention, as this degree of hemorrhage is poorly tolerated. Balancing this are the realizations that most intrathoracic hemorrhages will cease when pleural apposition is achieved, and that if one drains 1500 ml and the bleeding stops, if the patient is stable, and if the chest x-ray demonstrates expansion of the lung, then operative intervention is not necessary. Postoperatively the guidelines are only general as to how much pleural drainage should prompt a return to the operating room. These vary according to the procedure, coagulation status of the patient, and how much irrigation was left in the chest upon closure. In general, more than 800 ml in 1 hour, 400 ml/hr for 2 consecutive hours, 200 ml/hr for 4 consecutive hours, or 800 ml over 8 hours should make one consider returning to the operating room.

BIBLIOGRAPHY

1. Brunner RG, Vinsant GO, Alexander RH, et al: The role of antibiotic therapy in the prevention of empyema in patients with an isolated chest injury (ISS 9-10): A prospective study. J Trauma 30:1148, 1990.
2. Cullen DJ, Caldera DL: The incidence of ventilator-induced pulmonary barotrauma in critically ill patients. Anesthesiology 50:185, 1979.
3. Daly RC, Mucha P, Pairolero PC, Farnell MB: The risk of percutaneous chest tube thoracostomy for blunt thoracic trauma. Ann Emerg Med 14:865, 1985.

4. Fishman NH: Thoracic Drainage: A Manual of Procedures. Chicago, Year Book Medical Publishers, 1983.
5. Isaacson JJ, George LT, Brewer MJ: The effect of chest tube manipulation on mediastinal drainage. Heart Lung 15:601, 1986.
6. Kirby RR: Ventilatory support and pulmonary barotrauma (editorial). Anesthesiology 50:181, 1979.
7. LeBlanc KA, Tucker WY: Prophylactic antibiotics and closed tube thoracostomy. Surg Gynecol Obstet 160:259, 1985.
8. Lim-Levy F, Babler SA, De Groot-Kosolcharoen J, et al: Is milking and stripping chest tubes really necessary? Ann Thorac Surg 42:77, 1986.
9. Locorto JJ Jr, Tischler CD, Swan KG, et al: Tube thoracostomy and trauma—antibiotics or not? J Trauma 26:1067, 1986.
10. Miller TA: Physiologic Basis of Modern Surgical Care. St. Louis, C.V. Mosby, 1988.
11. Ray RJ, Alexander CM, Williams J, Marshall BE: Influence of the method of re-expansion of atelectatic lung upon the development of pulmonary edema in dogs. Crit Care Med 12:364, 1984.
12. Timby J, Reed C, Zeilender S, Glauser FL: "Mechanical" causes of pulmonary edema. Chest 98:973, 1990.
13. Wilkerson PD, Keegan J, Davies SW, et al: Changes in pulmonary microvalvular permeability accompanying re-expansion oedema: Evidence from dual isotope scintigraphy. Thorax 45:456, 1990.

16. BRONCHOSCOPY

Christopher Tyler, M.D.

1. What are the indications for bronchoscopy?

Bronchoscopy has a wide variety of diagnostic and therapeutic indications: (1) to assess airway patency, (2) to evaluate abnormal sputum cytology, (3) to stage lung cancer, (4) to evaluate for traumatic bronchial tear, (5) to evaluate suspected tracheoesophageal fistula, (6) to evaluate problems associated with endotracheal tubes, (7) to investigate abnormalities on chest x-ray, (8) to obtain selective cultures in pneumonia or abscess, (9) to evaluate unexplained recurrent laryngeal nerve or diaphragm paralysis, (10) to remove secretions, plugs, and foreign bodies not dislodged by conventional means, and (11) to carry out difficult or hazardous intubations in patients with head, neck, laryngeal, or facial trauma.

2. What airways are visually accessible by the bronchoscope?

The typical bronchoscope is 58 cm long with an external diameter of 3.5–6.0 mm. The smaller-diameter scope offers an extended range in the smaller airways, whereas the larger scope affords a larger suction channel for removal of secretions and the passage of biopsy tools. All subsegmental bronchi are accessible by either size bronchoscope.

3. What are the risks and complications of bronchoscopy?

Bronchoscopy by skilled physicians is reasonably safe. Risks include (1) death (< 1/10,000; 1/500 if transbronchial biopsy is performed), (2) hypoxia, (3) hypercarbia or respiratory failure, (4) aggravation of asthma, (5) bleeding (1–4%), (6) pneumothorax (< 1%; 5% if transbronchial biopsy is performed), (7) postbronchoscopy fever (16%), (8) arrhythmia (32% have atrial arrhythmias, 20% have ventricular arrhythmias), and (9) anesthetic complications related to atropine, lidocaine, morphine, or benzodiazepine. Anesthetic complications account for approximately half of all bronchoscopy-related complications.

High-risk situations include uremia (45% have significant hemorrhage after transbronchial biopsy), bleeding diathesis, emphysema, unstable asthma, refractory hypoxia or hypercarbia, uncooperative or combative patient, malignant arrhythmia or recent MI, pulmonary hypertension, and pulmonary abscess. Minor bleeding is the rule after transbronchial biopsy and is usually self-limited or easily controlled with topical dilute epinephrine (5 ml of 1:10,000). Patients should be alerted to the possibility of blood-streaked sputum for 12–48 hours.

4. What preparations are necessary for bronchoscopy?
The patient must not have eaten for 6 hours prior to the procedure. The patient must sign a consent form and understand the procedure. Supplemental oxygen and suction must be available during the procedure. The results of coagulation studies must be normal. Patients with bronchospasm or a history of asthma should receive inhaled beta-agonists prior to bronchoscopy, as bronchoscopy can exacerbate bronchospasms. EKG and oxygen saturation must be monitored continuously during the procedure.

5. What type of anesthesia is required for bronchoscopy?
The bronchoscopist can use either the nasal or oral route. Typically the patient is premedicated with morphine, 7–15 mg IM, and atropine, 0.6–0.8 mg IM, to blunt cough and vagal reflexes. Benzodiazepines can be used in anxious patients and will further diminish the cough reflex; however, these agents decrease the drive to breathe and will dramatically decrease ventilation in patients given narcotics. Topical anesthesia is achieved with nebulized lidocaine, and lidocaine-soaked pledgets are applied in each pyriform sinus to block the internal branch of the superior laryngeal nerve. The total dose of lidocaine is usually less than 400–600 mg and toxic serum levels (5–6 $\mu g/ml$) are rarely achieved.

6. What complications might be anticipated in the postbronchoscopy period?
Topical anesthesia lasts from 45 minutes to 1.5 hours. During this time, the patient is at risk for aspiration. The patient may also have an impaired level of consciousness related to premedication, an impaired gag reflex, or may be nauseated secondary to the narcotic administered. Patients should be given nothing by mouth, and the head of the bed should be elevated for 1–2 hours after the procedure. If the patient can tolerate small sips of water after 1–2 hours, the aspiration precautions can be terminated. Bronchoalveolar lavage (BAL) typically results in a drop in PaO_2 of 10–20 torr that reaches a maximum at 2–6 hours. Supplemental oxygen is usually required for several hours after the procedure. Postbronchoscopy fever is an occasional complication yet rarely indicates the development of pneumonia.

7. Is a chest x-ray required following fiberoptic bronchoscopy?
Chest x-ray following transbronchial biopsy is considered standard to evaluate for pneumothorax. However, the yield of routine chest x-ray remains low, and its routine use is questioned by some investigators.

8. What procedural modifications are necessary when performing bronchoscopy on ventilated patients?
Bronchoscopy can be safely performed in ventilated patients under most circumstances. Insertion of the bronchoscope through an endotracheal tube significantly increases the resistance to air flow. For this reason, an endotracheal tube 8.0 mm or larger is preferred. The level of PEEP should be reduced by 5–10 cm H_2O owing to the increased expiratory resistance. It is generally advisable to have an experienced respiratory therapist hand-ventilate the patient with 100% oxygen during the procedure to monitor pulmonary compliance, airway resistance, and oxygen saturation, and to ensure adequate ventilation. Hemodynamic monitoring is likewise critical, given the influence of changing ventilatory

dynamics on cardiac performance. BAL is well tolerated in ventilated patients, although drops in PaO_2 can be exaggerated in critically ill patients, especially in those whose hypoxic pulmonary vasoconstriction is impaired by the use of nitrates. Transbronchial biopsy can be performed in ventilated patients, although the risk of pneumothorax and tension pneumothorax is considerably higher.

9. What are the advantages and disadvantages of the rigid bronchoscope?
The rigid bronchoscope affords more effective control of the airway and a larger channel for instruments and suctioning, and patients can be ventilated through a rigid scope. Disadvantages include a limited range of view to the proximal mainstem bronchi and the need for general anesthesia. The rigid bronchoscope is preferred for removal of large foreign bodies, for control of massive hemoptysis, and for laser surgery.

10. What is the normal cellular composition of BAL fluid? In which diseases is an abnormal composition found?
Alveolar macrophages compose 90–96% and lymphocytes compose 6–8% of the cells obtained. Neutrophils, eosinophils, basophils and mast cells make up 1% of the cells obtained. An abnormal cellular composition of BAL is useful in categorizing inflammatory lung diseases into lymphocytic or neutrophilic alveolitis. Typical examples of lymphocytic alveolitis include sarcoidosis and hypersensitivity pneumonitis, whereas examples of neutrophilic alveolitis include collagen vascular disease, idiopathic pulmonary fibrosis, and bacterial pneumonias.

11. What is the value of bronchoscopy in the evaluation of pulmonary infiltrates in immunocompromised patients?
In a recent series the usefulness of the protected brush catheter together with BAL was studied in 96 immunocompromised patients.[18] Protected brush cultures detected pulmonary bacterial infections in 22% of cases but showed a high frequency of false-positive results (27%). BAL had an overall diagnostic yield of 49%. Combining protected brush and BAL diagnostic values, 69% of pulmonary infiltrates were diagnosed. However, the results obtained by both techniques resulted in modification of treatment in only 31% of cases. Of patients with nondiagnostic bronchoscopy, approximately half have treatable disease diagnosed by open lung biopsy.

12. What is the diagnostic yield of bronchoscopy for lung cancer?
The yield depends on the location and size of the tumor. In general the diagnostic accuracy for malignancy is up to 90% for endobronchial lesions and 60–70% for parenchymal lesions.

13. What is the utility of bronchoscopy in the diagnosis of *Pneumocystis carinii* pneumonia?
The yield for Pneumocystis on sputum induction varies widely between institutions, probably because of variable technical experience. The sensitivity in experienced hands is approximately 60%. The sensitivity of bronchoalveolar lavage in most series is 90–93%. The sensitivity of BAL and transbronchial biopsy combined is approximately 97%. Given the clinical importance of the diagnosis, the relatively low sensitivity of sputum induction, the high risk of side effects of empirical therapy, and the low morbidity of bronchoscopy, it is generally advisable to pursue a negative sputum examination with bronchoscopy in patients with the appropriate clinical history.

14. What is the utility of fiberoptic bronchoscopy in the diagnosis of pulmonary tuberculosis?
In approximately 70% of patients, diagnoses can be established by sputum smears and cultures alone; however, only 50% of patients will have smear-positive sputum, allowing

immediate diagnosis. Findings in smears and cultures from fiberoptic bronchoscopy are of comparable sensitivity (80%) to those from sputum (70%). Among smear-negative patients, 70% have smear-positive diagnostic bronchoscopy, which provides an immediate diagnosis. The yield is similar in patients with smear-negative miliary tuberculosis. Transbronchial biopsy significantly improves the sensitivity for immediate diagnosis.

15. What is the value of bronchoscopy in the relief of malignant airway obstruction?
The ability to manage acute airway obstruction can be lifesaving. However, the prognosis in malignant airway obstruction is almost always fatal. Relief of proximal obstruction should be considered palliative and temporizing. Therapeutic options include resection, irradiation with or without chemotherapy, manual relief of the obstruction via rigid bronchoscopy or laser therapy, and occasionally the use of stents. Because most neoplastic airway obstructions recur after temporizing therapy, clinicians should understand that they are not "preventing" death by suffocation, but rather are delaying it. Unless prolonged survival can be anticipated after relief of airway obstruction, serious consideration should be given to the use of narcotic analgesics to relieve dyspnea as a terminal comfort measure.

16. What is the role of fiberoptic bronchoscopy in evaluating the causes of pleural effusions?
Bronchoscopy is more likely to reveal the etiology of pleural effusion in patients who have a pulmonary abnormality on chest x-ray films, whereas thoracentesis with closed pleural biopsy is more diagnostic when these features are absent.

CONTROVERSY

17. Do all patients with hemoptysis need to undergo bronchoscopy?
No, but deciding which patients do not is controversial. The differential diagnosis for hemoptysis includes bronchitis, cancer, bronchiectasis, infections (tuberculosis, fungal disease, bacterial pneumonias, and abscesses), pulmonary infarction, and all the entities associated with alveolar hemorrhage. The primary role of bronchoscopy is to diagnose malignancy and to localize the site of bleeding. In patients with clear-cut nonmalignant sources of bleeding (e.g., pulmonary infarction) and mild hemoptysis, bronchoscopy is not indicated. However, in patients with an unexplained abnormality on chest x-ray or with massive hemoptysis (> 600 ml/24 hr), bronchoscopy potentially would be very useful. The controversy comes in patients with hemoptysis and a normal chest x-ray. Although the most frequent cause of hemoptysis is bronchitis, up to 50% of patients with lung cancer will have at least one episode of hemoptysis. However, less than 5% of patients with hemoptysis and a normal chest x-ray will have lung cancer. Virtually all of those patients have identified risks for lung cancer, including age > 40 and/or a significant smoking history or hemoptysis of greater than one week's duration.

BIBLIOGRAPHY

1. Barrio JL, Harcup C, Baier HJ, Pitchenik AE: Value of repeat fiberoptic bronchoscopies and significance of nondiagnostic bronchoscopic results in patients with the acquired immunodeficiency syndrome. Am Rev Respir Dis 135:422–425, 1987.
2. Chang SC, Perng RP: The role of fiberoptic bronchoscopy in evaluating the causes of pleural effusions. Arch Intern Med 149:855–857, 1989.
3. Davenport RD: Rapid on-site evaluation of transbronchial aspirates. Chest 98:59–61, 1990.
4. George R, Light R, Matthay MA, Matthay RA (eds): Chest Medicine, 2nd ed. Baltimore, Williams & Wilkins, 1990.
5. Ghows MB, Rosen MJ, Chuang MT, et al: Transcutaneous oxygen monitoring during fiberoptic bronchoscopy. Chest 89:543–544, 1986.

6. Jackson CV, Savage PH, Quinn DL: Role of fiberoptic bronchoscopy in patients with hemoptysis and a normal chest roentgenogram. Chest 87:142–144, 1985.
7. Marsh BR: Bronchoscopic brachytherapy. Laryngoscope 99(Pt. 2, Suppl 47):1–13, 1989.
8. Mehta J, Krish G, Berro E, Harvill L: Fiberoptic bronchoscopy in the diagnosis of pulmonary tuberculosis. Am Rev Respir Dis 133:962, 1986.
9. Murray JF, Nadel J (eds): Textbook of Respiratory Medicine. Philadelphia, W.B. Saunders, 1988, pp 1921–1930.
10. Neff TA: Bronchoscopy and Bactec for the diagnosis of tuberculosis: State of the art, or a brief dissertation on the efficient search for the tubercle bacillus? Am Rev Respir Dis 133:962, 1986.
11. Olopade CO, Prakash UB: Bronchoscopy in the critical-care unit. Mayo Clin Proc 64:1255–1263, 1989.
12. Pincus PS, Kallenbach JM, Hurwitz MD, et al: Transbronchial biopsy during mechanical ventilation. Crit Care Med 15:1136–1139, 1987.
13. Russell MD, Torrington KG, Tenholder MF: A ten-year experience with fiberoptic bronchoscopy for mycobacterial isolation: Impact of the Bactec system. Am Rev Respir Dis 133:1069–1071, 1986.
14. Van Gundy K, Boylen CT: Fiberoptic bronchoscopy: Indications, complications, contraindications. Postgrad Med 83:289–294, 1988.
15. Vesco D, Kleisbauer JP, Orehek J: Attenuation of bronchofiberscopy-induced cough by an inhaled beta 2-adrenergic agonist, fenoterol. Am Rev Respir Dis 138:805–806, 1988.
16. Wagner ED, Ramzy I, Greenberg SD, Gonzalez JM: Transbronchial fine-needle aspiration: Reliability and limitations. Am J Clin Pathol 92:36–41, 1989.
17. Winterbauer RH, Bass JB Jr: Controversies in pulmonary medicine: Fiberoptic bronchoscopy with protected brush catheterization should be used for the specific diagnosis of nosocomial pneumonia. Am Rev Respir Dis 138:1072–1074, 1988.
18. Xaubet A, Torres A, Marco F, et al: Pulmonary infiltrates in immunocompromised patients: Diagnostic value of telescoping plugged catheter and bronchoalveolar lavage. Chest 95:130–135, 1989.

17. PACEMAKERS

Mari McQuitty, R.N.

1. The Inter-Society Commission for Heart Disease (ICHD) has developed a three-letter pacemaker code. What is the ICHD code?

1st letter	2nd letter	3rd letter
Chamber paced	Chamber sensed	Mode of response
A–atrial	A–atrial	O–nonapplicable
V–ventricular	V–ventricular	I–inhibited
D–dual	D–dual	T–triggered
		D–I&T

Example: VVI: ventricular paced, ventricular sensed, inhibited mode

2. What are the major indications for cardiac pacing?
- Acquired atrioventricular (AV) block
- AV block associated with myocardial infarction
- Bifascicular and trifascicular block
- Sick sinus syndrome
- Hypersensitive carotid sinus syndrome

3. What are the indications for temporary pacemaker therapy?
- Heart block with myocardial infarction
- Sick sinus syndrome in patients presenting with symptomatic bradycardia prior to permanent pacemaker insertion
- Suppression of atrial and ventricular tachyarrhythmias
- After cardiac surgery for control of bradycardia and suppression of tachycardias

4. Which access sites are most commonly used for transvenous pacing? How is the catheter electrode passed?
The preferred sites are the jugular and subclavian veins, although the antecubital and femoral sites can be cannulated. The catheter is advanced slowly to the SVC, into the right atrium, through the tricuspid valve, and to the RV, where it is positioned against the endocardial surface.

5. Which two methods can the physician use to guide the catheter electrode?
1. By direct visualization of the radiopaque catheter passage with fluoroscopy.
2. By electrocardiographic means—the free end of the electrode can be attached to the chest lead terminal of the ECG machine, and the intracavitary ECG records (with differing configurations) its passage from the vena cava, through the atrium, and into the RV.

6. Which four conditions must be met for optimal pacing?
1. A conduction catheter (electrode) must be in contact with the heart muscle.
2. The electrode must be connected to a power source.
3. There must be absence of anoxia or electrolyte or acid-base imbalance.
4. There must be minimal damage to the myocardium.

7. The AV sequential temporary pulse generator is used with increasing frequency in the critical care setting. What is the advantage of AV synchrony during pacing?
By maintaining AV synchrony, the normal mechanical sequence of atrial pumping followed by ventricular filling is uninterrupted. The atria are responsible for 25–30% of ventricular filling. Loss of "atrial kick" can cause pooling of blood and resultant pulmonary and peripheral venous congestion.

8. When is AV sequential pacing not effective?
AV sequential pacing cannot be used in the presence of atrial tachycardia, flutter, or fibrillation, or in dilated, "electrically silent" atria.

9. What are the advantages and limitations of atrial pacing?
Atrial pacing preserves atrial contribution to cardiac output. Hemodynamic studies have demonstrated that an appropriate atrial contraction at end-diastole abruptly increases ventricular filling and lowers mean arterial pressure, particularly in patients with decreased ventricular compliance. Atrial pacing with rate increase can also be beneficial in suppressing atrial ectopic beats. Atrial pacing is possible only if AV conduction is intact.

10. How is the AV sequential temporary pulse generator set for atrial pacing?
Atrial pacing is performed in the asynchronous or fixed mode. Demand pacing of the atria is generally not successful, because the pulse generator mechanism is not sensitive enough to detect p-waves. The ventricular rate is set to the desired pacing rate; the atrial output is set to the desired current for atrial capture; and the ventricular output, AV interval, and ventricular sensitivity controls are not used and should be set to their minimum.

11. What is pacing threshold? How does the caregiver test for this threshold?
Threshold is the amount of energy needed to capture the atrium and/or ventricle expressed in milliamperes (mA). The threshold level is determined by gradually decreasing the output until 1:1 capture is lost, then increasing the output until capture is regained. The threshold should then be sent at mA 2 to 3 times the threshold.

12. What is pacemaker sensing?
Sensing is the ability of the pacemaker to detect the heart's intrinsic electrical activity. The pacemaker can be programmed to sense ventricular depolarization.

13. How is the appropriate sensitivity setting determined for demand pacing?
The appropriate setting can be determined by decreasing the pacing rate until the patient's underlying rhythm is evident; the dial is then turned counterclockwise (from 1.0 millivolt toward asynchronous) until the pacing escape interval is reached. The dial should then be set slightly to the right of this point, thus ensuring demand functioning.

14. What action should be taken when the temporary pacemaker fails to discharge?
Check the connections at the generator terminal and replace the batteries. If this does not correct the problem, replace the generator itself. If none of these efforts works, the pacing wire itself may be fractured.

15. What action should be taken when a pacemaker artifact appears within the escape interval?
This can usually be corrected by increasing the sensitivity, i.e., turning the sensitivity dial clockwise toward 1.0 millivolt. If this does not work, the generator battery should be replaced.

16. What is oversensing?
Oversensing is the absence of a pacing artifact during a pause greater than the escape interval. The pacemaker is inhibited when it should be firing, usually the result of a high sensitivity setting.

17. What are some complications associated with temporary cardiac pacing?
- Ventricular irritation
- Perforation of the ventricular wall or septum
- Retrograde migration of the RV catheter into the RA
- Abdominal twitching or hiccups
- Infection and phlebitis
- Tamponade

BIBLIOGRAPHY

1. ACC/AHA Task Force: Guidelines for the implantation of cardiac pacemakers and antiarrhythmia devices. J Am Coll Cardiol 18:1–13, 1991.
2. Benotti JR: Temporary cardiac pacing. In Rippe JM, et al (eds): Intensive Care Medicine. Boston, Little, Brown and Co., 1985.
3. Douglas MK, Shinn JA: Advances in Cardiovascular Nursing. Rockville, MD, Aspen, 1985.
4. Finkelmeier BA, O'Mara SR: Temporary pacing in the cardiac surgical patient. Crit Care Nurs Jan–/Feb 1984, pp 108–113.
5. Gillette PC, Griffin JC: Practical Cardiac Pacing. Baltimore, Williams & Wilkins, 1986.
6. Hauser RG, Vicari RM: Temporary pacing: Indications, modes and techniques. Med Clin North Am 70:813–827, 1986.
7. Meltzer LE, Pinneo R, Kitchell JR: Intensive Coronary Care—A Manual for Nurses, 3rd ed. Bowie, MD, Charles Press, 1977.
8. Mond HG, Strathmore NF: The technique of using cardiac pacemakers: Implantation, testing and surveillance. In Hurst JW, et al (eds): The Heart, 7th ed. New York, McGraw-Hill, 1990.
9. Moses HW, Taylor GJ, Schweiner JA, Dove JT: A Practical Guide to Cardiac Pacing, 2nd ed. Boston, Little, Brown and Co., 1987.
10. Silver MD, Goldschlager N: Temporary transvenous cardiac pacing in the critical care setting. Chest 93:607–613, 1988.

III: Pulmonary Medicine

18. ACUTE PNEUMONIA

Marvin I. Schwarz, M.D.

1. What normal defense mechanisms protect against the development of pneumonia?
Normal lung defense mechanisms include (1) filtration and humidification of the inspired air as it passes through the upper airway; (2) an intact cough reflex; (3) mucus secretion and mucociliary transport by the tracheobronchial respiratory epithelium; (4) normal macrophage lymphocyte function (cellular immunity); (5) adequate function of B-lymphocytes, immuno-globulin, and complement (humeral immunity); and (6) adequate numbers of functioning neutrophils.

2. In the immunocompetent host, what factors predispose to acute pneumonia?
Basically, in a patient with normal defense mechanisms, either there is an overwhelming exposure to an infectious agent or the agent is particularly virulent. Both of these situations can lead to pneumonia. However, factors known to predispose to acute bacterial pneumonia include a previous viral upper respiratory infection, gastroesophageal reflux, chronic alcohol consumption, cigarette smoking, alteration in level of consciousness, anesthesia, tracheobronchial intubation, preexisting lung disease, diabetes mellitus, and corticosteroid medication.

3. Under what circumstances will a community-acquired pneumonia result in respiratory failure and require an ICU admission?
Under ordinary circumstances, the majority of viral, mycoplasmal, and bacterial pneumonias do not require ICU admission. Situations that alter this are (1) pneumonia superimposed upon preexisting lung disease (e.g., COPD or cystic fibrosis); (2) pneumonia complicated by septicemia and the superimposition of the adult respiratory distress syndrome (ARDS); (3) extensive aspiration pneumonia usually following an alteration in the level of consciousness; (4) pneumonia in the alcoholic patient; (5) infrequently, a viral, mycoplasmal, or bacterial pneumonia is very diffuse and leads to respiratory failure; and (6) that the elderly in general are predisposed to more severe bacterial pneumonias.

4. Which noninfectious diseases occur acutely and have symptoms, signs, and radiographic findings similar to those of acute diffuse pneumonia?
(1) ARDS secondary to sepsis, toxic inhalations (chlorine), massive trauma, air embolism, near drowning, high altitude, neurogenic pulmonary edema, and excessive blood product replacement; (2) acute immunologic pneumonia (systemic lupus erythematosus); (3) hypersensitivity pneumonitis; (4) drug-induced pneumonitis or pulmonary edema; (5) diffuse alveolar bleeding (Goodpasture's syndrome); (6) bronchiolitis obliterans organizing pneumonia; (7) acute interstitial pneumonia (Hamman-Rich syndrome); and (8) eosinophilic pneumonia.

5. Which bacteria are responsible for acute community-acquired pneumonias that can lead to ICU admission?
Streptococcus pneumoniae (pneumococcus) is the most common pathogen causing pneumonia and is most frequently seen in patients with COPD, in demented patients, in

elderly patients, and in patients with congestive heart failure. Next most frequent is *Haemophilus influenzae,* which occurs in the same setting as *S. pneumoniae.* Staphylococcus is generally more common in the elderly, but following influenza, all age groups are affected. Community-acquired gram-negative pneumonias occur in nursing home residents. *Branhamella catarrhalis* is another important cause of pneumonia in elderly patients and in patients with COPD.

6. How does the clinical presentation of acute pneumonia differ in the elderly?

A typical presentation of pneumonia includes productive cough, chills, fever, and pleurisy. In the elderly, however, this clinical symptom complex is often absent; fever, altered mental status (confusion), and dehydration are more common in the elderly. On the other hand, leukocytosis and a leftward shift of the white blood cell count are to be expected in all patients with bacterial pneumonia.

7. What is the significance of leukopenia in the immunocompetent patient with acute pneumonia?

The failure to incite leukocytosis in response to a bacterial infection is associated with a very poor prognosis and increased mortality. This situation is more likely to occur in the alcoholic at any age and in the elderly patient generally.

8. What constitutes an adequate sputum Gram stain?

The sputum Gram stain is the most important diagnostic technique for the identification of the causative agent of an acute pneumonia in the nonintubated patient. An adequate sample is one in which the neutrophil count is ≥ 25 and the epithelial cell count ≤ 10 cells per low power field. Any sample that does not fulfill the above requirements probably represents oropharyngeal secretions and should be discarded.

9. How sensitive is the sputum Gram stain for the diagnosis of a community-acquired bacterial pneumonia?

The finding of gram-positive lancet-shaped diplococci ($> 10/$HPF) is 85% specific and 62% sensitive for *S. pneumoniae.* Gram-negative coccobacillary stains typify *H. influenzae.* *Staphylococcus aureus* is a gram-positive organism that occurs in clusters. The sputum Gram stain influences the initial choice of antibiotic.

10. Which laboratory tests are most definitive for the diagnosis of acute bacteria pneumonia?

Because 25–30% of patients with community-acquired pneumonia are bacteremic, a positive blood culture is diagnostic. The same can be said for bacterial growth from the pleural fluid. Sputum cultures, on the other hand, are notoriously inaccurate in proven cases of pneumonia, and often give false-positive results because of oropharyngeal contamination.

11. What is nosocomial pneumonia? What is its significance?

Nosocomial pneumonia is acquired while in the hospital and is associated with different organisms that are often more resistant to antibiotic therapy compared with the bacteria responsible for community-acquired pneumonia. The mortality rate for nosocomial pneumonia is significantly higher (20–50% vs. 3–5%).

12. How common are nosocomial pneumonias?

Approximately 2 million nosocomial infections occur annually in the United States. Nosocomial pneumonia accounts for 15% of these, or 300,000 cases yearly.

13. How does bacteriology of nosocomial pneumonias differ from that of community-acquired pneumonias?

As opposed to community-acquired pneumonias, nosocomial pneumonias are most often caused by aerobic gram-negative rods (Klebsiella species, Pseudomonas species, Enterobacter species, *E. colli,* Proteus, Serratia and enterococcus), *Staphylococcus aureus,* and group B streptococcus. Contamination of the hospital water supply can result in Legionella species pneumonia.

14. What is the pathogenesis of nosocomial pneumonia?

Nosocomial pneumonia results from colonization of the oropharynx and subsequent repeated small aspirations of oropharyngeal secretions. There is also retrograde oropharyngeal contamination from the gastrointestinal tract, which is thought to play an important role. This is particularly significant because of the recent trend toward gastric alkalinity in critically ill ICU patients. Increasing the pH in the stomach allows for bacterial overgrowth.

15. What conditions are conducive to nosocomial pneumonia?

The two most important predisposing factors are admission to the ICU and endotracheal intubation. When both exist, up to 20% of patients will develop a nosocomial pneumonia. Other factors that contribute significantly include previous use of antibiotics, which allows for preselection of antibiotic-resistant stains, postsurgical state (50% of all nosocomial pneumonias), preexisting chronic lung disease, azotemia, and advanced age.

16. How is the development of a nosocomial pneumonia suspected by clinical criteria?

This is a difficult problem because oropharyngeal growth on sputum culture and the presence of purulent sputum do not necessarily equate with pneumonia. In addition, the appearance of radiographic infiltrates can have other etiologies. Although the clinical diagnosis of nosocomial pneumonia is far from precise, the existence of persistent fever, an increased number of infiltrates on the chest radiograph, purulent airway secretions, and increasing problems with oxygenation raises the suspicion.

17. What other conditions can cause fever and pulmonary infiltrates in an ICU setting?

Besides nosocomial pneumonia, one has to consider atelectasis, pulmonary embolism, pulmonary edema secondary to congestive heart failure or volume overload, and sepsis causing ARDS.

CONTROVERSY

18. Is the culture and Gram stain of endotracheal secretions of significant importance in the bacteriologic diagnosis of nosocomial pneumonia?

For:

1. Endotracheal secretions are easily accessible. A change in the amount and color is often the first sign of nosocomial pneumonia and therefore will reflect the etiologic agent.

2. Growth of an organism, particularly if supported by a positive blood culture, indicates the diagnosis.

Against:

1. Contamination of suctioned endotracheal secretions occurs frequently and does not reflect the underlying cause of the pneumonia.

2. Only 10% of nosocomial pneumonias are associated with bacteremia.

3. Other diagnostic methods are available that bypass the tracheobronchial tree such as bronchoscopy with bronchoalveolar lavage and the use of a plugged protected brush for culture of secretions from the lower respiratory tract.

BIBLIOGRAPHY

1. Breitenbucher RB, Peterson PK: Infections in the elderly. In Mandel GL, Douglas RG, Bennett JE (eds): Principles and Practice of Infectious Diseases, 3rd ed. New York, Churchill Livingstone, 1990, p 2316.
2. Driks MR, Craven DE, Celli BR, et al: Nosocomial pneumonia in intubated patients given sucralfate as compared with antacids or histamine type 2 blockers. N Engl J Med 317:1376–1382, 1987.
3. Faling JL: New advances in diagnosing nosocomial pneumonia in intubated patients. Part 1. Am Rev Respir Dis 137:253–255, 1988.
4. Lambert RS, George RB: Diagnosing nosocomial pneumonia in mechanically ventilated patients: Which techniques offer the most reliability and the least risk? J Crit Illness 2:57–62, 1987.
5. Murphy TF, Fine BC: Bacteremic pneumococcal pneumonia in the elderly. Am J Med Sci 288:114–118, 1984.
6. Penn RL: Choosing initial antibiotic therapy in pneumonia patient. J Crit Illness 1:57–67, 1986.
7. Pennington JE: Nosocomial pneumonia. In Mandel GL, Douglas RG, Bennett JE (eds): Principles and Practice of Infectious Diseases, 3rd ed. New York, Churchill Livingstone, 1990, pp 2099–2105.
8. Perlino CA, Rimland D: Alcoholism, leukopenia, and pneumococcal sepsis. Am Rev Respir Dis 132:757–760, 1985.
9. Toews GB: Southwestern internal medicine conference: Nosocomial pneumonia. Am J Med Sci 29:355–367, 1986.
10. Torres A, De La Bellacasa JP, Rodriquez-Roisin R, et al: Diagnostic value of telescoping plugged catheters in mechanically ventilated patients with bacterial pneumonia: Using the Metras catheter. Am Rev Respir Dis 138:117–120, 1988.
11. Verghese A, Berk SL, Boelen LJ, et al: Group B streptococcal pneumonia in the elderly. Arch Intern Med 142:1642–1645, 1982.

19. LUNG ABSCESS AND NECROTIZING PNEUMONIA

Thomas A. Neff, M.D.

1. What is a lung abscess?

A lung abscess is the collection of pus in a cavity in the lung tissue. Strictly speaking, any process that causes necrosis of lung tissue with suppuration, i.e., pus formation, is a lung abscess. Unless otherwise stated or qualified, a lung abscess is caused by a pyogenic bacterial infection.

2. Which organisms are the most common cause of lung abscess?

Mixed mouth flora, most frequently anaerobic organisms such as streptococci, fusobacteria, spirochetes, and bacteroides. This form of lung abscess is often called primary lung abscess.

3. What is the difference between a lung abscess and necrotizing pneumonia?

Their distinction is made on descriptive radiologic terms. The process is called a lung abscess when there is a single or dominant large cavity, usually 2 cm or greater, within a well-demarcated focal infiltrate. The process is called necrotizing pneumonia when there are multiple small areas of cavitation in a larger area of diffuse pneumonic infiltrate. Both processes often have a similar etiology (mixed mouth anaerobic organisms); however, the incidence of specific necrotizing *aerobic* bacteria, such as staphylococci, gram-negative bacilli, and even occasionally pneumococci, is more likely with necrotizing pneumonia.

4. What are the most frequent factors predisposing to a lung abscess?
Aspiration of mouth flora secondary to decreased level of consciousness for any reason (e.g., alcoholism, drug overdose, head trauma, stroke, or general anesthesia) is the first and most frequent basic cause. Other factors leading to aspiration are those that interfere with normal swallowing such as neuromuscular disease of the bulbar cranial nerves or pharynx and disease of the esophagus itself such as stricture, major reflux, and vomiting.

5. In what body position are patients at greatest risk for a major aspiration?
Flat on their backs.

6. What are the signs and symptoms of lung abscess?
Early on, small lung abscesses, especially those caused by mouth flora, may be quite indolent, with minimal symptoms and no signs. Malaise, fever with or without chills, weight loss, pleuritic pain, and cough eventually occur. The expectoration of foul-smelling, putrid, purulent sputum is highly suggestive of lung abscess and should always prompt a chest x-ray.

7. What are the other major differential diagnoses of an air-fluid level cavity on chest x-ray besides lung abscess?
- Cavitated bronchial carcinoma or other malignancies such as lymphoma
- Tuberculosis and specific fungal infections
- Infected pulmonary bullae with an air-fluid level
- Infected lung cysts (e.g., bronchogenic cyst)
- Lacerated lung with liquefying hematoma
- Infected sequestration
- Necrobiotic nodules or masses (e.g., rheumatoid arthritis or Wegener's granulomatosis)
- Cavitated pulmonary infarct
- Reinfected quiescent or previously sterile cavities (e.g., inactive tuberculosis cavity or sarcoidosis)
- Hiatus hernia

8. It is often stated that "edentulous patients do not develop a primary lung abscess." True or false? Why?
Edentulous patients *rarely* develop a primary (mouth flora) lung abscess, because most such aspirated organisms come from the infected gingival and periodontal tissues and spaces that toothless patients no longer have.

9. What complications may develop in patients with lung abscesses?
Hemoptysis, sometimes life-threatening, brain abscess, rupture with pyopneumothorax or empyema, and endobronchial spread of pus to new lung areas.

10. If one sees several or more small, 1- to 3-cm cavities in the lung on a chest x-ray, especially in multiple lobes, what should be considered?
This clinical picture should immediately raise the likelihood of a hematogenous (vs. endobronchial) mechanism. Therefore bacteremia or fungemia secondary to pyophlebitis or right-sided endocarditis must be considered. Cryptic intravenous drug abuse must not be overlooked in this setting when a more obvious cause is not apparent.

11. Why is a lung abscess or necrotizing pneumonia sometimes belatedly diagnosed in an ICU patient?
ICU patients are often in the recumbent position when chest x-rays are done, so that air-fluid levels signifying cavitation are not appreciated.

12. What is the main treatment for a lung abscess?
Specific antibiotic therapy. Because the majority of patients with lung abscess have mixed mouth flora as the cause of the abscess, good anaerobic coverage is crucial.

13. What is the preferred antibiotic regimen today?
Although penicillin and even tetracycline have had excellent clinical track records—90% success in the past—new data show the increasing emergence of penicillin-resistant organisms. Therefore, initial empirical therapy should be started with either clindamycin, 300 to 600 mg four times daily, or metronidazole, 400 mg three times daily, and penicillin, 500–750 mg four times daily. In sick, toxic, febrile patients, intravenous administration is indicated; however, oral therapy is usually appropriate in non-toxic afebrile patients. Oral therapy should be continued for 2–8 weeks or until the process is resolved.

CONTROVERSIES

14. All patients with a lung abscess should have a sterile invasive procedure, such as transtracheal aspiration (TTA), protected brush bronchoscopy (PBB), or percutaneous transthoracic needle aspiration (TTNA), for diagnosis before antibiotic therapy is initiated.
For the typical patient with out-of-hospital-acquired lung abscess with putrid sputum and a history of coma, most experts would not recommend an invasive procedure before trying empirical antibiotic therapy. For patients presenting with an unusual risk profile, however, such as a hospital-acquired infection, severely ill state, or immunodeficiency and for those failing to respond to initial empirical antibiotic treatment, the use of one of the invasive microbiologic "collection procedures" is indicated. Which technique (TTA, PBB, or TTNA) is selected depends on the experience, expertise, and bias of each consultant.

15. Bronchoscopy should be performed in patients with lung abscess to promote drainage and to avoid missing lung cancer, foreign bodies, etc.
Again, as argued in #14, it is impractical to suggest that one should routinely recommend an expensive invasive procedure with intrinsic risks in a patient with a disease that has such good outcome with empirical safe therapy in the majority of instances. Ill-advised, poorly performed bronchoscopy during the first few days of treatment may actually put a patient at risk for endobronchial spread of the infection. If radiographic evidence suggests lung cancer, bronchial obstruction, or whatever, then obviously diagnostic bronchoscopy may become indicated.

16. The indications or need for aggressive surgical resection (e.g., lobectomy) is still a controversial issue.
Here again, each patient's circumstances are more important than any predetermined dictum. Severe or recurrent hemoptysis, especially in a patient with a large, thick-walled cavity, certainly is one of the more compelling indications for aggressive surgical resection. Additional factors sometimes tipping the balance toward surgical resection include large areas of devitalized lung tissue secondary to infarction and large amounts of undrainable suppuration secondary to bronchostenosis. In patients for whom general anesthesia and thoracotomy pose an extremely high risk, an image-directed percutaneous pigtail catheter drainage approach may be effective and even safer than thoracotomy.

BIBLIOGRAPHY

1. Bartlett JG: Anaerobic bacterial infections of the lung. Chest 91:901–909, 1987.
2. Bartlett JG, Gorbach SL: Penicillin or clindamycin for primary lung abscess? Ann Intern Med 98:546–548, 1983.

3. Bartlett JG, Gorbach SL, Tally FP, Finegold SM: Bacteriology and treatment of primary lung abscess. Am Rev Respir Dis 109:510–517, 1974.
4. Finegold SM: Anaerobic pleuropulmonary infections. Chest 97:1–2, 1990.
5. Grinan NP, Lucena FM, Romero JV, et al: Yield of percutaneous needle lung aspiration in lung abscess. Chest 97:69–74, 1990.
6. Gudiol F, Manresa F, Pallares R, et al: Clindamycin vs. penicillin for anaerobic lung infections: High rate of penicillin failures associated with penicillin-resistant *Bacteroides melaninogenicus*. Arch Intern Med 150:2525–2529, 1990.
7. Levinson ME, Mangura CT, Lorber B, et al: Clindamycin compared with penicillin for the treatment of anaerobic lung abscess. Ann Intern Med 98:466–471, 1983.
8. Palmer DL, Davidson M, Lusk R: Needle aspiration of the lung in complex pneumonia. Chest 78:16–21, 1980.
9. Parker LA, Melton JW, Delany DJ, Yankaskas BC: Percutaneous small bore catheter drainage in the management of lung abscesses. Chest 92:213–218, 1987.
10. Wimberley NW, Bases JB, Boyd BW, et al: Use of a bronchoscopic protected catheter brush for the diagnosis of pulmonary infection. Chest 81:556–562, 1982.

20. EMPYEMA

Thomas A. Neff, M.D.

1. What is an empyema?

Literally, pus in a body space. The most common form of empyema is pus in the pleural space, sometimes called a thoracic or pleural empyema to distinguish it from rare forms such as subdural empyema.

2. Why do clinicians (e.g., thoracic surgeons, pulmonary disease specialists, infectious disease specialists) often disagree as to whether a patient really has an empyema?

The crux of such disagreements is the lack of a universally accepted qualitative and quantitative definition of pus. Whether the aspirated pleural fluid is pus or a parapneumonic effusion is in the eyes of the beholder. See Controversies.

3. What is the most common cause of empyema?

The most common cause is bacterial pneumonia. Empyemas are essentially a complication of a more basic underlying medical problem or process that should always be sought and identified, if possible, for successful management.

4. What factors make the risk of developing an empyema more likely in a patient with pneumonia?

- Delay in the diagnosis of the original pneumonia
- Delay of effective treatment of the original pneumonia
- Virulent, relatively resistant bacterial organisms
- A compromised host

5. What are the two most common pitfalls or errors leading to a delayed diagnosis of empyema in an ICU patient?

(1) Relying on a portable AP chest x-ray, often of poor quality, to "show or rule out" an empyema. (2) Delay in performing a diagnostic thoracentesis once pleural fluid is identified.

6. If a portable chest x-ray is inadequate or nondiagnostic and an empyema is still considered possible, what tests should be considered next?

Better and complete thoracic imaging of the pleural space is the key to accurate diagnosis and to selection of the appropriate drainage approach. High-quality PA and lateral chest x-rays may be all that is necessary. Portable bedside ultrasound may be most appropriate for an unstable patient at too high a risk to leave the ICU. Finally, a complete CT scan, including subdiaphragmatic upper abdomen cuts, is often required and usually invaluable. A timely diagnostic tap (thoracentesis), sometimes without a perfect x-ray, may be an expeditious approach.

7. What type of pleural fluid on gross examination may mimic an empyema?
Chylothoracic fluid.

8. What three principles must be followed for the appropriate and successful treatment of a patient with empyema?
1. Adequate drainage of the pus.
2. Specific effective antibiotic therapy.
3. Identification and management of basic underlying disease(s).

9. List the major techniques used to drain an empyema and/or a "complicated" parapneumonic effusion.
1. Thoracentesis* with a large-bore (#14 to #16) needle or catheter
2. Closed-chest tube (#28 to #40) thoracostomy,* usually with suction
3. Mini-thoracotomy with or without rib resection and a large-bore empyema tube
4. Formal thoracotomy with decortication and/or empyemaectomy.

 * Often adequate for parapneumonic effusion, usually not for a true (i.e., thick, viscous pus) empyema.

10. What are two acute major risks or morbidities of inadequate management of empyema?
1. Most frequently, uncontrollable sepsis and its sequelae.
2. Occasionally, respiratory failure.

11. What is the major chronic sequel to inadequate management of empyema?
Fibrothorax with a significant restrictive ventilatory defect that may require decortication.

CONTROVERSIES

12. How is an empyema differentiated from a complicated parapneumonic effusion?
The answer really depends on the criteria that each physician accepts in the definition of each entity. Besides the gross visual appearance of the fluid, the following additional characteristics of pleural fluid and/or "numbers" have been proposed to separate these two diagnoses: odor, viscosity, bacterial culture and/or Gram stain, WBC, glucose, and pH. To most physicians, a thick viscous fluid with or without bacteria signifies an empyema. The WBC ($> 20,000$ or $> 50,000$), the glucose (< 20 mg/dl), or the pH (<7.0) is an arbitrary "cutoff" that some use to define an empyema versus a complicated parapneumonic effusion.

13. Do all "complicated" parapneumonic effusions need immediate drainage?
Since pleural effusions have first been subjected to chemical and microscopic analysis, physicians have been trying to find predictive formulas to answer this question. The answer that usually emerges from careful objective studies is that no single test of pleural fluid is uniformly accurate, but rather all pleural fluid data must be used along with each patient's

specific clinical picture (e.g., fever, systemic symptoms, WBC, size of effusion, type of organism, underlying process, clinical course) to make the best decision for each patient.

14. Is there a role for streptokinase or other enzymatic "lytic" therapy in the treatment of empyema and complicated parapneumonic pleural effusion?
In the 1950s and 1960s, intrapleural enzymes such as streptokinase and chymotrypsin were used with mostly poor results and therefore were abandoned. However, with the recent advent of more available purified thrombolytic enzymes and the improved technique of CT-scan-directed chest tube placement, there now appears to be a definitive role for such therapy in selected patients.

BIBLIOGRAPHY

1. Berger HA, Morganroth ML: Immediate drainage is not required for all patients with complicated parapneumonic effusions. Chest 97:731–735, 1990.
2. Ferguson MK: The healing hand. Chest 97:4–5, 1990.
3. Lemmer JH, Botham MJ, Orringer MJ: Modern management of adult thoracic empyema. J Thorac Cardiovasc Surg 90:849–855, 1985.
4. Light RW: Management of parapneumonic effusions. Arch Intern Med 141:1339–1341, 1981.
5. Moulton JS, Moore PT, Mencini RA: Treatment of loculated pleural effusions with transcatheter intracavitary urokinase. AJR 153:941–945, 1989.
6. Orringer MB: Thoracic empyema—back to the basics. Chest 93:901–902, 1988.
7. Taryle DA, Potts DE, Sahn SA: The incidence and clinical correlates of parapneumonic effusions in pneumococcal pneumonia. Chest 74:170–173, 1978.
8. Varkey B, Rose HD, Kutty CP, Politis J: Empyema during a ten-year period. Arch Intern Med 141:1771–1776, 1981.

21. PNEUMONIA IN IMMUNOCOMPROMISED PATIENTS

Elizabeth L. Aronsen, M.D.

1. Who are immunocompromised patients?
This is actually a very large and diverse group that, for the purposes of discussion, can be divided into four major (and sometimes overlapping) subsets: patients with (1) malignancy; (2) solid organ or bone marrow transplant; (3) congenital or acquired primary immunodeficiency; and (4) chronic systemic illness (e.g., malnutrition, uremia, alcoholism, collagen vascular disease, chronic obstructive pulmonary disease, steroid therapy, or asplenia). Patients with human immunodeficiency virus (HIV) disease could be included under acquired immunodeficiency but will be discussed elsewhere in this book.

2. What are the normal host defenses against lung disease?
To understand why immunocompromised patients are at increased risk for pulmonary disease, it is helpful to appreciate the normal host defenses of the lung and which of these are impaired in various immunodeficiency states. This, in turn, allows us to better predict the most likely infectious or noninfectious pulmonary pathology for a given patient. For example:
    Upper airway defenses include air filtration and humidification by nasal ciliated epithelia.

Cough reflexes are triggered by activation of neural and chemoreceptors and are powered past an intact epiglottis. The closed epiglottis provides additional protection against aspiration.

Mucociliary clearance is provided by specialized cells of the upper airway.

Normal oral flora of low virulence make it difficult for pathogens to establish a foothold.

Nonspecific antimicrobial factors include immunoglobulins (Ig) A and G, complement components, surfactant, and alveolar macrophages.

Specific systemic host responses to pathogens are established via humoral or cell-mediated immunity (CMI).

3. What are abnormal host defenses in immunocompromised patients?

Impairment can occur at any point in the normal host defense for a given patient and depends not only on the underlying associated disease, but often also on specific therapies for that disease. For example:

Upper airway defenses are bypassed altogether by intubation.

Cough reflex is decreased and aspiration increased with changes in mental status (e.g., encephalopathy, coma, or secondary to drugs or alcohol).

Mucociliary clearance is reduced by aspirin therapy.

Alterations in oral flora occur in uremia, alcoholism, or as a consequence of prior antibiotics or other medications.

Nonspecific antimicrobial factors are impaired in a variety of immunocompromised patients. Malnutrition is linked to decreases in complement and secretory IgA. Hypocomplementemia has also been demonstrated in various collagen vascular diseases, uremia, and alcoholism. Calcium channel blockers inhibit phagocytic properties of alveolar macrophages.

Congenital or acquired defects in humoral immunity likely to be encountered in an adult population include multiple myeloma, common variable (acquired) hypogammaglobulinemia, thymoma with hypogammaglobulinemia, and selective IgA or IgG subclass deficiencies, and are associated with recurrent pneumonias and bronchiectasis.

CMI is the predominant or only systemic immune defect in hairy cell leukemia, acute lymphocytic leukemia, and cartilage hair hypoplasia syndrome as well as during therapy with corticosteroids or cyclosporine. Malnutrition and alcoholism also depress CMI.

Both CMI and humoral immunity are significantly affected by age, uremia, following solid organ transplantation or bone marrow transplant, and as a part of Job's syndrome (hypergammaglobulinemia E). Hodgkin's disease and chronic lymphocytic leukemia are among malignancies associated with defects in both humoral immunity and CMI, as is cytotoxic therapy with azathioprine or cyclophosphamide.

4. What kinds of infectious pneumonias should I look for in my immunocompromised patients?

Of those infectious causes diagnosed, *Streptococcus pneumoniae* remains the number-one causative organism, followed by *Hemophilus influenzae,* Legionella spp., *Staphylococcus aureus*, protozoans, fungi, viruses (especially the herpesviruses), and mycobacteria. Organisms previously considered to be of low virulence or of no consequence in humans must now be included in the differential diagnosis of infectious etiologies in the immunocompromised patient.

5. What are noninfectious causes of pulmonary infiltrates in immunocompromised patients?

Noninfectious causes include cardiac and noncardiac pulmonary edema, embolism, hemorrhage, lymphangitic or other metastatic spread of malignancy, primary intrathoracic malignancy, chemical (aspiration) pneumonitis, and cytotoxic or radiation pneumonitis.

Many noninfectious and infectious causes of pulmonary infiltrates present with similar signs and symptoms, including cough, dyspnea, tachycardia, and fever, making diagnosis difficult.

6. How do I diagnose the cause of a pulmonary infiltrate in an immunocompromised patient?

A minimum workup of the immunocompromised patient who presents with pulmonary infiltrates includes the following:

History. As always, the history will provide important clues to the etiology. What is the time course of the illness? What are the associated symptoms? What underlying disease does (or might) the patient have? What occupational, travel, or other exposure history is there? What medications is the patient currently taking or has recently been given? (*Note:* Some pulmonary effects of medications can be delayed as long as 6 months or more.)

Physical examination and chest x-ray. The physical exam is often less helpful than the history and often is nonspecific. Roentgenographic findings on chest x-ray are diverse for any given illness. However, both of these can be helpful in prioritizing the differential diagnosis and should not be neglected. For example, signs of consolidation suggest bacterial over viral etiology or hemorrhage over drug-associated pneumonitis.

Laboratory examination and cultures. Beyond the complete blood cell count and possibly coagulation studies, laboratory analysis of blood rarely narrows the differential but will likely be helpful in the acute care of the patient and may also provide prognostic significance. All patients should be extensively cultured prior to initiation of any antibiotic therapy if possible. Respiratory samples should be examined by Gram stain and cultured for routine bacterial, viral, mycobacterial, and fungal pathogens. The lab should be alerted to suspected organisms and to the nature of the patient's underlying disease, and requested to keep the cultures longer before ruling out more fastidious organisms such as Nocardia. Special stains for Pneumocystis may be employed on induced sputum in suspected cases. Immunocytochemical techniques are helpful and provide rapid diagnosis if available at your institution.

Invasive diagnostic techniques. In general, the more acutely and seriously ill your patient is, the more invasive the diagnostic techniques you will employ. These range from transtracheal or transthoracic needle aspiration (rarely used anymore in this population because of the unacceptably high associated morbidity), to fiberoptic bronchoscopy with bronchoalveolar lavage and/or transbronchial biopsy, to open-lung biopsy. Since lung tissue is often required for definitive diagnosis and since open-lung biopsy virtually guarantees sufficient tissue to make a diagnosis if one is possible, many experts advocate early and aggressive use of this procedure. Others counsel a more cautious approach and advise using open-lung biopsy as a procedure of last resort since most immunocompromised patients will experience recurring lung disease and will not tolerate repeated surgical procedures. In this latter view, it is better to treat a patient based on one's clinical impression without a diagnosis, rather than completely satisfy one's academic curiosity. Finally, pulmonary artery (PA) catheters may provide additional diagnostic information as well as guide therapy.

7. What percentage of immunocompromised patients will have a definitive diagnosis?

Despite our best efforts, as many as one-third of pulmonary infiltrates remain undiagnosed.

8. What therapy should I initiate in my immunocompromised patient?

Several principles, based on good judgment and common sense, should always prevail. Assessing the severity of the patient's illness with appropriate triage to the ICU or general ward is paramount. The patient must have sufficient respiratory support, including mechanical ventilation if necessary. Antimicrobial therapy is often wisely initiated early; again, in general, the more acutely and seriously ill your patient is, the broader the initial spectrum of antibiotics you are likely to use. These can be tailored somewhat to the specific circumstances of your patient. For example, asplenia or defects in humoral immunity should alert you particularly to encapsulated bacteria, whereas abnormal cell-mediated immunity increases the risk of viruses, fungi, protozoans, and other intracellular organisms such as Mycoplasma. A reasonable broad-spectrum initial antibiotic choice might be a semisynthetic penicillin or a third-generation cephalosporin plus an aminoglycoside.

Timing of the acute illness with respect to the underlying disease will increase the likelihood of specific diagnoses and, therefore, the need for specific and directed therapy. For example, following bone marrow transplant, early infectious pulmonary complications are more likely to be bacterial or fungal, with viral or protozoal infections occurring somewhat later (on average about 8 weeks after transplant). Recent hospitalization increases the risk of gram-negative organisms and *Staph. aureus.* Certain fungi are endemic to various areas of the country (e.g., Histoplasma in the Midwest or Cryptococcus in the Southwest United States), and should alert physicians to consider them in patients with an appropriate travel history. Diarrhea is more commonly associated with atypical (20%) than typical (4%) pneumonias. Thrombocytopenia or an abnormal coagulation profile may suggest pulmonary hemorrhage or disseminated intravascular coagulopathy (DIC). Placement of a PA catheter can help in fluid management, as well as support a diagnosis of cardiovascular dysfunction or sepsis. In any case, therapy should be quickly tailored to the specific diagnosis as soon as it is available so as to avoid iatrogenic complications.

9. What is the mortality of immunocompromised patients in the ICU with pulmonary disease?

Obviously this varies as a function of the underlying disease, the severity and type of acute illness, and associated nonprimary organ system dysfunction. Statistics reveal average mortalities in the range of 60–80% for most scenarios. Only early intervention and conscientious care by the health care team will have any significant effect on these odds for your patient.

BIBLIOGRAPHY

1. Fang G-D, et al: New and emerging etiologies for community-acquired pneumonias with implications for therapy. Medicine 69:307–316, 1990.
1a. Gross TJ, et al: Noninfectious pulmonary diseases masquerading as community-acquired pneumonia. Clin Chest Med 12:363–393, 1991.
2. Grossman J, Kahn F: Noninfectious pulmonary disease in the immunocompromised host. Semin Respir Med 10:78–88, 1989.
3. Krowka MJ, et al: Pulmonary complications of bone marrow transplantation. Chest 87:237–246, 1985.
4. Marcy TW, et al: Pulmonary consequences of congenital and acquired immunodeficiency states. Clin Chest Med 10:503–519, 1989.
5. Skerrett SJ, et al: Respiratory infections and acute lung injury in systemic illness. Clin Chest Med 10:469–502, 1989.
6. Stover DE: Diagnosis of pulmonary disease in the immunocompromised host. Semin Respir Med 10:89–100, 1989.
7. Williams DM, et al: Pulmonary infection in the compromised host. Am Rev Respir Dis 114:359–394, 1976.

22. ASTHMA

Robert A. Bethel, M.D.

1. What historical factors are important to determine in patients with acute severe asthma?
One usually cannot take a complete history from a patient with acute, severe asthma before therapy must begin. Nevertheless, some historical factors are important to obtain as soon as possible, as they may affect treatment. A cardiac history may help determine whether wheezing and shortness of breath are due to left ventricular failure instead of asthma. An appropriate history for pulmonary emboli should be obtained, as pulmonary emboli can masquerade as acute asthma. A medication history should be obtained, as some medications induce asthma attacks and alter appropriate therapy. For example, attacks precipitated by beta-adrenergic blockers (including glaucoma medications) often do not respond well to beta-agonists. Other bronchodilators (anticholinergic agents, methylxanthines) should be considered. In the rare case of asthma precipitated by cholinesterase inhibitors, inhaled anticholinergic drugs may be especially useful. It is helpful to identify specific and nonspecific triggers of an acute asthma attack (for example, aspirin, other nonsteroidal anti-inflammatory drugs, food additives such as sulfites, inhaled antigens such as animal danders, molds and pollens, air pollutants, fumes, and smoke) to allow one to counsel patients to avoid the same triggers in the future.

2. What physical findings indicate a severe asthma attack?
Heart rate > 130 beats/min, pulsus paradoxus > 20 mm Hg, respiratory rate > 30 breaths/min, use of accessory respiratory muscles, silent chest, lethargy, somnolence, and advancing fatigue.

3. What laboratory tests should be done in acute asthma?
1. An objective measurement of airway obstruction (FEV_1 or peak flow) allows determination of the severity of an attack and the response to therapy. A forced expiratory maneuver may exacerbate asthma in some persons, but most patients can perform this maneuver without difficulty.
2. Arterial blood gases should be obtained in patients with severe attacks. Acute asthma decreases PaO_2. If PaO_2 is normal, central airway obstruction mimicking asthma should be considered. An increased or even normal $PaCO_2$ indicates potential fatigue, and close observation is needed for possible mechanical ventilation.
3. A chest radiograph should be obtained when the history or physical exam raises the question of pulmonary infection, heart failure, pulmonary embolus, or a complication of acute asthma, such as pneumothorax. Without evidence in the history or physical exam of these disorders, the yield of chest radiographs is small.
4. A CBC should be obtained if acute asthma is thought possibly to be secondary to bacterial infection.
5. Serum theophylline concentration should be measured if the patient is taking theophylline. A low theophylline level may contribute to an acute attack. An acute asthma attack or recent change in medication may alter theophylline metabolism and induce theophylline toxicity.

4. Which patients develop near-fatal or fatal asthma?
Patients who develop sudden, severe attacks or who have severe, slowly progressive disease. Although it is difficult to identify such patients prospectively, some risk factors have been postulated: a marked circadian variation in lung function, recurrent hospitalization or emergency room visits, previous life-threatening attacks, or the use of three or more medications.

5. What are the important differential diagnoses to make immediately in the treatment of acute, severe asthma?

The differential diagnosis of asthma is large. However, asthma is misdiagnosed most significantly in the acute situation in patients with left ventricular failure or central airway obstruction (as may be due to epiglottitis, laryngeal edema, laryngeal spasm, vocal cord paralysis, or vocal cord dysfunction). It is important to differentiate these disorders, as they are common and require significantly different therapy from asthma.

6. How important is CO_2 retention in acute asthma?

$PaCO_2$ is decreased in most patients with acute asthma. Some authors suggest that when $PaCO_2$ is normal or increased, fatigue is likely and mechanical ventilation should be instituted. Recent studies indicate, however, that most patients with CO_2 retention at initial evaluation do not require mechanical ventilation. Spontaneous ventilation improves with time in most patients with conventional therapy. Because mechanical ventilation in severe asthma is hazardous and difficult, it is wise not to begin mechanical ventilation in acute asthmatics merely because of an elevated $PaCO_2$ (unless it is quite high and associated with significant respiratory or metabolic acidosis). If CO_2 retention increases or if a patient appears progressively fatigued or lethargic, mechanical ventilation should be instituted.

7. How should beta-adrenergic agonists be used in acute asthma?

Beta-2 selective adrenergic agonists are usually the drug of first choice to treat acute asthma. In general, they should be given by the inhaled route. Usually, they are as effective when inhaled as when taken subcutaneously or intravenously. If they cannot be delivered adequately to airways by inhaled techniques (which may be a problem in a patient with very low FEV_1), then subcutaneous administration or, at times, even intravenous infusion (terbutaline) should be considered. Inhaled beta-adrenergic agents should be used repeatedly to tolerance.

8. How should corticosteroids be used in acute asthma?

Systemic corticosteroids should be given early to almost all patients admitted to hospital for acute asthma. Corticosteroids hasten recovery from an acute attack. They take several hours to have a clearcut effect. Recommended doses vary considerably, but typical doses for a severe attack might be 60–125 mg of methylprednisolone intravenously every 6 hours. As a patient improves, the corticosteroid dose can be consolidated to once daily and tapered rapidly to lower levels (for example, prednisone 60 mg orally once a day). The dose can be further tapered as indicated by the patient's condition. Traditionally, corticosteroids have been given intravenously during acute, severe asthma attacks, but the oral route is probably just as effective and is less costly.

9. How should aminophylline be used in acute asthma?

Aminophylline is of questionable usefulness in acute asthma. Several good studies have shown that the addition of aminophylline to good beta-agonist and corticosteroid therapy adds nothing but adverse effects. It possibly could be reserved for patients not responding to beta-agonist and corticosteroid therapy.

10. What other drugs are helpful in acute asthma?

Supplemental oxygen is indicated in almost all severe asthma attacks. Inhaled ipratropium bromide or glycopyrrolate may add to the bronchodilator effects of beta-agonists. These nonabsorbable anticholinergic drugs are well tolerated.

11. What other drugs are harmful in acute asthma?

Several inhaled agents may irritate airways in acute asthma and should be avoided: inhaled corticosteroids, cromolyn, acetylcysteine, cool mist, and ultrasonic mists. Sedatives should be avoided, as they may precipitate respiratory failure.

12. Is magnesium therapy useful to treat refractory asthma?

Intravenous magnesium sulfate ($MgSO_4$) to treat acute refractory asthma has been studied only minimally. It should not yet be a routine part of one's acute asthma armamentarium. The long-term efficacy is unknown, and the short-term efficacy is uncertain. Nevertheless, intravenous $MgSO_4$ may be tried in severe asthma attacks refractory to conventional therapy. The emergency room dose for an average size adult is 1–2 gm in 50 ml of normal saline infused over 20 minutes. To treat **status asthmaticus**, the above loading dose should be followed by continuous intravenous infusion of 1–2 gm/hr. Magnesium can cause significant muscle weakness and respiratory depression, especially in patients with renal insufficiency. One should observe for these adverse effects. Serum magnesium levels and deep tendon reflexes should be monitored. $MgSO_4$ therapy is probably safest in mechanically ventilated patients. This therapy should not interrupt the frequent use of inhaled beta-agonists, systemic corticosteroids, or supplemental oxygen, and should not delay needed intubation and mechanical ventilation. If $MgSO_4$ is used, it is advisable to measure FEV_1 or peak flow at the beginning and end of infusion to determine whether $MgSO_4$ causes bronchodilation, and to measure the baseline serum magnesium level to determine whether it is low.

The mechanisms by which $MgSO_4$ may improve acute asthma are unknown. Proposed mechanisms include (1) relaxation of bronchial smooth muscle (through blocking calcium channels); (2) improvement of underlying hypomagnesemia with consequent improvement in respiratory muscle function (where $MgSO_4$ has been found most effective, baseline serum magnesium concentration has been low-normal; beta-adrenergic drugs may lower serum magnesium; (3) inhibition of neural release of acetylcholine; and (4) sedation.

13. How does one know when an asthmatic is in trouble?

- $FEV_1 < 30\%$ predicted and still $< 40\%$ predicted after 1 hour of therapy
- Use of accessory muscles of respiration
- Pulsus paradoxus > 20 mm Hg
- $PaCO_2$ normal or increased
- Heart rate > 130
- Silent chest
- Lethargy, somnolence, fatigue

14. What are the indications for intubation and mechanical ventilation in acute asthma?

- Apnea, near apnea, or cardiopulmonary arrest
- Progressive increase in $PaCO_2$
- Lethargy and somnolence
- Advancing fatigue and impending exhaustion
- Deterioration in airflow despite vigorous medical therapy, with the development of the above findings

Possible indications
- Myocardial ischemia
- Life-threatening arrhythmias
- Metabolic acidosis
- Pneumothorax

15. What are the problems associated with mechanical ventilation in asthma? How are they overcome?

Difficult intubation. Endotracheal intubation of patients with acute severe asthma often is difficult because patients are in distress and not fully cooperative, and because intubation may increase bronchospasm and induce laryngospasm. Intubation should be attempted by the most experienced person available. This is not a time for training inexperienced personnel. In an alert patient, thorough local anesthesia of the pharynx and larynx is necessary. Sometimes sedation (midazolam or diazepam) and possibly paralysis (pancuronium, vecuronium, or succinylcholine) may be necessary. One may use blind nasotracheal intubation, orotracheal intubation, or intubation over a bronchoscope, whichever method the physician feels most confident with. I think intubation over a bronchoscope gives the greatest control and blind nasotracheal intubation is the most difficult in this acute situation. Oral intubation is indicated for the the apneic, cyanotic patient.

High airway pressure and barotrauma. High airway pressures cause pneumothorax, pulmonary interstitial emphysema, pneumomediastinum, subcutaneous emphysema, pneumoperitoneum, and tension lung cyst. A pneumothorax or tension pneumothorax can be catastrophic. Mechanical ventilation in asthma is usually performed with a volume cycle mode, although investigation with pressure support modes is under way. Maximal therapy with inhaled beta-agonists and with corticosteroids and attention to suctioning airway secretions will help decrease airway pressures. Ventilation with Heliox (a helium-oxygen mixture) can be used to decrease airway pressures and improve ventilation. If airway pressures are significantly high, one can use controlled hypoventilation, allowing decreased minute ventilation and carbon dioxide retention (possibly with supplemental intravenous sodium bicarbonate) to decrease complications and deaths. A sudden increase in airway pressure suggests plugging of the endotracheal tube or airways with secretions, atelectasis, migration of the endotracheal tube into a mainstem bronchus, or pneumothorax.

Hyperinflation, intrinsic PEEP, and hypotension. In severe airway obstruction, exhalation is often incomplete at the end of a respiratory cycle, causing intrinsic PEEP, hyperinflation, decreased cardiac return, and hypotension. One needs to observe for these complications, especially when mechanical ventilation is first initiated. Hyperinflation and intrinsic PEEP are treated with low respiratory rates (allowing greater time for exhalation), by increasing inspiratory flow rate and thereby decreasing T_I/T_{TOT} (this also allows greater time for exhalation), by using as large an endotracheal tube as possible (to decrease expiratory resistance), and occasionally by adding low levels of extrinsic PEEP. Hypotension is treated by trying to decrease hyperinflation and intrinsic PEEP, and by intravenous volume expansion.

Agitation, dyspnea, and dyssynchrony with the ventilator. These problems frequently complicate mechanical ventilation in asthmatic patients and contribute significantly to the hazards of mechanical ventilation. It is preferable to avoid sedation and paralysis of mechanically ventilated patients as much as possible because of the increased ventilator dependence these agents cause. Nevertheless, sedation and paralysis are frequently needed in asthmatics. Agitation and dyssynchronous breathing also contribute to increased airway pressure and hyperinflation. Sedation and paralysis may improve these problems.

Weaning. Few studies report the relative efficacy of various weaning modes from mechanical ventilation in asthmatic patients. Because severe airway obstruction usually improves considerably with treatment and time, weaning is seldom a problem.

Problems associated with mechanical ventilation in general. Airway obstruction, intubation of a mainstem bronchus, endotracheal-tube-induced trauma, pneumonia, atelectasis, upper gastrointestinal hemorrhage, sepsis, etc. should be prevented and treated, as in all mechanically ventilated patients.

16. What are additional unconventional therapies that may help patients with severe refractory asthma?
In general, the therapies described above plus time will suffice to allow enough improvement for discontinuation of mechanical ventilation. Other therapies that have been used include general anesthesia, neuroleptic tranquilizers, extracorporeal membrane oxygenation, and bronchoscopy with lavage. Often, as consultants ruminate over the advisability of these

more invasive therapies, time passes, the patient improves, and additional therapy is no longer required.

BIBLIOGRAPHY

1. Darioli R, Perret C: Mechanical controlled hypoventilation in status asthmaticus. Am Rev Respir Dis 129:385–387, 1984.
2. Fanta CH, Rossing TH, McFadden ER Jr: Treatment of acute asthma: Is combination therapy with sympathomimetics and methylxanthines indicated? Am J Med 80:5–10, 1986.
3. Gluck EH, Onorato DJ, Castriotta R: Helium-oxygen mixtures in intubated patients with status asthmaticus and respiratory acidosis. Chest 98:693–698, 1990.
4. Littenberg B, Gluck EH: A controlled trial of methylprednisolone in the emergency treatment of acute asthma. N Engl J Med 314:150–152, 1986.
5. Mansel JK, Stogner SW, Petrini MF, Norman JR: Mechanical ventilation in patients with acute severe asthma. Am J Med 89:42–48, 1990.
6. Marini JJ: Should PEEP be used in airflow obstruction? (Editorial) Am Rev Respir Dis 140:1–3, 1989.
7. Menitove SM, Goldring RM: Combined ventilator and bicarbonate strategy in the management of status asthmaticus. Am J Med 74:898–901, 1983.
8. Siegal D, Sheppard D, Gelb A, Weinburg PF: Aminophylline increases the toxicity but not the efficacy of an inhaled beta-adrenergic agonist in the treatment of acute exacerbations of asthma. Am Rev Respir Dis 132:283–286, 1985.
9. Skobeloff EM, Spivey WH, McNamera RM, Greenspan L: Intravenous magnesium suflate for the treatment of acute asthma in the emergency department. JAMA 262:1210–1213, 1989.

23. CHRONIC OBSTRUCTIVE PULMONARY DISEASE

Enrique Fernandez, M.D.

1. What is COPD?

Chronic obstructive lung disease (COLD) or chronic obstructive pulmonary disease (COPD) is a clinical term referring to a group of diseases "characterized by persisting slowing of airflow during expiration." Most experts would exclude patients with upper airways obstruction and some specific lung diseases associated with chronic airflow obstruction (CAO). These diseases would include some of the pneumoconioses, sarcoidosis, advanced tuberculosis, etc. In these cases, the underlying lung disease is the primary diagnosis. More recently the term "chronic airflow limitation" has been proposed, with the thought that "limitation" describes more precisely the physiologic impairment than does "obstruction." In general, patients who die of symptomatic COPD have pathologic characteristics of emphysema, chronic bronchitis, or small airways disease, or a variable mix of them. With better physiologic evaluations, the various contributions of emphysema, chronic bronchitis, and small airways disease to CAO now may be better appreciated during life. However, as a general designation, CAO is still appropriate, and, if known, the form or type of CAO would then be indicated.

2. What are the criteria for diagnosis of COPD?

1. There should be an obstructive ventilatory abnormality on spirometry: low-percent predicted FEV_1 plus a low FEV_1/FVC ratio. FEV_1 should be below the limit of normal ($< 75\%$ of predicted).

2. The obstruction should persist despite normal maximal therapy given over a period of time. (The failure to correct the airway obstruction with the administration of one dose of inhaled bronchodilator is not sufficient evidence to exclude reversible asthma.) At the same time, a significant response to bronchodilator "but not reversal to normal" might be found in patients with COPD, indicating that these patients might have some reversible bronchospastic component.

3. Upper airway lesions should be excluded (by physical examination, using inspiratory and expiratory flow volume curves, or by laryngoscopy, bronchoscopy, or special reontgenographic procedure). A chest x-ray serves more to rule out specific lung diseases that may lead to CAO than to make the diagnosis of COPD.

4. History, physical examination, and work-up will help to assess the severity of the disease as well as provide a diagnosis. Important points in the history are smoking habits, presence and duration of cough and sputum, and degree of dyspnea and exercise limitation, as well as history of atopic disease, intermittent wheezing, or seasonal variation of symptoms. The measurement of flows and lung volumes before and after administration of bronchodilators as well as after maximal therapy will help to assess degree of obstruction and reversibility. Arterial blood gases on room air are obtained to assess the degree of hypoxemia if present, the need for supplemental oxygen, and the presence or absence of respiratory failure (CO_2 retention). Measurement of serum alpha$_1$-antitrypsin is recommended for subjects with CAO, and phenotyping should be done if the serum level is < 80 mg/dl. This is important for replacement therapy, mainly in patients with PiZ phenotype, and for epidemiologic counseling. Other tests that might be clinically indicated to assess the disease include measurement of lung elastic recoil, pulmonary diffusing capacity, computed tomography, and right cardiac catheterization to evaluate right heart and pulmonary hemodynamics.

3. What are the major pathologic changes in COPD?

The major changes are found in the airways and in the parenchyma. The bronchitic elements consist mainly of airway mucosal inflammation and edema together with enlargement of the submucosal glands. The submucosal glands are enlarged and the goblet cells are hyperplastic and extend down to lower levels of the respiratory tract than is usual. Possibly because of mucus hypersecretion, the airways are chronically colonized with saprophytes. Airways of all sizes may be affected. At the end of the spectrum is pure emphysema, with predominant abnormalities being in the parenchyma. Destruction of alveolar septa leads to the confluence of adjacent alveoli and enlarged terminal air spaces. Most patients have a combination of the two diseases. These disorders appear to be closely related to chronic irritation of the airways from either cigarette smoking or atmospheric pollutants, possibly in association with genetic factors such as deficiency of alpha$_1$-antitrypsin. Only a small percentage of smokers develop chronic bronchitis, pure emphysema or a combination of both; why the majority do not develop disease is not yet understood.

4. What is the physiology of COPD?

The bronchitic patient has moderate to severe increases in airway resistance with little increase in lung volume or decrease in gas transfer capacity (DLCO). Arterial blood gases usually reveal moderate-to-severe hypoxemia sometimes with hypercapnia, indicating ventilation/perfusion inequality—universal in all COPD patients—along with a tendency for hypoventilation. The abnormality in arterial blood gases puts the bronchitic patient at risk for cor pulmonale and other hypoxemic complications. The pathologic abnormalities of emphysema have two principal consequences: loss of gas exchange surface and the loss of radial traction on small airways, which leads to an increase in physiologic dead space, impairment in gas exchange, and the tendency of small, unsupported airways to collapse. Their premature closure during expiration traps air in the distal air space, which leads to hyperinflation. The patient breathes at very high lung volume, placing chest wall and respiratory muscles at a disadvantage. In spite of marked inequality in ventilation/perfusion matching and impairment in gas exchange, some alveolar hyperventilation is common in emphysematous patients, which makes hypoxemia and hypoxic complications such as cor pulmonale less common or severe in these patients compared with chronic bronchitis.

5. What is the therapeutic approach to COPD?

The fifth leading cause of death in the United States, chronic obstructive respiratory conditions cannot be cured but can be alleviated considerably by appropriate management. Although the damage due to emphysema is permanent, many of the pathophysiologic changes of small airways disease, chronic bronchitis, and chronic asthma can be reversed to some extent, and such reversal should be a goal of therapy. Because the smoking habit is the main epidemiologic factor in these conditions, smoking cessation will help the patient more than any other medical treatment. Other measures are the use of beta-adrenergic agents, anticholinergics, methylxanthines, corticosteroids, antibiotics, expectorants and mucolytics, oxygen, and treatment of respiratory failure.

6. Should theophylline be used in the treatment of COPD?

Long-acting forms of methylxanthines might provide bronchodilatation for at least 12 hours; however, they are weak bronchodilators and their use requires careful supervision. They also have an inotropic effect on diaphragmatic strength and reduce muscle fatigue in vitro and in experimental animals. Through a randomized, double-blind, placebo-controlled, crossover trial, Murciano and colleagues evaluated the effects of theophylline in COPD. After 2 months of theophylline therapy, patients had significant improvement in dyspnea, pulmonary gas exchange, partial pressure of arterial carbon dioxide, vital capacity, and forced expiratory volume in one second. No significant changes in airway resistance or functional residual capacity were found. There was also an improvement in respiratory muscle performance, which may have accounted for the improvement in respiratory function and level of dyspnea. Unfortunately, methylxanthines have a very narrow therapeutic margin as well as serious toxic effects if the acceptable blood level is exceeded. Side effects such as sleep changes, changes in mood, and loss of short-term memory are not infrequent; the most dangerous side effects include ventricular arrhythmias and convulsions, which can be fatal.

In patients who benefit from theophylline, a long-acting preparation in a dose that keeps the blood level at about 10 mg/L should be used. This level provides almost all the bronchodilation achievable and is still far from the maximal permissible level (20 mg/L). A second use of methylxanthines is in the control of nocturnal symptoms. A dose of 250–500 mg of a long-acting preparation at bedtime minimizes the diurnal fluctuation in airflow that causes many patients with COPD to experience their worst dyspnea in the early hours of the morning. Metabolism of these agents can vary with the clinical condition of the patient and with use of concomitant drugs.

7. What common drugs and diseases may increase serum theophylline concentration?

Drugs	Diseases
Cimetidine	Cirrhosis
Troleandomycin	Congestive heart failure
Erythromycin	Pneumonia
Calcium channel blockers: Single case reports	Hypothyroidism
Nifedipine	Herpes simplex infection:
Verapamil	Further study required
Oral contraceptives	
Vaccines:	
Influenza	

Drugs
    BCG: Further study required
    Beta blockers: Further study required
    Allopurinol: High doses (600 mg/dl)
    Vidarasine: Single case report

8. What common drugs and diseases may decrease serum theophylline concentration?

Drugs	Diseases
Barbiturates	Hyperthyroidism
Carbamazepine	Cystic fibrosis
Isoniazid	Pancreatitis
Rifampin	
Sulfinpyrazone	
Activated charcoal	

9. What is the role of beta-adrenergic drugs?

Inhalation of beta-adrenergic drugs has an increased benefit-to-toxicity ratio compared with oral administration. Acute administration of beta-2 agonists results in a fall in airflow resistance, and improvement in function is often seen after a period of time, even though no benefits are seen initially. Because of this, an aerosolized bronchodilator is usually prescribed whether or not the spirogram improves on initial testing following inhalation of bronchodilators. Delivery of bronchodilators by intermittent positive pressure breathing (IPPB) has no greater beneficial effect than a metered dose inhaler (MDI), which is the preferred method of delivery; however, the technique of inhalation is a major determinant in the effectiveness of aerosolized bronchodilators. Many bronchodilators are also available in solution form for nebulization, which is useful in patients who are too dyspneic or uncoordinated to use an MDI correctly. Connecting extension tubes or aerochambers to the MDI is another way to help patients who are unable to master the right technique of inhalation. There is little to recommend one over another of the various options for MDI beta-adrenergic therapy. Albuterol, metaproterenol, terbutaline, pirbuterol, and bitolterol are similar in their actions, selectivity, side effects, and potency. The technique of administration is much more important than minor differences between specific beta$_2$-adrenergic agonists. Oral, slow-release beta-agonists, such as albuterol, may improve airflow in COPD patients with nocturnal exacerbation.

10. What is the value of anticholinergic agents?

Inhaled atropine reduces the resistance to airflow in patients with chronic bronchitis. Its derivative, ipratropium bromide, is the only anticholinergic agent available by MDI. Most studies show that for patients with COPD, it is more effective and lasts longer as a bronchodilator than do adrenergic agents. It is poorly absorbed, so side effects are minimal. Tachyphylaxis has not been demonstrated. The recommended dose of 2 puffs four times daily is probably too small to achieve maximal bronchodilation and can be increased in patients with severe airflow obstruction who show response. Beta-adrenergic agents can be taken along with anticholinergic agents. This combination provides the rapid onset of action of the beta-adrenergic agent with the prolonged action of the anticholinergic.

11. When should antibiotics be used?

Production of excessive secretions in COPD patients may result from acute respiratory infections. Most of the acute flareups are due to viral or mycoplasma infections, but *Hemophilus influenzae* or *Streptococcus pneumoniae* have also been implicated. It is accepted now that long-term administration of antibiotics provides no benefit to the stable patient and, when given for acute exacerbations, its results are controversial and difficult to assess. In general, antibiotics should be used when there is reasonable evidence of bacterial infection. Tetracycline, ampicillin, amoxicillin, or the combination of trimethoprim and sulfamethoxazole for 10–20 days is generally effective. Other antibiotics should be reserved for the treatment of infections due to organisms that are resistant to the usual antimicrobial agents. It is acceptable to provide patients with a course of antibiotics acceptable for self-administration when sputum or symptoms suggest that an exacerbation is beginning.

12. What are the role and efficacy of mucolytic therapy in the treatment of COPD?

This question is difficult to answer, as there is no specific test to quantify the presence of mucus in the lower airways. Pulmonary function tests are not helpful, and it is difficult to assess sputum volumes, rheology, and clearance. The literature has not been objective and reliable. Recently, a randomized, double-blind, placebo-controlled, multicenter study has demonstrated the effectiveness and safety of iodinated glycerol, 60 mg qid, given to patients with chronic obstructive bronchitis. As compared with placebo, there was improvement in cough frequency and severity and in chest discomfort after 8 weeks of therapy. Mucolytic therapy is a useful adjunct in treating COPD patients with mucus production.

13. What is the role of oxygen therapy in COPD?

Chronic arterial hypoxemia is a feature of most advanced chronic lung diseases, almost always because of $\dot{V}/\dot{Q}$ maldistribution. Arterial hypoxemia may cause dysfunction in a number of organs, increasing morbidity and mortality. The British Medical Research Council (MRC) Trial and the Nocturnal Oxygen Therapy Trial Group (NOTT) are two controlled studies that have provided data on which are based the current recommendations and justification for the use of long-term oxygen (LTO$_2$) in hypoxemic COPD patients. Combining the results from the two studies makes it clear that oxygen therapy has a clear survival advantage over no oxygen therapy and that continuous oxygen therapy (19+ hr/day) results in the greatest benefit in terms of improved survival. The mechanisms by which LTO$_2$ therapy improves survival in patients with COPD is unclear. High pulmonary artery pressure, high pulmonary vascular resistance, and low stroke volumes are associated with increased mortality, and the effects of oxygen on hemodynamics might influence survival; the beneficial effects of oxygen therapy on pulmonary hemodynamics have been confirmed. Beneficial effects of oxygen therapy have been demonstrated conclusively only in hypoxemic patients.

14. What are the indications for long-term oxygen therapy in COPD patients?

If the patient, when at rest on room air and in stable condition, has:

1. PaO$_2$ < 55 mm Hg	2. PaO$_2$ = 56–59 mm Hg
or	or
SaO$_2$ < 85%	SaO$_2$ = 86–89%

and the patient has evidence of one of the following secondary diagnoses:

- Dependent edema suggesting congestive heart failure or "P" pulmonale on EKG, or erythrocytosis with hematocrit > 56%
- During sleep:
  PaO$_2$ drops to or below 55 mm Hg, or drops more than 10 mm Hg, or
  SaO$_2$ drops to or below 85%, or drops more than 5%
- During exercise:
  PaO$_2$ drops to or below 55 mm Hg, or
  SaO$_2$ drops to or below 85%

When a patient fulfills the criteria for continuous oxygen therapy, oxygen should be prescribed in a dose sufficient to raise the PaO$_2$ to 65 to 80 mm Hg at rest during wakefulness. This PaO$_2$ usually is achieved with a 1- to 4-L/min oxygen flow through nasal prongs. The dose of O$_2$ should be increased by 1 L/min during sleep or exercise in order to prevent hypoxemic episodes. Oxygen should be given continuously at least 19 hours per day.

15. Is alpha$_1$-antitrypsin replacement worthwhile?

In the few patients with emphysema related to deficiency of alpha$_1$-antitrypsin with phenotype PiZ, long-term replacement of this agent can be given. At a dose of 60 mg/kg body weight intravenously weekly, it has been found that the enzyme appears in bronchoalveolar lavage fluid. However, this treatment is very expensive and still requires to be proved beneficial. In the future it may prove practical to administer the product by aerosol. Danazol, 200 mg three times daily, may also increase the level of the enzyme.

16. What are the reasons for hypoxemia in COPD patients during sleep?

Sleep depresses ventilation in healthy persons, producing an increase in arterial carbon dioxide pressure ($PaCO_2$) and a decrease in arterial oxygen pressure (PaO_2). Because many patients with severe COPD have reduced alveolar ventilation with hypoxemia and hypercapnia while awake, one would predict that they will have more profound alterations in arterial blood gases than healthy persons during sleep. In fact, these abnormalities occur, and the mechanisms of hypoxemia during sleep in COPD include:
1. Hypoventilation (the most important one)
2. Decrease in functional residual capacity ⎫
3. Ventilation/perfusion imbalance   ⎬ Contributing factors
4. Abnormal ventilatory control   ⎭

17. What are the consequences of hypoxemia during sleep in COPD patients?

Hemodynamics. Hypoxemia at night causes an increase in pulmonary arterial pressure

Cardiac dysrhythmias. Patients with COPD have an increased frequency of premature ventricular complexes (PVCs) during sleep, which decreases with supplemental oxygen treatment.

Polycythemia. Serum erythropoietin values rise at night in patients with COPD with modest hypoxemia.

Quality of sleep. Patients with COPD sleep poorly compared with matched normal controls. Arousals are common during episodes of desaturation.

Death during sleep. Death in COPD patients occurs more often at night, and death at night is more common in those with hypoxemia and CO_2 retention.

18. What are the causes of acute respiratory failure in COPD?

Bronchial infection, pulmonary emboli, cardiac failure, pneumonia, pneumothorax, respiratory depression (usually by the injudicious use of sedatives or narcotic analgesic drugs), surgery (especially of chest and upper abdomen), stopping of medications, or occasionally, malnutrition. In general, the criteria for the diagnosis of acute respiratory failure in COPD patients include hypoxemia ($PaO_2 < 60$ mm Hg), hypercapnia ($PaCO_2 > 50-70$ mm Hg), and respiratory acidosis (pH < 7.35) associated with worsening of the patient's respiratory symptoms compared with baseline.

19. What is the treatment of acute respiratory failure secondary to COPD?

- Use a conservative approach if at all possible (i.e., avoid an artificial airway and mechanical ventilation)
- Apply immediate lifesaving measures (treat hypoxemia and airflow obstruction)
- Determine and correct the precipitating factors
- Treat underlying condition
- Avoid complications
- Monitor in intensive care unit

Oxygen therapy is the cornerstone of treatment. Death or irreversible brain damage results within minutes when severe hypoxemia is present, whereas hypercapnia may be well tolerated. The appropriate amount of oxygen is that which satisfies tissue oxygen needs: usually a $PaO_2 > 60$ mm Hg, without worsening the respiratory acidosis and/or further depressing sensorium.

20. Should mechanical ventilation be used in COPD?

Except in life-threatening conditions, it seems reasonable to recommend ventilation when conservative aggressive treatment, including controlled oxygen therapy, has failed. This would be indicated by progressive worsening of hypoxia, by acidosis, by increased respiratory muscle fatigue, and by onset of nonarousable somnolence. Still, the need for mechanical ventilation remains a subjective judgment in spite of numerous proposed biologic criteria. Some recommend close monitoring of arterial PaO_2 and pH, and regard controlled oxygen therapy as having failed if PaO_2 could not be maintained over 50 mm Hg without the pH falling below 7.26. Intubation should be done with a tube at least 8 mm in internal diameter or greater, because of the frequent need for suctioning thick secretions. Ventilation should be maintained for at least 24–48 hours to allow recovery of fatigued respiratory muscles.

A frequent result of error in management is hyperventilation: the goal should be to maintain the patient's baseline arterial blood gases. These patients are frequently hypercapnic and have developed renal compensation. Hyperventilation will result in metabolic alkalosis (pH $>$ 7.50) with all its side effects—decreased cardiac output, impaired cerebral blood flow, cardiac arrhythmias, decreased ventilatory drive, and prolonged ventilation because of difficulty in weaning.

21. What is the prognosis for COPD patients after an episode of acute respiratory failure?
Several studies have indicated that respiratory intensive care can have a marked effect on the survival rate of patients with acute respiratory failure. However, the prognosis remains controversial. Hospital mortality has varied from 6–38% and the 2-year survival rate from 25–68%.

The cause of the acute respiratory failure is important in prognosis: mortality in patients presenting with infection (20%) is very different from that of patients presenting with heart failure (40%). The severity of acidosis on admission, expressed as arterial pH, correlates better with survival than does the absolute level of PaO_2; mortality increases markedly if pH is below 7.32.

The influence of mechanical ventilation on outcome remains unclear. Hudson divided several series of COPD patients complicated by acute respiratory failure into two groups: those treated before 1975 had a survival of 72%; those treated after 1975 had a survival of 91%. Thus, most patients with COPD survive an episode of acute respiratory failure, even if the subsequent prognosis for survival is poor and similar to that of other patients with COPD without episodes of acute respiratory failure. However, both are strongly related to the severity of the underlying process.

CONTROVERSIES

22. Are steroids indicated in the emergency treatment of acute exacerbations of COPD?
It is almost a universal practice to use steroids for acute exacerbations of COPD. This comes from the work of Albert and associates, who treated these patients with prednisone, 0.5 mg/ Hg every 6 hours for 3 days; however, there was only modest improvement in spirometric values after 72 hours of treatment. Emerman and associates used the intravenous administration of methylprednisolone in a randomized, controlled, double-blind study early in the treatment of acute exacerbations of COPD. Ninety-six patients without a history of asthma and all aged 50 years or more were given aminophylline and hourly aerosolized isoetharine. Thirty minutes after arrival in the emergency room, methylprednisolone, 100 mg, or physiologic saline solution was given. There were no better improvements in FEV_1 measured by spirometry initially and after the third and fourth aerosol treatment in patients receiving steroids than in the control group, nor was there a difference between groups in the rate of hospital admissions. So, the use of steroids in this situation is still controversial. However, it is doubtful that steroids are harmful when given only for a few (2–3) days.

23. Are steroids indicated in the chronic treatment of COPD?
Their use is still controversial. The number of "responders" cited varies between 6% and 25%; however, some patients do derive unequivocal benefit from corticosteroids. In general,

there is no way to predict who will respond to corticosteroids other than to perform a therapeutical trial. Some experts contend that patients who have an increase in FEV_1 of 15% or more from bronchodilator drugs might respond the best. The steroids are given at a dose equivalent to 40 mg/day of prednisone for 2 weeks, and then FEV_1 is re-measured. Unless the control measurements are markedly reproducible, only increases of FEV_1 greater than 30% are considered to indicate a positive response. In patients who respond, an attempt to maintain the response with high doses of inhaled steroids (1200–1500 mg daily) is made. Unfortunately only a small number of patients can be maintained on inhaled steroids. In patients in need of oral steroids, a dose larger than 20 mg/day of prednisone should be avoided, because complications such as osteoporosis, diabetes, and myopathy, which are disastrous in elderly sick patients, might occur.

BIBLIOGRAPHY

1. Albert RK, Martin TR, Lewis SW: Controlled clinical trial of methylprednisolone in patients with chronic bronchitis and acute respiratory insufficiency. Ann Intern Med 92:735–758, 1980.
2. American Thoracic Society: Standards for the diagnosis and care of patients with chronic obstructive pulmonary disease (COPD) and asthma. Am Rev Respir Dis 136:225–244, 1987.
3. Bone RC: Symposium on respiratory failure. Med Clin North Am 67:549–750, 1983.
4. Cherniack RM, Irvin C (eds): Chronic Respiratory Failure. 32nd Annual Aspen Lung Conference. Chest 97(Suppl): 1990.
5. Douglas NJ, Flenley DC: Breathing during sleep in patients with obstructive lung disease. Am Rev Respir Dis 141:1055–1070, 1990.
6. Emerman CL, Connors AF, Lukens TW, et al: A randomized controlled trial of methylprednisolone in the emergency treatment of acute exacerbations of COPD. Chest 95:563–567, 1989.
7. Fernandez E: Beta-adrenergic agonists. Semin Respir Med 8:353–365, 1987.
8. Hubbard RC, Brantley ML, Sellers SE, et al: Anti-neutrophil-elastase defenses of the lower respiratory tract in α_1-antitrypsin deficiency directly augmented with aerosol of α_1-antitrypsin. Ann Intern Med 111:206–212, 1989.
9. Mendella LA, Manfreda J, Warren CPW, Anthonisen NR: Steroid response in stable chronic obstructive pulmonary disease. Ann Intern Med 96:17–21, 1982.
10. Murciano D, Auclair M-H, Pariente R, Aubier M: A randomized, controlled trial of theophylline in patients with severe chronic obstructive pulmonary disease. N Engl J Med 320:1521–1525, 1989.
11. Nocturnal Oxygen Therapy Trial Group: Continuous or nocturnal oxygen therapy in hypoxemic chronic obstructive lung disease: A clinical trial. Ann Intern Med 93:391–398, 1980.
12. Pierson DJ: Acute respiratory failure. In Sahn SA (ed): Pulmonary Emergencies. New York, Churchill Livingstone, 1982.
13. Watanabe S, Kanner RE, Cutillo AG, et al: Long-term effect of almitrine bismesylate in patients with hypoxemic chronic obstructive pulmonary disease. Am Rev Respir Dis 140:1269–1273, 1989.
14. Ziment T: Pharmacologic therapy of obstructive airway disease. Clin Chest Med 11:461–486, 1990.

24. COR PULMONALE

Enrique Fernandez, M.D.

1. What is cor pulmonale?

The World Health Organization defines cor pulmonale as "enlargement of the right ventricle (dilation and/or hypertrophy) due to increased right ventricular overload from diseases of the lungs or pulmonary circulation." Right heart failure need not be present. The definition of cor pulmonale excludes right heart abnormalities that are secondary to left heart failure or congenital heart disease.

2. What is the differential diagnosis of cor pulmonale?

Differential Diagnosis of Cor Pulmonale

Category	Example
Secondary Pulmonary Hypertension	
Pulmonary interstitial disease	Sarcoidosis, interstitial fibrosis, scleroderma, asbestosis, etc.
Occlusive disorders of pulmonary arteries	Pulmonary embolism
Alveolar hypoventilation	
With normal lungs	Central hypoventilation Kyphoscoliosis
Ventilation/perfusion abnormalities	Chronic airway disease, emphysema, chronic bronchitis
Primary Pulmonary Hypertension	Idiopathic

3. What is the pathophysiology?

The normal right ventricle is a thin-walled, distensible muscular pump that accommodates considerable variations in systemic venous return without large changes in filling pressure. The initial pathophysiologic event in the production of cor pulmonale is an elevation of the pulmonary vascular resistance due to a primary pulmonary disorder. With increase in resistance, pulmonary arterial pressure rises to a degree that maintains cardiac output. The rise in pulmonary arterial pressure increases the workload on the right ventricle. Acute increases in workload lead to right ventricular dilation; chronic increases, to right ventricular hypertrophy.

4. What are the symptoms and signs?

Clinical detection of cor pulmonale is difficult for two main reasons: (1) history and physical findings are often dominated by the underlying disease; and (2) the symptoms and signs of pulmonary hypertension per se are subtle until they become far advanced, and the symptoms are most often those of the primary disease. On physical examination, the clues for pulmonary hypertension are:

- Accentuation of the pulmonic closure sound (increased P_2)
- Palpable closure "tap" in the second left interspace
- Right-sided S_4
- Accentuated A wave in the jugular pulse
- Right ventricular hypertrophy may cause palpable left parasternal lift
- Murmurs of pulmonary and tricuspid insufficiency and palpable right ventricular heave
- Prominent jugular V waves, indicating the development of tricuspid regurgitation.

When right ventricle failure occurs:

- Right-sided gallop (S_3)
- Tricuspid regurgitation murmur
- Neck vein distention–hepatomegaly–dependent peripheral edema.

5. What are the EKG criteria of right ventricle hypertrophy?

- qR pattern in leads V_1 or V_3 R
- An R wave in V_1 or V_3 R > 1.0 in V_5 or V_6
- An R/S ratio > 1.0 in V_1 or < 1.0 in V_5 or V_6
- An R' in V_1 or V_3 R > 6 mm or an R's in V_1 > 1.0 (QRS duration < 0.10 second)
- Delayed intrinsicoid deflection of right precordial leads
- Right axis deviation
- ST-T changes in the right precordium

6. What tests can help determine the diagnosis?

Chest radiograph. Usually shows the signs of the primary pulmonary disease (e.g., hyperinflation in emphysema). When pulmonary hypertension is present, there may be enlargement of the right pulmonary artery shadow in anterior projection ($>$ 17 mm in diameter) and of the left pulmonary artery shadow in lateral projection ($>$ 18 mm in diameter).

Echocardiography. Often technically difficult because of the large lungs. It might show right ventricular wall thickening and enlargement of its cavity in relation to that of the left ventricle. Doppler flow studies often allow for accurate assessment of pulmonary artery pressure.

Radionuclide angiography (gated blood pool scan). Measures right and left ventricular ejection fraction.

Right heart cardiac catheterization. Is the best and the most definitive procedure for the diagnosis and etiology of pulmonary hypertension.

7. What is the treatment of cor pulmonale?

Oxygen. A large, controlled study of oxygen therapy demonstrated that long-term oxygen therapy improves the survival of hypoxemic COPD patients. This increased survival might be explained as follows: (1) Oxygen relieves pulmonary vasoconstriction, decreasing pulmonary vascular resistance and improving right ventricle stroke volume and cardiac output. (2) Oxygen therapy improves arterial oxygen content, improving the delivery of oxygen to vital organs (heart, brain, etc.).

Diuretics. This therapy may be needed in congestive cardiac failure to take care of the excess water that the lungs share and to improve alveolar ventilation and gas exchange. However, the use of diuretics might produce hemodynamic side effects, such as volume depletion, decreased venous return to the right ventricle, and decreased cardiac output. Another complication is the production of hypokalemic metabolic alkalosis, which diminishes the CO_2 stimulus to the respiratory center, decreasing ventilatory drive.

Phlebotomy. It may provide symptomatic relief in the patient with marked polycythemia (hematocrit $>$ 60%). Blood volume has a more important influence than blood viscosity on pulmonary artery pressure. In the resting patient, phlebotomy produces mild decrease in mean pulmonary artery pressure and pulmonary vascular resistance, with no significant change in cardiac output. In polycythemic COPD patients, phlebotomy might also improve exercise tolerance with increasing workload, duration of exercise, and maximal oxygen consumption. There are no long-term benefits with repeated phlebotomies.

8. When should vasodilator therapy be recommended?

Vasodilators should be considered when conventional therapies, including oxygen, have failed to improve signs of right ventricular failure or pulmonary hypertension. Right heart catheterization should be performed to assess hemodynamics and oxygenation, before vasodilator use. The following guidelines have been recommended to define a beneficial hemodynamic response to vasodilators:

1. Pulmonary vascular resistance is reduced by at least 20% and
2. Cardiac output is increased or unchanged.
3. Pulmonary arterial pressure is decreased or unchanged and
4. Systemic blood pressure is not significantly reduced.

After a therapeutic regimen has been used continuously for 4–6 months, right heart catheterization should be repeated to assess whether the hemodynamic benefits persist.

9. Is there impairment of the left ventricle in chronic cor pulmonale?

The impairment of left ventricle function has been documented in some patients with chronic cor pulmonale. In patients with severe chronic cor pulmonale, left ventricular end-diastolic pressure increases, and left ventricle ejection fraction is depressed both at rest and with exercise. This impairment of left ventricular function has been thought to be produced by sustained hypoxia and/or interventricular septal bulging toward the left ventricle owing to right ventricular pressure overload. Pathologically the walls of both ventricles are thicker; myocyte diameters of both ventricles are significantly greater in patients with COPD than in controls; and the percentage of fibrosis in the left ventricle is significantly greater only in patients with right ventricular hypertrophy.

10. Should digoxin be used for COPD?

Recently, it has been reported that digoxin might improve transdiaphragmatic twitch response to phrenic nerve stimulation and increase blood flow to the diaphragm in patients with COPD. This may give digoxin a role in the treatment of the acute decompensated patient. Clinical studies, however, support the use of digitalis in cor pulmonale only if left ventricular failure is present. In well-done studies, right ventricular ejection fraction showed improvement only in patients who had an initial reduction in left ventricular ejection fraction. In addition, digoxin may itself cause arrhythmias, another argument against its routine use.

11. What are the effects of vasodilator agents in the treatment of pulmonary hypertension?

Vasodilators produce a beneficial response in hemodynamic parameters in some patients with primary pulmonary hypertension; its use in COPD (when pulmonary hypertension has other etiologic factors) is still under investigation. The main potential adverse effects include (1) systemic hypotension—vasodilators are potent dilators of the systemic circulation, which might lead to hypotension, failure, and circulatory collapse—and (2) decreased arterial oxygen saturation—by disrupting pulmonary vascular tone with mismatching of ventilation-perfusion in the lung.

BIBLIOGRAPHY

1. Berger HJ, Matthay RQ, Loke J, et al: Assessment of cardiac performance with quantitative radionuclide angiography: Right ventricular ejection fraction with reference to findings in chronic obstructive pulmonary disease. Am J Cardiol 41:897–905, 1978.
2. Berglund E, Widimsky J, Malmberg R: Lack of effect of digitalis in patients with pulmonary hypertension with and without heart failure. Am J Cardiol 11:477–482, 1963.
3. Fishman AP: Chronic cor pulmonale. Am Rev Respir Dis 114:775–794, 1976.
3a. Klinger JR, Hill NS: Right ventricular dysfunction in chronic obstructive pulmonary disease. Chest 99:715–723, 1991.
4. Kohama A, Tarauchi J, Hori M, et al: Pathologic involvement of the left ventricle in chronic cor pulmonale. Chest 98:794–800, 1990.
5. Mathur PN, Powles ACP, Pugsley SO, et al: Effect of digoxin on right ventricular function in severe chronic airflow obstruction. Ann Intern Med 95:283–288, 1981.
6. McFadden ER Jr, Braunwald E: Cor pulmonale and pulmonary thromboembolism. In Braunwald E (ed): Heart Disease: A Textbook of Cardiovascular Medicine. Philadelphia, W.B. Saunders, 1987, pp 1572–1598.
7. Reeves JT: Approach to the patient with pulmonary hypertension. In Weir EK, Reeves JT (eds): Pulmonary Hypertension. New York, Futura Publishing Co., 1984, p 30.
8. Weir EK, Rubin LJ, Ayres SM, et al: The acute administration of vasodilators in primary pulmonary hypertension. Am Rev Respir Dis 140:1623–1630, 1989.
9. Weitzenbaum E, Sautegeau A, Ehzhart M, et al: Long term course of pulmonary arterial pressure in chronic obstructive pulmonary disease. Am Rev Respir Dis 130:993–998, 1984.
10. Wiedemann HP, Matthay RA: Cor pulmonale in chronic obstructive pulmonary disease: Circulatory pathophysiology and new concepts of therapy. In Simmons DH (ed): Current Pulmonology. Volume 8. Chicago, Year Book Medical Publishers, 1987, pp 127–162.
11. World Health Organization: Chronic cor pulmonale. A report of the expert committee. Circulation 27:594–615, 1963.

25. ACUTE RESPIRATORY FAILURE

Martin Zamora, M.D.

1. What is meant by acute respiratory failure (ARF)?
ARF is a physiologically defined condition that may result from a variety of disease processes. It occurs when the respiratory system is unable to adequately exchange oxygen and carbon dioxide between the environment and the tissues of the body. It may develop over the course of minutes, hours, or days in patients with previously normal lung function or patients with preexisting disease.

2. How is ARF defined by arterial blood gas analysis?
Although no rigid criteria apply for all patients, it is generally accepted that respiratory failure is present when the arterial PO_2 is less than 50 mm Hg and/or the PCO_2 is greater than 50 mm Hg, with a decrease in arterial pH to 7.30 while the patient is breathing room air.

3. ARF may occur via two primary processes.
(a) What are the two primary types of ARF?
ARF may be due to failure of oxygenation (hypoxemia) or failure of ventilation (hypercapnia). Both processes may be present in a given patient but generally one type predominates.
(b) What physiologic mechanisms may cause hypoxemia? What are their responses to supplemental oxygen?
- alveolar hypoventilation
- ventilation perfusion mismatch
- right-to-left shunt
- diffusion limitation
- low inspired oxygen fraction (e.g., high altitude)

The hypoxemia caused by all these mechanisms is reversible with supplemental oxygen with the exception of shunt. Due to continued perfusion of unventilated lung units, increasing the partial pressure of inspired oxygen has little or no effect on shunt.
(c) What physiologic mechanisms may cause hypercapnic ARF?
Hypercapnia is the result of alveolar hypoventilation. Mechanisms responsible may be:
- central—decreased normal respiratory drive
- neuromuscular—decreased neural transmission or muscular translation of the drive signal
- abnormalities of the chest wall
- abnormalities of the lungs and airways

4. Which disease processes are associated with each type of ARF? Which are reversible?
The differential diagnosis of hypoxemic ARF can be delineated based on whether there is concomitant hypercapnia and whether the lung fields on chest x-ray are "black" (normal or hyperlucent) or "white" (radiopaque). If the patient is normocapnic and the chest x-ray is black, pulmonary embolus, circulatory collapse, or right-to-left shunt is likely. If the chest x-ray is diffusely white, adult respiratory distress syndrome (ARDS), cardiogenic pulmonary edema, or pulmonary fibrosis is possible. If the abnormality is localized, the patient may have pneumonia, atelectasis, or pulmonary infarction. If the chest x-ray is black in patients with hypercapnia, then status asthmaticus, chronic obstructive pulmonary disease (COPD), or alveolar hypoventilation secondary to drug overdose, neuromuscular weakness, paralysis, or sleep apnea syndrome is likely. If the chest x-ray is diffusely white, end-stage pulmonary fibrosis or severe ARDS is possible, whereas if the findings are localized, the patient could

have pneumonia with underlying COPD or respiratory depression secondary to drugs or oxygen therapy.

In general, most of the above are reversible. However, severe COPD, sleep apnea syndrome, diseases of the respiratory muscles, cervical fracture leading to paralysis, and kyphoscoliosis may lead to chronic carbon dioxide retention and chronic respiratory failure. In patients with these underlying disorders, ARF due to other etiologies may occur and should be investigated.

5. What empirical therapy should be employed emergently in patients with ARF?

Raising the PO_2 to greater than 50 mm Hg is the first goal of therapy. If the patient is alert and cooperative, supplemental oxygen with a repeat arterial blood gas within 20–30 minutes and close observation in the ICU may be adequate. If the patient is stuporous, comatose, or has a decreased gag reflex with shallow respirations, then control of the airway by endotracheal intubation is warranted. In the case of suspected opiate overdose (respiratory depression, pinpoint pupils, and coma), intubation followed by naloxone (Narcan, 1–5 ampules IV) is indicated.

6. What are the indications for endotracheal intubation?

- Cardiopulmonary resuscitation with the need for complete control of the airway
- Airway protection from aspiration of gastric contents
- Need for mechanical ventilation
- Control of copious airway secretions
- Complete upper airway obstruction

7. What are the indications for mechanical ventilation?

Mechanical ventilation is required whenever the patient is unable to maintain adequate alveolar ventilation ($PCO_2 < 50$ mm Hg and pH of 7.35). It is more difficult to determine when mechanical ventilation is indicated in patients with hypoxemic ARF and normal alveolar ventilation. However, excessive work of breathing to maintain a normal PCO_2 may lead to respiratory muscle fatigue and failure, requiring mechanical ventilation. The decision for intubation and mechanical ventilation must be based on the clinical appearance of the patient and blood gas analysis, and must take into account whether or not the underlying process is reversible. Mechanical ventilation may also be used to provide hyperventilation to head trauma patients in order to reduce cerebral edema for the first 24–48 hours.

8. What is PEEP? When should it be used?

Positive end-expiratory pressure (PEEP) is a technique to mechanically correct hypoxemia by increasing lung volume. PEEP increases the expiratory threshold pressure, which prevents the patient's airway pressure from falling below that preset level during the respiratory cycle. This increases the volume of gas in the patient's chest at end-expiration (functional residual capacity). The treatment would therefore be expected to be beneficial in patients with restrictive lung diseases such as ARDS, because the hypoxemia in this disorder may be due to alveolar collapse, filling, or both. PEEP should not be used routinely in all hypoxic critically ill patients, particularly those with obstructive airway disease, as it may lead to high intrapulmonary pressures that predispose the patient to barotrauma (pneumothorax).

9. What is the significance of the patient who is "fighting the ventilator"?

The sudden onset of agitation and distress in a patient who previously was tolerating mechanical ventilation is a medical emergency and signifies acute deterioration in the underlying disease, malfunction of the ventilator, or obstruction of the airway or endotracheal tube. The patient should be disconnected from the ventilator and manually ventilated. Vital signs should be obtained, the chest examined, the airway suctioned, and arterial blood gas analysis and chest x-ray performed. If no etiology is found after these measures, the ventilator setup may be incorrect for the patient's needs. Changes in the ventilator settings are in order so as to more closely match the machine to the patient's requirements.

10. When can patients be weaned from mechanical ventilation?

Patients should be clinically improved with stabilization and correction of any underlying conditions that may interfere with weaning (electrolyte disturbances, fluid overload, severe anemia, or severe pain requiring analgesics or sedatives). Patients should be alert, with stable vital signs, and have an intact gag reflex. Physiologic guidelines are: $PO_2 > 60$ mm Hg with the $FiO_2 < 50\%$ and PEEP = 0–5 cm H_2O, respiratory rate < 20, vital capacity > 10–15 ml/kg, tidal volume > 5 ml/kg, minute ventilation (VE) < 10 L/min, maximum ventilator volume $> 2 \times$ VE, and negative inspiratory force of > -25 cm H_2O.

11. What are some postextubation complications?

- Hoarseness
- Difficulty swallowing and risk of aspiration
- Severe glottic edema leading to laryngospasm (may be treated with racemic epinephrine 0.5 ml/3ml saline via nebulized aerosol)

BIBLIOGRAPHY

1. Bone RC: Symposium on respiratory failure. Med Clin North Am 67:549–750, 1983.
2. Irwin RS: A Physiologic Approach to Managing Respiratory Failure. In Rippe JM (ed): Intensive Care Medicine, 2nd ed. Boston, Little, Brown and Co., 1991.
3. Kaminski MJ, Young RR: Neuromuscular and neurological disorders affecting respiration. In Roussos C, Macklem PT (eds): The Thorax (Lung Biology in Health and Disease, Vol. 29). New York, Marcel Dekker, 1985.
4. King TE: Acute respiratory failure. In Schrier RW (ed): Current Medical Therapy. New York, Raven Press, 1984.
5. Pierson DJ: Acute respiratory failure. In Sahn SA (ed): Pulmonary Emergencies. New York, Churchill Livingstone, 1982.
6. Sahn SA, Lakshminarayan S, Petty TL: Weaning from mechanical ventilation. JAMA 235:2208, 1976.
7. Stauffer JL: Tracheal intubation. In Sahn SA (ed): Pulmonary Emergencies. New York, Churchill Livingstone, 1982.
8 Weisman IM, Rinaldo JE, Rogers RM: Positive end-respiratory pressure in acute respiratory failure. N Engl J Med 307:1381, 1982.
9. Zwillich CW, Pierson DJ, Creagh CE, et al: Complications of assisted ventilation: A prospective study of 354 consecutive episodes. Am J Med 57:161, 1974.

26. ADULT RESPIRATORY DISTRESS SYNDROME

Polly E. Parsons, M.D.

1. What is adult respiratory distress syndrome (ARDS)?

A noncardiogenic pulmonary capillary leak syndrome characterized clinically by the development of rapidly progressive hypoxemia, diffuse alveolar infiltrates on chest x-ray, and decreased lung compliance following a known predisposing insult. Pathologically the syndrome is characterized acutely by alveolar and interstitial edema and flooding of the alveoli with a proteinaceous exudate and inflammatory cells, including neutrophils and macrophages, followed by the development of pulmonary fibrosis.

2. What conditions predispose to the development of ARDS?

Several at-risk conditions have been identified, such as sepsis, pulmonary aspiration, pulmonary contusion, long bone fractures, pancreatitis, multiple blood transfusions, near drowning, and drug toxicity. The most common predisposing conditions are sepsis and pulmonary aspiration of gastric contents, in which the incidence of ARDS is 20–40%.

3. Explain the pathogenesis of ARDS.

The pathogenesis of ARDS is not known, but there are theories based on data from clinical studies and animal models. It is likely that ARDS results from a combination of events beginning with the systemic release of mediators (such as complement fragments, endotoxin, tumor necrosis factor) that activate/stimulate neutrophils and macrophages (and perhaps other cell types) to become sequestered within the pulmonary capillaries and release toxic products such as oxygen metabolites, proteases, and leukotrienes. The inability to clearly delineate the pathogenesis of ARDS has significantly hampered efforts to treat the syndrome.

4. Why do patients with ARDS die?

Less than 10% of deaths in patients with ARDS are due to hypoxic respiratory failure. The majority of deaths that occur within 72 hours result from the original precipitating insult, whereas after 72 hours death is caused by infection.

5. What is the mortality from ARDS?

When ARDS was first described in 1967, the mortality rate was 58% (7/12 patients). Despite significant advances in critical care since then, the mortality rate is still greater than 50%. Recent studies suggest that mortality is influenced by some factors such as patient age, presenting diagnosis, and fluid requirements.

6. How fast does ARDS develop?

Very fast: 80% of patients develop ARDS within 24 hours of onset of a predisposing condition and 95% develop it within 72 hours. Preliminary data suggest that many patients develop the syndrome within less than 6 hours.

7. Can ARDS be prevented?

No. The precipitating clinical disorder must be prevented.

8. What therapy is available for ARDS?

Currently no specific therapy is effective for ARDS, although several agents, including steroids, prostaglandin E1 (PGE_1), and N-acetylcysteine, have been tried. However, some therapeutic modalities that have significant potential are being developed or studied. These include surfactant replacement, anti-endotoxin antibodies, anti-tumor necrosis factor antibodies, and anti-proteinases.

9. How can pneumonia be diagnosed in a patient with ARDS?

This is an area of intense discussion. The clinical diagnosis is generally based on the development of new infiltrates on chest x-ray, purulent sputum, fever, and peripheral leukocytosis. However, in an autopsy study of patients with ARDS, it was shown that 80% of patients without pneumonia had fever and leukocytosis; 70% had purulent sputum. Thus, clinical parameters alone do not appear to be adequate. The other tools available include bronchoscopy with lavage, protected brush sampling, transbronchial biopsy, and open lung biopsy. The sensitivity and specificity of these procedures in patients with ARDS are not well defined. The keys to diagnosis are constant surveillance and a low threshold for evaluating and treating the patient.

10. What are the pulmonary sequelae in survivors of ARDS?
Surprisingly, some survivors are virtually unimpaired 1 year after an episode of ARDS despite evidence of pulmonary fibrosis early in the disease course and prolonged mechanical ventilation with high PEEP and FiO_2. The percentage of survivors that returns to normal pulmonary function is difficult to ascertain from the literature. Although more than 25 studies of ARDS survivors have been published, they have been hampered by inconsistent definitions of ARDS, different methods of assessing pulmonary function, varying duration of follow-up, and variable attention to pre-ARDS pulmonary status, length of ventilation, severity of ARDS, and in-hospital complications of ARDS. It appears that there is a spectrum of pulmonary impairment, with the majority of survivors having mild to moderate impairment, a very few patients having severe impairment, and a small but significant group of patients who are normal.

11. How should patients with ARDS be ventilated?
The current mainstay of ventilatory support of ARDS patients is positive end-expiratory pressure (PEEP). PEEP improves oxygenation by recruiting collapsed alveoli and, thus, restoring the functional residual capacity toward normal. The amount of PEEP used should be that which allows the greatest reduction in FiO_2 with the least amount of cardiopulmonary compromise ("best PEEP").

Other ventilatory strategies have been tried with varying degrees of success. The ones that have received the most attention are high-frequency jet ventilation (HFJV), extracorporeal membrane oxygenation (ECMO), and inverse ratio ventilation (IRV). HFJV has been studied extensively and has not been shown to offer additional benefit to conventional ventilation. ECMO was also found to be ineffective initially, but in current trials using modified strategies, patient survival appears to be improved. IRV is beneficial in some patients, although there is no way to predict which patients will respond, and patients have to be monitored carefully for evidence of hemodynamic compromise.

12. What are the major complications of ventilation in these patients?
Barotrauma (often manifested by pneumothorax), oxygen toxicity, and large airway trauma from prolonged intubation.

13. ARDS is frequently complicated by multiple organ failure (MOF). Which organs are typically involved?
Kidneys, liver, brain, gastrointestinal tract, hematologic system, and heart.

14. Is there a role for steroids in ARDS?
No role for steroids in ARDS has been established.

CONTROVERSY

15. What is appropriate fluid management for a patient with ARDS?
A. Fluid administration should be minimized to avoid increased alveolar flooding:

This has been the dogma for years and is supported by the concept that the primary problem in ARDS is capillary leak. It follows then that if intravascular pressure is decreased, the extrusion of fluid into the alveoli will be minimized. Accordingly, pulmonary capillary wedge pressure (PCWP) is kept below 10 cm H_2O by avoiding volume infusion and using diuretics if necessary. If the patient becomes hypotensive in the face of a low PCWP, some physicians will start pressors whereas others will increase the PCWP with volume administration.

B. Fluids should be administered to increase the PCWP to the level necessary to maximize oxygen delivery:

Some data suggest that the mortality from ARDS and the development of MOF may be related to inadequate oxygen delivery to the tissues. Because oxygen delivery is partly dependent upon cardiac output, it follows that increasing ventricular filling to maximize cardiac output would be beneficial in ARDS, especially if done prior to the development of ARDS in high-risk patients or early in the course of ARDS. This approach requires vigilant physiologic monitoring to be certain that the infusion of volume to maximize cardiac output does not exacerbate hypoxemia secondary to additional alveolar flooding.

BIBLIOGRAPHY

1. Ashbaugh DG, Bigelow DB, Petty TL, Levine BE: Acute respiratory distress in adults. Lancet 2:319–323, 1967.
2. Bernard GR, Luce JM, Sprung CL, et al: High-dose corticosteroids in patients with the adult respiratory distress syndrome. N Engl J Med 317:1565–1570, 1987.
3. Dorinsky PM, Gadek JE: Mechanisms of multiple nonpulmonary organ failure in ARDS. Chest 96:885–892, 1989.
4. Elliott CG: Pulmonary sequelae in survivors of the adult respiratory distress syndrome. Clin Chest Med 11:789–800, 1990.
5. Fowler AA, Hamman RF, Good JT, et al: Adult respiratory distress syndrome: Risk with common predispositions. Ann Intern Med 98:593–597, 1983.
6. Hudson LD: The prediction and prevention of ARDS. Respir Care 35:161–172, 1990.
7. Pepe PE: The clinical entity of adult respiratory distress syndrome. Crit Care Clin 2:377–403, 1986.
8. Pepe PE, Potkin RT, Reus DH, et al: Clinical predictors of the adult respiratory distress syndrome. Am J Surg 144:124–128, 1983.
9. Shoemaker WC: Circulatory pathophysiology of ARDS and its fluid management. In Shoemaker WC, et al (ed): Textbook of Critical Care, 2nd ed. Philadelphia, W.B. Saunders, 1989.
10. Stoller JK, Kacmarek PM: Ventilatory strategies in the management of the adult respiratory distress syndrome. Clin Chest Med 11:755–772, 1990.
11. Suchyta MR, Elliott CG, Colby T, et al: Open lung biopsy does not correlate with pulmonary function after the adult respiratory distress syndrome. Chest 99:1232–1237, 1991.

27. ASPIRATION

Robert M. Cook, M.D., and York E. Miller, M.D.

1. What is aspiration?
Aspiration is the penetration of foreign material past the vocal cords and into the airways.

2. What are the major consequences of aspiration?
This depends on both the volume and nature of aspirated material. Large volumes of sterile, nonirritating fluid can be introduced into the airways with minor sequelae. Small volumes of oral secretions are universally aspirated during sleep in healthy individuals. Four major groups of clinically significant aspirations are defined by the material aspirated: (1) Foreign bodies or thick particulate fluids can cause airway obstruction. (2) Acidic gastric contents cause a chemical pneumonitis or adult respiratory distress syndrome (ARDS). (3) Aspiration of infected material can result in infectious pneumonia or lung abscess. (4) A syndrome of aspiration occurs in drowning. Overlaps or combinations of these four often occur.

3. Which patients are at risk for aspiration?
Patients with conditions that increase gastric volume, decrease gastric pH, decrease lower esophageal sphincter tone, or lower the normal airway protective mechanisms are at

increased risk for aspiration. Obesity, pregnancy, trauma (particularly orofacial with loss of teeth), emergent surgical procedures, and the use of agents such as drugs or alcohol that depress consciousness all predispose to aspiration.

4. When should airway obstruction by a foreign body be suspected?

Stridor or localized wheezing can occur in this situation. Chest x-rays are helpful to demonstrate radiopaque foreign bodies, such as teeth or bone fragments, or localized areas of atelectasis. CT scans can be helpful. Bronchoscopy (either rigid or fiberoptic) allows the identification and removal of foreign objects and should be performed in all patients in whom aspiration is suspected.

5. What are the results of aspiration of gastric acid?

Aspiration of gastric acid causes immediate and intense injury to the airway and alveolar epithelium. Bronchospasm, pulmonary edema, alveolar collapse due to loss of surfactant, and loss of intravascular fluid volume all occur. ARDS can evolve. Although treatment by neutralization of airway fluids has been attempted, acid instilled into the airways is rapidly absorbed and neutralized, rendering these therapies futile. Despite a better understanding of aspiration of acid, mortality is still 55–70%.

6. What organisms commonly produce infectious complications of aspiration?

This depends on the patient population. In normal, healthy individuals who develop aspiration pneumonia, oral anaerobes are usually responsible: Bacteroides species, anaerobic streptococci, and Fusobacterium species. Hospitalized or debilitated individuals may also have oropharyngeal colonization with *Staphylococcus aureus* or gram-negative organisms. Treatment should be designed to provide first-line anaerobic coverage with high-dose penicillin or clindamycin; additional antibiotics to cover staphylococci or gram-negative organisms should be added in high-risk patients.

7. Does intubation or tracheostomy prevent aspiration?

No. Both intubation and tracheostomy actually breach some of the normal upper airway defenses. Balloon insufflation does not totally protect against fluid entering the airway. In patients with depressed consciousness or neuromuscular disease, however, intubation or tracheostomy may be indicated to decrease the volume of aspiration and to allow suctioning of airway contents.

8. What preventive measures can be used prior to endotracheal intubation?

Aspiration of gastric contents during intubation can be catastrophic. Several precautions can be taken. Awake intubation, without sedation, can be performed. Fiberoptic intubation may be superior if available. Pressure on the cricoid cartilage (Sellick's maneuver) occludes the esophagus and can prevent aspiration. Excessive assisted ventilation with an Ambu bag prior to intubation often dilates the stomach and predisposes to emesis. Ascertainment of correct placement of the endotracheal tube (both by presence of breath sounds and by absence of gastric sounds during ventilation) should be rapidly accomplished.

Maneuvers designed to decrease gastric pH, increase lower esophageal sphincter tone, and decrease gastric volume using H_2 blockers with or without metoclopramide can be undertaken in high-risk individuals, with intubations planned several hours in advance. Particulate antacids can produce pulmonary damage upon aspiration and should be avoided.

9. Should antibiotics be administered prophylactically to hospitalized patients at risk for aspiration?

Prophylactic antibiotics should be avoided in order to decrease the risk of colonization by resistant organisms.

CONTROVERSIES

10. How does one differentiate between chemical pneumonitis and infectious pneumonitis caused by aspiration?

This can be very difficult. Fever, leukocytosis, purulent sputum, and pulmonary infiltrates occur in both disorders. Gram stain and culture of expectorated sputum is not helpful because of contamination by oropharyngeal flora. If indicated, aerobic and anaerobic cultures of lower airway secretions can be obtained by fiberoptic bronchoscopy and protected brush techniques. Transtracheal aspiration, formerly frequently carried out, is now rarely performed because of a greater complication rate than with fiberoptic bronchoscopy. Many clinicians prefer to err on the side of empirical antibiotic treatment of possible infectious aspiration pneumonia.

11. Are corticosteroids indicated in the treatment of gastric acid aspiration?

The use of corticosteroids in this situation is attractive because of the theoretical potential of blocking lung injury; however, no clinical studies have demonstrated benefit. Certainly, the administration of corticosteroids for aspiration has little support at the present.

BIBLIOGRAPHY

1. Bartlett JG, Gorsbach SL, Finegold SM: The bacteriology of aspiration pneumonia. Am J Med 56:202–207, 1974.
2. Blitzer A: Approaches to the patient with aspiration and swallowing disabilities. Dysphagia 5:129–137, 1990.
3. Dal Santo G: Acid aspiration pathophysiologic aspects, prevention, and therapy. Int Anesthesiol Clin 24:31–52, 1986.
4. Joyce TH: Prophylaxis for pulmonary acid aspiration. Am J Med 83(Suppl 6A):46–52, 1987.
5. LoCicero J: Bronchopulmonary aspiration. Surg Clin North Am 69:71–76, 1989.
6. Lode H: Microbiological and clinical aspects of aspiration pneumonia. J Antimicrobiol Chemother 21(Suppl C):83–87, 1988.
7. Mendelson C: The aspiration of stomach contents into the lungs during obstetric anesthesia. Am J Obstet Gynecol 52:191–205, 1946.
8. Pennza PT: Aspiration pneumonia, necrotizing pneumonia and lung abscess. Emerg Clin North Am 7:279–307, 1989.
9. Ruffalo RL: Aspiration pneumonitis: Risk factors of the critically ill patient. DICP 24:S12–S16, 1990.

28. HEMOPTYSIS

Michael E. Hanley, M.D.

1. What is hemoptysis?

Hemoptysis is the expectoration of blood originating from the lower respiratory tract (trachea, bronchi, or lung parenchyma). It is further classified as massive or frank (gross). Massive hemoptysis is expectoration of greater than 600 cc of blood in a 24-hour period. Frank or gross hemoptysis is expectoration of less than 600 cc of blood in a 24-hour period but more than blood streaking. True hemoptysis must be differentiated from pseudohemoptysis. The latter is expectoration of blood originating from a source other than the lower respiratory tract. Pseudohemoptysis may result from either aspiration of blood from the gastrointestinal tract in patients with hematemesis or blood draining into the larynx and trachea from bleeding sites in the oral cavity, nasopharynx, or larynx.

2. What is the differential diagnosis of hemoptysis?

Although hemoptysis may be associated with many conditions (see table below), it results in general from either focal or diffuse pulmonary parenchymal processes or tracheobronchial, cardiovascular, or hematologic disorders. The frequency with which hemoptysis is associated with these conditions is determined by the age of the patient, the population being studied (surgical versus medical, veterans' hospital versus city/county indigent hospital), and amount of blood expectorated. Lung neoplasms, a common cause of hemoptysis in elderly patients, rarely occur in patients younger than 40 years of age. The most common causes of hemoptysis are also different when hemoptysis is scant or frank as opposed to massive. Scant or frank hemoptysis most commonly results from either bronchitis/bronchiectasis (40%) or lung neoplasms (25%). Other common conditions associated with scant or frank hemoptysis include active pulmonary tuberculosis, chronic necrotizing pneumonia, pulmonary infarction, congestive heart failure, and bleeding diathesis.

Causes of Hemoptysis

TRACHEOBRONCHIAL DISORDERS	LOCALIZED PARENCHYMAL DISEASES
Acute tracheobronchitis	Nontuberculous pneumonia
Amyloidosis	Actinomycosis
Gastric aspiration	Amebiasis
Bronchial adenoma	Ascariasis
Bronchial endometriosis	Aspergilloma
Bronchial telangiectasia	Bronchopulmonary sequestration
Bronchiectasis	Coccidioidomycosis
Bronchogenic carcinoma	Congenital and acquired cyst
Broncholithiasis	Cryptococcosis
Chronic bronchitis	Lipoid pneumonia
Cystic fibrosis	Histoplasmosis
Endobronchial hamartoma	Hydatid mole
Endobronchial metastasis	Lung abscess
Endobronchial tuberculosis	Lung contusion
Foreign body aspiration	Metastatic cancer
Bronchial mucoid impaction	Mucormycosis
Tracheobronchial trauma	Nocardiosis
Tracheoesophageal fistula	Paragonimiasis
	Pulmonary endometriosis
CARDIOVASCULAR DISORDERS	Pulmonary tuberculosis
Aortic aneurysm	Sporotrichosis
Congenital heart disease	
Congestive heart failure	DIFFUSE PARENCHYMAL DISEASES
Fat embolism	Disseminated angiosarcoma
Mitral stenosis	Farmer's lung
Postmyocardial infarction syndrome	Goodpasture's syndrome
Pulmonary arteriovenous malformation	Idiopathic pulmonary hemosiderosis
Pulmonary artery aneurysm	IgA nephropathy
Pulmonary embolus	Legionnaires' disease
Pulmonary venous varix	Mixed connective tissue disease
Schistomiasis	Mixed cryoglobulinemia
Superior vena cava syndrome	Polyarteritis nodosa
Tumor embolization	Scleroderma
	Systemic lupus erythematosus
HEMATOLOGIC DISORDERS	Viral pneumonitis
Anticoagulant therapy	Wegener's granulomatosis
Disseminated intravascular coagulation	
Leukemia	OTHER
Thrombocytopenia	Idiopathic
	Iatrogenic

Adapted from Irwin RS, Hubmayr R: Hemoptysis. In Rippe JM, Irwin RS, Alpert JS, Dalen JE (eds): Intensive Care Medicine. Boston, Little, Brown, 1985.

3. What are common causes of massive hemoptysis?

The most common cause of massive hemoptysis in patients who are not intubated when hemoptysis begins is inflammatory lung disease. This category includes tuberculosis (40%), bronchiectasis (30%), necrotizing pneumonitis (10%), lung abscess (5%), and fungal infection (5%). Pulmonary neoplasm and arteriovenous malformation constitute only about 10% of all cases.

When massive hemoptysis begins after endotracheal intubation, upper airway trauma secondary to the intubation procedure or trauma from the endotracheal tube or endotracheal suction catheters must be considered in addition to the processes listed above. If hemoptysis begins after a latent period of one or more weeks after intubation, a tracheoinnominate artery fistula may be the source of hemorrhage. This possibility is increased if a tracheostomy tube is present. Pulmonary artery rupture and pulmonary infarction should be considered when hemoptysis occurs in a patient with a pulmonary artery catheter. The latter diagnosis should be suspected if a wedge-shaped infiltrate is present distal to the catheter on the chest roentgenogram.

4. What is the significance of massive hemoptysis?

Massive hemoptysis is generally due to hemorrhaging from the bronchial artery (systemic pressure) circulation as opposed to the low-pressure pulmonary artery circuit, and therefore may be life-threatening. Mortality from massive hemoptysis in some studies is 75–100%.

5. What is the initial approach to evaluation of critical care patients with hemoptysis?

After the patient has been hemodynamically stabilized, the site, etiology, and extent of bleeding should be determined. In addition to a thorough history and physical examination, complete blood counts, coagulation studies, and arterial blood gases should be obtained. Identifying the site of bleeding requires visualization of the airways, including the nasopharynx and oropharynx, and examination of the chest roentgenogram. Nasal fiberoptic bronchoscopy allows examination of the nasopharynx, larynx, and major airways and may reveal if hemorrhaging is focal or diffuse. When presence of an endotracheal tube compromises this examination, upper airway bleeding may be detected by aspirating the trachea free of blood with a bronchoscope, while the endotracheal balloon is expanded, and then observing fresh blood flow down from above the balloon when it is decompressed. Rigid bronchoscopy may be required if hemorrhaging is massive, such that blood cannot be adequately removed with a flexible bronchoscope.

Examination of the chest roentgenogram often gives clues to both the site and etiology of hemoptysis. Presence of an infiltrate suggests the existence of a pulmonary parenchymal process. However, occasionally an infiltrate may occur after aspiration of blood coming from the upper airway. Similarly, presence of diffuse infiltrates suggests diffuse parenchymal disease, although this roentgenographic pattern may also occur with localized bleeding associated with severe coughing (coughing disperses the blood diffusely).

6. What is the immediate management of massive hemoptysis?

Immediate management includes maintaining airway patency, stopping ongoing hemorrhage, and preventing rebleeding. Maintenance of airway patency is of paramount importance, as death from massive hemoptysis is more commonly due to asphyxiation secondary to major airway obstruction than to exsanguination. Several approaches have been advocated to maintain airway patency. If hemorrhage is occurring from a focal site and the site of hemorrhage is known, the patient should be positioned with the bleeding site dependent to prevent contamination of noninvolved airways. If the site of hemorrhage is unknown or diffuse, the patient should be placed in the Trendelenburg position. Airway patency may also be maintained by bronchoscopically guided selective intubation of the nonbleeding mainstem bronchus or placement of a double-lumen (Carlen's) endotracheal tube. The latter should be placed only by physicians experienced in its use.

If the etiology of hemorrhage is known, specific therapy (such as antibiotics for bronchiectasis) should be instituted to stop ongoing hemorrhage. Blood products should also be administered to correct any coagulopathy that is present. Life-threatening hemorrhage from a focal site may require more aggressive strategies. Surgical resection should be considered in patients with adequate underlying lung function; however, the mortality associated with this approach is high. Hemoptysis in patients with severe underlying respiratory disease has been successfully treated by tamponade with Fogarty catheters placed under bronchoscopic guidance and by cautery with bronchoscopic laser photocoagulation. Limited success in stopping parenchymal hemorrhaging has also been achieved by bronchial artery embolization, occlusion of the involved pulmonary artery with a Swan-Ganz catheter, iced normal saline lavage of hemorrhaging lung segments, topical administration of epinephrine, and administration of intravenous vasopressin.

Once active hemorrhaging has been arrested, efforts should be made to prevent rebleeding. This usually includes adequate cough suppression with antitussives such as high-dose codeine or morphine and avoidance of chest percussion.

CONTROVERSIES

7. Should antitussives be aggressively administered to patients with massive hemoptysis?
For:

Excessive, harassing, violent cough aggravates and stimulates hemorrhaging, promoting continued bleeding or rebleeding in patients in whom hemorrhaging has stopped.

Against:

1. Aggressive administration of narcotic antitussives may result in oversedation and narcosis.

2. An effective cough is required to clear blood from the airways and avoid asphyxiation.

3. Oversuppression of the cough reflex may result in retention of blood in the lungs and/or aspiration, both of which may contribute to development of pneumonia or atelectasis.

8. Do patients with massive hemoptysis benefit from early resectional surgery?
For:

1. Older literature suggests that surgical mortality is 9–23%, with mortality related to magnitude of resection (pneumonectomy worse than lobectomy). Mortality of conservative (medical) therapy in these studies (using historical controls) is estimated at 75–80%.

2. A recent study of 123 patients with massive hemoptysis revealed a surgical mortality of 18% compared to 32% with conservative therapy. No distinction was made as to whether conservatively treated patients were operative candidates or inoperative due to advanced underlying lung disease.

Against:

1. Surgical mortality in a recent retrospective review of 73 patients with massive hemoptysis was 13% compared with 2% for patients who were operative candidates but treated conservatively.

2. Mortality of patients with massive hemoptysis treated conservatively is related to the etiology of hemoptysis, operability, and rate of hemorrhaging. Hemoptysis due to neoplastic processes or tuberculosis, in inoperative patients, or at a rate greater than 600–1000 cc per 24 hours is associated with higher mortality.

3. Recent studies indicating superior survival with conservative therapy may be due to advances in nonsurgical care or changes in relative frequencies of etiologies of massive hemoptysis.

9. Does evaluation of massive hemoptysis require rigid bronchoscopy?

For:

1. Higher suctioning capacity of rigid bronchoscopy allows superior clearing of blood from the tracheobronchial tree, permitting better evaluation of airways.

2. Rigid bronchoscopy permits superior maintenance of an adequate airway and minute ventilation.

Against:

1. Rigid bronchoscopy is poorly tolerated both subjectively and physiologically in acutely ill patients and allows only limited evaluation of the bronchial tree because only proximal portions of the bronchial tree are visualized. This results in insufficient time and maneuverability to permit effective lavage and evaluation of individual lung segments.

2. Increased range of flexible fiberoptic bronchoscopy permits evaluation at the level of segmental and subsegmental bronchi, resulting in increased diagnostic accuracy in both localization and visualization of bleeding site (especially the upper lobes).

3. Flexible fiberoptic bronchoscopy permits selective lavage and selective placement of Fogarty catheters in segmental and subsegmental bronchi.

BIBLIOGRAPHY

1. Bookstein JJ, Moser KM, Kalafer ME, et al: The role of bronchial arteriography and therapeutic embolization in hemoptysis. Chest 72:658–661, 1977.
2. Brobowitz ID, Ramakrishna S, Shim YS: Comparison of medical v surgical treatment of major hemoptysis. Arch Intern Med 143:1343–1346, 1983.
3. Conlan AA, Hurwitz SS, Krige L, et al: Massive hemoptysis: Review of 123 cases. J Thorac Cardiovasc Surg 85:120–124, 1983.
4. Corey R, Hla KM: Major and massive hemoptysis: Reassessment of conservative management. Am J Med Sci 294:301–309, 1987.
5. Crocco JM, Rooney JJ, Fankushen DS, et al: Massive hemoptysis. Arch Intern Med 121:495–498, 1968.
6. Gong H Jr, Salvatierra C: Clinical efficacy of early and delayed fiberoptic bronchoscopy in patients with hemoptysis. Am Rev Respir Dis 124:221–225, 1981.
7. Gourin A, Garzon AA: Control of hemorrhage in emergency pulmonary resection for massive hemoptysis. Chest 68:120–121, 1975.
8. Gourin AG, Garzon AA: Operative treatment of massive hemoptysis. Ann Thorac Surg 18:52–60, 1974.
9. Imgrund SP, Goldberg SK, Walkenstein MD, et al: Clinical diagnosis of massive hemoptysis using the fiberoptic bronchoscope. Crit Care Med 13:438–443, 1985.
10. Irwin RS, Hubmayr R: Hemoptysis. In Rippe JM, Irwin RS, Alpert JS, Dalen JE (eds): Intensive Care Medicine. Boston, Little, Brown, 1985.
11. McCollum WB, Mattox KL, Guinn GA, Beall AC: Immediate operative treatment for massive hemoptysis. Chest 67:152–155, 1975.
12. Saw EC, Gottlieb LS, Yokoyama T, Lee BC: Flexible fiberoptic bronchoscopy and endobronchial tamponade in the management of massive hemoptysis. Chest 70:589–591, 1976.
13. Sehhat S, Oreizie M, Moinedine K: Massive pulmonary hemorrhage: Surgical approach as choice of treatment. Ann Thorac Surg 25:12–15, 1978.
14. Smiddy JF, Elliott RC: The evaluation of bronchoscopy with fiberoptic bronchoscopy. Chest 64:158–162, 1973.
15. Wolfe JD, Simmons DH: Hemoptysis: Diagnosis and management. West J Med 127:383–390, 1977.

29. PULMONARY EMBOLISM

Polly E. Parsons, M.D., and Thomas A. Neff, M.D.

1. What is the primary source of pulmonary emboli (PE)?
Greater than 90% of PE arise from clots in the deep veins of the pelvis and legs.

2. How good is the physical exam for deep venous thrombosis (DVT)?
Poor. Only about 50% of patients in whom a DVT is suspected on clinical exam will have a positive venogram, and less than 50% of patients with a DVT will have the classic findings of erythema on clinical exam.

3. How should patients in whom a DVT is suspected be evaluated?
The key is to detect clots in the thigh and pelvis, as it is rare for clots in the calf to produce large or fatal PE. The gold standard for diagnosis is the venogram, which may be an uncomfortable invasive procedure that is difficult to perform in a critically ill patient. Less invasive measurements are now available. Impedance plethysmography can detect a major proximal DVT with 95% accuracy. Doppler ultrasound combined with real-time B-mode imaging (Duplex scanning) has an accuracy of 95%. Radiofibrinogen leg scanning is most accurate for the diagnosis of clot in the calf and distal thigh veins and, therefore, is less helpful as well as cumbersome and time-consuming.

4. What are some of the risk factors for PE?
Cancer

Obesity

Congestive heart failure

Prolonged immobilization

Oral contraceptive agents

Major surgical procedures (e.g., hip replacement)

Pregnancy

Trauma

Myocardial infarction with prolonged bed rest

Nephrotic syndrome

Previous history of DVT

5. What is the recommended prophylactic therapy for patients at risk for the development of DVT/PE?
Prophylaxis is recommended. The most commonly used regimen is low-dose heparin, 5000 units subcutaneously every 8–12 hours. This regimen is less effective in patients who have a fractured hip or are undergoing hip or prostatic surgery, so additional measures such as intermittent pneumatic compression stockings are used. These stockings are also used in patients who cannot tolerate anticoagulation.

6. How do patients with PE usually present?
Patients with PE can present with symptoms ranging from mild shortness of breath to cardiogenic shock. The two most common symptoms are chest pain and shortness of breath. The most common clinical signs, tachypnea and tachycardia, are also nonspecific.

7. When should the diagnosis of PE be suspected in a critically ill patient?
Many patients in the ICU are at risk for the development of PE, so the clinician has to have a high index of suspicion for the diagnosis and watch carefully for subtle clues such as:

Acute onset of tachypnea

Tachycardia

Unexplained agitation or anxiety

Changes in chest x-ray such as atelectasis, basilar infiltrate, or elevated hemidiaphragm

Hypotension

Nonspecific back or side pain	Pulmonary hypertension
Unexplained hypoxia	Asymmetric leg swelling
Respiratory alkalosis	Unilateral leg pain

8. Are there specific findings on chest x-ray in PE?

No. In many patients the chest x-ray will be normal or have subtle abnormalities such as slight elevation of a hemidiaphragm, focal hyperlucency of the lung parenchyma, or atelectasis. Some patients will have small pleural effusions or focal parenchymal infiltrates.

9. What are the EKG findings in PE?

The EKG findings are variable and relatively nonspecific. Sinus tachycardia and nonspecific ST segment and T wave changes occur frequently. The classic EKG findings of S_1, Q_3, T_3 or right bundle branch block occur in less than 15% of patients. The development of a new rightward axis shift from an admission or preoperative EKG in a critically ill patient should raise concern about potential PE.

10. How is the diagnosis of PE confirmed?

The first test is a ventilation/perfusion (V/Q) scan. A normal V/Q scan effectively rules out the diagnosis of PE, although there are rare instances of large saddle emboli extending from the main pulmonary artery that may be associated with a normal lung scan. The key here is the index of clinical suspicion. A high-probability lung scan supports the diagnosis of PE, although the false-positive rate is as high as 15% in some clinical series. The problem occurs when the scan is read as indeterminate, which happens frequently when the chest x-ray is abnormal. Pulmonary angiography is often required in these instances to confirm the diagnosis and is considered to be the gold standard for the diagnosis of PE. An adequate negative pulmonary angiogram effectively rules out the diagnosis of clinically significant PE and a positive angiogram confirms the diagnosis. However, technical limitations may prevent an adequate study from being performed, so the physician may have to rely on clinical judgment and studies of the lower extremities for decision making.

11. What percentage of patients with DVT without symptoms of PE will have a positive V/Q scan?

Approximately 50%.

12. On a perfusion lung scan, is the complete absence of perfusion to one whole lung with preserved perfusion to the opposite lung diagnostic of PE?

Always remember that most PE are multiple and/or bilateral. Therefore, the scenario described above would be unusual. The other diagnoses to consider would be mediastinal/ hilar adenopathy, fibrosing mediastinitis, tumor infiltration of a vessel, congenital absence of a pulmonary artery, or ascending aortic aneurysm dissection.

13. What is massive PE?

Massive PE is occlusion of more than 50% of the segmental pulmonary vasculature or an equivalent amount of central clot. This is the level of occlusion that would be expected to cause hemodynamic compromise in most patients. However, in patients with underlying cardiac or pulmonary disease, there may be significant hemodynamic compromise with less loss of the pulmonary vasculature. Most experts would define massive PE clinically as PE complicated by systemic hypotension with or without syncope and severe "refractory" hypoxemia.

14. What are the goals of treatment for PE? How are they achieved?
The major goals of PE therapy are to prevent further clot, promote resolution of existing clot, and prevent sequelae. These goals are achieved in the majority of patients with intravenous heparin therapy acutely, followed by oral warfarin for 3–6 months.

15. Which patients with PE should be treated with thrombolytic therapy?
This is generally reserved for patients with massive PE and hypotension. Although some data suggest that long-term sequelae may be diminished with lytic therapy, there is no evidence that morbidity or mortality is significantly altered.

16. When should the placement of an intravenous filter be considered?
When a patient has a documented (i.e., by repeat angiogram) recurrent embolism on "adequate" anticoagulation therapy or when a patient cannot be anticoagulated, a filter can be placed in the inferior vena cava to prevent propagation of clots from the pelvis/lower extremities. These filters can be placed under local anesthesia, so they are useful even in critically ill patients.

17. Are pulmonary embolism and pulmonary infarction the same?
No. Only 10% of patients with pulmonary embolism will have the clinical diagnosis of pulmonary infarction, although the incidence at autopsy may be much higher. Pulmonary infarction should be suspected in the patient with acute pleuritic chest pain, hemoptysis, and a parenchymal infiltrate on chest x-ray.

18. When should a fever in a patient with PE be of concern?
Patients with PE alone may have temperatures > 39° C early in the disease course, and low-grade fevers may persist for 4–6 days. Persistent high-grade fevers should arouse suspicion of superinfection.

BIBLIOGRAPHY

1. Kelley MA, Carson JL, Palevsky HI, Schwartz JS: Diagnosing pulmonary embolism: New facts and strategies. Ann Intern Med 114:300–306, 1991.
2. Marder VJ, Sherry S: Thrombolytic therapy: Current status. N Engl J Med 318:1585–1595, 1988.
3. Mohr DN, Ryu JH, Litin SC, Rosenow EC: Recent advances in the management of venous thromboembolism. Mayo Clin Proc 63:281–290, 1988.
4. Moser KM: Thromboembolic disease. In Bordow RA, Moser KM (eds): Manual of Clinical Problems in Pulmonary Medicine, 2nd ed. Boston, Little, Brown, 1986, pp 249–257.
5. Murray HW, Ellis GC, Blumenthal DS, Sos TA: Fever and pulmonary thromboembolism. Am J Med 67:232–235, 1979.
6. Novelline RA, Baltarowich OH, Athanasoulis CA, et al: The clinical course of patients with suspected pulmonary embolism and a negative pulmonary arteriogram. Radiology 126:561, 1978.
7. PIOPED Investigators: Value of the ventilation/perfusion scan in acute pulmonary embolism: Results of the prospective investigation of pulmonary embolism diagnosis (PIOPED). JAMA 263:2753–2795, 1990.
8. Rosenow ED, Osmundson PJ, Brown ML: Pulmonary embolism. Mayo Clin Proc 56:161–178, 1981.
9. Rutherford R, Norton D: Venous disease. In Abernathy CM, Harken AH (eds): Surgical Secrets, 2nd ed. Philadelphia, Hanley & Belfus, 1991, pp 248–251.
10. Sahn SA, Heffner JE: Pulmonary medicine. In Sahn SA, Heffner JE (eds): Critical Care Pearls. Philadelphia, Hanley & Belfus, 1989, pp 12–14.

IV: Cardiology

30. CHEST PAIN

Carter Willis, M.D.

1. Define angina pectoris.

Angina pectoris is a clinical syndrome resulting from myocardial ischemia characterized by episodes of precordial pain or pressure typically precipitated by exertion and relieved by sublingual nitroglycerin (SL NTG) or rest.

2. What questions should you ask a patient with suspected new onset of angina pectoris to characterize the chest pain? What are the customary answers?

Intensity   Duration
Character   Initiating and alleviating factors
Location   Associated symptoms
Radiation

Angina is typically described as being of variable intensity and dull character, with a deep, diffuse location either substernal or involving the left precordium. Pain may radiate to the left shoulder, the left arm, the head, the neck, the back, or even the right arm or upper abdomen. The pain may be referred to as tightness, heaviness, or pressure. Angina rarely lasts more than 20 minutes unless it is associated with acute myocardial infarction (MI) or is caused by persistent dysrhythmia. Associated symptoms include dyspnea, diaphoresis, lightheadedness, and fatigue or weakness. Response to therapy is generally dramatic—within 1–3 minutes after treatment with SL NTG 0.3–0.6 mg.

3. What are the risk factors for development of atherosclerotic coronary artery disease (CAD)?

Hypertension   Family history
Diabetes   Hyperlipidemia
Smoking   Obesity
Male > 40 years old   Type A personality

Although alcohol abuse may be related to the development of a cardiomyopathy, it is not a risk factor for atherosclerotic disease.

4. What is the differential diagnosis in new-onset acute chest pain?

Few disorders truly mimic classic angina, and a good history will help to direct the evaluation. Pleuritic chest pain that increases with inspiration is unlikely to be anginal in nature but may be due to pleuritis, pericarditis, myocarditis, pulmonary embolism with infarction, or even spontaneous pneumothorax or pneumomediastinum (Hamman's disease). Changes in body position may bring on nonanginal, sharp, lancinating pain in the arm, shoulder or chest due to cervical or thoracic nerve root compression in patients with thoracic outlet obstruction. Superficial, nonanginal chest pain associated with tenderness to palpation may reflect local inflammation in the form of xiphodynia, pectoral myofasciitis, costochondritis (Tietze's syndrome), or precordial vein thrombophlebitis. A thoracic aortic aneurysm may cause sustained chest pain that radiates to the back and might be diagnosed by chest x-ray or aortic angiogram. Cholecystitis due to cholelithiasis may cause epigastric pain that may be confused with angina. Pain that is rapidly relieved by swallowing food, water, or antacids is typically caused by gastritis, peptic ulcer, achalasia, esophagitis due to hiatal hernia, or esophageal spasm. However, these "clinical tests" may be misleading, as 5–10% of patients with angiographically demonstrated CAD may obtain relief from oral antacids (perhaps due to placebo effect), and SL NTG frequently alleviates pain associated with esophageal spasm. Finally, patients with anxiety or depression may complain of chest pain with associated hyperventilation, but again a careful history should reveal distinct nonanginal features.

5. Is chest pain more frequent in patients with mitral valve prolapse than in those without this condition?
No.

6. What causes the pain of pericarditis?
The pericardium is relatively insensitive to pain. Pain in pericarditis is likely to be caused by inflammation of adjacent structures, namely the parietal pleura. Noninfectious pericarditis (e.g., from MI or uremia) is relatively painless or characterized by mild pain, whereas infectious pericarditis is painful.

7. What is "atypical angina" or "atypical chest pain"?
This poorly defined term is often used loosely to describe a symptom complex that is not entirely consistent with classic angina, i.e., there may be one or more unusual characteristics or nonanginal features as described above. As many as 80% of patients with atypical angina have been found to have normal coronary angiograms.

8. What are "anginal equivalents"? Why are they important?
Some patients with myocardial ischemia may present without chest discomfort and instead have referred pain to the mandible, maxilla, cheek, ear, tongue, wrist, or elbow, or combinations of these areas. Symptoms typically associated with angina may be present.

9. How is angina related to myocardial ischemia?
Angina occurs shortly after the onset of myocardial ischemia, which results whenever the metabolic oxygen demand exceeds the available oxygen supply.

Ischemia: myocardial O_2 demand $\gg$ myocardial O_2 supply

10. What are some typical initiating factors for angina?
Exertion is the most common cause; others include abrupt exposure to cold, emotional stress, pain due to an injury, fever with rigors, or a large meal (angina may occur postprandial). Certain medical conditions such as aortic stenosis, thyrotoxicosis, and anemia may initiate or aggravate anginal symptoms. A transient or sustained acute tachydysrhythmia may cause or worsen angina.

11. What are the major determinants of myocardial oxygen consumption?
Heart rate, contractility, mean arterial pressure (afterload), and left ventricular chamber size (a function of preload).

12. What organ in the body normally has the largest arteriovenous oxygen difference (A-V DO$_2$), i.e., the greatest oxygen extraction at rest?
You got it. The gradient across the heart is normally about 8–12 ml O_2/dl. This is significant because it indicates that **oxygen extraction is near maximum at rest**, which means that extraction can change only moderately and an increase in myocardial oxygen demand must be matched by an increase in myocardial oxygen supply by increasing coronary blood flow. **Autoregulation** is the homeostatic process by which myocardial oxygen consumption (MVO$_2$) is matched precisely with coronary blood flow in essentially a linear relationship.

13. How severe must the degree of stenosis be in a coronary artery to interfere significantly with coronary flow during routine exercise?

Coronary stenosis generally must reduce luminal diameter by 50% or more to be considered significant. This is equivalent to a 75% decrease in lumen cross-sectional area and an even greater decrease in flow. You may recall that flow through a pipe is proportional to the fourth power of the radius:

$$\textit{Poiseuille's Equation}\quad \text{Flow} = \frac{3.14\ (\text{pressure difference})(\text{radius})^4}{8\ (\text{vessel length})(\text{fluid viscosity})}$$

14. What is stable angina? How would you manage a patient presenting with an acute episode?

Stable angina refers to chronic anginal pain that occurs at a reproducible level of exercise without recent change in severity or frequency and is relieved reliably with rest and/or a standard dose of NTG. Coronary angiograms of patients with a classic history of stable angina have shown that $> 95\%$ of patients will have one or more coronary vessels with $> 50\%$ stenosis.

First and foremost, **place the patient at rest** with the **head elevated** and then treat with SL NTG, 0.3–0.6 mg, repeated at 5-minute intervals as necessary, or use cutaneously applied 2% Nitropaste, 0.5–2 inches (nitropaste has the advantage of being readily removable if the patient suddenly develops hypotension). In a patient with previously diagnosed stable angina, by definition rapid resolution of the chest pain will occur within 1.5–5 minutes. Prophylactic therapy would include use of a longer-acting oral or transdermal nitrate preparation, possibly in combination with an oral beta blocker or calcium channel blocker.

15. What is unstable angina?

Unstable angina is also sometimes called accelerated angina, crescendo angina, preinfarction angina, or intermediate coronary syndrome. It may be one of several types:

1. Previously stable angina that has worsened in severity, increased in frequency, become prolonged in duration (> 20 minutes), or no longer responds to SL NTG therapy.

2. Angina that occurs at rest or awakens the patient from sleep (so-called "angina decubitus" and "nocturnal angina").

3. New-onset angina in a patient with no prior symptoms should be considered unstable until it can be better defined.

16. How is the management of unstable angina different from that of stable angina?

The unstable subset of angina is associated with a notably higher rate of acute MI and sudden death secondary to malignant dysrhythmias. Thus, intervention and monitoring are more aggressive, as this constitutes a medical emergency. As before, initially **place the patient at rest and treat with nitrates.** Begin **supplemental oxygen** by nasal cannula or face mask. Check the patient's **blood pressure and pulse rate** to rule out potentially treatable hypotension, hypertension, or a tachydysrhythmia. Do a **12-lead EKG** to look for the ST-segment depression and T-wave inversion that typically occur during angina and to rule out variant angina or acute MI manifested as ST-segment elevation. Place an intravenous (IV) catheter and start an **NTG drip** at 10–30 μg/min with titration up or down as needed. These patients may initially need small doses of **IV morphine** to achieve rapid control of pain. The addition of an oral **calcium channel blocker** should be considered for patients with rest or nocturnal pain as a primary feature. An IV **beta blocker** such as metoprolol would be advocated for patients with excessive heart rates, although an **esmolol infusion** may be preferred because of its 9-minute half-life, allowing rapid titration to changing conditions. **Aspirin,** 325 mg orally per day, should be started routinely. Patients with unstable angina require admission to a coronary care unit for continuous telemetry and hemodynamic monitoring.

Controversial: A heparin infusion may be started if there are no contraindications. Two studies have found this to be beneficial in patients with unstable angina, but this is not yet universally accepted as standard therapy.

17. What diagnostic studies are indicated in patients presenting with unstable angina?

Early coronary angiography is indicated immediately following pharmacologic stabilization, because in up to 30% of patients with unstable angina, a nonoccluding "labile" thrombus or a "complex" atherosclerotic plaque (one with fissuring or hemorrhage) may be identified and thrombolytic therapy or angioplasty may be indicated. Additionally, if pharmacologic therapy is not adequate, the patient may require emergent coronary artery bypass surgery, and a coronary angiogram is helpful in that it outlines the relevant anatomy.

Angiographically, 10–20% of patients will have left-main disease, 40% will have triple-vessel disease, and another 40% will have double- or single-vessel disease. Up to 50% of patients with unstable angina may also have a component of **vasospasm** contributing to their dynamic stenosis. However, less than 10% of patients presenting with unstable angina will have vasospasm alone as the cause of ischemia.

18. What is variant angina? How is it diagnosed and managed?

Also known as **Prinzmetal's angina**, variant angina is frequently attributable to vasospasm alone (> 75% of patients), although many patients will also have significant fixed proximal coronary lesions. Patients typically present with nonexertional chest pain, with the 12-lead EKG showing ST-segmental elevation instead of the typical ST-depression. The diagnosis may be suggested by history and EKG, but early coronary angiography is indicated. The key to diagnosis is **provocative testing** using a spasm-inducing agent such as ergonovine or methacholine given in a cardiac catheterization lab with spasm visualized on angiogram. Rescue is performed with IV or intracoronary NTG. An alternative method of diagnosis is the **cold pressor test**, which involves immersing the patient's hand in cold water while monitoring for symptoms. In this case SL, transdermal, or IV NTG is used for reversal of symptoms. Therapy centers on the aggressive use of nitrates, both acutely and for chronic control, with calcium channel blockers advocated as adjuncts.

19. Are there nonpharmacologic ways to treat medically refractory myocardial ischemia?

An intraaortic balloon pump (a form of left ventricular assist device) may be temporarily used to manage a patient with medically refractory angina. It functions to augment diastolic coronary artery flow by diastolic inflation of a 30–40 cc balloon placed in the thoracic descending aorta. Additionally, left ventricular (LV) afterload is reduced by systolic deflation of the balloon, resulting in augmentation of LV stroke volume, reduction of LV wall stress, and reduction of myocardial oxygen consumption.

20. What is the neuroanatomic pathway involved in development of angina?

Afferent impulses are initially detected by chemoreceptive and mechanoreceptive visceral cardiac nociceptors that stimulate primary afferents traveling back to the middle and inferior cervical ganglia and the upper four thoracic sympathetic ganglia. Cell bodies are located in the dorsal root ganglia with projections into the ventral spinothalamic tract. Second-order neurons ascend to the ventroposterior thalamus and then on to the frontal and somatosensory cortex.

21. Which patients are at risk for "silent ischemia" (myocardial ischemia without chest pain)?

Patients who have an interruption of the neural pathway at any point along its course may have ischemia without the conscious sensation of chest pain. For instance, diabetics and the elderly are two groups at risk for autonomic neuropathy, and consequently these patients may not have pain with ischemia. Cardiac transplant recipients have complete denervation of the transplanted organ and will not have chest pain with ischemia. Also, patients with reinfarction of a previously incompletely infarcted area may not experience chest pain.

BIBLIOGRAPHY

1. Buda A, Levene DL: The influence of inspiration on angina pectoris: A clue to right coronary disease. Am Heart J 92:537, 1976.
2. Constant J: The clinical diagnosis of nonanginal chest pain: The differentiation of angina from nonanginal chest pain by history. Clin Cardiol 6:11, 1983.
3. Hurst JW: The Heart, 7th ed. New York, McGraw-Hill, 1990.
4. Lewis HD: Protective effects of aspirin against acute myocardial infarction and death in men with unstable angina. N Engl J Med 309:396, 1983.
5. Maccioli GA: The intraaortic balloon pump: A review. J Cardiothorac Anesth 2:365, 1988.
6. Plotnick GD: Approach to the management of unstable angina. Am Heart J 98:111, 1979.
7. Telford AM: Trial of heparin vs. atenolol in prevention of myocardial infarction in intermediate coronary syndrome. Lancet i:1225, 1981.
8. Theoux P: ASA, heparin, or both to treat acute unstable angina. N Engl J Med 319:1105, 1988.
9. Willerson JT: Conversion from chronic to acute coronary artery disease: Speculation regarding mechanism. Am J Cardiol 54:1350, 1984.
10. Williams MR: Coronary artery spasm: A current review. Anesthesiol Rev 16:21, 1989.

31. MYOCARDIAL INFARCTION

Carter Willis, M.D.

1. How soon does myocardial ischemia begin after coronary artery occlusion?
At rest, the heart has the highest metabolic rate of any organ in the body at approximately 6–10 ml O_2/100 gm of tissue/minute. It also has the highest arteriovenous oxygen difference (A-V DO_2) at rest, reflecting near maximal oxygen extraction. Consequently, after coronary occlusion, **the onset of ischemia occurs within 60 seconds**, leading to anaerobic metabolism and subsequent impairment of systolic myocardial contraction.

2. What is the most sensitive indicator of myocardial ischemia/infarction? How should we monitor for it? *Controversial*
In the conscious individual, reporting of anginal symptoms by the patient in combination with continuous EKG and hemodynamic monitoring remains the standard. However, we must resort to other means for early detection of myocardial ischemia in the unconscious patient (undergoing general anesthesia, for instance).

Under normal conditions, the heart is a net lactate extractor and may use this as an energy source in addition to oxygen, but with the onset of ischemia net lactate production begins. The rapid transition to lactate production may be detected by serial blood sampling from the coronary sinus in cardiac catheterization labs, but has not yet found its way into operating room practice.

3. How soon does cell death occur after the onset of ischemia?
Myocardial cell death will occur within 20–40 minutes in the presence of complete occlusion; however, collateral flow may prolong this period to several hours. Transmural

cellular necrosis is generally a late finding and yields deep Q waves on EKG due to the absence of depolarization current from the dead tissue.

Transmural infarction → Absence of electrical depolarization → Deep Q waves on EKG

4. Why is the early recognition of myocardial ischemia important?

The initial myocardial dysfunction is generally reversible if blood flow is restored within 15 minutes. Additionally, infarction does not occur uniformly and simultaneously throughout the jeopardized area of myocardium. Instead, an initial small zone of irreversible infarction is surrounded by a larger border zone of reversible ischemia. Part of this larger zone can be salvaged with proper intervention. An infarct is said to be **evolving** if < 4–6 hours have elapsed since the onset of symptoms. A **completed infarct** is one in which the symptoms of myocardial ischemia have been present for > 4–6 hours. It is well established that infarct size may be reduced by as much as 30% by early administration of IV beta blockers during the evolving infarct stage. Treated patients also have fewer ventricular dysrhythmias and reduced mortality. Trials using intravenous nitroglycerin (IV NTG) have demonstrated similar favorable results for reduction of infarct size and improved survival. However, studies using calcium channel blockers such as verapamil and nifedipine have been disappointing. Positive results have only been obtained using diltiazem in patients with non-Q-wave infarction with ejection fractions > 40% without congestive heart failure. Fibrinolytic/thrombolytic therapy represents another physiologically appealing method for restoring blood flow and salvaging border zone myocardium; it has been shown to be clearly beneficial with early application.

5. What causes chronic atherosclerotic coronary artery disease to suddenly convert to acute occlusion, leading to infarction? *Controversial*

A large body of angiographic data indicate that a transiently occlusive "labile thrombus" may play a role in the conversion of chronic atherosclerotic coronary disease to acute coronary occlusion in > 85% of patients suffering transmural infarction. Angiograms done within 4–6 hours of the onset of infarction show vessel occlusion, with follow-up angiograms after 12 hours showing resolution of the thrombus.

6. What is fibrinolytic/thrombolytic therapy?

Streptokinase is the prototypic enzyme that is used as a plasminogen activator. It binds to plasminogen or plasmin to form an activated complex that can then diffuse into a thrombus and convert thrombus-bound plasminogen to plasmin. Plasmin is a proteolytic enzyme that acts on fibrin, causing fibrinolysis with resultant thrombolysis and reperfusion of the obstructed vessel.

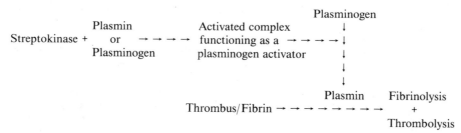

7. What are the available thrombolytic agents? When are they indicated?

Clot lysis may be achieved using streptokinase, urokinase, tissue plasminogen activator (TPA), anisoylated plasminogen streptokinase activator complex (APSAC), or oral aspirin. Initial studies centered on the use of intracoronary (IC) thrombolytics, but the limited availability of staff and facilities restricted application of this therapy to a relatively small group of patients. IC thrombolytics have the disadvantage of delaying therapy for 1–2 hours to perform cardiac catheterization during a crucial period while the patient continues to infarct border-zone myocardium. Thus, the focus has been redirected toward systemically administered IV thrombolytics that can be started promptly in the emergency room. Efficacy of IC and IV thrombolytics is similar (about 75%). The rate of hemorrhagic complications is also similar (< 5%). Successful recanalization with IV thrombolytics typically occurs within 30–60 minutes. In the GISSI trial, patients treated with IV streptokinase within 1 hour had mortality at 21 days reduced as much as 47% compared with controls. The results were less dramatic, although still substantial, when therapy was initiated later. Similar results have been found by other investigators using urokinase, TPA, and APSAC. In the ISIS-2 trial, which treated patients up to 24 hours after onset of symptoms, IV streptokinase reduced mortality 26% and aspirin reduced mortality 21%, with a 46% mortality reduction being achieved using combination therapy.

8. What is a typical dose of streptokinase?
Practices vary, but a typical loading dose of streptokinase would be 250,000 units infused over 30 minutes followed by a continuous infusion of 100,000 units per hour.

9. When is thrombolytic therapy not indicated? Contraindicated?
Absolute contraindications include active bleeding, known presence of intracranial lesions with potential for hemorrhage (such as a tumor, previous cerebrovascular accident, arteriovenous malformation, or aneurysm), and uncontrolled severe hypertension.

Relative contraindications include major surgery within 10 days, postpartum state, hypocoagulable state (liver disease), recent cardiopulmonary resuscitation, and recent needle biopsy.

Controversial: Because thrombolytic therapy is associated with hemorrhagic risks and therapeutic benefit depends on early intervention, most investigators have recommended that a cutoff time be set at 6 hours after onset of symptoms. However, this notion is being challenged by new study data suggesting reduced short-term mortality even with later administration. **Thrombolytics may be indicated up to 24 hours after onset of symptoms.**

10. What other adverse effects are associated with the use of thrombolytics?
Transient ventricular irritability may occur with recanalization of the occluded artery. Generally, a lidocaine bolus and/or infusion is given prior to beginning thrombolytic therapy.

Allergic reaction to streptokinase has been described with manifestations including rash, urticaria, hypotension, bronchospasm, and angioneurotic edema. Patients previously treated with streptokinase (within 6 months) and patients with recent streptococcal infections are at increased risk. Antibodies in these patients may also inactivate streptokinase and render it ineffective. Urokinase or TPA may be preferred under these circumstances.

Fevers may occur in up to 30% of patients receiving streptokinase. Pretreatment with acetaminophen and hydrocortisone greatly reduces this problem.

11. What is the role of emergent percutaneous transluminal coronary angioplasty (PTCA) in the setting of acute MI? *Controversial*
In the past, emergent PTCA has been done **primarily** (without thrombolytic therapy), **adjunctively** (used immediately after starting thrombolysis to assist recanalization), or **secondarily** (following failed thrombolysis). Primary PTCA is unacceptable because of the inherent time delay and high incidence of dysrhythmias. PTCA used immediately with thrombolysis may be associated with a high mortality, more frequent bleeding complications, a higher rate of emergency coronary artery bypass grafts (CABGs), frequent reocclusions (30%), and no clear improvement in myocardial salvage. The current philosophy dictates that immediate use of PTCA should be reserved for thrombolytic failures (10–30% of

treated patients). Otherwise, PTCA should be delayed for 24–48 hours after thrombolysis. The one exception to this rule is the patient presenting with cardiogenic shock. In this situation, early, aggressive intervention is warranted, including PTCA and intraaortic balloon pump (IABP), in an attempt to reduce the excessively high mortality seen in this group of patients (50–80%).

12. What is the role of emergency CABG in acute MI?
This is essentially never indicated or utilized without a preceding attempt at medical therapy. Two exceptions to this rule would include (1) patients experiencing a complication while undergoing PTCA, such as perforation or total occlusion of a coronary artery; facilities for emergent CABG should always be immediately available for patients undergoing PTCA, and (2) patients with acute MI complicated by papillary muscle necrosis leading to severe mitral regurgitation and fulminant pulmonary edema, who may require surgical mitral valve replacement and CABG.

13. What is Laplace's law? Why is it important?

$$\text{Wall tension} = \frac{\text{Distending pressure}}{2} \times \frac{\text{Chamber radius}}{\text{Wall thickness}}$$

This law is important to know in order to understand the cardiac effects of changing preload. It is easy to see that wall tension increases with increases in distending pressure (central venous pressure) or chamber radius (dilate the ventricle). Consequences of increased wall tension include decreased subendocardial coronary artery blood flow and increased myocardial oxygen consumption (MVO_2) leading to ischemia.

14. Why does NTG have an antianginal/anti-ischemic effect? *Controversial*
- Significant venodilation → decreases wall tension (preload) → decreases MVO_2
- Minimal systemic arterial vasodilation → decreases afterload → decreases MVO_2
- Relaxing effect on stenotic and collateral coronary arteries → increases O_2 delivery

The predominant effect of NTG appears to be venodilation, systemically and in the pulmonary circulation, resulting in an increase in venous capacitance leading to decreased ventricular volume and wall tension (decreased preload). This, in turn, may decrease MVO_2 and improve subendocardial blood flow (increasing oxygen delivery).

15. What are the onset and duration of action of NTG?
After sublingual administration, onset of action occurs in < 60 seconds, the peak effect is achieved at about 2 minutes, and the duration of effect is about 15–30 minutes. In angina lasting longer than 15 minutes despite repeated doses of SL NTG, an IV NTG infusion should be considered. Onset of action is < 30 seconds, with the effect being rapidly terminated several minutes after discontinuation. Infusions should be started at 10–30 μg/min and titrated as needed.

16. What are Killip classes?
In 1967, Killip reported on 250 acute MI patients treated in a CCU. Patients were classified into four clinical groups by severity of myocardial derangement:

	Mortality
1. Absence of heart failure	6%
2. Presence of heart failure–S_3 + basilar rates	17%
3. Severe heart failure/gross pulmonary edema	38%
4. Cardiogenic shock with hypoperfusion/hypotension, oliguria, peripheral cyanosis, and cool extremities	81%

Killip found that the incidence of dysrhythmias, cardiac arrests, and short-term hospital mortality increased as cardiac function decreased. After treatment of 100 patients, a protocol mandating early defibrillation was introduced that allowed nurses to cardiovert if a physician was not available within 60 seconds. It was subsequently noted that mortality was significantly decreased for patients in groups 1–3.

17. Can patients with acute MI be classified based on directly measured hemodynamic variables?

In 1976, Forrester divided patients with acute MI into four subsets based on directly measured hemodynamic variables. These hemodynamic subsets of patients had clinical features similar to those of Killip's groups:

	Mortality
1. No pulmonary congestion + no hypoperfusion (PCWP < 18, CI > 2.2)	3%
2. Pulmonary congestion + no hypoperfusion (PCWP > 18, CI > 2.2)	9%
3. Hypoperfusion + no pulmonary congestion (PCWP < 18, CI > 2.2)	23%
4. Pulmonary congestion + hypoperfusion (PCWP > 18, CI < 2.2)	51%

PCWP = pulmonary capillary wedge pressure; CI = cardiac index.

Again, comparative mortality among subsets was shown to correlate with diminishing cardiac function. The parameters used to derive these subsets are also helpful in optimizing therapy. For instance, a patient in subset #1 would likely require only basic therapy in the form of rest, supplemental O_2, IV NTG, IV morphine sulfate for pain control, continuous telemetry, and hemodynamic monitoring. However, patients in subset #2 would additionally need restriction of fluids combined with a diuretic (IV furosemide) ± a carefully titrated low-dose vasodilator (NTG or nitroprusside) to unload the LV ± a low-dose inotrope (dopamine or dobutamine) to increase contractility. Patients in subset #3 would need basic therapy with supplemental IV fluid boluses to maximize cardiac output (CO) ± a low-dose inotrope to increase CO. Subset #4 patients require basic therapy and maximal emergent therapy, including combinations of vasopressors/inotropes ± intubation with mechanical ventilation ± IABP ± emergent PTCA ± CABG.

Clinical estimation of the patient's hemodynamic subset in acute MI is correct only about 70% of the time. In order to avoid this type of error, hemodynamic variables can be measured directly using a pulmonary artery (PA) catheter and arterial line.

18. Has the use of the PA catheter–derived data been shown to favorably influence outcome in patients with acute MI? *Controversial*

Improved long-term survival has been noted in patients with acute MI since the advent of the CCU. Many factors are felt to have contributed to this trend, including precise assessment of hemodynamic status using invasive monitoring, rapid dysrhythmia recognition and treatment with immediate defibrillation, and improved pharmacologic therapy. It is the opinion of many experts that PA monitoring is invaluable in selected patients with acute MI, as it may allow tailoring of specific therapy. However, studies have failed to document improved outcome, and some investigators argue that use of the PA catheter is associated with a deleterious effect on outcome.

19. What are the indications for a PA catheter in acute MI? *Controversial*

Patients presenting without pulmonary edema or peripheral hypoperfusion do not require a PA catheter. Patients with peripheral hypoperfusion/hypotension, but not pulmonary edema, do not need a PA catheter unless hypoperfusion does not readily correct with IV fluids. Patients presenting with acute MI and pulmonary edema will frequently require a PA catheter to assist in titrating fluids, afterload reducing agents, and inotropes, unless they rapidly improve with diuretics alone. Indications for a PA catheter immediately in patients with acute MI include:

1. Cardiogenic shock
2. Physical exam suggesting cardiac tamponade, ventricular septal defect, or acute mitral regurgitation (may be diagnosed using 2-D precordial cardiac echocardiography)
3. Oliguria or hypotension that is unresponsive to fluid boluses

Use of the PA catheter has declined in recent years, and significant controversy remains regarding its use in a variety of situations.

20. What are the potential complications of a PA catheter?

- Catheter-related sepsis
- Injuries related to insertion (vascular damage, pneumothorax, air embolus)
- Pulmonary infarction (extremely rare)
- Pulmonary artery rupture (extremely rare)
- Dysrhythmias with insertion

21. What is the Fick equation? How is it used?

This is a commonly used principle centered on the fact that delivered O_2 minus O_2 consumed equals O_2 returning to the heart, or, stated another way:

DO_2 (O_2 delivery) = CO × CaO_2 (arterial O_2 content)

O_2 returning to the heart = CO × CvO_2 (mixed venous O_2 content)

VO_2 (O_2 consumption) = O_2 delivery – O_2 returning to the heart

Fick Equation VO_2 = CO ($CaO_2 - CvO_2$) = CO (A-V DO_2)

All of these variables can be determined by using a PA catheter and an arterial line.

22. What are the major complications of acute MI?

Cardiac dysrhythmias/arrest	Renal failure
Venous thrombosis and pulmonary embolism	Pericarditis
Ventricular septum rupture	Hypotension
Ventricular free wall rupture (tamponade)	Ventricular dysfunction
Papillary muscle + mitral valve dysfunction	Cardiogenic shock
LV mural thrombosis with arterial embolism	Mental status changes

23. Should patients with acute MI be anticoagulated prophylactically? *Controversial*

The idea behind anticoagulation of patients with acute MI is based on prevention of deep venous thrombosis/pulmonary embolism, prevention of LV mural thrombi with embolization → CVA, and prevention of progression or reformation of intracoronary thrombus. However, it has not been convincingly demonstrated that mini-dose subcutaneous heparin (5000 units two or three times daily) confers any real benefit. It is also unclear whether the risk of these potential complications outweighs the risks associated with full-dose IV heparin in large groups of MI patients. However, we can identify select patients at increased risk for LV thrombi (LVT), including those with transmural anterior MI (30–40% incidence of LVT) and apical akinesis/dyskinesis. These patients may be considered for prophylactic IV heparinization. Two-dimensional echocardiography is the procedure of choice for the detection of LV mural thrombus.

24. How are cardiac enzymes helpful in the diagnosis of acute MI?

Creatine kinase (CK) is a dimeric enzyme with an MB subfraction that is highly specific for myocardial tissue. It reliably starts to rise 4–8 hours after an MI begins, peaks at about 12–24 hours, and returns to baseline at 48–60 hours. Some labs use the actual CK-MB concentration to define the normal limit, with thresholds ranging from 5–25 IU/L. However, it is more common to use the percentage of total CK (MB/M total), with normal thresholds ranging from 3–8%. Levels above this range are diagnostic of acute MI in the absence of certain processes known to elevate levels. Hypothyroidism is associated with reduced CK-MB clearance and high levels. Certain skeletal muscle disorders, including rhabdomyolysis, dermatomyositis, Duchenne's muscular dystrophy, alcoholic myositis, and viral myositis, are associated with increased production of CK-MB and high levels. Patients with diabetes or seizures may also have falsely high levels.

Lactate dehydrogenase (LDH) is also useful for confirming acute MI. It begins to rise at 8–12 hours, peaks at 72–144 hours, and declines by 8–14 days. For patients presenting in a delayed fashion, this may be a useful test. LDH has five isomers, with the normal ratio of LD_1 to LD_2 being < 0.7. A ratio of > 1.0 in the absence of hemolysis is diagnostic of subacute MI.

25. What is Dressler's syndrome?

Also called the **post-MI syndrome**, it occurs days to weeks after an acute MI and comprises pleuritic chest pain, pericardial friction rub, fever, leukocytosis, and sometimes a pulmonary infiltrate. It usually responds to nonsteroidal anti-inflammatory agents (NSAIDs), but more resistant cases may need a course of steroid therapy. It may be confused with unstable post-infarction angina.

26. When do right ventricular (RV) infarctions occur? How are they managed?

RV infarct complicates inferior MI in about 30–35% of cases, whereas less than 10% of anterior MIs have associated RV infarcts. The most reliable EKG evidence is ST-segment elevation in the right precordial leads (particularly R V_4) with associated ST-elevation in left precordial leads II, III, and AVF. Clinical signs include a high central venous pressure with systemic hypotension and a clear chest on physical exam. With a large infarction, the RV may essentially become a conduit from the systemic veins to the pulmonary circulation. Management is centered upon volume loading (CVP = 16–20) and early use of inotropes (dopamine or dobutamine) to maintain blood flow to the LV (preload) and to maximize CO.

BIBLIOGRAPHY

1. Forrester JS: Medical therapy of acute MI by application of hemodynamic subsets. N Engl J Med 293:1358, 1976.
2. Gibson RS: Diltiazem and reinfarction in patients with non-Q wave MI. N Engl J Med 315:423, 1986.
3. GISSI: Effectiveness of IV thrombolytic treatment in acute MI. Lancet i:397, 1986.
4. Gomez-Marino O: Improvement in long-term survival among patients hospitalized with acute MI, 1970 to 1980. N Engl J Med 316:1353, 1987.
5. Hurst JW: The Heart, 7th ed. New York, McGraw-Hill, 1990.
6. ISIS-2 Collaborative Group: Randomized trial of IV streptokinase, oral aspirin, both, or neither among 17,187 cases of suspected MI. Lancet ii:349, 1988.
7. Kandel G: Mixed venous O_2 saturation: Its role in the assessment of the critically ill patient. Arch Intern Med 143:1400, 1983.
8. Kaplan K: Prophylactic anticoagulation following acute myocardial infarction. Arch Intern Med 146:593, 1986.
9. Killip T: Treatment of MI in the coronary care unit. Am J Cardiol 20:457, 1967.
10. Lee L: Multicenter registry of angioplasty therapy of cardiogenic shock: Initial and long-term survival. Circulation 76(Suppl 6):261, 1987.
11. Lee TH: Serum enzyme assays in the diagnosis of acute MI. Ann Intern Med 105:221, 1986.
12. Leung JM: Prognostic importance of postbypass regional wall motion abnormalities in patients undergoing coronary artery bypass surgery. Anesthesiology 71:16, 1989.
13. Mangano D: Association of perioperative myocardial ischemia with cardiac morbidity and mortality in men undergoing noncardiac surgery. N Engl J Med 323:1781, 1990.
14. Matthay M: PA catheterization: Risks compared with benefits. Ann Intern Med 15:826, 1988.
15. Passimani E: TIMI-2 Pilot Study: TPA followed by PTCA. J Am Coll Cardiol 10:51B, 1987.
16. Resnekov L: Cardiogenic shock. Chest 83:893, 1983.
17. Topol EJ: Coronary angioplasty for acute MI. Ann Intern Med 109:970, 1988.

18. Willerson JT: Conversion from chronic to acute coronary artery disease: Speculation regarding mechanism. Am J Cardiol 54:1350, 1984.
19. Wolf PL: Common causes of false-positive CK-MB test for acute MI. Clin Lab Med 6:577, 1986.
20. Yusuf S: Reduction of infarct size, arrhythmias, and chest pain by early IV beta-blockade in suspected acute MI. Circulation 67(Suppl I):I-32, 1983.

32. ACUTE DYSRHYTHMIAS

Carter Willis, M.D.

1. Can you outline the normal cardiac conduction system?

First, pacemaker cells in the **sinoatrial (SA) node** spontaneously depolarize. Impulses are then conducted through nondiscrete atrial conduction tracts to the **atrioventricular (AV) node.** The **common bundle of His** is a thick, discrete tract that conducts from the AV node to the ventricles until it bifurcates into the **right** and **left bundle branches.** The left bundle branch is the larger of the two and divides again into a thick **anterior fascicle** and a thin **posterior fascicle.**

2. What are three fundamental mechanisms for generation of dysrhythmias?

Reentry, enhanced automaticity, and afterpolarizations → triggered activity.

3. How does reentry occur? What are some examples?

Reentry may occur on a large or small scale, i.e., **macroreentry** or **microreentry,** depending on the size of the circuit. Atrial and ventricular flutter and fibrillation are probably examples of microreentry circuits due to dispersion of refractoriness. Two frequently seen examples of macroreentry might include paroxysmal nodal supraventricular tachycardia (PSVT) and orthodromic Wolff-Parkinson-White (WPW) syndrome. The common elements in these examples include:

1. The existence of two parallel pathways with slightly different conduction speeds and recovery times (or refractory periods) allowing . . .

2. An atrial premature beat to establish unidirectional conduction block in one (beta-fast) pathway while anterograde conduction occurs in the other (alpha-slow) pathway.

3. Ventricular activation occurs and the **same action potential** is conducted retrograde by the fast pathway such that the tissue proximal to the block is reexcited and conducted anterograde again.

4. A macroreentrant loop has been established that will perpetuate itself.

4. What is enhanced automaticity?

The cardiac conduction system consists of two populations of physiologically different cells. The primary **pacemaker cells** of the SA and AV nodes may generate slow-response action potentials (APs) and have the ability to spontaneously depolarize, thus demonstrating automaticity. The **conducting cells** generate fast-response APs and also may spontaneously depolarize, but are normally overdriven by the dominant SA node. Under conditions of hypokalemia, hypoxemia, or catecholamine stress, phase 4 depolarization and threshold potential may be altered in the conducting cells (and myocardial cells), allowing them to develop enhanced automaticity and become **secondary ectopic pacemakers.** A good example of an automatic dysrhythmia would be a multifocal atrial tachycardia (MAT), which is usually due to multiple secondary ectopic atrial pacemakers associated with hypoxemia in patients with COPD.

5. What is the Vaughan-Williams classification of antidysrhythmic drugs?

In 1975 a scheme was devised by Vaughan-Williams whereby agents were grouped based on their effects on the intracellular AP. Some of the more commonly used agents are summarized below.

Commonly Used Antidysrhythmic Drugs

CLASS	SUBCLASS	AP EFFECT	EKG EFFECT	CARDIAC EFFECTS	USES
1. Membrane stabilizers (fast-channel sodium blockers)	A. Quinidine, procainamide, disopyramide	↓ phase 0 ↓ phase 4 ↑ duration ↑ threshold potential ↓ RMP	↑ QRS ↑↑ Q-T	↓ automaticity ↓ conductivity ↓ contractility	SVT VT WPW
	B. Lidocaine, tocainide, mexilitene, phenytoin	sl ↓ phase 0 ↓ phase 4 ↓ duration ↑ threshold potential	sl ↓ Q-T	↓ automaticity sl ↓ contractility sl ↑ AV conduction ↑ Fib threshold	VT
	C. Flecainide, encainide	↓↓ phase 0	↑↑ P-R ↑↑ QRS sl ↑ Q-T	↓ automaticity ↓↓ conductivity ↓ contractility ↓ AV conduction	VT WPW
2. Beta blockers	Propranolol, metoprolol, atenolol, esmolol	↓ phase 4 ↓ duration ↓ RMP	↑ P-R sl ↓ Q-T	↓ automaticity ↓ conductivity ↓↓ contractility ↓↓ AV conduction	SVT VT WPW
3. Neural adrenergic antagonists	Bretylium, amiodarone	↓ phase 0 ↓ phase 4 ↑↑ duration	↑ P-R sl ↑ QRS ↑ Q-T	↓ automaticity ↓ conductivity ↑ Fib threshold	SVT VT WPW
4. Slow-channel calcium antagonists	Verapamil, diltiazem	↓ phase 4 ↓ duration ↓ RMP	↑ P-R sl ↑ Q-T	↓ automaticity ↓ conductivity ↓ contractility ↓↓ AV conduction	SVT WPW

AP = action potential; RMP = resting membrane potential; sl = sublingual.

6. How would you rapidly evaluate a patient with an acute onset of a new dysrhythmia?

The first thing to do is to take 10 seconds to talk with the patient (if he or she is conscious). If **mentation** is compromised or syncope has occurred, this implies inadequate cerebral perfusion and the patient should be cardioverted emergently. If mentation is acceptable, then **check blood pressure and heart rate and apply oxygen** while asking about **chest pain and dyspnea.** Do a 12-lead EKG, listen to the chest, and attach a pulse oximeter. If the patient is having angina or developing pulmonary edema, cardioversion is urgently needed, preferably after an amnestic agent has been given (if the clinical situation will allow this). If the patient is just sensing **palpitations,** then provide reassurance and take a quick history while examining the 12-lead EKG.

7. When should physical maneuvers be employed to terminate a dysrhythmia?

Vagotonic maneuvers such as Valsalva, carotid massage, and the diving reflex are indicated as first-line therapy for SVTs in conscious, cooperative patients. For paroxysmal SVTs, the Valsalva maneuver in the supine position may be highly effective (54%), whereas the diving reflex may be less effective (17%) but equal to carotid massage (17%). Carotid massage should not be used in patients with known or suspected carotid vascular disease. Use of the diving reflex involves complete facial immersion in a pan or bucket of ice cold water, and some patients may find this unappealing.

8. When is direct current (DC) cardioversion indicated?
Elective DC cardioversion is frequently used to treat **atrial fibrillation.** An initial energy level would be 50–100 joules, with higher levels occasionally required. **Atrial flutter** is readily responsive to cardioversion, often requiring only 10–50 J. **Microreentrant SVTs** frequently respond to cardioversion at levels of 25–100 J. Cardioversion using 50–100 J may be used for patients with stable **ventricular tachycardia (VT)** who have reasonable perfusion. **R-wave synchronization** should be used for all of these elective/urgent cardioversions. **Pulseless VT** is treated like **ventricular fibrillation (VF),** i.e., with emergent nonsynchronized cardioversion with 200–300 J; if no immediate response, then 360 J should be administered.

9. Under what circumstances is DC cardioversion either not indicated or contraindicated?
- Any nonsustained tachycardia
- AV block
- MAT or other automatic tachycardias—not effective due to rapid recurrence
- Digitalis toxicity (cardioversion may lead to VF/VT asystole)

10. What are the potential complications of cardioversion?
- Chest wall soreness
- Elevation of serum enzymes (LDH, SGOT, CPK), reflecting myocardial damage
- Induced dysrhythmias—ectopic beats and short pauses are common, but VT, VF, and asystole are rare with the use of synchronization
- Systemic and pulmonary embolism have been reported.

11. When should you treat patients with premature ventricular complexes (PVCs)?
In survivors of myocardial infarction (MI), patients with complex PVCs have been shown to have an increased risk of sudden death for up to 24 months after infarction. **Lown's grading system** is commonly used as an approximate means of correlating the severity of this ectopy with the risk of sudden death.

Lown's Grading System

GRADE	DESCRIPTION OF PVCs
0	None
1	Uniform $< 30/hr$
2	Uniform $> 30/hr$
3	Multiform
4a	Couplets
4b	Triplets or greater
5	R-on-T phenomena

Studies suggest that suppression of ectopy in post-MI patients may lessen the risk of sudden death. Thus, oral antidysrhythmic therapy is generally indicated for grade 3 ectopy or greater.

Controversial: It is unclear whether similar chronic ectopy has any prognostic value in non-MI patients, and thus the value of treatment also remains unclear.

12. Distinguish PVCs from premature atrial contractions (PACs).
PVCs typically yield a bizarre, wide (> 0.12) QRS complex, with the ST segment usually sloping off in an opposite direction from the main QRS vector. Because a PVC may occur

simultaneously with atrial activity, the P wave can be lost in the QRS complex, although rarely you may see retrograde conduction in the form of an inverted P wave following the PVC. PVCs are often followed by a fully compensatory pause; the SA node is not reset, such that the next sinus beat occurs in rhythm with the preceding atrial activity (you can march out the P waves).

PACs are often preceded by an abnormal, inverted, premature P wave. The QRS complex is generally narrow and similar to that of the preceding sinus beats. PACs reset the SA node, such that the next sinus beat does not occur in synchrony with the preceding atrial activity (you cannot march out the P waves).

13. Is prophylaxis for ventricular fibrillation indicated in the setting of an acute MI?

VF is the most dreaded dysrhythmic complication of acute MI; 50% of deaths in acute MI occur within the first 2 hours due to VF. VF may be heralded by warning dysrhythmias such as uniform PVCs, multiform PVCs, R-on-T PVCs, or VT. However, primary VF occurring without warning dysrhythmias may also develop in up to 20% of patients, so prophylactic therapy is used for the first 24–48 hours in some centers. The most commonly used agent is lidocaine (50–100 mg IV bolus followed by infusion of 1–4 mg/min).

14. How is lidocaine metabolized? What are the risk factors for toxicity?

Lidocaine undergoes oxidative dealkylation in the **liver** and has a plasma half-life of 1.5–2 hours. Any condition that decreases hepatic function or reduces hepatic blood flow may reduce elimination and increase half-life, resulting in potential accumulation and toxicity, including:

Hepatitis or cirrhosis
Age > 65 years
Congestive heart failure
Shock (cardiogenic, septic, hypovolemic)
Major abdominal surgery

Serum levels should be checked regularly in patients at risk for accumulation and toxicity. Therapeutic effect is achieved at levels of 1.5–6 $\mu g/ml$, and toxicity is generally avoided if levels are kept < 6 $\mu g/ml$.

15. What are the signs and symptoms of lidocaine toxicity?

The first symptom is often confusion, agitation, or euphoria. Other early findings might include dizziness, tinnitus, nausea ± vomiting, diplopia, and tremors or twitching. Toxic patients may deteriorate to unconsciousness and convulsions, with respiratory and cardiac depression leading to full arrest.

16. What are afterdepolarizations? How do they result in triggered activity?

Afterdepolarizations (ADs) are depolarizations following the action potential. They are also referred to as **oscillatory afterpotentials.** Early ADs may occur in phase 3 of the cardiac AP and late ADs may occur in phase 4 of the AP. Each of these may result in **triggered activity.** A triggered focus differs from an automatic focus in that it **does not initiate spontaneous APs, but may result from an AP.** ADs are normally subthreshold, but under certain conditions they may exceed threshold potential, leading to repetitive cycles of **nondriven impulses.** These are different from the driven impulses that originate from a pacemaker cell. Typical conditions that may increase the amplitude of ADs include hypokalemia, hypomagnesemia, hypercalcemia, ischemia, catecholamine excess, premature beats, slow heart rate, and drugs (such as type 1A antidysrhythmics). Triggered activity has been implicated as a cause of polymorphic VT and monomorphic VT, but may also cause SVTs.

Sustained, triggered dysrhythmias are not caused by reentry or enhanced automaticity, but instead appear to be perpetuated by repetitive ADs.

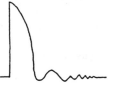

or

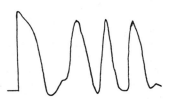

Subthreshold afterdepolarizations

Afterdepolarizations giving rise to multiple nondriven impulses

17. What is torsade de pointes?
First described in 1966, it literally means "twisting of the points." This is an appropriate description for polymorphic VT that rotates around the isoelectric line of the EKG, thus continually changing its axis.

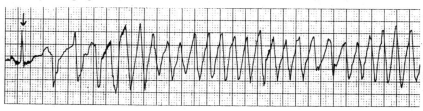

18. What causes torsade de pointes?
It is associated with the congenital prolonged Q-T syndromes (Romano-Ward and Lange-Nielsen) and underlying ischemic cardiac disease. It may be caused by bradycardia (Q-T interval is heart rate dependent) and electrolyte imbalances that prolong Q-T (hypomagnesemia, hypocalcemia, hypokalemia). Drug therapy that prolongs Q-T is a common cause (types 1A, 1C, and 3 antidysrhythmics, phenothiazines, and tricyclic antidepressants). Quinidine and procainamide are most commonly implicated in drug-induced torsade, and this may be the underlying mechanism of so-called quinidine syncope.

19. How is the treatment of torsade different from that of other VTs?
Torsade is generally self-terminating and tends to subside spontaneously after some seconds or minutes unless coronary perfusion is compromised, in which case there may be secondary degeneration to VF. If the episode of torsade is sustained, emergent DC cardioversion with 100 J or more is the treatment of choice. Follow up immediately with rapid overdrive transcutaneous pacing at 100+ or use isoproterenol as a pacing agent until a temporary transvenous pacemaker can be placed. Pacing will shorten the Q-T and prevent recurrence of torsade while you isolate and treat the underlying problem. Any potential offending drug should be discontinued and electrolyte disorders should be corrected.

20. How can you differentiate VT from a wide-complex SVT?
The clinical presentation may not always be helpful. Both may be regular in rhythm, have paroxysmal onset, or cause hypotension. The 12-lead EKG should be closely examined, as the following features may help to clarify the diagnosis:
- Presence of atrioventricular dissociation indicates VT.
- QRS width > 0.14 favors VT in the absence of preexisting bundle branch block or accessory conduction pathway. QRS width < 0.12 favors SVT.

- Left-axis deviation $> 30°$ favors VT in the absence of preexisting bundle branch block or accessory conduction pathway.
- Presence of fusion or capture beats favors VT.
- QRS configuration in V_1:

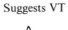

Suggests VT   Suggests SVT

21. Why is it therapeutically important to differentiate VT from SVT?

Misdiagnosis of wide-complex tachycardia may lead to misdirected therapy and consequent poor outcome. Administration of verapamil to patients with VT is frequently followed by hypotension ($> 85\%$ of patients) or degeneration of the rhythm to ventricular fibrillation or asystole (20% of patients). When in doubt, some physicians recommend using **procainamide** (100 mg IV q 5 min up to 1 gm loading dose followed by an infusion of 1–4 mg/min).

22. What is Ashman's phenomenon?

In 1947, a case was reported in which a man with atrial fibrillation (AF) was treated with quinidine and developed aberrantly conducted beats in a right bundle branch block (RBBB) pattern that mimicked VT. The aberrantly conducted beats occurred as singlets, couplets, and in long runs, but were always preceded by a long R-R interval followed by a short R-R interval.

Ashman's phenomenon occurs when a descending impulse finds one of the bundle branches still in its effective refractory period (ERP) and is blocked on that side while conducting down the other side (usually the right side is blocked). This phenomenon can be perpetuated by the impulse being conducted through the septum from LV to RV and then back up the right bundle to the His bundle, where it is blocked because the main bundle is now refractory. A second, atrial-driven impulse descends and the same conduction pattern is encountered. The fact that the refractory period varies with cycle length accounts for the long-short initiation sequence.

23. What is preexcitation? How do patients present with it?

Preexcitation exists when, in relation to atrial events, the whole or some part of the ventricular muscle is activated earlier by the impulse originating in the atria than would be expected if the impulse reached the ventricles by way of the normal cardiac conduction system alone. Patients with preexcitation dysrhythmias typically present with recurrent paroxysmal tachycardias, but are at risk for sudden death.

24. How frequently does WPW occur?

The reported incidence of the classic WPW electrocardiogram is 1–3 per 1000 population, and paroxysmal tachycardias are noted in about 40–80% of patients with this abnormal EKG pattern.

25. What are the three most common types of preexcitation?

1. The typical anatomy seen in the WPW syndrome first described in 1930 involves an electrically conductive muscle bridge (Kent bundle) connecting the atria and ventricle that bypasses the AV node. During sinus rhythm, the surface EKG will show a shortened P-R interval ($< .12$ msec), a slurred QRS upstroke (delta wave), and a widened QRS

complex (> .12 msec; fusion beat). These occur because the accessory bypass tract (BT) conducts more rapidly than the normal system and ventricular activation occurs from two separate points in an anomalous fashion. WPW is by far the most common type of preexcitation.

2. In the Lown-Ganong-Levine syndrome (LGL), first reported in 1952, James fibers create an atrio–His bundle tract, which bypasses the AV node, leading to a shortening of the P-R interval without a delta wave or widened QRS.

3. A third type of preexcitation involves a His bundle–ventricular bypass tract called a Mahaim fiber. All known Mahaim fibers have extended from the His bundle to the right ventricular myocardium, resulting in a normal P-R interval with a widened QRS in the configuration of a left bundle branch block. A slurred QRS upstroke (delta wave) may also be seen.

26. How many conduction patterns are possible with WPW?

Obviously, there are two possible conduction patterns, and the direction in which conduction occurs may be based on the conduction speeds and ERPs of the two possible paths. The normal cardiac conduction system is generally the slow pathway, and the BT is usually the fast pathway. If the AP is conducted anterograde down the AV node and back through the BT, you will usually see a narrow-complex SVT (rate 120–220, usually < 200) without the stigmata of preexcitation (so-called orthodromic conduction). Inverted, retrograde P waves following the QRS in the inferior leads are typical of this conduction pattern and may be one clue to the diagnosis. Patients with slower rates may present only with palpitations, but even in the absence of coronary artery disease or cerebrovascular disease, when the rate of SVT is > 180, up to 50% of patients may experience syncope, dyspnea, or chest pain. So this rhythm can cause some problems.

On the other side of things, if the AP is conducted down the BT to the ventricle and back up the AV node (so-called antidromic conduction) you can see wide-complex, very fast (rate 220–300) rhythms that may mimic VT and usually cause some immediate symptoms. If you look closely, the rhythm may be slightly irregular, as this conduction pattern is often seen with atrial fibrillation . . . and the delta wave may be present.

To complicate matters, patients with WPW may also have sinus tachycardias. Take a look at the following table for a quick summary.

	ONSET	DELTA WAVE	QRS	REGULAR
Sinus tachycardia	gradual	+	wide	+
Orthodromic PSVT	paroxysmal	–	narrow	+
Antidromic PSVT	paroxysmal	+	wide	±

27. Can you identify WPW patients at risk for sudden death?

Sudden death probably occurs as a consequence of induced VF. The pathogenesis of the VF is unclear, but is probably related to an impulse entering the ventricle during the vulnerable period or simply 1:1 conduction of AF via the BT. Klein examined 31 WPW patients with documented prior VF and noted several common elements in these patients when compared to a control group of 73 WPW patients without a history of VF:

1. AF with rapid ventricular response preceded VF in 25 of 31 patients.
2. The VF group had a significantly higher incidence of multiple bypass tracts.
3. Patients in the VF group had significantly faster conduction times and shorter ERPs.
4. VF occurred shortly after digitalis was used for treatment of AF in 6 patients.

Use of digoxin is contraindicated in WPW patients with a history of AF and an antidromic conduction pattern.

28. How do you treat WPW acutely?

Recommendations for initial therapy in the acute setting depend on the presenting dysrhythmia. The narrow-complex, regular tachycardia should be treated first with **vagal maneuvers** in the awake, cooperative patient. If this fails, then drugs are the next step, and **adenosine** (Adenocard) would be a good choice, although other drugs that block the AV node can be used such as verapamil, propranolol, and digoxin. Adenosine has an extremely high success rate for treatment of this dysrhythmia. Procainamide, quinidine edrophonium bromide (Tensilon), and phenylephrine have also been used successfully.

The wide-complex, irregular tachycardia is unlikely to respond to vagal maneuvers and generally requires rapid, aggressive treatment as this rhythm may herald the onset of VF. Group 1A drugs such as **procainamide** and **quinidine** have been the drugs of choice in the past, acting to slow conduction and increase ERP in the BT. Adenosine, 6–12 mg IV, is also highly effective for this reentrant dysrhythmia but it will not convert the AF. It may just temporarily break the reentry cycle. **Digoxin and verapamil are contraindicated in this setting.** McGovern reported on a small series of WPW patients with AF degenerating to VF after receiving verapamil. Long-term oral drug therapy often consists of procainamide, quinidine, amiodarone, or flecainide.

Always remember that cardioversion can be effectively used for WPW as outlined previously.

29. What are the indications for transvenous pacing in acute MI?

- Profound sinus bradycardia resistant to atropine with hypoperfusion
- Junctional rhythm with hypoperfusion
- Mobitz type I block (may be observed)
- Mobitz type II block
- New LBBB
- New RBBB with anterior MI
- New RBBB with inferior MI—often transient and may be observed
- New bifascicular block (new RBBB + LAFB or new RBBB + LPFB)
- Complete heart block

30. What is adenosine? Its mechanism of action?

Adenosine (Adenocard) remains unclassified as an antidysrhythmic drug. It is an endogenous purine nucleotide occurring in all cells of the body. The mechanism of action of exogenously administered adenosine probably involves binding to extracellular purine receptors, resulting in inhibition of adenylate cyclase and leading to decreased intracellular cAMP. Phosphodiesterase inhibitors, which elevate cAMP, will oppose the effects of adenosine and, in fact, theophylline and caffeine are adenosine antagonists. Exogenously administered adenosine has a half-life of < 10 seconds. Its effects are terminated by cellular uptake (by RBCs and endothelial cells) and enzymatic degradation (adenosine kinase converts to AMP; adenosine deaminase converts to inosine). Adenosine is not dependent on any organ system for metabolism. In the cardiovascular system, it has been shown to:

- Depress SA node automaticity
- **Suppress AV node conduction**
- Depress ventricular automaticity
- Attenuate the stimulatory effects of catechols on ventricular myocardium
- Reduce ADs and triggered activity due to catecholamines
- Cause coronary and systemic vasodilatation

31. Is adenosine useful for dysrhythmia termination?

Comparison of large numbers of patients presenting with various types of PSVTs shows that response rates for adenosine, 12 mg IV (93%), are similar to those for verapamil, 7.5 mg IV (91%). Time to conversion with adenosine is considerably shorter than with verapamil (seconds compared to minutes). Adenosine is highly effective and somewhat specific for macroreentrant SVTs involving the AV node or an accessory BT. It will not convert atrial fibrillation/flutter, but it will produce transient high-grade AV block. It is not effective for ventricular dysrhythmias. Adverse effects with adenosine are transient (< 60 seconds) and include flushing, dyspnea, and chest pain or pressure. Transient dysrhythmias may be seen in up to 45% of patients, including PVCs, bradycardias, complete AV block, asystole, and atrial fibrillation/flutter.

32. What is the dysrhythmia in the following 12-lead EKG?

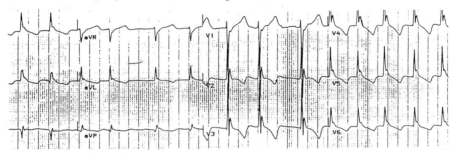

This is not a dysrhythmia. These are Osborne waves, which may be seen with varying degrees of hypothermia. They resolve gradually with rewarming and do not require any specific treatment.

33. What is the conduction pattern in the following EKG?

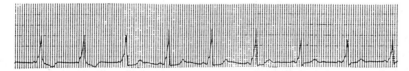

This is the classic WPW EKG, as evidenced by the presence of a short P-R interval, delta wave, and widened QRS. This patient also had episodes of paroxysmal tachycardia.

34. What is the dysrhythmia in the following EKG?

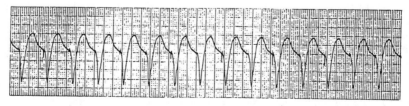

This patient has a functional ventricular pacemaker. Notice the pacer spikes preceding each QRS complex.

35. What is the dysrhythmia in the following EKG?

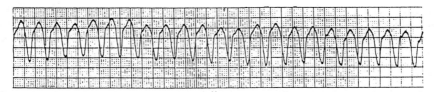

This patient had pulseless VT, which was successfully cardioverted. The rhythm is fast (about 160–180), regular, and monomorphic.

BIBLIOGRAPHY

1. Dessertenne F: La tachycardie ventriculaire a deux foyers opposés variables. Arch Mal Coeur 59:263–272, 1966.
2. DiMarco JP: Adenosine for pSVT: Dose ranging and comparison with verapamil. Assessment in placebo-controlled, multicenter trial. Ann Intern Med 113:104, 1990.
3. Gallagher JJ: The Wolfe-Parkinson-White syndrome and the preexcitation dysrhythmias. Med Clin North Am 60:101, 1976.
4. Gouaux JL, Ashman R: Auricular fibrillation with aberration simulating ventricular tachycardia. Am Heart J 30:366, 1947.
5. Hurst JW: The Heart, 7th ed. New York, McGraw-Hill, 1990.
6. Kay GN: Torsade de pointes: The long-short initiating sequence and other clinical features: Observations in 32 patients. J Am Coll Cardiol 2:806, 1983.
7. Klein GJ: Ventricular fibrillation in the WPW syndrome. N Engl J Med 301:1080, 1979.
8. Lown B: Approaches to sudden death from coronary heart disease. Circulation 48:130, 1971.
9. McGovern B: Precipitation of cardiac arrest by verapamil in patients with WPW syndrome. Ann Intern Med 104:791, 1986.
10. Mehta D: Relative efficacy of various physical maneuvers in the termination of junctional tachycardia. Lancet 1988, p 1181.
11. Stewart RB: Wide-complex tachycardia: Misdiagnosis and outcome after emergent therapy. Ann Intern Med 104:766, 1986.
12. Vaughan-Williams EM: Classification of antiarrhythmic drugs. J Pharmacol Ther 1:115, 1975.
13. Wellens JJ: The value of the electrocardiogram in the differential diagnosis of a tachycardia with a widened QRS complex. Am J Med 64:27, 1978.

33. AORTIC DISSECTION

David E. Schwartz, M.D.

1. What is aortic dissection?

Dissection of the aorta occurs with a tear in the intima of the artery. Blood is propelled under pressure through the tear and dissects into the media of the aorta. The hematoma can progress along the course of the aorta and occlude any of the arterial branches of the aorta, including branches of the arch of the aorta or the mesenteric arteries. Retrograde dissection can involve the coronary arteries. The right coronary artery is more frequently involved than the left. Retrograde dissection can also result in loss of commissural support for one or more of the aortic valve cusps and result in acute aortic insufficiency.

The false channel that is created is located in the outer half of the aortic media. The outer wall of this channel is only one-fourth as thick as the original media. This explains the high frequency of rupture of the aorta in patients with aortic dissection. Rupture of the aortic arch occurs most frequently into the mediastinum, the descending thoracic aorta into the left pleural space, and the abdominal aorta into the retroperitoneum. Because the parietal pericardium is attached to the ascending aorta just proximal to the origin of the innominate artery, rupture of any portion of the ascending aorta can lead to cardiac tamponade from hemopericardium.

2. Where is the intimal tear located?
In approximately 70% of patients, the intimal tear, which is the beginning of the dissection, is located in the ascending aorta. In 10% of patients, the laceration is located in the aortic arch, and in approximately 20% of patients the tear is in the descending thoracic aorta. Only rarely is an intimal tear identified in the abdominal aorta.

3. What are the frequency and mortality of aortic dissection?
There are at least 2,000 new cases of aortic dissection in the United States every year. If untreated, aortic dissection has a mortality rate of 90% in three months.

4. What factors predispose to aortic dissection?
Hypertension is the most important etiologic factor; it is present in 70–90% of patients who develop dissection. **Congenital disorders** associated with aortic dissection include Marfan syndrome, Ehlers-Danlos syndrome, a congenitally bicuspid aortic valve, aortic coarctation, Turner syndrome, giant-cell aortitis, and relapsing polychondritis. There is also an association with **pregnancy**. Half of all dissections in women under the age of 40 have been reported to occur during pregnancy, most frequently in the third trimester. In addition, aortic dissection **following medical or surgical procedures** has been described. These include procedures in which the aorta has been entered, in which aortic counterpulsation devices have been inserted, and in which the aorta or its main branches have been cannulated. Trauma is an infrequent cause of aortic dissection. Pathologically aortic dissection is associated with cystic medial necrosis. Dissections are more frequent in males, with a male to female ratio of 3:1.

5. How has aortic dissection been classified?
The first classification system for aortic dissection was that of DeBakey. He described three types of aortic dissection. In Type I the dissection begins in the aortic root and extends beyond the ascending aorta. Type II is confined to the ascending aorta. Type III dissections begin distal to the takeoff of the left subclavian artery. In Type IIIA the dissection is limited to the thoracic aorta, whereas a Type IIIB dissection descends below the diaphragm. Rarely Type III dissections progress retrograde toward the aortic arch and ascending aorta. A simpler classification system has more recently been described. Type A dissections involve the ascending aorta, and Type B dissections are distal to the left subclavian artery.

6. What are the clinical features of aortic dissection?
The most striking clinical manifestation of acute aortic dissection is the abrupt onset of symptoms. Some features of the pain of aortic dissection may be helpful in differentiating it from other causes of acute pain, including myocardial infarction. The onset of sudden severe chest pain usually heralds aortic dissection. Pain may be present in up to 90% of patients. Patients with aortic dissection often localize the pain in the anterior chest with extension to the back. They frequently describe the pain as ripping or tearing in quality. The pain is usually of maximal intensity from its inception and is frequently unremitting. The pain may migrate along the path of the dissection. This contrasts to the pain of myocardial infarction, which has more of a crescendo nature and is frequently described as pressure or a crushing sensation.

Symptoms of heart failure may be due to the development of acute aortic insufficiency. Patients may also present with neurologic symptoms such as syncope, stroke, a peripheral neuropathy from ischemia, and lower-extremity weakness due to compromise of arterial blood flow to the spinal cord. Syncope is felt to be an ominous sign. It is frequently associated with rupture of the dissection into the pericardial space.

7. What physical findings and clinical manifestations are suggestive of aortic dissection?
On physical examination patients with aortic dissection may appear to be in shock. However, more than half of patients with distal dissection are hypertensive. Hypotension suggests cardiac tamponade, rupture of the dissection into the intrapleural or intraperitoneal spaces, or occlusion of the brachial arteries resulting in "pseudohypotension." The loss of peripheral pulses is an important clue to presence of an aortic dissection. This occurs in approximately one-half of patients with proximal dissection and signifies involvement of the brachiocephalic vessels. Only one-sixth of patients with a distal dissection have diminution of a peripheral pulse.

Acute aortic regurgitation may be present in 50% of patients with proximal dissection and can be due to simple widening of the aortic annulus or actual disruption of the aortic valve leaflets. Cardiac tamponade and pleural effusions may indicate rupture of the aortic dissection. These findings portend a poor prognosis and should be searched for carefully. Pleural effusions, which occur most frequently in the left chest, can be caused by rupture of the dissection into the pleural space or from weeping of fluid from the aorta as the result of an inflammatory reaction to the dissection.

Additional physical findings include Horner's syndrome, caused by compression of the cervical sympathetic ganglion, mottling of the flanks, which suggests rupturing of the aneurysm into the retroperitoneal space, and myocardial infarction due to dissection of the coronary arteries. The right coronary artery is most frequently involved, and myocardial infarction is seen in 1–2% of patients with dissection. Mesenteric ischemia or infarction occurs in less than 1% of patients. Severe hypertension with diastolic pressure as high as 160 mm Hg has been encountered in patients with distal dissections. This severe hypertension may be secondary to renal ischemia. Hypotension is an ominous finding and is detected in approximately one-fifth of patients with an ascending aortic dissection. It is suggestive of external rupture or cardiac tamponade.

Other less frequent manifestations of aortic dissection include vocal cord paralysis from compression of the left recurrent laryngeal nerve, compression of the pulmonary arteries by the expanding aorta, and complete heart block from extension of the aortic hematoma into the area of the atrioventricular node. Hemoptysis from rupture into the tracheal bronchial tree and hematemesis from perforation into the esophagus have been reported.

8. What laboratory and radiologic data are helpful in confirming the diagnosis of aortic dissection?
Laboratory data are usually unrevealing. Patients may be anemic due to loss of blood into the false lumen of the dissection. Patients may have moderate leukocytosis with white blood cell counts of 10,000–14,000 white cells/ml. Lactic acid dehydrogenase and bilirubin levels are sometimes elevated because of hemolysis within the false lumen. Disseminated intravascular coagulation has been reported. The electrocardiogram may be helpful because it shows no signs of ischemia in a patient with severe chest pain. This should suggest the diagnosis of aortic dissection.

Radiographic examination of the chest often provides valuable information. In 90% of patients there is an abnormality in the aorta seen on chest x-ray. Most frequently this is simply widening of the aorta and the mediastinum. The most specific sign on chest x-ray may be separation of calcium that is present in the intima of the aorta from the outer border of the false channel. Normally this distance is no more than 0.5 cm. A distance greater than 1 cm is highly suggestive of aortic dissection—the so-called calcium sign.

9. Which techniques are useful in making the diagnosis of aortic dissection?

Angiography is the definitive modality for diagnosing aortic dissection. It has a diagnostic accuracy of 95–99%. The site of the origin of the dissection, the extent of the dissection, and the integrity of the principal arterial trunks that arise from the aorta can be derived from an angiogram. Frequently both the true and false aortic channels can be identified. Other clues to the presence of an aortic dissection include a linear lucency, which represents the aortic intima and media separating the two channels, distortion of the contrast column, and flow reversal or stasis in the aorta. Insufficiency of the aortic valve can also be demonstrated by angiography. Although aortography remains the gold standard, there is a false-negative rate of approximately 2%.

Other imaging techniques include computed tomography (CT), two-dimensional echocardiography, transesophageal echocardiography, and magnetic resonance imaging (MRI). When CT scans are obtained with contrast material, aortic dissection can be demonstrated as two channels within the aortic silhouette. The diagnostic accuracy of CT scanning is about 90%. CT scans have occasionally shown aortic dissections that were not visible on angiography. However, CT scanning does not reveal the point of origin of the dissection or quantify the aortic insufficiency that may be present. CT scanning is most helpful in following patients in whom the diagnosis has already been made and who are being treated medically.

Two-dimensional echocardiography is also useful in diagnosing aortic dissection.

Transesophageal echocardiography, a recently described technique, may prove to be useful in the diagnosis of dissecting thoracic aneurysms. The entire descending thoracic aorta, portions of the aortic arch, and the aortic root can be readily visualized. Combining this technique with transthoracic echocardiography should allow both the ascending and descending aorta to the level of the diaphragm to be well visualized.

MRI can be used in the diagnosis of aortic dissection. It shows not only the anatomy of the aorta itself but also its major arterial branches. The usefulness of MRI may be limited by the inability of critically ill patients to tolerate the long duration required to obtain the image.

10. What should be considered in the differential diagnosis of aortic dissection?

The differential diagnosis of acute aortic dissection includes acute myocardial infarction, pulmonary embolism, cerebrovascular accidents, acute aortic regurgitation, thoracic nondissecting aneurysm, mediastinal cysts or tumors, pericarditis, cholecystitis, pleuritis, musculoskeletal pain, and atherosclerotic emboli.

11. How should patients in whom acute aortic dissection is suspected be managed?

The initial management is directed at halting the progression of the dissection. The patient's condition should be stabilized prior to additional studies to confirm the diagnosis. A cardiothoracic surgeon should be consulted immediately. Patients should be admitted to an intensive care unit for monitoring and therapy. The patient's clinical condition and symptoms, as well as blood pressure, cardiac rhythm, and urine output, should be monitored carefully. It may be necessary to monitor central venous pressure and/or pulmonary artery pressures and cardiac output. An intraarterial catheter should be placed to monitor blood pressure.

The initial goals of medical therapy are to treat hypertension, decrease the velocity of left ventricular ejection, and treat the patient's pain. Most authorities believe that systolic blood pressure should be lowered to 100–120 mm Hg, a mean pressure of 60–65 mm Hg, or to the lowest level that is compatible with perfusion of the vital organs. Wheat and associates were the first to describe the successful reduction in the frequency of aortic rupture by aggressively lowering arterial blood pressure. These investigators pointed out the importance of the rate of rise of aortic pressure as the component of stress on the aortic wall that may cause and propagate a dissection.

In addition to management of blood pressure, supportive care should include determining if the patient has myocardial ischemia or infarction, and making sure that sufficient blood is available in the blood bank in case of rupture of the dissection.

12. What is the role of sodium nitroprusside in management of acute aortic dissection?
Sodium nitroprusside is a potent vasodilator and is recommended as the initial therapy to lower blood pressure. However, this drug alone can cause an increase in the velocity of left ventricular ejection and could potentially contribute to worsening of the dissection. Thus therapy with this drug should be combined with the use of a beta-adrenergic blocking agent. The most commonly employed beta blocker is propranolol, and the recommended dose is 0.05–0.15 mg/kg of body weight every 4–6 hours. A test dose of 0.5 mg should be administered intravenously, and then doses of 1 mg administered intravenously to obtain a heart rate of 60–80 beats per minute. Propranolol may be contraindicated in the presence of bradycardia, asthma, and heart failure. There is not as much experience with other beta blockers in the treatment of aortic dissection, but there is no reason to believe that they would not be effective in this condition.

Sodium nitroprusside acts directly on smooth muscles, causing both arterial and venous dilatation. It lowers blood pressure within 1–2 minutes of beginning the infusion, and the effect dissipates within 2 minutes after the infusion has stopped. The initial dose is 0.25–0.5 μg/kg/min, titrated slowly to control blood pressure. The side effects of this drug include nausea, restlessness, somnolence, and hypotension. The potential for cyanide and/or thiocyanate toxicity exists.

13. Are there alternatives to sodium nitroprusside?
Yes. If nitroprusside is ineffective or poorly tolerated by a patient, then most authorities believe that trimethaphan, a ganglionic blocking agent, should be used. The initial infusion rate is 1 mg/min, and the dose should be titrated to blood pressure. This drug has the advantage of decreasing left ventricular ejection, and beta blockade is not necessary. Complications of this drug include profound hypotension, tachyphylaxis to its effect, somnolence, and sympathoplegia with constipation, urinary retention, ileus, and pupillary dilatation. This drug is usually not effective for more than 48 hours. Other agents that have been used to treat acute aortic dissection include reserpine and calcium channel antagonists.

14. What are the toxic complications of sodium nitroprusside therapy? How are they recognized and treated?
Cyanide and thiocyanate toxicity. It is recommended that doses no larger than 10 μg/kg/min be administered to patients and that the total dose given not exceed 3–3.5 mg/kg. Cyanide toxicity can be recognized by increasing tolerance to the drug, elevated mixed venous oxygen content, and the development of lactic acidosis. Thiocyanate toxicity is characterized by muscle weakness, hyperreflexia, confusion, delirium, and coma. When the drug is being infused at rates higher than 3 μg/kg for periods exceeding 72 hours, thiocyanate levels should be measured. Thiocyanate levels below 10 mg/100 ml are generally well tolerated. Cyanide poisoning can be treated with amyl nitrite, sodium nitrite, and sodium thiosulfate. For patients with severe thiocyanate toxicity, hemodialysis has been performed.

15. Once the patient has been stabilized medically, what are the options for therapy?
There is now general agreement that patients with a proximal (Type A) dissection should be treated surgically, whereas patients with acute distal (Type B) dissections may be

managed medically. The goals of surgical therapy are to resect the aortic segment containing the proximal intimal tear, to obliterate the false channel, and to restore aortic continuity by employing a graft or reapproximating the transected ends of the aorta. In most cases of proximal aortic dissection, cardiopulmonary bypass is employed. For patients with aortic insufficiency, it may be possible to resuspend the aortic valve, but in some cases, replacement of the aortic valve is necessary. In some cases of proximal dissection, reimplantation of the coronary arteries may be required. The surgical mortality for patients with Type A dissection is approximately 15–20% in the medical centers with the most experience.

Definitive therapy for Type B dissection is usually medical. Wheat and colleagues in 1965 described a series of patients with distal dissections who were successfully treated medically. Surgery is indicated if medical therapy is failing. This would include evidence of continued dissection, rupture, ischemia of an organ or extremity due to the dissection, and pain that is not relieved with medical therapy. It is felt that patients with distal dissection do better with medical therapy than with surgical therapy because they tend to be older, have extensive atherosclerotic vascular disease, and have complicating medical conditions including cardiac and pulmonary disease. Most patients with distal dissection can be managed medically; however, one-third of patients will eventually require surgery for an enlarging aneurysm and/or dissection. Patients with distal dissection are treated chronically with beta blockers and other standard antihypertensive medications. They should be followed closely for progression of their dissection, with frequent visits to their physician and noninvasive assessment of the extent of the dissection.

BIBLIOGRAPHY

1. Chaudhry A, Romereo L, Pugatch RD, et al: Diagnosis of aortic dissection by computed tomography. Ann Thorac Surg 35:322–325, 1983.
2. DeSanctis RW, Doroghazi RM, Austen WG, Buckley MJ: Aortic dissection. N Engl J Med 317:1060–1067, 1987.
3. Doroghazi RM, Slater EE, DeSanctis RW, et al: Long-term survival of patients with treated aortic dissection. J Am Coll Cardiol 3:1026–1034, 1984.
4. Eagle KA, Quetermous T, Kritzer GA, et al: Spectrum of conditions initially suggesting acute aortic dissection but with negative aortograms. Am J Cardiol 57:322–326, 1986.
5. Granato JE, Dee P, Gibson R: Utility of two-dimensional echocardiography in suspected ascending aortic dissection. Am J Cardiol 56:123–129, 1985.
6. Larson EW, Edwards WD: Risk factors for aortic dissection: A necropsy study of 161 cases. Am J Cardiol 53:849–855, 1984.
7. Pumphrey CW, Fay T, Weir I: Aortic dissection during pregnancy. Br Heart J 55:106–108, 1986.
8. Roberts WC: Aortic dissection: Anatomy, consequences, and causes. Am Heart J 101:195–214, 1981.
9. Slater EE, DeSanctis RW: The clinical recognition of dissecting aortic aneurysm. Am J Med 60:625–633, 1976.
10. Tinker JH, Michenfelder JD: Sodium nitroprusside: Pharmacology, toxicology and therapeutics. Anesthesiology 45:340–354, 1976.
11. Wheat MW, Palmer RF, Bartley TD, Seelman RC: Treatment of dissecting aneurysms of the aorta without surgery. J Thorac Cardiovasc Surg 50:364–373, 1965.

34. VALVULAR HEART DISEASE

David E. Schwartz, M.D.

MITRAL STENOSIS

1. What are the causes of mitral stenosis?
Rheumatic heart disease is the most common cause. Congenital forms of mitral stenosis do occur in infants. Infrequently mitral stenosis is a complication of systemic lupus erythematosus, rheumatoid arthritis, and malignant carcinoid.

2. Does mitral stenosis usually occur alone?
Mitral stenosis is the sole valvular lesion in approximately 25% of patients with rheumatic heart disease, whereas an additional 40% have combined mitral stenosis and mitral regurgitation. Mitral stenosis and aortic regurgitation may also occur together.

3. Does mitral stenosis affect men or women more frequently?
Women are affected twice as frequently as men.

4. What is the latency period?
The latency period is between three and four decades between patients' initial episode of rheumatic fever and the development of symptomatic valvular heart disease.

5. What is the normal mitral valve area?
The normal mitral valve area is approximately 4 to 6 cm². When the valve area decreases to approximately 2 cm², mild mitral stenosis exists and an abnormal pressure gradient is generated between the left atrium and left ventricle.

6. What is critical mitral stenosis?
Mitral stenosis is considered critical when the valve area is less than 1 cm². With critical mitral stenosis there is usually a gradient of approximately 20 mm Hg between left atrial pressure and left ventricular diastolic pressure.

7. What are the pathophysiologic abnormalities associated with mitral stenosis?
As valve area decreases, a larger pressure gradient between the left atrium and the left ventricle is needed to generate flow, resulting in substantial elevations in left atrial pressure. This elevated pressure in turn raises pulmonary venous and capillary pressures. As pulmonary capillary pressure exceeds plasma oncotic pressure, fluid is filtered into the interstitium. As the pressure continues to rise, the pulmonary lymphatic system can no longer pump out this fluid and it begins to fill the lung interstitium and alveoli. Pulmonary arteriolar resistance increases and impedes right ventricular ejection. The right ventricle hypertrophies to meet this increased load. Eventually the ventricle dilates and fails. As left atrial pressure rises, the left atrium also dilates and becomes substantially enlarged, predisposing to the development of atrial fibrillation and the loss of effective atrial contraction. In most patients left ventricular diastolic pressure and volume are normal.

8. Why do patients with mitral stenosis tolerate tachycardia poorly?
As heart rate increases, diastole shortens more than systole. This decreases the time available for flow across a stenotic mitral valve. Left ventricular filling is impaired. In addition, patients with mitral stenosis do not tolerate atrial fibrillation. When atrial contraction is lost, cardiac output may be decreased by 20%. Thus, it is desirable to maintain both sinus rhythm and a slow heart rate.

9. What are the signs and symptoms of mitral stenosis?

Most patients report dyspnea and progressive limitations of physical exertion. Orthopnea, paroxysmal, nocturnal dyspnea, fatigue, weakness, and hemoptysis are also common. As mitral stenosis advances, symptoms of right heart failure occur, including nausea, anorexia, right upper quadrant pain, ascites, and peripheral edema. Hoarseness has also been described (Ortner's syndrome), and is thought to be due to compression of the left recurrent laryngeal nerve by a dilated left atrium or an enlarged pulmonary artery. Chest pain may occur and may be difficult to distinguish from classic angina pectoris. Thromboembolism is a serious complication of mitral stenosis and, prior to the development of surgical therapy, occurred in 20% of patients. Risk factors for embolization include age over 40 years, low cardiac output, and atrial fibrillation. Anticoagulation should be considered in such patients.

10. Describe the typical physical examination of a patient with mitral stenosis.

Patients characteristically have ruddy cheeks, a normal or reduced left ventricular impulse, and often a right ventricular heave. A prominent S_1 is heard, as is a loud P_2, signifying pulmonary hypertension. An opening snap occurring after S_2 is a classic finding. The murmur of mitral stenosis, typically a low-pitched diastolic rumble that begins with the opening snap of the mitral valve, is best heard at the apex with the bell of the stethoscope and the patient in the left lateral decubitus position.

11. How is the diagnosis of mitral stenosis established?

Electrocardiographic evidence includes left atrial enlargement (P mitrale), right-axis deviation, and right ventricular hypertrophy. Atrial fibrillation may also be seen. A chest x-ray may show signs of left atrial enlargement such as an elevated left main stem bronchus, a double cardiac density, and a prominent left heart border. Evidence of increased lung water may also be seen on chest x-ray. This includes pulmonary vascular redistribution, interstitial edema, and Kerley B lines. Signs of pulmonary hypertension may be present.

Echocardiography is the diagnostic method of choice. Two-dimensional (2-D) echocardiography is more useful than M-mode. Physical findings on 2-D echocardiography include doming of the mitral valve leaflets and restriction of their motion. Thickening of the mitral valve is also frequently seen. An enlarged left atrium is expected. The valve orifice can often be imaged and measured directly. The extent of calcification and pliability can also be assessed by 2-D echocardiography, which may allow selection of appropriate patients for mitral valvulotomy. Echocardiography allows the other cardiac valves to be assessed for abnormalities. Doppler echocardiography is also useful in assessing the severity of mitral stenosis. Cardiac catheterization is not required for the diagnosis of mitral stenosis but may be performed to evaluate the extent of coronary artery disease either in patients who have symptoms suggestive of angina or in elderly patients.

12. How should patients with mitral stenosis be managed?

Patients who are asymptomatic or minimally symptomatic can be managed medically. Medical management should be directed at prophylaxis against endocarditis, management of atrial fibrillation, prophylaxis against systemic embolization, and treatment of right heart failure. In patients with an abnormal mitral valve, prophylaxis with antibiotics prior to dental or surgical procedures is mandatory. Atrial fibrillation with rapid ventricular response is poorly tolerated by patients with mitral stenosis and should be aggressively treated with agents to decrease ventricular response. Digoxin is the drug of choice, but it is much less effective when patients exercise. The combination of digoxin and a beta-adrenergic blocking agent is effective in controlling ventricular rate when digoxin alone fails. However, beta blockers should not be used alone, as they may reduce exercise capacity. Calcium channel blockers such as verapamil and diltiazem have also been used to control ventricular response in atrial fibrillation. Problems exist with verapamil both because of its negative inotropic effect and because it can decrease renal clearance of digoxin, which may lead to elevated serum digoxin concentrations and digoxin toxicity. Diltiazem may be a better choice when combined with digoxin to control ventricular response in atrial fibrillation because diltiazem does not alter digoxin clearance. Combination therapy with diltiazem and digoxin has been shown to adequately control ventricular response at rest and with exercise in patients with atrial fibrillation.

Pharmacologic or electrical cardioversion to restore sinus rhythm is desirable if at all possible. Frequently this will involve the administration of quinidine or a similar antiarrhythmic agent. Patients should be anticoagulated for 2–3 weeks prior to the attempt at cardioversion. Patients who remain in atrial fibrillation, who have heart failure, or have previously experienced embolic phenomena should be maintained on oral anticoagulation with coumadin unless it is contraindicated.

Diuretic therapy and digoxin may help to relieve the symptoms of right heart failure. However, when patients become more symptomatic, surgical therapy should be considered. Once symptoms are severe, patients have a rapid downhill course. Options include catheter balloon valvuloplasty, mitral commissurotomy (either open or closed), and mitral valve replacement.

13. How is balloon mitral valvuloplasty performed?
This technique presents an alternative to the surgical treatment of mitral stenosis. The procedure is performed by advancing a small balloon flotation catheter across the intraatrial septum and advancing the catheter with the balloon through the stenotic mitral valve. The balloon is then inflated for short periods of time to enlarge the mitral valve area. The mechanisms responsible for improvement in valvular function are thought to include fracture of calcium deposits and commissural separation. This procedure can be done with a single- or double-balloon technique.

14. What options exist for surgical therapy for patients with mitral stenosis?
Surgical therapy consists of open commissurotomy or mitral valve replacement. Closed commissurotomy is rarely performed in the United States. Indications for mitral valve replacement or commissurotomy include patients with symptomatic heart failure that is New York Heart Association Class II or higher, pulmonary hypertension, or a mitral valve area of less than 1 cm^2. In addition, patients who have had systemic embolization from the stenotic mitral valve should undergo valve replacement even though they are without other significant symptoms.

15. What types of valves are available for valve replacement?
Two types of prosthetic valves are available for replacement in both the mitral and the aortic position: mechanical prostheses and bioprostheses. Mechanical valves can be cate-gorized into the ball-and-cage valves, such as the Starr-Edwards valve, and valves that use a tilting disk design. The Starr-Edwards valve remains the standard in that it has the longest record of durability. Its disadvantages include its bulky design and a higher incidence of hemolysis. The valve ring has been covered with cloth to reduce the incidence of thromboembolism. Because of its bulky design, it may be inappropriate for patients with a small aortic annulus or small left ventricular cavity. Tilting disk valves are now made of pyrolite, which is almost diamond-hard. Differences in the mode of retention of the disk allow for varying degrees of valve opening. The Björk-Shiley valve is the prototypic tilting disk valve. This valve is less bulky and has a lower profile than the Starr-Edwards valve. Two serious problems with the valve have been reported: one is thrombosis and the other is strut fracture. Changes in the design of the valve have been made in an attempt to overcome these problems. The St. Jude Medical valve is constructed of pyrolite and consists

of two semicircular disks that pivot between open and closed positions without the need for supporting struts. It is believed by some surgeons that this valve has more favorable flow characteristics and produces lower gradients across the prosthetic valve. Other disk valves include Medtronics, Omniscience, Duromedics, and Carbomedics. All of these mechanical prosthetic valves appear to be very durable. However, no study has prospectively compared the advantages and disadvantages of the various tilting disk valves.

Patients should be anticoagulated for life when a mechanical valve is used in either the mitral or aortic position. Anticoagulation decreases the risk of thromboembolism by one-third. Thromboembolism is more common with mechanical valves in the mitral position.

Tissue valves were developed to overcome the risk of thromboembolism. The most common tissue valves available are porcine heterografts. These include porcine valves that are fixed and sterilized using glutaraldehyde, which greatly decreases the antigenicity of the valves. The valves are then mounted on manufactured frames. Biologic valves have also been manufactured from porcine pericardium. Examples of tissue valves include the Carpentier-Edwards porcine valve, Carpentier-Edwards pericardial valve, the Ionescu-Shiley valve, and the Hancock valves. All these biologic valves are minimally thrombogenic. Patients should be anticoagulated for the first three months following surgery while the valve sewing ring becomes endothelialized, because this period is associated with a high likelihood of thromboembolism. Patients can then safely discontinue anticoagulation. The major problem with tissue valves is their limited durability; degeneration and calcification can become sufficiently severe that the patient requires repeat valve replacement. Failures usually begin to appear within the fourth or fifth postoperative year. By 10 years, the rate of valve failure requiring replacement may be 20–30%.

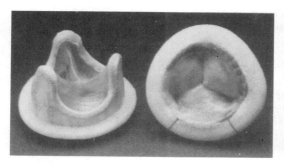

Carpentier-Edwards porcine valve

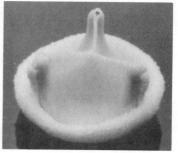

The Ionescu-Shiley
pericardial valve

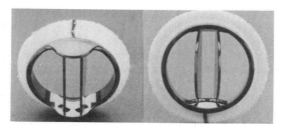

The St. Jude Medical heart valve prosthesis

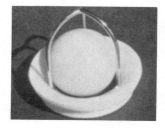

Starr-Edwards aortic
Silastic ball prosthesis

MITRAL REGURGITATION

16. Describe the mitral valve apparatus.
The mitral valve apparatus consists of two leaflets, approximately 120 chordae tendineae, two papillary muscles, an annulus, and portions of the left ventricular and atrial walls. The anterior leaflet of the mitral valve is more mobile than the posterior leaflet and accounts for roughly two-thirds of the valve area. However, the anterior leaflet is attached to only one-third of the mitral valve annulus.

17. What are the possible causes of mitral regurgitation?
Mitral regurgitation can be caused by many processes. Because the mitral valve complex is composed of a number of different structures, any abnormality in one of the structures may lead to insufficiency of the valve. The causes may be acute or chronic. Acute causes include ruptured chordae tendineae, papillary muscle rupture or dysfunction, endocarditis, and trauma. Conditions that lead to the insidious development of mitral insufficiency include rheumatic heart disease, mitral valve prolapse, such as with the click-murmur syndrome, myxomatous degeneration as seen in Marfan's syndrome, endocarditis, and left ventricular enlargement with dilatation of the mitral valve annulus.

18. What is the pathophysiology of mitral regurgitation?
Mitral insufficiency leads to volume overload of the left ventricle. With each ventricular contraction, a portion of left ventricular output is ejected backward into the left atrium. The greater the regurgitant fraction, the lower will be the forward cardiac output. The regurgitant volume of blood is returned to the left ventricle, resulting eventually in enlargement of both the left ventricle and atrium. Increases in left ventricular size lead to enlargement of the mitral annulus and can increase regurgitation. With significant regurgitation into the left atrium, pulmonary venous pressure rises and leads to an increase in pulmonary venous pressure and eventually pulmonary edema.

19. What is the presentation in acute versus chronic mitral regurgitation?
The presentations are very different because of differences in left atrial size. With acute mitral regurgitation, left atrial size is small and cannot accommodate the increase in volume that occurs during mitral regurgitation. This leads to an elevation in left atrial pressure that is reflected into the pulmonary vasculature. The low compliance of the left atrium causes these high pulmonary pressures, and for a given regurgitant flow, more pulmonary congestion is produced during acute mitral regurgitation than chronic mitral regurgitation. With chronic mitral regurgitation, the left atrium has an opportunity to dilate and better accommodates the regurgitant load. In chronic mitral regurgitation, symptoms are most likely due to the fall in forward cardiac output.

20. What are the symptoms and signs of mitral regurgitation?
Signs and symptoms vary with the severity of regurgitation and its rate of onset. Symptoms usually do not develop in patients with chronic mitral regurgitation until the left ventricle fails. Many patients with mild mitral regurgitation remain asymptomatic for their entire lives. Patients with acute mitral regurgitation quickly develop pulmonary hypertension and pulmonary edema. Right heart failure may also develop, and is characterized by hepatomegaly, peripheral edema, and ascites. Angina pectoris is rare unless the patient has coexistent coronary artery disease. When left ventricular ejection is normal, the carotid pulse is also normal, as is the left ventricular impulse. Generally, S_1 is soft and S_2 widely split. In patients with congestive heart failure, an S_3 may be present. Characteristically the murmur of mitral regurgitation is a high-pitched holosystolic murmur that is most prominent at the cardiac apex with radiation to the axilla. With abnormalities of the posterior leaflet of the mitral valve, the murmur may radiate to the sternum or the aortic area.

21. Which studies aid in the diagnosis of mitral regurgitation?
The **electrocardiogram** (EKG) in a patient with mitral regurgitation will show left atrial enlargement and, in one-third of patients, evidence of left ventricular enlargement. The EKG may also show atrial fibrillation. The chest x-ray typically shows enlargement of both the left atrium and ventricle and signs of pulmonary congestion. Calcification of the mitral valve annulus may be seen in elderly patients.

Two-dimensional echocardiography will reveal an enlarged left atrium and a dilated hyperdynamic left ventricle in cases of chronic mitral insufficiency. Echocardiography also helps to determine the underlying cause of mitral regurgitation. A ruptured papillary muscle or chordae tendineae may be seen. Other causes that can be detected with echocardiography include mitral valve prolapse, a flail leaflet, and vegetations on the mitral valve.

Doppler echocardiography will show a jet into the left atrium with systole. Severity of regurgitation is related to the penetration into the left atrium. Severe mitral regurgitation is present when the high-velocity jet penetrates into the pulmonary veins. Doppler echocardiography allows noninvasive assessment of the severity of mitral regurgitation that correlates well with angiography.

In patients with **pulmonary artery catheters** in place, a large V wave detected when the catheter is in the wedge position is felt to indicate the presence of mitral insufficiency. However, in a study of 50 patients with large V waves on pulmonary capillary wedge pressure (PCWP) tracings, 36% had no or trace mitral regurgitation as determined by angiography. Conditions that produced large V waves without mitral regurgitation included mitral stenosis, a mitral valve prosthesis, coronary artery disease with congestive heart failure, aortic valve disease with congestive heart failure, and ventricular septal defects. In addition, of the patients with documented severe mitral regurgitation, 32% had only trivial V waves on the PCWP tracing. Thus the finding of V waves on a PCWP tracing is neither highly sensitive nor specific for severe mitral regurgitation.

22. How should patients with mitral regurgitation be managed in the intensive care unit?
Most patients who present to the intensive care unit will have acute mitral regurgitation and congestive heart failure. The goals of medical care are hemodynamic stabilization and identification of the etiology of the acute mitral insufficiency. Afterload reduction is the mainstay of therapy. By reducing the afterload to ejection of the left ventricle, forward flow is encouraged while regurgitation is decreased. Left atrial pressure decreases, as does pulmonary congestion. Left ventricular volume also falls, which may decrease the size of the mitral annulus and further decrease mitral insufficiency. Afterload reduction with intravenous nitroprusside is the treatment of choice in patients with papillary muscle rupture and other causes of acute severe mitral regurgitation. Nitroprusside should be started at 3–6 $\mu g/kg/min$ and the dose increased until symptoms are relieved or systolic pressure falls below 100 mm Hg. Toxicity from nitroprusside is unusual during the first 24 hours of therapy. If patients are hypotensive with acute mitral insufficiency, they may benefit from inotropic agents such as dopamine or dobutamine. However, because of its alpha agonist activity, dopamine may elevate systemic vascular resistance and increase the regurgitant fraction. These patients are probably best managed by early insertion of an intra-aortic balloon pump. By decreasing afterload, the balloon pump allows aortic ejection to increase and decreases the regurgitant fraction. In patients whose mitral insufficiency is associated with ischemia, the increase in coronary perfusion accomplished with intraaortic balloon counterpulsation may decrease mitral insufficiency. If patients remain in cardiogenic shock, emergency catheterization and valve replacement must be performed.

23. What are the surgical options for patients with mitral insufficiency?
Surgical therapy for mitral insufficiency includes mitral valve replacement and a reconstructive procedure such as annuloplasty. A Carpentier ring can be inserted to reinforce the

annulus. Additional attempts at repair of the valve include shortening of the chordae tendineae or plication of the leaflets themselves. This has been shown to be a valuable technique in selected patients with mitral insufficiency. The advantage of repair of the mitral valve as opposed to replacement with a prosthetic valve is that there is no need to anticoagulate the patient, as the risk of thromboembolism is lower. The mainstay of surgical therapy is mitral valve replacement, as discussed previously.

AORTIC STENOSIS

24. What are the etiologies of aortic stenosis?

Aortic stenosis may be the result of a congenitally abnormal aortic valve. Unicuspid valves usually produce severe obstruction in infancy. More common is the congenitally bicuspid valve. Premature calcification of a bicuspid valve is the single most common cause of isolated aortic stenosis in the Western world, accounting for approximately 50% of cases. The abnormal architecture of the valve induces turbulent flow, which causes trauma to the leaflets and ultimately leads to fibrosis and calcification of the leaflets. Patients usually become symptomatic in the fourth or fifth decade of life. Congenitally malformed valves can also be tricuspid, with the cusps of unequal size. There may be commissural fusion. Abnormal flow characteristics through these valves may predispose to premature calcification. Rheumatic heart disease accounts for 30% of cases of aortic stenosis. In most patients with rheumatic aortic stenosis, there is associated mitral valve disease. Rheumatic disease is an unlikely cause of isolated aortic stenosis. Degenerative disease of the aortic valve may also lead to stenosis. This usually occurs on a relatively normal tricuspid valve. With senile-calcific aortic stenosis, calcium accumulates in the pockets of the aortic cusps, which leads to eventual fibrosis and commissural fusion. Patients' symptoms usually do not occur until the ages of 60–70. Obstruction to outflow of the left ventricle can also be caused by hypertrophic obstructive cardiomyopathy and supravalvular or subvalvular stenosis. Discussion of these subjects is beyond the scope of this chapter. Aortic valvular stenosis without accompanying mitral valve disease is more common in men than women. There is also an association between gastrointestinal bleeding and aortic stenosis.

25. When is aortic stenosis considered critical?

Obstruction to outflow of the left ventricle is considered critical when the aortic valve area is either less than 0.75 cm^2 in the average-size adult or approximately 0.4 cm^2/m^2 body surface area. This also corresponds to a peak systolic pressure gradient between the aorta and the left ventricle of 50 mm Hg in the presence of a normal cardiac output. Normal aortic valve area is 3 to 3.5 cm^2.

26. How is valve area calculated?

When evaluating a patient with a stenotic valve in either the aortic or mitral position, calculation of valve area is based on a measurement of the pressure gradient and the flow across the valve. These formulas are referred to as the Gorlin equations.

$$\text{Aortic valve area (cm}^2) = \frac{F}{44.3 \sqrt{\Delta P}}$$

$$\text{Mitral valve area (cm}^2) = \frac{F}{37.7 \sqrt{\Delta P}}$$

For these formulas, flow (F) is equal to flow across the valve in milliliters/second, and change in pressure (ΔP) is equal to the mean pressure gradient in mm Hg across the orifice.

The constants 44.3 and 37.7 relate to turbulence of flow across the valves and differ between the aortic and mitral valves. Flow is derived by the equation:

$$\text{Flow (F) (ml/sec)} = \frac{\text{Cardiac output (ml/min)}}{\text{DFP (sec/min) or SEP (sec/min)}}$$

For the mitral valve, diastolic filling period (DFP) is derived by measuring the time from mitral valve opening to closure per beat and multiplying by the heart rate. For the aortic valve, systolic ejection period (SEP) is equal to the systolic ejection time (aortic valve opening to closure) multiplied by the heart rate.

It is apparent from these formulas that calculation of valve area depends on flow rates and that with low flows, these estimates may be in error. If regurgitation coexists with stenosis of a valve, valve area calculations will be falsely lowered. This occurs because the actual flow across a valve per beat is greater than that calculated using the systemic cardiac output.

27. What is the pathophysiology of aortic stenosis?
Obstruction to aortic outflow at the aortic valve results in a pressure gradient developing from the left ventricle to the aorta. The left ventricle compensates by developing concentric hypertrophy. The consequences of left ventricular hypertrophy include reduced diastolic compliance, a rise in left ventricular end-diastolic pressure, and an increase in myocardial oxygen consumption. This increase in oxygen consumption is related mainly to increased left ventricular wall tension. Potential imbalances in myocardial oxygen demand-supply relationships can result because of compromised subendocardial coronary blood flow related to high subendocardial intramural pressure. This explains why patients may develop signs of coronary ischemia without having concomitant coronary artery disease.

As left ventricular hypertrophy increases and ventricular compliance falls, there is an increase in left ventricular pressure. With time this leads to elevations of left atrial pressure, and pulmonary venous and capillary pressures. This may lead to transudation of fluid into the lungs with resulting dyspnea and other signs of congestive heart failure. In addition, because of the decrease in left ventricular compliance, patients with aortic stenosis are dependent on organized atrial contraction for ventricular filling. Atrial fibrillation with the loss of "atrial kick" is poorly tolerated by patients with aortic stenosis. Also, because there is a limitation of cardiac outflow through a stenotic valve, patients with aortic stenosis do not tolerate reductions in afterload.

28. What are the signs and symptoms of aortic stenosis?
On physical examination, a patient with significant aortic stenosis will have a delayed carotid upstroke with a prominent anacrotic notch. With left ventricular failure the cardiac impulse is displaced inferiorly and laterally and is sustained. Auscultation will usually reveal a normal S_1 and a single S_2 because of calcification of the aortic valve. There is also frequently an S_4 gallop. The murmur of aortic stenosis is characteristically a crescendo-decrescendo murmur maximal at the second right intercostal space. This murmur is often well transmitted along the cardiac vessels and to the apex of the heart. It is best heard at the base of the heart.

The traditional triad of symptoms in patients with aortic stenosis includes angina, syncope, and heart failure. Congestive heart failure may occur in 60% of patients, angina in 50%, and syncope in 40% of patients. On cardiac catheterization 60% of patients with aortic stenosis will have coexisting coronary artery disease. However, patients with angina may or may not have significant coronary stenosis. Once angina develops, life expectancy is approximately 5 years. Syncope is frequently exertional and may result from peripheral vasodilatation with exertion. Because of the relatively fixed cardiac output in patients with aortic stenosis, there is ineffective compensation for this vasodilation. Once syncope develops, survival is approximately 3 years. With the onset of left ventricular failure, survival averages 2 years.

29. Which studies aid in the diagnosis of aortic stenosis?

With significant aortic stenosis, an enlarged cardiac silhouette on **chest x-ray** will be seen because of a prominent left ventricle. A dilated ascending aorta may also be seen. This results from poststenotic dilatation. With left ventricular failure, pulmonary venous congestion and pulmonary edema can be seen.

EKG evidence of aortic stenosis includes left ventricular hypertrophy, left atrial enlargement, left-axis deviation, and conduction defects. With severe aortic stenosis atrial fibrillation can occur.

Echocardiography using both the two-dimensional mode and Doppler techniques is helpful in diagnosis and management. With two-dimensional echocardiography, doming of the leaflets occurs with valvular aortic stenosis. The valve may also be heavily calcified and immobile. Doppler echocardiography can be used to measure the peak and mean transvalvular gradients, the latter of which corresponds well to the information obtained at cardiac catheterization.

Cardiac catheterization allows valve area to be calculated and coronary arteries to be visualized.

30. How should patients with aortic stenosis be managed medically?

Patients should have prophylaxis for endocarditis with dental and surgical procedures. They should be counseled to report the symptoms of syncope, heart failure, and angina quickly to their physician. Although atrial arrhythmias occur in less than 10% of patients with isolated aortic stenosis, patients with frequent atrial premature contraction should receive agents to maintain a normal sinus rhythm. If atrial fibrillation does occur, patients may experience significant symptoms, including congestive heart failure, angina, and significant hypotension. These may necessitate emergency electrical cardioversion. Medications should then be administered to preserve normal sinus rhythm.

Patients with aortic stenosis may be asymptomatic for many years. However, once symptoms do develop, life expectancy is shortened unless surgical intervention is performed. The timing of surgery is critical. If the operative procedure is carried out in patients with left ventricular failure or a depressed ejection fraction, the operative mortality is from 10–25%, which is nearly 5 times higher than in patients with normal ventricular function.

31. Is percutaneous balloon valvuloplasty an option to surgical therapy in patients with critical aortic stenosis?

Aortic balloon valvuloplasty has had less success in patients with aortic stenosis than in patients with mitral stenosis. In patients with critical aortic stenosis, there is an increase in valve area and a reduction in the gradient across the aortic valve following percutaneous balloon valvuloplasty. Patients do show an improvement in functional classification. However, restenosis is common, and valve area increases on the average by only 50%. The final valve area after balloon valvuloplasty averages 0.9 to 1.0 cm^2 in most series. Most authorities recommend balloon valvuloplasty of the aortic valve only in specific patients. These include patients who are inoperable because of extremely high surgical risk and patients who decline valve replacement. In most other patients, aortic valve replacement remains the standard of therapy. The operative mortality for aortic valve replacement in most centers ranges from 2–8%. Risk factors include impairment of left ventricular function, age, and the presence of other valvular lesions. Following successful valve replacement, symptoms and hemodynamics are improved. Ventricular performance may return to normal in most patients after successful aortic valve replacement for aortic stenosis. There also may be regression of left ventricular mass. In patients with aortic stenosis and coronary artery disease, valve replacement and myocardial revascularization should be performed at the same time.

During the surgical procedure, the calcified aortic valve must be removed carefully because of the risk of embolization. There is some evidence that the consequences of systemic embolization can be lessened by anesthetic techniques that include high doses of sodium thiopental.

AORTIC INSUFFICIENCY

32. What are the causes of aortic insufficiency?

Aortic insufficiency can be caused by processes that involve either the aortic valve leaflets themselves or the aortic root. Rheumatic fever is a common cause. Fusion of the commissures may restrict the opening of a valve, resulting in combined aortic stenosis and aortic insufficiency. Other conditions that may affect the valve leaflets themselves include infective endocarditis, connective tissue diseases such as Marfan syndrome and Ehlers-Danlos syndrome, and myxomatous degeneration of the aortic valve. Diseases of the aortic root result in aortic regurgitation. Processes that dilate the ascending aorta prevent proper coaptation of the aortic valve leaflets. These conditions include cystic medionecrosis of the aorta, syphilitic aortitis, ankylosing spondylitis, other connective tissue disorders, systemic hypertension, and Marfan syndrome. Additional causes of aortic insufficiency are trauma and aortic dissection. Aortic insufficiency can be acute or chronic. Most patients presenting to intensive care units will have acute severe aortic insufficiency, most likely due to infective endocarditis, dissection of the ascending aorta, trauma, and malfunction of a prosthetic aortic valve.

33. What is the pathophysiology of aortic insufficiency?

The basic pathophysiologic abnormality in aortic insufficiency is volume overload of the left ventricle because of leakage during diastole of some portion of the previously ejected stroke volume back into the left ventricle. In patients with acute aortic insufficiency, there is an abrupt increase in left ventricular end-diastolic volume, which results in marked elevations of left ventricular end-diastolic pressure. This occurs because the left ventricle does not have time to dilate and accommodate the elevated volume load. As left ventricular end-diastolic pressure rises, left atrial pressure rises, and eventually pulmonary congestion appears with signs and symptoms of congestive heart failure.

Chronic aortic insufficiency differs from acute aortic insufficiency in that the left ventricle has time to compensate for the increased volume load by dilating. There is also hypertrophy of the ventricle. Aortic insufficiency results in the largest end-diastolic volumes of any form of heart disease—so-called cor bovinum. Left ventricular muscle mass is also greatly elevated and may exceed 1,000 gm. The ejection fraction in patients with severe aortic insufficiency is often within normal limits, both at rest and during exercise, even when myocardial function is depressed. This may be because exercise results in peripheral vasodilatation and because an increase in heart rate decreases the regurgitant fraction per beat. Ultimately left ventricular function deteriorates, leading to elevations in left ventricular end-diastolic volumes and pressure that are reflected into the pulmonary circulation.

34. What are the signs and symptoms of chronic aortic insufficiency?

Patients with chronic aortic insufficiency may be asymptomatic for many years and may have many physical findings consistent with aortic insufficiency. There is a widened pulse pressure due to elevated systolic pressures and a relatively low diastolic pressure. This is created by the rapid runoff of blood from the aorta back into the left ventricle. Diastolic pressures may be recorded close to 0 mm Hg. Carotid pulses are bounding and may have a bisferious quality with a double systolic impulse. Other physical findings include:

- Corrigan's pulse, which is described as rapid upstroke and collapse of the pulse in peripheral arteries.
- De Musset's sign, which is head bobbing with each heartbeat.
- Duroziez's sign, which is the diastolic murmur auscultated when the stethoscope compresses the femoral artery.
- Quincke's pulse, which refers to the visible pulsation in the capillaries of the nail bed.

With chronic aortic regurgitation there is inferior and lateral displacement of the left ventricular impulse. S_1 and A_2 may be diminished. S_3 and S_4 gallops are frequently heard. The hallmark of aortic insufficiency is a high-pitched, blowing, diastolic murmur heard at the right upper sternal border, the left sternal border, and the cardiac apex. This murmur is best heard with the patient sitting up and leaning forward. A mid-diastolic rumble is frequently heard at the cardiac apex, simulating mitral stenosis. This Austin Flint murmur is due to turbulent flow across the mitral valve, which is partially closed by the regurgitant jet from the incompetent aortic valve.

35. What are the signs and symptoms of acute aortic insufficiency?

The presentation is very different from that of chronic aortic insufficiency because of a precipitous rise in left atrial pressure as well as a reduction in forward cardiac output. Patients classically have dyspnea with exertion, orthopnea, and paroxysmal nocturnal dyspnea. Tachycardia and marked peripheral vasoconstriction with a normal pulse pressure are present. Patients appear acutely ill, with decompensated heart failure and pulmonary edema. The first heart sound is diminished because of absent or premature mitral valve closure. S_3 and S_4 gallops are common. In acute aortic regurgitation, the murmur may be difficult to appreciate. It is a short, low-frequency diastolic murmur. In patients with acute aortic insufficiency, other physical findings may provide clues to the cause of aortic valve dysfunction. With infective endocarditis, fever, petechiae, purpura, and arterial embolic events may be seen. Chest or back discomfort or unequal pulses suggests the possibility of aortic dissection. In patients with a marfanoid appearance, the possibility of Marfan syndrome with aortic dissection should also be entertained.

36. What studies aid in the diagnosis of aortic insufficiency?

In patients with chronic aortic insufficiency, a **chest x-ray** will show impressive cardiomegaly. The ascending aorta may be dilated. Signs of pulmonary congestion will be present if the patient has congestive heart failure.

An **EKG** will show left ventricular hypertrophy and left atrial enlargement. In patients with acute aortic insufficiency, sinus tachycardia is usually seen.

Two-dimensional and Doppler echocardiography are useful. Doppler echocardiography is the primary noninvasive method used to diagnose the presence of aortic insufficiency. Color-flow Doppler imaging is especially useful. With echocardiography, early mitral valve closure may be seen, and this is due to marked elevation of left ventricular diastolic pressure in acute aortic regurgitation. Color-flow Doppler imaging allows the detection of mild degrees of aortic insufficiency that may be inaudible. Regurgitant flow can be quantified.

37. How should patients with acute, severe aortic insufficiency be managed in the intensive care unit?

Surgical therapy is the treatment of choice for patients who are hemodynamically unstable. Until the surgical procedure can be performed, medical management serves to stabilize the patient. General supportive measures include supplemental oxygen to maintain an adequate arterial oxygen content. Urine output should be carefully monitored. Pulmonary edema can be treated with diuretics, nitrates, and morphine sulphate. However, some patients require mechanical ventilation to maintain adequate gas exchange. Patients frequently need pulmonary artery catheterization as well as systemic arterial catheterization for optimal management. Vasodilator therapy with sodium nitroprusside is ideally suited for treating patients with aortic insufficiency. By decreasing afterload, forward output is improved. There is a reduction in ventricular filling pressures, with an improvement in pulmonary congestion. Should a patient's cardiac index be less than 2 L/min/m^2 with a nitroprusside infusion, then it may be necessary to improve cardiac performance. Dobutamine, which is devoid of intrinsic alpha-adrenergic agonist activity, may be useful in this situation. A dobutamine infusion can be started at 3–5 μg/kg/minute and titrated to improve cardiac output. The side effect of tachycardia may be helpful in patients with aortic insufficiency because of the decrease in diastole, which may further reduce the regurgitant volume per beat. In patients with severe pulmonary edema and hypoxemia, vasodilators such as nitroprusside can worsen hypoxemia by overcoming hypoxic pulmonary vasoconstriction. This may require the administration of higher oxygen concentrations and/or the use of higher levels of end-expiratory pressure.

In the intensive care unit, the etiology of aortic insufficiency should also be diagnosed. For patients with infective endocarditis, appropriate antibiotic therapy should be instituted as soon as possible. For patients with aortic insufficiency due to dissection, surgical therapy as quickly as possible is indicated. Patients with aortic dissection should have blood pressure controlled and should receive therapy to decrease the shear force in the ascending aorta (left ventricular dp/dt). Management is aimed at preparing these patients for surgical valve replacement, which is the mainstay of therapy for patients with acute aortic insufficiency.

BIBLIOGRAPHY

1. Assey ME, Spann JP: Indications for heart valve replacement. Clin Cardiol 13:81–88, 1990.
2. Braunwald E: Valvular heart disease. In Braunwald E (ed): Heart Disease: A Textbook of Cardiovascular Medicine. Philadelphia, W.B. Saunders, 1988, p 1023.
3. DePace NL, Nestico PF, Morganroth J: Acute severe mitral regurgitation. Am J Med 78:293–306, 1985.
4. Fuchs RM, Heuser RR, Yin FCP, Brinker JA: Limitations of pulmonary wedge V waves in diagnosing mitral regurgitation. Am J Cardiol 49:849–854, 1982.
5. Nishimura RA, Holmes DR, Reeder GS: Percutaneous balloon valvuloplasty. Mayo Clin Proc 65:198–220, 1990.
6. Rahimtoola SH: Perspectives on valvular heart disease: An update. J Am Coll Cardiol 14:1–23, 1989.
7. Safian RD, Berman AD, Diver DJ, et al: Balloon aortic valvuloplasty in 170 consecutive patients. N Engl J Med 319:125–130, 1988.

35. PERICARDIAL DISEASE
(Pericarditis and Cardiac Tamponade)
David E. Schwartz, M.D.

1. What is the pericardium?

The pericardium is an invaginated sac that extends from the great vessels to enclose the heart. This sac is composed of a fibrous outer layer and an inner serous membrane formed from a single layer of mesothelial cells. The visceral pericardium adheres to the epicardial surface of the heart and reflects back upon itself to form the parietal pericardium. The space between the serous layers of the visceral and parietal pericardium normally holds up to 50 ml of an ultrafiltrate of plasma. The protein concentration of this fluid is one-third that of plasma, and this fluid also contains phospholipids that serve as a lubricant. Normally, as well as in disease, the visceral pericardium is the source of pericardial fluid.

2. What is the function of the pericardium?

The pericardium functions to reduce friction between the heart and the other structures of the mediastinum. It also serves as a barrier to protect the heart from inflammatory processes that involve the lungs or pleura. The pericardium limits acute cardiac dilatation and may prevent kinking of the great vessels. Pericardial pressure is a determinant of the transmural distending pressure of the cardiac chambers. This pressure is the difference between intracardiac and intrapericardial pressure. The pressure in the pericardial space is similar to intrapleural pressure and varies from –5 to +5 cm H_2O during respiration. The relationship between pressure and volume in the pericardial space is exponential. Once the pericardium is filled, any further increase in volume is accompanied by a sharp rise in intrapericardial pressure. Normally the pericardial space can acutely accommodate only 100–200 ml of fluid before there is a significant increase in pressure. However, if fluid accumulates slowly, the pericardium can stretch to accommodate 1–2 liters of fluid without reaching the steep portion of the pressure-volume curve. Although the pericardium serves many functions, congenital absence of the pericardium is associated with no significant functional abnormalities.

3. What is acute pericarditis?

Acute pericarditis is inflammation of the pericardial sac. Pathologically, pericarditis involves influx of leukocytes, deposition of fibrin, and an increase in vascularity of the pericardium with increased permeability. This inflammatory process may also involve the myocardium and can lead to adhesions between the epicardium and the pericardium. The visceral pericardium may produce excess fluid in reaction to the injury. This leads to effusive pericarditis.

4. What causes acute pericarditis?

The most common causes of pericarditis are viral and bacterial infections, tuberculosis, uremia, myocardial infarctions, trauma, and malignancies. Even after appropriate evaluation, many cases are of unknown etiology. Pericarditis is more common in men than in women. The incidence ranges from 2–6% in autopsy series, although it is diagnosed in only 1 of 1000 hospital admissions.

5. What are the clinical manifestations of acute pericarditis?

Clinically, the syndrome of acute pericarditis is characterized by chest pain, a pericardial friction rub, and frequently fever. Often there is no clinical evidence of pericardial fluid, but small effusions may be detected by echocardiogram. These usually do not progress to produce hemodynamic embarrassment.

The pain of pericarditis is sharp and pleuritic and is located retrosternally or in the left precordial region. Pain with swallowing is frequently described. The pain is exacerbated by the supine position and lessened by sitting up and leaning forward. Radiation of the pain to the trapezius ridge may be helpful in differentiating pericarditis from acute myocardial infarction (MI).

A pericardial friction rub is pathognomonic for acute pericarditis. These rubs are evanescent and best detected with the diaphragm of the stethoscope placed firmly at the lower left sternal border while the patient is sitting up and leaning forward. The classic rub is described as having three components that are related to the motion of the heart during a cardiac cycle. The components of the rub are produced by atrial contraction, ventricular systole, and rapid ventricular filling during diastole. The loudest sound is that of ventricular contraction, while the least commonly detected is the early diastolic sound of rapid ventricular filling. With atrial fibrillation the presystolic component due to atrial contraction is absent, and only a two-component rub is heard. Pericardial friction rubs can be detected in the presence of pericardial effusions.

6. What are the typical electrocardiographic (EKG) changes of acute pericarditis?

EKG abnormalities appear in approximately 90% of cases of acute pericarditis. There are four recognized stages of ST and T wave abnormalities in pericarditis: Stage I changes are diagnostic of pericarditis and usually occur with the onset of pain. These consist of ST segment elevation, in which the ST segment is concave upward and is present in all leads except aVr and V_1. The T waves are usually upright. These features distinguish the stage I changes of pericarditis from the EKG changes seen in acute MI. Stage II follows in several days when the ST segments return to baseline. Stage III is inversion of the T waves. In stage IV the T waves revert to normal. Almost 50% of patients with acute pericarditis will have all four EKG stages. PR-segment depression can occur during stage I or II, and may be seen in over 70% of patients. However, in patients with acute MI and pericarditis detected by the development of a pericardial friction rub, only 1 of 31 patients had EKG changes diagnostic of pericarditis.

In patients with pericarditis and a pericardial effusion, low voltage of the ventricular complex may be seen in association with a normal amplitude of the P wave in the limb leads. This is explained by the absence of an effusion over the posterior surface of the atria, which is partially without a pericardial covering. Electrical alternans, which is variation in the amplitude of the ventricular complexes due to changes in cardiac position with rotation of the heart, is also seen in patients with pericarditis and a pericardial effusion.

Sinus tachycardia is often seen in patients with pericarditis who are not febrile or hemodynamically unstable. Atrial arrhythmias are infrequent in uncomplicated cases of pericarditis.

7. What other laboratory findings are helpful in diagnosing pericarditis?

Pericarditis is associated with signs of inflammation, including an elevation of the erythrocyte sedimentation rate and an elevated white blood cell count. Slight increases of the MB fraction of creatine phosphokinase have been described when epicardial inflammation occurs in acute pericarditis. In uncomplicated cases of pericarditis, the chest x-ray is nonspecific. If there is a large pericardial effusion in association with pericarditis, the chest x-ray will show enlargement and changes in shape of the cardiac silhouette. In one-fourth of patients with pericarditis, pleural effusions are found. These are usually left-sided, or, if bilateral, are larger on the left. In contrast, right-sided pleural effusions are the rule in patients with congestive heart failure. The chest x-ray may also reveal an etiology for the development of pericarditis such as a malignancy or an infection.

Echocardiography is the most sensitive method of detecting the presence of a pericardial effusion in patients with pericarditis. With small effusions, fluid is first detected posterior to the left ventricle during systole. With larger effusions, the fluid can be seen during both systole and diastole and may be present anteriorly. In massive effusions, the heart may "swing" within the pericardium. This may be responsible for the phenomenon of electrical alternans.

8. Is pericardial biopsy or pericardiocentesis helpful in the diagnosis of the etiology of acute pericarditis?

If, after a routine history and physical examination and laboratory studies, the common etiologies of pericarditis have been ruled out and the illness has lasted over 1 week, it may be appropriate to obtain pericardial tissue or fluid. In 231 consecutive patients with acute pericardial disease, this approach yielded a diagnosis in only 14% of patients. However, when pericardiocentesis or pericardectomy was done to relieve cardiac tamponade, a diagnosis was made in up to 54% of patients. These results suggest that in the patient with tamponade, if tissue or fluid is carefully evaluated, a diagnosis may be made that will affect therapy. However, for uncomplicated cases of acute pericarditis, invasive diagnostic techniques are not helpful.

9. How should the patient with acute pericarditis be managed?
The first determination to be made is whether the patient has hemodynamic compromise from the presence of a pericardial effusion. Next, the etiology of the pericarditis should be determined if possible, and appropriate treatment instituted. If, on echocardiogram, the patient has no evidence of an effusion or has an effusion that is not of hemodynamic significance, then the patient is best managed conservatively. (The management of patients with tamponade is discussed later.) The patient should be hospitalized to exclude MI or an infectious etiology. Careful observation is warranted because of subsequent development of a pericardial effusion that could cause hemodynamic embarrassment. Patients should be kept on bed rest. Oral anticoagulants should be discontinued. If anticoagulation is absolutely necessary, it is safest to administer intravenous heparin, which can be quickly reversed by discontinuing the infusion or by administering protamine. The treatment of viral or idiopathic pericarditis includes pain relief with nonsteroidal anti-inflammatory agents (NSAIDs) or, in severe cases, a short course of corticosteroids.

10. What is the natural history of acute pericarditis?
Most patients with viral or idiopathic pericarditis recover with only symptomatic therapy. In others, recurrent or relapsing pericarditis may follow acute pericarditis. Often these patients require therapy with corticosteroids. Management of this syndrome includes slowly tapering the steroid dose. In extreme cases that require steroids for prolonged periods, pericardectomy has been performed to relieve pain. The prognosis for patients with other forms of pericarditis varies with the prognosis of the underlying disease.

There are life-threatening complications of pericarditis, including the development of a pericardial effusion under pressure, which can result in cardiac tamponade. Pericarditis can also become chronic and lead to the development of fibrosis and calcification of the pericardium. This may result in constriction of the heart.

11. What is cardiac tamponade?
Cardiac tamponade is the accumulation of pericardial contents to the point that there is hemodynamically significant compression of the cardiac chambers.

12. What are the characteristics of cardiac tamponade?
It is characterized by elevated intracardiac pressures, a decrease in filling of the ventricles, and a reduction in stroke volume. In patients with acute cardiac tamponade from penetrating cardiac wounds, Beck described, in 1935, the triad of (1) falling arterial blood pressure, (2) elevated systemic venous pressure, and (3) a small quiet heart. Patients in whom the cardiac compression developed more slowly usually presented with ascites, a small quiet heart, and high central venous pressure.

13. What causes cardiac tamponade?
Cardiac tamponade can occur from any cause of either acute or chronic pericarditis. In a review of 56 medical patients at a city hospital, the most frequent etiologies for cardiac tamponade were neoplastic and viral or idiopathic disease. In patients with tamponade, the pericardium can contain transudative or exudative fluid, blood, frankly infected material, or gas. Pneumopericardium under tension has been well described in children and adults. This is a life-threatening complication of mechanical ventilation. The mortality for patients with tension pneumopericardium has been reported to be as high as 56%. Cardiac tamponade also occurs from trauma to the heart, most commonly from stab wounds. It is thought that after a stab wound to the heart, the pericardium is able to seal itself, allowing the accumulation of blood in the pericardial space. Pacemaker insertion, cardiac catheterization, and placement of central venous lines have all been associated with cardiac tamponade. Tamponade associated with central venous line placement is usually due to

perforation of the right atrium, usually occurs 24 hours following placement of the line, and has a mortality approaching 80%. It is recommended that the tips of central venous catheters be positioned in the superior vena cava to avoid this potentially lethal complication.

14. What is the pathophysiology of cardiac tamponade?

The addition of fluid to the pericardium at a rate exceeding the ability of the pericardium to stretch will increase intrapericardial pressure. As pericardial pressure rises, it approaches atrial and ventricular diastolic pressures. When these pressures are equal, the transmural pressure distending the cardiac chambers approaches zero. Increases in pericardial pressure are reflected by a rise in central venous pressure. In hypovolemic patients the rise in central venous and pericardial pressures is less prominent, and the diagnosis of cardiac tamponade may be difficult to make.

As intrapericardial pressure rises further, the heart is compressed and ventricular diastolic volumes fall. Stroke volume also falls, and cardiac output is maintained by activation of the sympathetic nervous system. With cardiac tamponade, mean arterial pressure is reduced, as is the pulse pressure, because of this fall in stroke volume. Increased adrenergic tone results in an increase in heart rate and contractility. With severe tamponade, blood pressure is maintained by an increase in systemic vascular resistance, which allows blood pressure to be maintained at the expense of a fall in cardiac output. As tamponade progresses, systemic arterial pressure cannot be maintained and organ perfusion declines. Reduction in coronary perfusion leads to ischemia of the endocardium. Sinus bradycardia, which has been described in cases of severe pericardial tamponade, may be due to sinoatrial node ischemia and heralds cardiovascular collapse and death.

15. What changes are seen in the arterial and venous pulses with cardiac tamponade?

With cardiac tamponade, characteristic phasic changes occur in arterial and venous pressure wave forms. Normally with inspiration there is an increase in venous return that results in an increase in preload of the right ventricle and a small decrease in left ventricular volume. This leads to a decrease in systolic blood pressure of no more than 10 mm Hg. Pulsus paradoxus is a hallmark of cardiac tamponade and there is a fall in arterial systolic pressure with inspiration of greater than the normal value of 10 mm Hg. In patients with pericardial tamponade, pulsus paradoxus is seen because of an exaggerated increase in venous return to the right heart during inspiration. This increase in right ventricular volume shifts the intraventricular septum leftward, decreasing left ventricular end-diastolic volume, which results in a fall in output of the left ventricle and of systolic arterial pressure. On physical examination pulsus paradoxus can be detected by a decrease in strength or, in severe cases, loss of a patient's pulse with inspiration. Pulsus paradoxus is not specific to cardiac tamponade and is seen in patients with severe heart failure, asthma and obstructive lung disease, and massive pulmonary embolism.

There are also characteristic changes in the venous wave forms with cardiac tamponade. Normally the venous system has three positive waves forms. The **a wave** is related to atrial contraction, and the **c wave** to closure of the tricuspid valve. The **v wave** results from filling of the atrium during ventricular contraction with the tricuspid valve closed. The **X descent** represents atrial relaxation. The **Y descent** occurs when the tricuspid valve opens and the atrium empties into the ventricle during diastole. In patients with cardiac tamponade, the X descent is preserved, whereas the Y descent is abolished (see figure at top of next page). These changes occur because the decreased cardiac volume during systole allows atrial pressure to fall and preserves the X descent. However, in diastole the increase in intrapericardial pressure prevents diastolic filling of the ventricle and the Y descent is truncated.

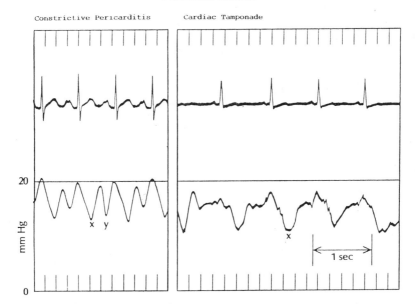

Pressure tracings from the right atrium illustrate the different wave forms in constrictive pericarditis and cardiac tamponade. In chronic constrictive pericarditis, an "M" or "W" contour is formed by prominent dips in both systolic (X descent) and diastolic (Y descent) pressure. In cardiac tamponade, only the systolic dip (X descent) is prominent.

16. What is helpful in making the diagnosis of cardiac tamponade?

The presence of jugular venous distention was the most common physical finding in 56 medical patients with cardiac tamponade. Pulsus paradoxus was present in over 70% of these patients. Kussmaul's sign, an increase in central venous pressure with inspiration, is not seen in patients with pericardial tamponade unless there is a component of pericardial constriction. In patients with tension pneumopericardium, shifting tympany can be demonstrated over the precordium, and a characteristic murmur, *"bruit de moulin,"* due to the presence of air and fluid in the pericardium is heard.

Findings on chest x-ray and EKG are nonspecific. Echocardiography is most helpful in diagnosing the presence of a hemodynamically significant pericardial effusion. Cardiac tamponade can be demonstrated on echocardiogram by finding compression of the right ventricular free wall during early diastole. Diastolic collapse of the right atrial and ventricular free walls is also seen on echocardiogram during tamponade.

Hemodynamic monitoring and cardiac catheterization are invaluable in making the diagnosis of tamponade. The typical finding of loss of the Y descent in the right atrial pressure tracing with preservation of the X is suggestive of tamponade. Intraarterial pressure measurement can help to document the presence of pulsus paradoxus. If pericardial pressure is measured at the time of cardiac catheterization, it should equal atrial and ventricular diastolic pressures. Placement of a pulmonary artery catheter will show elevation and equilibration of diastolic pressures within 3–4 mm Hg of each other.

17. What should be considered in the differential diagnosis of tamponade?

Clinical conditions that can be confused with cardiac tamponade include massive pulmonary embolism, tension pneumothorax, severe exacerbation of obstructive lung disease, constrictive pericarditis, restrictive cardiomyopathy, and cardiogenic shock from right ventricular infarction.

18. How should the patient with tamponade be treated?

In the acute setting, medical stabilization of the patient involves maintaining filling pressures with volume expansion to try to prevent diastolic collapse of the heart. Hemodynamic support of the patient with tamponade may also be required. Because the compensatory activation of the sympathetic nervous system results in an increase in systemic vascular resistance, some authorities have recommended inotropic support with isoproterenol to maintain heart rate and contractility as well as to lower afterload. This may be dangerous in patients with marginal blood pressure or inadequate preload. Agents such as dopamine or norepinephrine, which increase the inotropic state of the heart and maintain blood pressure, may be useful in the medical stabilization of the patient. Positive-pressure ventilation in patients with cardiac tamponade is associated with a fall in cardiac output, because the decrease in venous return is associated with increased intrathoracic pressure. If at all possible, spontaneous ventilation should be maintained for patients with tamponade. If supportive measures do not result in improvement, drainage of pericardial fluid needs to be performed emergently.

Definitive therapy for patients with cardiac tamponade involves drainage of the pericardium so that cardiac compression is relieved. This can be done percutaneously or surgically. Percutaneous pericardiocentesis can be performed blindly or guided by two-dimensional echocardiography. The use of echocardiography to guide pericardiocentesis has improved the safety of the procedure. In a series of 117 patients undergoing 132 pericardiocenteses, there were no deaths related to the procedure. Patients who have tamponade from a traumatic cause are unlikely to benefit from pericardiocentesis for a prolonged period of time because of the rapid reaccumulation of pericardial fluid. These patients require surgical management.

Surgical therapy for effusive pericardial disease can involve complete pericardectomy, partial pericardectomy, or creation of a pericardial window. In unstable patients, a pericardial window can be performed using only local anesthesia. This allows the maintenance of spontaneous ventilation. If an unstable patient requires a more extensive procedure, then pericardiocentesis may need to be performed prior to the induction of anesthesia. Limited pericardectomy allows drainage of the pericardial fluid into the left hemithorax. Complete pericardectomy is performed using either a left anterior thoracotomy or a median sternotomy. Cardiopulmonary bypass is frequently used for complete pericardectomy.

19. Following cardiac surgery, can a patient in whom the pericardium is open suffer cardiac tamponade?

Yes. Although the pericardium may be left open after cardiac surgery, patients are still at risk for the development of cardiac tamponade. The accumulation of blood in the mediastinum can compress the heart, which can occur because of occlusion of thoracostomy tubes placed during the surgical procedure in 2% of patients following cardiac surgery. Patients with hypotension, low cardiac output, elevated intravascular pressures, and a fall in the output of mediastinal drainage tubes should be suspected of having cardiac tamponade. Marked widening of the mediastinum on chest x-ray may be seen. Obtaining a chest x-ray should not delay therapy. Emergency thoracotomy in the intensive care unit for patients with cardiac tamponade after cardiac surgery is the treatment of choice. The incidence of wound infection is 5% and is not increased by closing the patient's chest in the ICU.

20. What is constrictive pericarditis?

Constrictive pericarditis is the restriction of diastolic filling of the heart produced by the adhesion of a thickened, often calcified, pericardium to the heart. This usually affects all chambers of the heart equally. In most cases the visceral and parietal pericardium are fused. Patients frequently present with dyspnea and the symptoms and signs of elevated venous pressures. Those with long-standing constriction will have peripheral edema, ascites, and a wasted appearance. Elevation of jugular venous pressure is nearly always present, and Kussmaul's sign (a paradoxical increase in venous pressure with inspiration) may be found in patients with constriction. If the patient's neck is examined carefully, the rapid Y descent in the jugular venous wave form can often be seen. On auscultation, an early systolic sound called the pericardial knock may be heard and is fairly specific for constrictive pericarditis.

21. What are the causes of constrictive pericarditis?

Anything that can cause acute pericarditis can result in constrictive pericarditis. The major causes include infections, connective tissue disorders, neoplastic diseases, trauma, metabolic abnormalities, radiation therapy, and myocardial infarction. Worldwide, tuberculosis is the most common etiologic agent, but it accounts for less than 20% of cases in the developed world.

22. How does the cardiac compression due to constrictive pericarditis differ from that of cardiac tamponade?

With thickening of the pericardium, there is restriction of the diastolic enlarging of the ventricles that limits ventricular filling. Filling is normal during the first third of diastole. However, in the last two-thirds of diastole, continued ventricular filling is abruptly halted by the thickened pericardium. This pattern of filling is exemplified by the classic dip and plateau pressure waveform seen in constrictive pericarditis. There is an early diastolic fall in pressure that is immediately followed by a steep rise in pressure to a plateau level.

The presence of Kussmaul's sign and the absence of pulsus paradoxus helps to distinguish constrictive pericarditis from pericardial tamponade. In addition, a prominent Y descent in the right atrial pressure waveform (see figure on p. 157) is seen in constrictive pericarditis and is absent in tamponade. Thickening or calcification of the pericardium seen on echocardiogram or computed tomography may help in making the diagnosis of constrictive pericarditis.

BIBLIOGRAPHY

1. Callaham M: Pericardiocentesis in traumatic and nontraumatic cardiac tamponade. Ann Emerg Med 13:924–945, 1984.
2. Callahan JA, Seward JB, Nishimura RA, et al: Two-dimensional echocardiographically guided pericardiocentesis: Experience in 117 consecutive patients. Am J Cardiol 55:476–479, 1985.
3. Cummings RG, Wesly RL, Adams DH, Lowe JE: Pneumopericardium resulting in cardiac tamponade. Ann Thorac Surg 37:511–518, 1984.
4. Edwards H, King TC: Cardiac tamponade from central venous catheters. Arch Surg 117:965–967, 1982.
5. Griffin S, Fountain W: Pericardio-peritoneal shunt for malignant pericardial effusion. J Thorac Cardiovasc Surg 98:1153–1154, 1989.
6. Guberman BA, Fowler NO, Engel PJ, et al: Cardiac tamponade in medical patients. Circulation 64:633–640, 1981.
7. Fairman RM, Edmunds LH: Emergency thoracotomy in the surgical intensive care unit after open cardiac operation. Ann Thorac Surg 32:386–391, 1981.
8. Fowler NO: Constrictive pericarditis: New aspects. Am J Cardiol 50:1014–1017, 1982.
9. Fowler NO, Gabel M: The hemodynamic effects of cardiac tamponade: Mainly the result of atrial, not ventricular, compression. Circulation 71:154–157, 1985.
10. Hancock EW: On the elastic and rigid forms of constrictive pericarditis. Am Heart J 100:917–923, 1980.
11. Krainin FM, Flessas AP, Spodick DH: Infarction-associated pericarditis: Rarity of diagnostic electrocardiogram. N Engl J Med 311:1211–1214, 1984.
12. Krikorian JG, Hancock EW: Pericardiocentesis. Am J Med 65:808–814, 1978.
13. McCaughan BC, Schaff HV, Piehler JM, et al: Early and late results of pericardiectomy for constrictive pericarditis. J Thorac Cardiovascular Surg 89:340–350, 1985.

14. McGregor M: Pulsus paradoxus. N Engl J Med 301:480–482, 1979.
15. Permanyer-Miralda G, Sagrista-Sauleda J, Soler-Soler J: Primary acute pericardial disease: A prospective series of 231 consecutive patients. Am J Cardiol 56:623–630, 1985.
16. Surawicz B, Lasseter KC: Electrocardiogram in pericarditis. Am J Cardiol 26:471–474, 1970.
17. Weiss JM, Spodick DH: Association of left pleural effusions with pericardial disease. N Engl J Med 308:696–697, 1984.

36. ECHOCARDIOGRAPHY IN INTENSIVE CARE

Olivia Vynn Adair, M.D.

1. Why has echocardiography emerged as an important imaging technique in the management of the intensive care patient?

Success in the management of patients in the intensive care unit (ICU) often depends on prompt and precise diagnosis. Echocardiography is, therefore, particularly advantageous, as it provides both anatomic and physiologic assessment of the heart noninvasively or minimally so with transesophageal echocardiography (TEE). The results are immediately available and serial examinations can easily be performed on unstable patients at the bedside with reliability.

2. Name the various echocardiographic imaging techniques.

The imaging techniques of echocardiography are M-mode, two-dimensional (2-D), TEE, color-flow mapping, and Doppler ultrasound. M-mode contributes information on wall motion, valve excursion, and chamber size, and aids in timing of events during the cardiac cycle. 2-D Echocardiography provides an image of all chambers, outflow tracts, valves, aortic root, descending aorta, and the great vessels. Color-flow and Doppler imaging provide information on blood velocity, direction, and turbulence across the valves, within the chambers, across any shunts, and in the thoracic aorta. TEE permits close evaluation of the heart and aorta from the esophagus and stomach.

3. What are some indications for echocardiographic imaging of the ICU patient?

Hemodynamic instability with suspected cardiac etiology (e.g., tamponade, cardiac dysfunction, low perfusion rate)
Chest pain
Chest trauma
Valve disease
Regurgitation or stenosis, especially with pulmonary edema or syncope
Cerebrovascular or systemic thromboembolic event
Aortic disease

4. Why is echocardiography an important diagnostic imaging technique in cardiac tamponade?

Cardiac tamponade has a high mortality rate if not accurately and promptly diagnosed and treated. Echocardiography is the most sensitive technique for the detection and localization of a pericardial effusion, and is highly valuable in evaluating the hemodynamic significance of the effusion. Echocardiography should be considered routinely when tamponade is suspected, as it is quickly performed at bedside, is very sensitive, and can identify effusions as small as 15 ml. Tamponade often may be detected echocardiographically in the absence of physical signs.

5. What are the findings on echocardiography in cardiac tamponade? How sensitive and specific is this imaging technique for tamponade?

The typical findings on echocardiography in tamponade are late diastolic collapse of the right atrial wall (the earliest change) and early diastolic right ventricular free wall collapse or indentation. These findings are highly sensitive, 80–92%, and specific, approximately 100%. The changes on echocardiography occur when the cardiac output has decreased as little as 20% and before a drop in systemic arterial blood pressure occurs. These echocardiographic findings may be absent in hypertrophy, in elevated right-sided pressures, and after cardiac surgery because of adhesions to the free walls of the heart chambers. If the echocardiogram is not diagnostic of tamponade, but clinical suspicion is high, especially with hemodynamic compromise, a Swan-Ganz catheter should be placed to evaluate for equalization of pressures, an indication of cardiac tamponade.

6. How is echocardiography useful in pericardiocentesis?

All patients undergoing pericardiocentesis should have a 2-D echocardiogram to determine whether the routine approach for the aspiration needle and catheter is appropriate. With an apical four-chamber view providing continuous imaging during the procedure, the needle is visualized as it enters the pericardial sac (agitated saline may be incorporated as an aid if needed). Catheter placement is then verified, and the decrease in pericardial fluid monitored with 2-D echocardiography.

7. Describe the technique of TEE and its risks.

TEE uses a modified flexible gastroscope with an ultrasound transducer mounted on the tip and has the capacities of M-mode and 2-D echocardiography as well as Doppler and color-flow imaging. After the patient has been premedicated with an oral topical anesthetic and a short-acting intravenous relaxant, the probe, 9 mm in diameter and 100 cm long, is introduced as an upper endoscope to approximately 50 cm (to the stomach). Although anesthesiologists quickly adopted TEE for intraoperative monitoring of left ventricular function and ischemia, it is now routinely used in ambulatory, critical care, and emergency room settings. The study can be completed in approximately 20 minutes at the bedside and with minimal risk to the patient. There have been only three reported associated fatalities— two secondary to perforation of the esophagus and one to bradycardia. Minor throat irritation is the most common complaint. Antibiotic prophylaxis is administered by most centers to patients with valvular or congenital heart disease (as prescribed by the American Heart Association), although the incidence of bacteremia is much less frequent than with the gastroscope. Because the probe is introduced blindly, a relative contraindication is esophageal disease, i.e., varices, strictures, diverticuli, or scleroderma.

8. What are the indications and benefits of transesophageal compared with transthoracic echocardiography in the critical care patient?

The retrocardiac vantage of TEE circumvents interference from interposing structures (skin, bone, lungs) and poor imaging windows that may be due to chest wall abnormalities, bandages, or injuries, thus negating the 10% of studies that are technically difficult with transthoracic echocardiography (TTE) to increase the success rate of TEE to > 98%. In studies of prosthetic valves, TEE eliminates the shadows and artifacts seen on TTE. Also, because of the angle of approach, color-flow Doppler evaluation of intraseptal shunts and valvular regurgitant flow are markedly improved with TEE. Evaluation of both native and prosthetic valve vegetations in endocarditis is much more sensitive with TEE; especially in smaller (< 5 mm) vegetations, TEE is four times more sensitive than TTE. Patients presenting with cerebrovascular events benefit from TEE imaging, as the entire left atrium is easily visualized, including the left atrial appendage, which is rarely viewed with TTE and is the major location of a cardiac emboli source. Another important use of TEE is imaging of the thoracic aorta for aneurysm, dissection, and an intimal flap. All areas of the aorta are accessible, and the accuracy of diagnosing an aortic dissection with TEE is 93–100%.

9. Is echocardiography an acceptable technique in the diagnosis and management of thoracic aorta dissection compared with other imaging techniques?
Aortic dissection is rapidly fatal if not promptly diagnosed and treated, and requires confirmation by a diagnostic imaging technique such as aortography, echocardiography, computed tomography (CT), or magnetic resonance imaging (MRI). Aortography used to be considered the gold standard, but its sensitivity and specificity in recent studies are only 88% and 94%, respectively, and aortography has the disadvantages of time delay, the invasiveness of aortic catheterization and contrast material, and radiation exposure, making the initial study and serial studies less desirable. In comparison, combined transesophageal and transthoracic echocardiography is rapid (study time 15–20 minutes), mobile, easily done at bedside, and accurate (sensitivity 99%, specificity 98%), and allows on-line, immediate interpretation. In addition, no contrast material is required, and the entry tear of the dissection is identified in > 87% of patients. Echocardiography also provides additional data (e.g., aortic insufficiency, other valve disease, cardiac function, pericardial effusion). CT, although relatively noninvasive, requires contrast material, involves a moderate time delay, often does not permit identification of entry tear, and has a low sensitivity, 83% (specificity 100%). MRI has the advantages of high sensitivity and specificity (95% and 98%, respectively), noninvasiveness, and provision of additional cardiac data. Disadvantages are that the patient must be relatively stable to be transported, support equipment may not be able to be brought into the imaging suite, a relative time delay, unavailability of equipment and emergency staff, and identification of entry tear identified in only 39% of patients. Therefore, echocardiography (combined transthoracic and transesophageal) should be performed when dissection of the thoracic aorta is suspected as the first study for diagnosis, for location of entry tear, and for identification of aortic insufficiency and other cardiac abnormalities.

10. Should all patients with blunt chest trauma undergo echocardiography?
Cardiac contusion from blunt chest trauma remains a challenge in ICU management because the picture is often complicated by major injuries and fractures. Cardiac complications associated with such trauma include myocardial contusion, laceration or rupture; valve damage or rupture, and marked myocardial depression. Although echocardiography offers immediate noninvasive imaging, the incidence of functional cardiac abnormalities due to blunt trauma is low (< 20%), even with a high incidence of major injuries and fractures (50%). Also, because the course is usually benign, even in patients sustaining contusion, the additional cost of echocardiography is not warranted routinely in patient management. The deaths in this group of patients in a large study were not related to cardiac abnormalities but rather to other injuries. Therefore, echocardiography should be based on clinical findings that suggest cardiac complications (murmur, rub, congestive heart failure, and unusual chest pain with associated symptoms) or unexpected deterioration in the clinical course of the patient.

11. Do patients with penetrating chest wall injury require echocardiography routinely?
A higher proportion of patients presenting with penetrating chest injury have cardiac complications than do those sustaining blunt chest trauma. For example, up to 33% of patients with penetrating chest wall injury have silent hemopericardium. Other findings include regional wall abnormalities, pneumopericardium, and foreign bodies. Therefore, a low threshold for echocardiography should be entertained in patients presenting with penetrating chest wall trauma.

12. What is the sensitivity of transesophageal versus transthoracic echocardiography in the diagnosis of endocarditis?

TEE improves detection of vegetation on both native and prosthetic valves. The sensitivities of TEE and TTE are 100% and 63%, respectively, whereas the specificities are the same (98%). Larger vegetations (> 10 mm) are visualized by both techniques, but only 25% of smaller vegetations (< 5 mm) are detected by TTE compared with 100% by TEE. Also, 20–30% of TTE studies are technically inadequate and the overall success rate of TTE in detection of vegetations, 50 to 80%. TEE has a > 98% success rate in diagnostic studies of patients presenting with possible endocarditis.

13. Is a baseline echocardiogram recommended for all patients with endocarditis?

Bacterial endocarditis results in high morbidity and a mortality rate of 33%. Specific high-risk patients are more likely to develop complications and require surgery, and therefore should have an echocardiogram. For example, patients with native aortic valve involvement in endocarditis and patients with a history of intravenous drug abuse have a 2.5 times increased risk of periannular infection and local extension of infection (occurring in 50%). Because of the seriousness of such sequelae, these patients should have serial echocardiography for follow-up. Other complications to be evaluated are the development of annular abscesses, aneurysms, and fistulous communications. Patients with echocardiographically evident vegetations vs. silent endocarditis (no vegetation visualized) require surgery 93% vs. 15%, have major embolic events 47% vs. 15%, and mortality is 35% vs. 23%. Therefore, it is reasonable to perform echocardiography early in the absence of an immediate response to appropriate therapy to evaluate for the presence of a vegetation. Also, because the initial study may be negative and clinical signs of complications (congestive heart failure, arrhythmias, heart block, pericarditis, and valve destruction) are late findings, serial echocardiograms may be required to plan early surgery, as emergent surgery is associated with high mortality.

14. What complications of endocarditis can be diagnosed by echocardiography?

Two complications that are identifiable echocardiographically are regurgitant flow and obstructive flow (with large vegetations) across the valves. These abnormal flow profiles may be associated with leaflet destruction or rupture. Perivalvular abscess and local extension of infection may be visualized, as may fistula formation, rupture or abscess of the sinus of Valsalva, myocardial or root abscess, mycotic aneurysm, pericardial effusions, and unexpected multiple valve involvement. Because increased morbidity and mortality are associated with the complications of endocarditis, their recognition is extremely important. Often TEE will be required to obtain the highest resolution, especially in prosthetic valve endocarditis.

15. What diagnostic role does echocardiography play in the evaluation of an AIDS patient admitted with respiratory distress and hemodynamic instability?

Recent studies have identified cardiac abnormalities in as many as 70% of patients with AIDS, and they are more common in hospitalized patients. These abnormalities include pericardial effusions, tamponade, pericardial and myocardial tumors, valve disease, myocarditis, and cardiomyopathy. Because the presenting symptoms may not be specifically pulmonary or cardiac in origin and because their management may be drastically altered, it is recommended that these patients undergo early echocardiography. Cardiac implications of AIDS (e.g., tamponade, endocarditis, and myocarditis) may be fatal if not treated promptly, and many are treatable or at least manageable.

16. What is the appropriate imaging modality for a patient admitted with acute pulmonary edema and a prosthetic valve?

Any patient with a prosthetic valve who presents with evidence of acute pulmonary edema or cardiac dysfunction should have prompt investigation of the valve for dysfunction or endocarditis with an echocardiogram. Failure rates of approximately 7% and 9% per year are expected for aortic and mitral prosthetic valves, respectively. The most sensitive imaging techniques for this purpose are TEE and color-flow Doppler imaging. Information desired includes regurgitant or stenotic flow, movement of leaflets or mechanical processes, paravalvular regurgitation, vegetations, dehiscence of valve ring, and atrial and ventricular thrombi.

17. What diagnostic benefits are gained from echocardiography for the patient admitted with a new cerebral embolic event?
Echocardiography plays an important role in the search for a potential cardiac source of the emboli in the evaluation of patients with transient ischemic attacks or strokes. Approximately one-sixth of all cerebral infarcts are due to cerebral embolism of cardiac origin. Thrombi may be located in the chambers, aorta, and great vessels. Also, possible myxoma, other cardiac tumors, valvular vegetations, intracardiac shunts, and patent foramen ovale may be the source of embolization and are identifiable with an echocardiogram. Echocardiography is particularly beneficial in identifying the source of embolism in younger patients (< 45 years of age), with one study demonstrating a positive echocardiogram in 37% of these patients presenting with a stroke. Likewise, patients with a history of cardiac disease are much more likely to have a cardiac source of cerebral emboli. In addition, other individuals without a known source of embolus should undergo echocardiography, and TEE may be required.

18. When should stroke patients undergo TEE?
TEE permits, with better resolution than TTE, detailed imaging of important areas that have a high potential for being a cardiac source of the emboli. These areas include the left atrium, especially the appendage (rarely visualized on TTE), and intraseptal defects, including patent foramen ovale. TEE has been shown to be four times more sensitive in imaging small valvular vegetations (< 5 mm), which serve as a source of emboli. A recent study demonstrated that in patients presenting with an unexplained stroke, a cardiac source was identified in 57% of cases by TEE compared with 15% by TTE. TEE also provided a diagnosis in 40% of patients without a cardiac history. Therefore, it is recommended that patients with a stroke of unknown etiology, even with a normal TTE, undergo TEE.

BIBLIOGRAPHY

1. Adair OV, Randive N, Krasnow N: Isolated toxoplasma myocarditis in acquired immune deficiency syndrome. Am Heart J 118:856–857, 1989.
2. Dressler FA, Roberts WC: Infective endocarditis in opiate addicts: Analysis of 80 cases studied at necropsy. Am J Cardiol 63:1240–1257, 1989.
3. Erbel R, Engberding R, Daniel W, et al: Echocardiography in diagnosis of aortic dissection. Lancet March 1989, pp 457–461.
4. Erbel R, Rohmann S, Drexler M, et al: Improved diagnostic value of echocardiography in patients with infectious endocarditis by transesophageal approach. Eur Heart J 9:43–53, 1988.
5. Fisher EA, Goldman ME: Transesophageal echocardiography: A new view of the heart. Ann Intern Med 113:91–93, 1990.
6. Himelman RB, Chung WS, Chernoff DN, et al: Cardiac manifestations of human immunodeficiency virus infections: A two-dimensional echocardiography study. J Am Coll Cardiol 13:1030–1036, 1989.
7. Hossack KF, Moreno CA, Vanway CW, Burdick DC: Frequency of cardiac contusion in nonpenetrating chest injury. Am J Cardiol 61:391–394, 1988.
8. Klodas E, Edwards WD, Khandheria B: Use of transesophageal echocardiography for improving detection of valvular vegetations in subacute bacterial endocarditis. J Am Soc Echo 2:386–389, 1989.
9. Moten M, Pandian NG: Echocardiography in cardiac tamponade. Cardiovasc Reviews & Reports 9(9):46–49, 1988.

10. Pavlides GS, Hauser AM, O'Neill WJ, Timmis GC: Transesophageal echocardiography: Current indications. J Intervent Cardiol 1:123–132, 1989.

11. Pearson AC, Labovitz AJ, Tatineni S, Gomez CR: Superiority of transesophageal echocardiography in detecting cardiac source of embolism in patients with cerebral ischemia of uncertain etiology. J Am Coll Cardiol 17:66–72, 1991.

12. Plummer D: Principles of emergency ultrasound and echocardiography. Ann Emerg Med 18:1291–1297, 1989.

13. Reid CL, Kawaniski DT, Rahimtoola SM, et al: Chest trauma: Evaluation by two-dimensional echocardiography. Am Heart J 113:971–976, 1987.

14. Scott PJ, Ettles DF, Wharton GA, Williams GJ: The value of transesophageal echocardiography in the investigation of acute prosthetic valve dysfunction. Clin Cardiol 13:541–544, 1990.

15. Singh S, Wann S, Schuchard G, et al: Right ventricular and right atrial collapse in patients with cardiac tamponade: A combined echocardiographic and hemodynamic study. Circulation 70:966–971, 1984.

16. Wilbers C, Carrol CL, Hnilica MA: Optimal diagnostic imaging of aortic dissection. Texas Heart Inst J 17:271–278, 1990.

17. Zenker G, Erbel R, Kramer G, et al: Transesophageal two-dimensional echocardiography in young patients with cerebral ischemic events. Stroke 19:345–348, 1988.

V: Infectious Disease

37. SEPSIS

Richard T. Ellison, III, M.D.

1. The term sepsis is used to describe overwhelming systemic disease caused by a microbial pathogen. What is the general management approach in patients with sepsis?

1. Identify and, when possible, eradicate any focus of infection.

2. Eliminate the underlying pathogen(s) both at infected sites and systemically.

3. Support the patient through the manifestations of organ dysfunction that arise as a consequence of the infection.

2. What are likely sources of serious nosocomial infection in ICU patients?

1. In the surgical ICU (SICU), the most common sources of infection are the urinary tract (affecting 15% of all SICU patients), wounds (10% of patients), pneumonia (8% of patients), and line-associated bacteremia (8% of patients). In medical ICU (MICU) patients, the common sites are the urinary tract (10% of all MICU patients), pneumonia (10% of patients), and line-associated bacteremia (5% of patients).[7]

2. Every site of an invasive device is a potential focus of infection. Nasotracheal tubes can predispose to nosocomial sinusitis, and nasogastric tubes to aspiration pneumonia.

3. What are the predominant pathogens in:
   a. Community-acquired sepsis?

Community-acquired sepsis is usually the result of systemic spread of a common focal bacteria infection. Common sources are pyelonephritis, pneumonia, intraabdominal infections, and severe cutaneous processes. The pathogens are related to the underlying processes and to the specific ability of the microorganism to spread from the local site to cause systemic disease. *Escherichia coli* and Klebsiella species predominate in urinary tract infections; *Streptococcus pneumoniae, Hemophilus influenzae,* and *Legionella pneumophila* in pneumonia; mixed enteric gram-negative rods and anaerobes in abdominal infections; and *Staphylococcus aureus* and *Streptococcus pyogenes* in cutaneous disease.

Less commonly, community-acquired sepsis is the primary manifestation of overwhelming systemic disease due to meningococcemia, Rocky Mountain spotted fever, tularemia, plague, or malaria. Also, the toxic shock syndrome due to *S. aureus* develops when apparently minor local infections with toxin-producing strains produce overwhelming systemic illness.

   b. Nosocomial sepsis?

As with community-acquired infections, the possible pathogens in nosocomial sepsis depend on the primary focus of the infectious process. Urinary tract infections, again, are most commonly due to enteric gram-negative rods such as *E. coli* and Klebsiella, but likely pathogens also include antibiotic-resistant Enterobacter, Serratia, and Pseudomonas species. Major pathogens found in nosocomial pneumonia, wound infection, and line infection include these same gram-negative pathogens and *S. aureus. Candida albicans* must be considered a cause of sepsis in patients with prolonged hospitalization who have received prior antibiotic therapy, have indwelling vascular access devices, have Candida isolated from a non-bloodstream site, have had intraabdominal surgery, have had hemodialysis, or have had chemotherapy-induced neutropenia.

c. Sepsis in the neutropenic patient?

The pathogens that cause sepsis in the oncology patient with chemotherapy-induced neutropenia are similar to those that routinely infect hospitalized patients. However, the incidence of *Pseudomonas aeruginosa* is increased in relation to the other gram-negative pathogens and *S. aureus*. In patients with permanent indwelling catheters, the incidence of *Staphylococcus epidermidis* sepsis also increases. In neutropenic patients who remain febrile on broad-spectrum antibacterial therapy, there is a high incidence of infections with fungi, particularly Candida species and Aspergillus.

4. What diagnostic studies should be performed to evaluate the patient with sepsis?

Diagnostic studies are done to define the site and etiology of the infectious process and to identify and quantitate secondary organ damage.

1. Two blood cultures should be obtained from separate venipuncture or central line sites. Depending on an individual institution's clinical microbiology laboratory, a single "blood culture" may involve from 1 to 3 tubes or bottles. Overall, the total blood volume cultured should be at least 30 ml. Additional cultures of urine, sputum, cerebrospinal fluid, or wounds should be taken as warranted by the clinical presentation.

2. Other studies to address the host response to infection, the potential site of infection, and potential organ involvement include CBC, differential, platelet count, PT and PTT, serum creatinine, serum liver function studies, and chest roentgenogram. Arterial blood gas determinations and additional biochemical and imaging studies are almost always necessary, but should be selected on the basis of the clinical situation.

5. What is appropriate antibiotic therapy for the patient with:

a. Community-acquired sepsis and a urinary tract focus?

The major pathogens in this setting are enteric gram-negative bacilli, *E. coli,* and Klebsiella, although enterococci are uncommonly identified. Intravenous trimethoprim-sulfamethoxazole given concurrently with an intravenous aminoglycoside (for 24 hours until the pathogen is identified) now appears to be safe and effective. Alternative acceptable regimens include intravenous ampicillin and an aminoglycoside, an intravenous third-generation cephalosporin, or intravenous ciprofloxacin.

b. Community-acquired sepsis and a lower respiratory focus?

The primary pathogens that cause both fulminant systemic infection and pneumonia in the U.S. include *S. pneumoniae, H. influenzae, L. pneumophila*. In the setting of recent influenza, *S. aureus* and *S. pyogenes* are also possible. The best immediate diagnostic test to discriminate between these pathogens is the sputum Gram stain, which can be used to select a narrow-spectrum antibiotic regimen. The moderately ill patient with pneumonia can be treated with oral agents, but the patient with pneumonia **and sepsis** initially requires broad-spectrum intravenous therapy. Ampicillin-sulbactam, or ticarcillin-clavulanic acid, or a second- or third-generation cephalosporin, or trimethoprim-sulfamethoxazole are all alternative regimens that will empirically cover *S. pneumoniae* and *H. influenzae* as well as the much less common *S. aureus* and *S. pyogenes*. Intravenous erythromycin provides the best coverage for *L. pneumophila*, although trimethoprim-sulfamethoxazole, imipenem/cilastatin, and ciprofloxacin also appear to be active against the pathogen.

c. Community-acquired sepsis with rash?

Major diagnostic concerns in overwhelming septicemia and rash are toxic shock syndrome, meningococcemia, and Rocky Mountain spotted fever, although characteristics of the rash and the clinical setting may help to narrow the differential. Empirical antibiotic treatment for toxic shock syndrome should be a semisynthetic antistaphylococcal penicillin or vancomycin; for meningococcemia, intravenous penicillin G or a third-generation cephalosporin; and for Rocky Mountain spotted fever, intravenous tetracycline or chloramphenicol.

d. Nosocomially acquired sepsis?

Empirical therapy in this setting should address both hospital-acquired enteric gram-negative bacteria and *S. aureus*. The gram-negative organism can be effectively treated with an intravenous aminoglycoside or third-generation cephalosporin, selection of the exact agent being dependent on known antimicrobial susceptibility patterns within a given institution. Empirical treatment of *S. aureus* may be with a semisynthetic antistaphylococcal penicillin, a first-generation cephalosporin, or vancomycin. Again, the precise agent used depends upon the institution's antimicrobial flora.

e. Sepsis in the neutropenic host?

In this setting, empirical antibiotic therapy should cover *Pseudomonas aeruginosa* as well as the other aerobic gram-negative pathogens. An antipseudomonal penicillin (ticarcillin, mezlocillin, or piperacillin) with an aminoglycoside, or either ceftazidime or cefoperazone with or without an aminoglycoside, is appropriate. If there is a strong suspicion of *S. aureus* infection, treatment with a semisynthetic antistaphylococcal penicillin, or a first-generation cephalosporin, or vancomycin should be added.

6. Is surgery of value in the management of sepsis?

Surgical drainage is required if there is a definable abscess. Although antimicrobial therapy can control the systemic spread of infection, it will not eradicate a focal abscess. The identification and subsequent elimination of such abscesses are essential components of therapy.

7. What further supportive measures are required in the patient with septic shock?

1. Vigorous resuscitation with intravenous fluids and hemodynamic monitoring should be performed to correct underlying deficits and to support the systemic blood pressure in the face of peripheral vasodilation and capillary endothelial leakage. Intravenous pressor therapy should be started. If systemic hypotension is not corrected in spite of increases in pulmonary capillary wedge pressures to 15 to 18 mm Hg, initial treatment should be with dopamine at levels up to 20 μg/kg/min. If hypotension persists, a second pressor such as norepinephrine should be added.

2. Respiratory function should be closely monitored for the development of the adult respiratory distress syndrome (ARDS). Elective intubation and mechanical ventilation may be necessary.

3. Renal and hepatic function should be monitored, as should the coagulation system, watching for disseminated intravascular coagulation (DIC).

8. Is there a role for corticosteroid therapy in patients with sepsis?

Studies performed in the 1950s, 1960s, and early 1970s suggested that high-dose corticosteroid therapy might be helpful in the treatment of septic shock. However, two placebo-controlled trials reported in 1987 found **no benefit** of high-dose steroid therapy in the treatment of sepsis in adults.[1,9] In contradistinction, recent work suggests that high-dose corticosteroids can decrease the complications of bacterial meningitis in children.

CONTROVERSY

9. Should adjunctive therapy directed at the direct inflammatory mediators of sepsis be used in routine therapy of septic shock?

For:

1. Evidence from multiple sources now indicates that the endotoxin of gram-negative bacteria (as well as components of other bacteria) induces macrophages to produce the cytokines tumor necrosis factor (TNF) and interleukin I (IL-1) that directly mediate the clinical manifestations of sepsis.

2. Recent human studies have found that monoclonal antibodies against endotoxin can prevent death due to gram-negative sepsis.[12] Monoclonal antibodies against TNF and IL-1 as well as innate antagonists of the cytokines can decrease mortality in experimental sepsis.

Against:

1. The benefit of antiendotoxin monoclonal antibody therapy appears to be limited to patients with sepsis due to gram-negative bacteria. Unfortunately, this represents only about 50% of patients with the sepsis syndrome. Thus, when the total population of patients presenting with sepsis is considered, the overall benefit is limited.[12] The potential benefit of using the monoclonal antibody therapy only after a diagnosis of gram-negative sepsis is confirmed has not yet been evaluated.

2. Both monoclonal antibodies against TNF and IL-1, a well as innate antagonists, should be active in sepsis of any origin and therefore circumvent the difficulties with the antiendotoxin preparations. However, no human studies of these agents have been completed.

BIBLIOGRAPHY

1. Bone RC, Fisher CJ Jr, Clemmer TP, et al: A controlled clinical trial of high-dose methylprednisolone in the treatment of severe sepsis and septic shock. N Engl J Med 317:653–658, 1987.
2. Craven DE, Kunches LM, Lichtenberg DA, et al: Nosocomial infection and fatality in medical and surgical intensive care unit patients. Arch Intern Med 148:1161–1168, 1988.
3. Harris RL, Musher DM, Bloom K, et al: Manifestations of sepsis. Arch Intern Med 147:1895–1906, 1987.
4. Jacobson M, Young LS: New developments in the treatment of gram-negative bacteremia. West J Med 144:185–194, 1986.
5. Johnson JR, Lyons MF II, Pearce W, et al: Therapy for women hospitalized with acute pyelonephritis: A randomized trial of ampicillin versus trimethoprim-sulfamethoxazole for 14 days. J Infect Dis 163:325–330, 1991.
6. McCabe WR, Treadwell TL, DeMaria AD Jr: Pathophysiology of bacteremia. Am J Med 75:7–18, 1983.
7. Parillo JE, Parker MM, Natanson C, et al: Septic shock in humans: Advances in the understanding of pathogenesis, cardiovascular dysfunction, and therapy. Ann Intern Med 113:227–242, 1990.
8. Parker MM, Parrillo JE: Septic shock: Hemodynamics and pathogenesis. JAMA 250:3324–3327, 1983.
9. The Veterans Administration Systemic Sepsis Cooperative Study Group: Effect of high-dose glucocorticosteroid therapy on mortality in patients with clinical signs of systemic sepsis. N Engl J Med 317:659–665, 1987.
10. Weinstein MP, Murphy JR, Reller LB, Lichtenstein KA: The clinical significance of positive blood cultures: A comprehensive analysis of 500 episodes of bacteremia and fungemia in adults. II. Clinical observations, with special reference to factors influencing prognosis. Rev Infect Dis 5:54–70, 1983.
11. Young LA, Martin WJ, Meyer RD, et al: Gram-negative rod bacteremia: Microbiologic, immunologic, and therapeutic considerations. Ann Intern Med 86:456–471, 1977.
12. Ziegler EJ, Fisher CJ Jr, Sprung CL, et al: Treatment of gram-negative bacteremia and septic shock with HA-1A human monoclonal antibody against endotoxin: A randomized, double-blind, placebo-controlled trial. N Engl J Med 324:429–436, 1991.
13. Ziegler EJ, McCutchan JA, Fierer J, et al: Treatment of gram-negative bacteremia and shock with human antiserum to a mutant *Escherichia coli*. N Engl J Med 307:1225–1230, 1982.

38. ENDOCARDITIS

Ira M. Dauber, M.D.

1. Who is at risk for endocarditis?

Patients with underlying valvular heart disease (rheumatic, other acquired valvular heart disease, mitral valve prolapse with regurgitation) and prosthetic heart valves (including bioprostheses) are at greatest risk. Congenital heart disease (ventricular septal defect, patent ductus arteriosus, tetralogy of Fallot), hypertrophic cardiomyopathy, and previous bacterial endocarditis (even without underlying heart disease) are also risk factors. These patients should receive endocarditis prophylaxis. Endovascular infections (septic thrombophlebitis, infected vascular prosthesis), intravenous (IV) drug abuse, and bacteremias of aggressive organisms (e.g., *Staphylococcus aureus*) present a risk for endocarditis even in patients without underlying heart disease. Fungal endocarditis is uncommon but can develop in immunocompromised patients and patients on long-term broad-spectrum antibiotics.

2. What are the common clinical features of endocarditis?

Endocarditis is usually a febrile illness. Both cardiac and extracardiac manifestations occur. Congestive heart failure due to valvular dysfunction (usually regurgitation), myocardial invasion with abscess formation (often signaled by bundle branch block or heart block), myocarditis and/or pericarditis can occur. Extracardiac manifestations are due to embolization (both septic and nonseptic emboli) and immune-complex manifestations (e.g., glomerulonephritis).

3. Are acute and subacute endocarditis different diseases?

No. Both are infectious/inflammatory diseases of heart valves. Endocarditis can vary in its time course and clinical features related to the aggressiveness of the underlying bacteriologic agent. Acute endocarditis has a rapid onset (days to weeks) and progression of an acute, toxic febrile illness with major cardiac symptoms, including congestive heart failure, valvular insufficiency, and conduction abnormalities. In contrast, subacute endocarditis is an indolent, chronic (weeks to months) illness with weight loss, malaise, persistent fever, heart murmur, and anemia, which may or may not present with cardiac manifestations. Peripheral manifestations such as splenomegaly, hematuria, Osler nodes, Janeway lesions, and Roth spots are more common with subacute endocarditis.

4. What type of heart murmurs are usually associated with endocarditis?

Regurgitant murmurs (aortic insufficiency, mitral or tricuspid regurgitation) secondary to valvular injury are the most common murmurs. Stenotic murmurs are rarely caused by endocarditis, although they may occur with prosthetic valve endocarditis. In many patients, a murmur may not be easily audible, as the murmurs of acute mitral regurgitation and aortic insufficiency can be short and obscured by tachycardia. Murmurs arising from tricuspid or pulmonic insufficiency may be difficult to appreciate on exam. Echocardiography with Doppler can be a valuable method for evaluating and detecting cardiac murmurs due to endocarditis.

5. How do right-sided and left-sided endocarditis differ?

In addition to the location of the infected valve and the underlying etiology (right-sided is more common with IV drug abuse), there are other important differences. Left-sided lesions are associated with systemic embolization (brain, kidney, spleen), whereas right-sided lesions embolize to the lung, presenting as lung abscess, pneumonia, or pulmonary emboli. Right-sided endocarditis may not be associated with an audible murmur (one-third of cases), usually have few peripheral manifestations (such as petechiae, Roth spots, hematuria), and may be culture negative. Right-sided valvular dysfunction is usually of less hemodynamic significance than left-sided valve lesions are.

6. How is the diagnosis of endocarditis made?
Positive blood cultures are the *sine qua non* of endocarditis. Two or more sets of blood cultures should be collected. In the absence of other sources of bacteremia, they are diagnostic. Endovascular infections such as endocarditis should be strongly considered with the combination of new-onset heart failure and a new heart murmur.

7. What is the role of echocardiography in the diagnosis and treatment of endocarditis?
Echocardiography is a useful adjunct in the diagnosis and treatment of endocarditis and can be used to determine the presence of regurgitant valvular lesions and/or vegetations; their presence, however, is not specific for active endocarditis. Echocardiography alone should not be used to rule out endocarditis. Although vegetations are strongly suggestive of endocarditis, their absence does not exclude the diagnosis, as small vegetations (< 3 mm) may be missed or they may not be present at the time the study is performed. Serial echocardiograms can be helpful for assessing the severity of valvular injury; cardiac dysfunction; the presence, size, and number of vegetations; and intramyocardial extension of the infection.

8. Do negative blood cultures rule out endocarditis?
Negative routine blood cultures do not absolutely rule out endocarditis. Approximately 10% of patients with endocarditis may have "culture-negative endocarditis." Prior antibiotic therapy is the most common cause of negative blood cultures. Slow-growing or fastidious organisms (nutritionally deficient bacteria, fungi, chlamydia) and right-sided endocarditis (up to 22% of cases) are also associated with culture-negative endocarditis. Some patients with culture-negative endocarditis are not infected and have marantic (thrombotic, nonbacterial) endocarditis.

9. Which valves are most commonly affected?
- Native valve (acute or subacute): mitral $>$ aortic $>$ tricuspid
- Prosthetic valve: aortic $>$ mitral
- Fungal: right $>$ left-sided valves
- IV drug abuse: right $>$ left-sided valves

10. What are the most common organisms causing endocarditis?
- Native valve (acute and subacute): Streptococcus (30–40%), *Staphylococcus aureus* (15–35%), Enterococcus (10–20%). Subacute usually due to *Streptococcus viridans*.
- Prosthetic valve: *S. aureus* and *Staphylococcus epidermidis*
- IV drug abusers: *S. aureus* and gram-negative organisms
- Fungal: Candida.

11. What is the initial therapy for endocarditis?
The hemodynamic consequences of endocarditis can be severe. Specific therapy tailored to the observed hemodynamic alterations should be initiated as soon as possible. Empirical antibiotic therapy can be started for acute endocarditis prior to the isolation of a causative organism. Initial IV therapy with penicillin, a beta-lactamase–resistant penicillin (e.g., nafcillin), and an aminoglycoside should provide effective therapy for the majority of patients. Because of the increased frequency of methicillin-resistant staphylococci in IV drug abusers and of *S. epidermidis* in prosthetic valve infections, vancomycin should be substituted for the penicillins in these patients. As the importance of obtaining a specific

microbiologic diagnosis cannot be overemphasized, therapy should be delayed until adequate numbers of blood cultures have been obtained.

12. How is endocarditis treated?

1. **Native valve bacterial endocarditis:** Usually responds to antibiotic treatment alone. Treatment is with bactericidal antibiotics for prolonged periods (4–6 weeks). Specific antibiotics are chosen based on the organism(s) isolated. Common choices are:

- Streptococci (nonenterococcal): penicillin G (10–20 million units qd)
- Enterococci: penicillin G + gentamicin
- Staphylococci: nafcillin or oxacillin ± gentamicin
- Staphylococci (methicillin-resistant): vancomycin
- Gram-negative: penicillin/cephalosporin + aminoglycoside (depends on organism)

2. **Fungal endocarditis:** Because of their poor outcome with medical therapy alone, patients with fungal endocarditis usually require surgical intervention. Intravenous antifungal therapy (amphotericin B ± 5-fluorocytosine) should be initiated and continued postoperatively.

3. **Prosthetic valve endocarditis:** "Early" (<2 months after insertion) and "late" prosthetic valve endocarditis are treated differently. Early infections are more commonly due to *S. epidermidis*, gram-negative bacteria, and diphtheroids. Initial therapy with vancomycin and gentamicin is indicated. Late infections have a spectrum similar to native valve endocarditis.

4. **Culture-negative endocarditis:** For acute endocarditis, initial therapy with vancomycin and gentamicin aimed at the bacterial causes of culture-negative endocarditis can be initiated. Further therapy is aimed at likely causes based on the clinical situation. In patients at risk for fungal endocarditis (immunosuppressed, prior broad-spectrum antibiotics, fungal infection elsewhere) or in whom there is no clinical improvement with empirical antibiotics, amphotericin B ± 5-fluorocytosine should be added. For subacute endocarditis, therapy should be withheld until there is a specific diagnosis.

Note: Therapy should be modified for penicillin-allergic patients or if renal dysfunction is present.

13. What are the indicators of a poor outcome with medical therapy?

Native valve infections usually respond to adequate antibiotic treatment, but prosthetic valve and fungal infections have a lower response rate. The presence of congestive heart failure, involvement of the aortic or a prosthetic valve, systemic embolization, large (>1.0 cm) vegetations, and an infecting organism other than streptococcus are associated with a worse outcome.

14. What are the signs and causes of treatment failure?

Treatment failure is evident as persistent infection, progressive cardiac dysfunction, or persistent hemodynamic instability. Failure to eradicate the infection may be due to emergence of resistant organisms, unsuspected multiple organisms (especially in IV drug abusers), inadequate drug levels, and/or the presence of a perivalvular or myocardial abscess. Fever usually resolves within 1 week of treatment, although persistent fever may be due to causes other than treatment failure (drugs, immune-complex nephritis, thrombophlebitis). Despite successful treatment of the infection, hemodynamic instability may continue due to the severity of valve injury and the limited ability of the heart to compensate for acute volume overload, as occurs with aortic or mitral regurgitation.

15. Are there late sequelae of endocarditis?

Risk of embolization can persist for up to 6 months (until there is full endothelialization of vegetations and injured endocardial surfaces). Mycotic aneurysms can present months or years after an episode of endocarditis. Congestive heart failure may develop due to persistent valve dysfunction.

CONTROVERSY

16. What are the role and optimal timing of surgery in the management of endocarditis?
Definite indications for surgery include hemodynamic instability (severe heart failure, valvular obstruction) and uncontrolled infection (persistent bacteremia, lack of an effective antimicrobial regimen, or fungal endocarditis). Relative indications are an organism other than streptococcus, intracardiac extension, repeated embolization, large (> 1.0 cm) vegetations, and early prosthetic valve endocarditis. The presence of vegetations on left-sided valves (mitral or aortic) has been considered to be an indication for early surgery, as systemic embolization (often cerebral) is one of the most feared complications of endocarditis. However, most patients with vegetations do not have emboli, and even patients without vegetations can have emboli. The procedure of choice is insertion of a prosthetic valve, although some tricuspid valve infections have been treated with valve removal without replacement.

Early surgery is necessary for hemodynamically unstable patients and has been suggested for patients with congestive heart failure or infections unlikely to respond to medical therapy alone (fungal or nonstreptococcal infections, prosthetic valves). Prolonged courses of ineffective antibiotic therapy are associated with poor survival if surgery is necessary (10% survival after 4–6 weeks of therapy vs. 83% if surgery is performed within 10 days of starting therapy). Hemodynamic status at the time of surgery is the most important predictor of outcome. Thus, early surgery can reduce the risks of progressive hemodynamic deterioration in patients who need (or will need) surgery. However, the placement of a foreign body into an infected surgical field is not without problems. Postoperative endocarditis occurs in up to 10% of patients with active infections at the time of surgery, and the incidence of valve dehiscence is higher without prior antibiotic therapy. In hemodynamically stable patients, a minimum of a 7- to 10-day course of antibiotics prior to surgery seems reasonable.

BIBLIOGRAPHY

1. Alsip SG, Blackstone EH, Kirklin JW, Cobbs CG: Indications for cardiac surgery in patients with active infective endocarditis. Am J Med 78(Suppl 6B):138–148, 1985.
2. American Heart Association: Prevention of bacterial endocarditis. JAMA 264:2919–2922, 1990.
3. Brandenburg RO, Giuliani ER, Wilson WR, Geraci JE: Infective endocarditis—A 25-year overview of diagnosis and therapy. J Am Coll Cardiol 1:280–291, 1983.
4. Buda AJ, Zotz RJ, LeMire MS, Bach DS: Prognostic significance of vegetations detected by two-dimensional echocardiography in infective endocarditis. Am Heart J 112:1291–1296, 1986.
5. Dinubile MJ: Surgery in active endocarditis. Ann Intern Med 96:650–659, 1982.
6. Mayer KH, Schoenbaum SC: Evaluation and management of prosthetic valve endocarditis. Prog Cardiovasc Dis 25:43–54, 1982.
7. O'Brien JT, Geiser EA: Infective endocarditis and echocardiography. Am Heart J 108:386–394, 1984.
8. Reisberg BE: Infective endocarditis in the narcotic addict. Prog Cardiovasc Dis 22:193–204, 1979.
9. Robbins MJ, Eisenberg ES, Frishman WH: Infective endocarditis: A pathophysiologic approach to therapy. Cardiol Clin 5:545–562, 1987.
10. Robbins MJ, Soeiro R, Frishman WH: Right-sided valvular endocarditis: Etiology, diagnosis and an approach to therapy. Am Heart J 111:128–135, 1986.
11. Sullam PM, Drake TA, Sande MA: Pathogenesis of endocarditis. Am J Med 78(Suppl 6B):110–115, 1985.
12. Van Scoy RE: Culture-negative endocarditis. Mayo Clin Proc 57:149–154, 1982.
13. Weinstein L: Infective endocarditis. In Braunwald E (ed): Heart Disease: A Textbook of Cardiovascular Medicine, 2nd ed. Philadelphia, W.B. Saunders, 1988, pp 1136–1178.
14. Wilson WR, Giuliani ER, Danielson GK: General considerations in the diagnosis and treatment of infective endocarditis. Mayo Clin Proc 57:81–85, 1982.

39. MENINGITIS

Randall Reves, M.D.

1. What are the clinical and pathophysiologic features that distinguish meningitis from other central nervous system infections?

Meningitis is an infection localized to the subarachnoid space. The inflammatory process may involve the entire leptomeningeal surface of the brain and spinal cord and spread through the foramina of Luscha and Magendie to produce ventriculitis. Neurologic dysfunction is usually limited to depressed sensorium and seizures; occasional cranial nerve defects result from the inflammation surrounding cranial nerves that traverse the subarachnoid space. Subdural empyema or epidural abscess within the cranium or spinal canal, brain abscess, encephalitis, myelitis, and neuritis tend to produce more localized signs or symptoms than those seen with meningitis.

2. What signs and symptoms should place meningitis in the differential diagnosis?

Symptoms of a recent upper respiratory infection followed by the development of headache, nuchal rigidity, vomiting, confusion, or lethargy should always prompt consideration of acute meningitis. Symptoms are often more subtle in infants, the elderly, or patients who develop meningitis associated with neurosurgical procedures.

3. What are the differences in acute, subacute and chronic presentations of meningitis?

Individuals presenting with a rapidly progressive illness of less than 24 hours' duration usually have bacterial meningitis. The acute presentation is seen in about 25% of cases of bacterial meningitis, and this group has a mortality rate of 50%. A subacute presentation of up to 7 days' duration is seen in nearly all cases of meningitis due to viruses and in three-quarters of cases due to bacteria. Bacterial meningitis presenting subacutely is associated with a mortality rate less than half that of those presenting with a fulminant course. The distinction between the acute and subacute presentations has important diagnostic, therapeutic, and prognostic implications. Chronic meningitis is usually due to tuberculosis or fungi and has a more gradual onset of meningeal symptoms or even presents as dementia.

4. When should one make an exception to the adage "If you think of doing a spinal tap, do one"?

Lumbar punctures generally should be avoided in the presence of brain abscess or other localized brain lesions in which the risk for herniation is deemed significant. Precautions should also be taken to avoid passing the spinal needle through an infected area such as infected skin or through an epidural abscess. In some situations, neurosurgical consultation may be required to sample cerebrospinal fluid (CSF) via cervical or cisternal approaches. Correction of severe coagulopathies or thrombocytopenia may be required before spinal tap.

5. When should a CT scan be done before a spinal tap in a patient presenting with meningitis?

Spinal taps should be preceded by CT scanning if brain abscess is suspected. When an individual presents with symptoms of meningitis associated with papilledema or focal neurologic defects, a localized CNS lesion should be ruled out before spinal tap. To avoid critical delays in therapy, empirical therapy for brain abscess and meningitis, such as chloramphenicol, can be initiated immediately after obtaining blood cultures. The spinal tap should be done after concerns about the presence of a mass lesion are resolved by CT scanning.

6. What is the goal in the approach to meningitis with an acute presentation?
The goal is to begin appropriate therapy within 30 minutes of patient contact. Because of the high case-fatality rate in patients with an acute presentation of meningitis, a rapid clinical assessment should be followed by empirical therapy appropriate for the clinical setting. Blood cultures and, unless a spinal tap is contraindicated, CSF samples should be obtained after a rapid clinical assessment, followed by empirical therapy. CSF Gram stains and other studies should then be examined promptly to assess the need for changes in therapy.

7. What is the goal in the approach to meningitis with a subacute presentation?
The goal is to complete the assessment and, if indicated, initiate therapy for bacterial meningitis within 2 hours of patient contact.

8. What CSF findings in meningitis should prompt initiation of antimicrobial therapy?
Patients with an acute, rapidly progressive course should receive empirical therapy, pending analysis of CSF results. In subacute presentations, indications for and choice of antimicrobial therapy should be based on prompt assessment of CSF studies as well as clinical and epidemiologic features. Gram stains of spun sediment of CSF are positive in 80–90% of culture-documented cases of meningitis and usually provide rapid information about likely etiologic agents. In the presence of negative Gram stain, analysis of other CSF parameters can be used to assist in the decision concerning empirical therapy. A CSF cell count of $> 1000/mm^3$, protein of > 150 mg/dl, or glucose of < 30 mg/dl would indicate a high probability of bacterial meningitis rather than a viral etiology and warrant appropriate antimicrobial therapy, pending the results of cultures and other studies. None of these guidelines alone or in combination can be used to rule out bacterial etiologies or preclude antimicrobial therapy; clinical judgment, frequent reassessment, and repeat spinal taps may be indicated. Latex agglutination tests for antigens of pneumococci, meningococci, or *Hemophilus influenzae* may be helpful, although not completely sensitive.

9. How are CSF findings interpreted in the setting of prior antimicrobial therapy?
Up to 50% of individuals with meningitis present after having received up to several days of antimicrobial therapy, usually by the oral route. Prior antimicrobial therapy will reduce the frequency of positive CSF Gram stains in culture-positive patients to 65% and will reduce the frequency of positive cultures. Several days of therapy are generally required to alter the high CSF cell count and the low glucose levels in patients with bacterial meningitis.

10. What is the role of empirical therapy in meningitis?
An etiologic diagnosis should be obtained in the great majority of cases of bacterial meningitis, and initial empirical therapy should be continued, altered, or discontinued after results of CSF studies and other clinical data are available.

11. What are the likely bacterial pathogens causing meningitis and recommended antimicrobial agents for empirical therapy?
For the usual case of community-acquired bacterial meningitis in the normal host, high-dose intravenous penicillin G is the drug of choice, or chloramphenicol for the penicillin-allergic patient; this is the case with gram-negative or positive diplococci present in CSF or pending results of smears or cultures. Meningitis in hospitalized or immunocompromised hosts may be due to *Hemophilus influenzae* or other gram-negative bacilli such as *Klebsiella pneumoniae* or *Escherichia coli*. A third-generation cephalosporin with high CSF penetration, such as cefotaxime, ceftriaxone, or ceftazidime, should be considered for empirical therapy. Staphylococci and nosocomial pathogens such as *Pseudomonas*

aeruginosa are more common in cases developing after neurosurgical procedures, so that empirical therapy should include vancomycin and ceftazidime, or an antipseudomonal penicillin, plus an aminoglycoside.

12. Why is chloramphenicol, often considered a bacteriostatic agent, the treatment of choice for the penicillin-allergic patient with pneumococcal or meningococcal meningitis?
Although chloramphenicol is bacteriostatic for enteric gram-negative bacilli, and therapy failure for meningitis due to such organisms is well documented, it is bactericidal for meningococci, pneumococci, and *H. influenzae* with the levels achievable in the CSF, and resistance to chloramphenicol among these organisms is rare. Because about 10% of individuals with true penicillin allergy will also be allergic to cephalosporins, chloramphenicol is considered the initial drug of choice in such patients; questionable histories of penicillin allergy can be sorted out while the patient is receiving effective therapy.

13. How long should therapy for bacterial meningitis be continued?
Pneumococcal or meningococcal meningitis should be treated for 7 days in most cases, and follow-up spinal taps are not routinely done. The recommended duration of therapy for other organisms varies up to several weeks.

14. What is the role for repeat spinal taps in the management of meningitis?
Routine follow-up spinal taps are not necessary for the typical cases of pneumococcal or meningococcal meningitis. Repeat taps are an integral part of the management of meningitis due to gram-negative bacilli because therapy should be continued for 10 days following negative CSF cultures. Intrathecal gentamicin (preservative-free) may be required in some cases of meningitis due to organisms such as *P. aeruginosa;* intraventricular gentamicin may be required in such cases with ventriculitis.

15. What are the causes of recurrent meningitis?
Recurrent bacterial meningitis can result from persistent unrecognized or undrained parameningeal foci. Recurrence can also result either from abnormal communications with the upper respiratory tract or skin or from immunologic defects. CSF leaks into the nasopharynx, middle ear, or paranasal sinuses can result from congenital defects or be acquired following trauma; pneumococcus is the usual etiologic organism, except in patients receiving antibiotics, who are more likely to acquire gram-negative bacilli. Recurrent meningitis from a variety of organisms, including gram-negative bacilli, can result from infected dermal sinuses that communicate with the subarachnoid space, usually in the lumbosacral region. Immunologic defects associated with recurrent meningitis include splenectomy, hypogammaglobulinemia, and inherited deficiencies of complement components.

16. Which studies are mandatory and which should also be considered in evaluation of the aseptic meningitis syndrome?
Aseptic meningitis is a syndrome of meningitis with negative Gram stains and cultures and typically a normal CSF glucose. It is not synonymous with viral meningitis. Secondary syphilis and "parameningeal foci" may produce CSF pleocytosis; parameningeal foci include localized suppurative processes in or adjacent to the meninges. Bacterial endocarditis may also present as aseptic meningitis. The evaluation of aseptic meningitis should always include blood cultures and serum RPR or VDRL (not just CSF). Sinus radiographs should be considered in all cases, and CT or MRI scans of the head or spine may be indicated in some instances to rule out brain abscess, epidural abscess, and subdural empyema as parameningeal foci.

Tuberculosis, fungi, and some fastidious organisms such as Leptospira, Borrelia, and Brucella may present with the aseptic meningitis syndrome and require specific additional testing for diagnosis. Individuals with aseptic meningitis and hypoglycorrhachia following fresh-water exposure may be at risk for parasitic meningitis due to Naegleria. Rocky Mountain spotted fever should be considered in patients presenting with symptoms of meningitis but with normal CSF studies.

17. What are the noninfectious causes of meningitis?
The clinical presentation of meningitis can result from inflammatory reactions to intrathecal medications or from systemically administered drugs such as trimethoprim/sulfamethoxazole or nonsteroidal anti-inflammatory agents. A murine monoclonal antibody, OKT3, and azathioprine have been associated with meningitis in transplant recipients. Other noninfectious causes include carcinomatosis (usually with hypoglycorrhachia), inflammatory reactions to necrotic tumors, Mollaret's syndrome, sarcoidosis, and connective tissue diseases. A slowly leaking cerebral aneurysm may be responsible for xanthochromic CSF in aseptic meningitis.

18. What form of empirical therapy should always be considered in chronic meningitis?
Acid-fast smears and cultures of CSF are negative in up to 90% and 60%, respectively, in case series of tuberculous meningitis. To avoid sequelae associated with delays in diagnosis and treatment of tuberculous meningitis, and pending 6-week culture results and evaluation of clinical response, empirical therapy should be considered in any chronic, undiagnosed cases of meningitis with declining or low CSF glucose levels.

19. How sensitive is India ink examination and cryptococcal antigen testing for cryptococcal meningitis?
The sensitivity of India ink examination of CSF for the diagnosis of cryptococcal meningitis is 50%. Cryptococcal antigen testing of CSF is positive in 85%, and the sensitivity is increased to 94% by testing both CSF and serum. Cryptococcus is the most common cause of meningitis in patients with AIDS, occurring in about 3% of such individuals. In the setting of AIDS, there may be little or no indication of inflammation in the CSF.

20. How contagious is meningitis?
Among adults, meningococcal meningitis is the only bacterial agent in which risk of disease transmission has been documented. Among household members, the risk of secondary cases within a month of onset of the index case has been determined to be < 1% (about 6 per 1000). Although cases have been reported among medical personnel caring for patients with meningococcal disease, the risk is probably considerably lower than that among household members. Two days' treatment with rifampin is recommended for household or other intimate contacts to interrupt nasopharyngeal carriage. Prophylactic therapy may be offered to those with intense exposure, such as occurs in performing intubation, but is not indicated for medical personnel in general. The enteroviruses that cause the majority of cases of viral meningitis are contagious, but most infected contacts are either asymptomatic or manifest febrile illnesses other than meningitis.

CONTROVERSIES

21. What is the optimal therapy for meningitis associated with CSF shunts?
Meningitis and/or ventriculitis associated with implanted ventriculoperitoneal shunts or with ventriculostomies used for temporary shunting may be due to a variety of nosocomial pathogens in the early postoperative period or to coagulase-negative staphylococci months later. Diagnosis may require the sampling of ventricular fluid. Antibiotics should be selected on the basis of susceptibility of the pathogens. Treatment failures occur in 30–40% of cases treated with antimicrobial therapy without removal of the prosthetic device. One

study found a higher risk of death among patients in whom the shunt was not immediately removed or replaced. It remains unclear whether an initial trial of medical therapy without removal of the shunt is warranted.

22. Should corticosteroids be given to individuals with meningitis?
A number of studies suggest that several days of dexamethasone therapy begun concomitantly with antimicrobial therapy reduces the frequency of neurologic complications of bacterial meningitis among infants and children. Most cases were due to *H. influenzae,* and the major complication prevented was hearing loss. The significance of these observations for adults with meningitis is unclear and clinical trials are in progress.

BIBLIOGRAPHY

1. Carpenter RR, Petersdorf RG: The clinical spectrum of bacterial meningitis. Am J Med 33:262–275, 1962.
2. Greenlee JE: Approach to diagnosis of meningitis: Cerebrospinal fluid evaluation. Infect Dis Clin North Am 4:583–598, 1990.
3. Kaufman BA, Tunkel AR, Pryor FC, Dacey RG Jr: Meningitis in the neurosurgical patient. Infect Dis Clin North Am 4:667–701, 1990.
4. McGee ZE, Baringer JR: Acute meningitis. In Mandell GL, Douglas R, Bennett JE (eds): Principles and Practice of Infectious Diseases, 3rd ed. New York, Churchill Livingstone, 1990, pp 742–754.
5. Odio CM, Faingezicht I, Paris M, et al: The beneficial effects of early dexamethasone administration in infants and children with bacterial meningitis. N Engl J Med 324:1525–1531, 1991.
6. Wispelwey B, Tunkel AR, Scheld WM: Bacterial meningitis in adults. Infect Dis Clin North Am 4:645–659, 1990.

40. URINARY TRACT INFECTIONS

Raymond N. Blum, M.D.

1. What are the risk factors associated with urinary tract infection (UTI) in the ICU?
Approximately 80% of nosocomial UTIs are associated with catheterization. The rate of acquisition of bacteriuria with a catheter in place is about 5–10% per day, with about 50% of patients bacteriuric by day 8. Other factors include female sex, diabetes, absence of systemic antibiotic use, and possibly diarrhea.

2. What is the pathogenesis of a catheter-related UTI?
Most catheter-related UTIs begin with colonization of the meatus and urethra, followed by an ascending infection. Some are related to colonization of the collection system and an intraluminal, ascending infection. Occasionally, bacteremic seeding of the kidneys can occur.

3. When should presence of a UTI be considered in a critically ill patient?
Signs and symptoms in a critically ill patient are often subtle but can include fever, leukocytosis, bacteremia, and lower abdominal and low-back pain. Of all nosocomial infections, 30% are infections of the urinary tract. Thus, in evaluating a hospitalized patient for infection, the clinician must pay attention to the urinary tract. The urinary tract is the source of nosocomial sepsis and bacteremia in 5–10% of cases.

4. How is the diagnosis of UTI established?

The gold standard of bacteriuria has been $\geq 10^5$ cfu/mm^3 in a urine culture. However, the presence of this level of bacteriuria may represent only colonization. Also, in ambulatory women, as few as 10^2 cfu/mm^3 has been associated with a true infection. In catheterized patients, most with low concentrations of bacteria will progress over a few days to $\geq 10^5$ cfu/ml. Supporting evidence of a true infection (in a non-neutropenic patient) is the presence of pyuria or hematuria as well as signs and symptoms.

5. What organisms are likely to be involved in UTI in catheterized patients?

The likely pathogens depend on the length of catheterization and the use of antimicrobial agents. Immediately after catheterization, gram-positive organisms such as *Staphylococcus epidermidis* and *Staph. aureus* can be seen. Otherwise, *E. coli*, Klebsiella, and enterococcus are more common. Resistant gram-negative organisms, such as those from the Serratia, Proteus, and Pseudomonas species, are more common in patients receiving broad-spectrum antimicrobials.

6. What are the complications of UTI?

Complications of nosocomial UTI include fever, pyelonephritis, perinephric abscess, bacteremia, sepsis, metastatic infections, and death. A three-fold increase in mortality is associated with UTI from an indwelling catheter in hospitalized patients. About 1% of hospitalized patients with nosocomial UTI will experience bacteremia. Catheter-associated UTI has been shown to increase hospital stays by 2–3 days. Metastatic infections can include endocarditis, especially in patients with valvular heart disease, osteomyelitis, and epidural abscess. In males, infections of the epididymis and testes can occur.

7. When is therapy indicated?

Therapy is indicated for all episodes of symptomatic bacteriuria. Treatment of episodes of asymptomatic bacteriuria without the removal of the catheter may lead to the emergence of resistant organisms. Therapy may be indicated for asymptomatic bacteriuria if catheter removal is anticipated within a few days.

8. What antimicrobial agents should be used?

Initial empirical therapy in patients with evidence of sepsis should include agents that are active against both gram-positive and gram-negative organisms, such as vancomycin or ampicillin, and a third-generation cephalosporin or an aminoglycoside. Therapy can be guided additionally by a Gram stain of the urine. Coverage should be narrowed as quickly as possible based on susceptibility testing. Therapy for mild symptoms may include oral agents such as trimethoprim/sulfamethoxazole.

9. What should be done with the catheter during infections?

If no longer required, the catheter should be removed. If there are leaks or evidence of obstruction in the catheter system, it should be replaced. Use of a condom cathether or intermittent catheterization should be considered.

10. What are the risk factors associated with candiduria?

Candiduria is associated with broad-spectrum antimicrobials, catheterization, diabetes, corticosteroids, female sex, and stasis of urine. A systemic fungal infection must always be considered when candiduria is found.

11. How should candiduria be managed?

Removal of the catheter is paramount to the elimination of candiduria. If this is not possible, bladder irrigation can be used. The role of systemic antifungal therapy, including amphotericin and fluconazole, should be reserved for serious infections or when there is evidence of systemic fungal infection. If candiduria does not resolve after catheter removal, the urinary tract is evaluated for obstruction. Treatment of asymptomatic candiduria in a catheterized patient may be replaced by bacteriuria.

12. What is role of bladder irrigation in managing candiduria?

Irrigation of the bladder with amphotericin using a triple-lumen catheter can help to decrease candiduria. This is usually done with a solution of 50 mg of amphotericin/L of D5W instilled either as a continuous infusion over 24 hours for 5–7 days or instilling 200–300 ml and clamping the catheter for 60–90 minutes at regular intervals for 5–7 days. It is especially useful when short-term catheterization is anticipated.

13. What are key features in preventing nosocomial UTI?

Elimination of unnecessary use of catheterization in the intensive care unit is the most important measure in decreasing the incidence of nosocomial UTIs. Aseptic insertion, meticulous care to avoid breaching the closed system, use of sterile technique in obtaining all urine specimens, and not changing the catheter unless obstruction or malfunction occurs can all help to decrease the risk of UTI. Follow-up urinalysis and culture should be done in all catheterized patients.

CONTROVERSIES

14. Is there a role for amphotericin bladder irrigations in treating candiduria?

For: Bladder irrigation with amphotericin is a safe and effective method for control of candiduria. Most episodes of candiduria will respond to a 5- to 7-day course of irrigations. The urine can be a source of both upper tract infections and dissemination of Candida.

Against: Candiduria often represents colonization in a catheterized patient on broad-spectrum antibiotics and will usually respond to removal of the catheter. Treatment of this colonization without catheter removal leads to replacement with bacteria (often more resistant organisms).

15. Should asymptomatic bacteriuria in short-term catheterized patients be treated?

For: There is a significant risk of bacteremia and sepsis in catheter-related bacteriuria. Hospital mortality is increased in patients with catheter-associated bacteriuria, and there is a 10–20% risk of UTI associated with an indwelling catheter even if it is removed. Absence of antimicrobial therapy is associated with bacteriuria sooner in catheterized patients.

Against: It is virtually impossible to maintain sterile urine in patients who require catheterization. Treating episodes of asymptomatic bacteriuria will lead to colonization with more resistant and perhaps more virulent organisms such as Pseudomonas and Serratia. If followed with daily urine cultures, most patients who develop symptomatic bacteriuria do so on the first day that bacteriuria is detected.

BIBLIOGRAPHY

1. Fisher JF, Chew WH, Shadomy S, et al: Urinary tract infections due to *Candida albicans*. Rev Infect Dis 4:1107–1118, 1982.
2. Garibaldi RA, Burke JP, Britt MR, et al: Meatal colonization and catheter-associated bacteriuria. N Engl J Med 303:316–319, 1980.
3. Garibaldi RA, Burke JP, Dickman ML, Smith CB: Factors predisposing to bacteriuria during indwelling urethral catheterization. N Engl J Med 291:215–219, 1974.
4. Givens CD, Wenzel RP: Catheter-associated urinary tract infections in surgical patients: A controlled study on the excess morbidity and costs. J Urol 124:646–648, 1980.

5. Krieger JN, Kaiser DL, Wenzel RP: Urinary tract etiology of bloodstream infections in hospitalized patients. J Infect Dis 148:57–62, 1983.
6. Kunin CM: Care of the urinary catheter. In Detection, Prevention and Management of Urinary Tract Infections, 4th ed. Philadelphia, Lea & Febiger, 1988.
7. Platt R, Polk BF, Murdock B, Rosner B: Risk factors for nosocomial urinary tract infections. Am J Epidemiol 124:977–985, 1986.
8. Platt R, Polk BF, Murdock B, Rosner B: Mortality associated with nosocomial urinary-tract infection. N Engl J Med 307:637–642, 1982.
9. Schaeffer AJ: Catheter-associated bacteriuria. Urol Clin North Am 13:737–747, 1986.
10. Turck M, Stamm W: Nosocomial infection of the urinary tract. Am J Med 70:651–655, 1981.
11. Warren JW: Catheter-associated urinary tract infections. Infect Dis Clin North Am 1:823–854, 1987.
12. Wise GJ, Kozinn PJ, Goldberg P: Amphotericin B as a urologic irrigant in the management of noninvasive candiduria. J Urol 128:82–84, 1982.

41. CANDIDIASIS

Susan R. Mason, M.D.

1. What risk factors are associated with the development of candidal infections?

- Long-term antibiotic therapy (risk increased further with broad-spectrum therapy)
- Hyperalimentation
- Steroid therapy
- Foreign bodies (intravascular catheters, prosthetic valves, Foley catheters)
- Malignancy
- Prolonged neutropenia
- HIV infection

2. What organs are most commonly involved in disseminated candidal infections?

The most common organs involved are the eyes, central nervous system, heart, and kidneys. Other organs frequently affected include the skin, bones, joints, respiratory tract, and GI tract. Hepatosplenic involvement is being recognized more commonly as well.

3. What are the diagnostic criteria for disseminated Candida infection?

- Positive blood cultures—may be absent in up to 80% of patients with Candida infection
- Endophthalmitis lesions
- Macronodular skin lesions with organisms seen on tissue biopsy
- Presence of Candida in biopsy of liver, spleen, or bone marrow

Note: The presence of oral candidiasis, candiduria, or sputum culture positive for Candida should be interpreted with caution, as it may represent colonization rather than infection.

4. What is the significance of a single blood culture positive for Candida?

A single positive culture of blood requires follow-up blood cultures, at a minimum. If an indwelling intravascular catheter is present, strong consideration should be given to removing it. If the patient is at risk for candidal infection (i.e., neutropenia, malignancy, steroids, etc.), then even one positive culture should be treated with antifungal medication such as parenteral amphotericin B.

5. What is appropriate therapy for disseminated candidiasis?

Amphotericin B is the mainstay of treatment. Unfortunately, the drug has many problematic side effects, including increasing serum creatinine, hypokalemia, hypomagnesemia, fever, and hypotension. Newer preparations of amphotericin B, with the drug incorporated into liposomes that have fewer severe side effects, are being investigated. Fluconazole, a newly licensed antifungal drug, is available for parenteral and oral use. Its role in the treatment of disseminated candidal infection appears promising but requires further study before becoming the drug of choice.

6. Does candiduria require antifungal therapy?

Candiduria is often eradicated upon removal of a Foley catheter or cessation of broad-spectrum antibiotic therapy. If candiduria persists or the patient continues to have fever, the bladder may be irrigated with amphotericin B for 3–5 days. Fluconazole is concentrated in the urine and may ultimately be the drug of choice for symptomatic or persistent candiduria.

7. How is the diagnosis of candidal pneumonia made?

Pulmonary infection with Candida is often the result of disseminated disease, so Candida may be cultured from multiple sites, including the lung. In the absence of documented disseminated disease, the diagnosis of candida pneumonia requires histopathologic evidence of tissue invasion and a positive culture for Candida.

8. If Candida is cultured from the drainage of an intraabdominal abscess, is systemic antifungal therapy required?

Usually in this circumstance, multiple bacterial organisms are cultured, and antibiotic therapy directed toward the bacterial pathogens is instituted. Antibiotics and adequate drainage usually suffice; however, if the patient remains febrile or otherwise unstable, systemic antifungal therapy may be indicated.

9. What is the outcome of disseminated candidal infection?

The overall mortality rates range from 37% to 62%, with lower mortalities in the nonleukemic population. Death rates are higher in patients with prolonged neutropenia and delayed antifungal therapy.

BIBLIOGRAPHY

1. Armstrong D: Problems in management of opportunistic fungal diseases. Rev Infect Dis 2(Suppl 7):S1591–S1599, 1989.
2. Gallis HA: Amphotericin B: Thirty years of clinical experience. Rev Infect Dis 12:308–329, 1990.
3. Kauffman CA, Bradley SF, Ross SC, et al: Hepatosplenic candidiasis: Successful treatment with fluconazole. Am J Med 91:137–141, 1991.
4. Meunier F: New methods for delivery of antifungal agents. Rev Infect Dis 2(Suppl 7):S1605–S1612, 1989.
5. Meunier-Carpentier F, Kiehn TE, Armstrong D, et al: Fungemia in the immunocompromised host: Changing patterns, antigenemia, high mortality. Am J Med 71:363–370, 1981.
6. Patel BCK, Kaye JB, Morgan LH, et al: Candidal endophthalmitis: A manifestation of systemic candidiasis. Postgrad Med J 63:563–565, 1987.
7. Thaler M, Pastakia B, Shauter TH, et al: Hepatic candidiasis in cancer patients: The evolving picture of the syndrome. Ann Intern Med 108:88–100, 1988.
8. Utz JP: Candidosis. Semin Respir Med 9:159–165, 1987.

42. CATHETER-RELATED INFECTIONS AND ASSOCIATED BACTEREMIA

Carlos E. Girod, M.D.

1. What are the different stages of catheter-related infections?
- **Catheter contamination:** Contamination with skin flora upon removal of catheter. Not true infection.
- **Catheter colonization:** Presence of organisms in the catheter by culture but absence of local or systemic infection.
- **Catheter-associated infection:** Recovery of more than a specific number of organisms in a catheter segment in association with clinical bacteremia or local infection.
- **Catheter-associated bacteremia:** Recovery of same organism in semiquantitative culture of catheter tip and blood cultures.

2. What is the incidence of catheter-related infections? (Is this a clinical syndrome rarely seen and associated only with inexperienced hands?)
No. Catheter-related infections remain among the top three causes of hospital-acquired infections, with an estimated incidence of 4–17%. Fatality rates in bacteremia and sepsis have been reported to be as high as 10–20%.

3. What are the portals of entry in catheter-related infections?
(1) Most studies have clearly shown that the skin around the insertion site is the most common portal of entry of infection. Analysis of catheter segments by Gram stain and semiquantitative cultures shows predominance of bacteria along the outer surface from tip to skin entry. Bacterial adherence followed by migration along catheter is the major mechanism. (2) The second most common portal of entry of bacteria is through contamination of the catheter hub during its manipulation. (3) Hematogenous dissemination from a distal infectious focus with colonization of catheter is less common and is associated with yeasts, enterococcus, and Klebsiella. Case reports of catheter colonization from the infused solution have been described with pathogens such as Pseudomonas and Enterobacter. (4) Other sources such as contaminated transducer kits and infusion lines are rare causes of catheter-related infections.

4. What are important risk factors for catheter-related infections?
Diabetes mellitus	Granulocytopenia
Altered host defense	Loss of skin integrity
Multiple medical problems	Presence of distal infection
Age < 1 year, > 60 years	Use of TPN
Immunosuppressive therapy	Sepsis

Review of the literature suggests that the presence of sepsis is the most important patient-related risk factor.

5. What are non–patient-related risk factors for catheter infections?
Alteration of skin flora	Inadequate maintenance
Lack of sterile procedure	Hypertonicity of infusate
Catheter adherence properties	Location and duration
Catheter size	Type of catheter
Lumen number	Skill of inserting physician

Duration of catheterization is the most important non–patient-related risk factor for catheter-related infection.

6. Is any specific type of catheter linked to increased infection?
Clinical trials have shown that tips of peripheral intravenous catheters have a significant risk for contamination 72 hours after insertion. Nevertheless, when changed every 72 hours, these catheters are less often associated with infection than are central, pulmonary, and arterial catheters. The insertion site should be upper extremity or external jugular. Use of a lower-extremity site carries a greater risk of infection.

Arterial catheters are associated with infection less than are pulmonary artery and central venous catheters. They are a rare source of bacteremia in ICU patients, probably because high arterial flow around the catheter decreases adherence of bacteria.

Central venous catheters carry a definite increased risk of related infection and bacteremia compared with peripheral and arterial catheters. Numerous studies have shown an incidence of bacteremia in triple-lumen catheters of 7–19% versus single-lumen of 3.7%. (Location of catheter and risk of infection are discussed in the Controversies section.)

Pulmonary artery catheters have a somewhat similar rate of infection: 5.8–12%. Others report even higher percentages attributed to the number of manipulations performed with these catheters.

7. Are physician's experience and timing at insertion important?
The skill and experience of the physician inserting the catheter are important factors. Fewer than 25 prior insertions carries an 18–20% incidence of catheter-related infection versus 8–12% for more than 25 prior insertions. Elective catheterization carries less risk of infection than emergency insertion. Increased incidence of catheter-related infection when placed after a 6-day ICU course has been described, and is probably a marker of severity of patient's illness.

8. How long can an intravascular catheter be used without risk of catheter-related infection?
Prolonged catheterization is the most important risk factor for related infection. No catheter should be left in place any longer than absolutely necessary. Recommended duration of catheter use prior to removal varies from as early as 48 hours to as long as 7 days.

Peripheral catheters require changing every 72 hours. Most careful clinical studies conclude that central venous and pulmonary artery catheters carry an increased risk of related infection 4 days after insertion. Changing of these catheters is recommended at that time.

9. Is changing an intravascular catheter over a guidewire associated with less risk of related infection than new site replacement?
Guidewire changes are recommended over new site insertion because of less risk of pneumothorax or bleeding complications. It is a safe and effective method for changing central venous catheters, ruling out catheter-related infection in a febrile, nonseptic patient, and placing pulmonary artery catheters at the site of previous central venous line. Every attempt must be made to sterilize the entire external portion of the catheter, guidewire, and surrounding skin. The removed catheter should be cultured and, if infected, the guidewire-placed catheter must be removed. This technique should not be performed in the setting of confirmed or clinically suspected sepsis.

10. What is the most sensitive and specific means of diagnosing catheter-related infections?
Physical exam is unreliable. Local inflammation or purulence at the entry site is seen in less than half of cases. Presence of fever, leukocytosis, and positive peripheral blood cultures are also not reliable indicators of catheter-related infection.

The most widely used and reliable test is removal of the catheter and culture of its tip by rolling it over a blood-agar plate as described by Maki et al. in 1977. Growth of >15 colonies per plate is associated with a specificity of 76–96% and a positive predictive value of 16–31%

for catheter-related bacteremia or sepsis. Other techniques such as Gram stain of the catheter surface and culture of the tip in broth are associated with high false-positive rates.

11. What organisms cause catheter-related infections?

Microbiology of Device-Associated Bacteremia

Staphylococcus aureus	Candida species[b]
Staphylococcus epidermidis	Pseudomonas aeruginosa[c]
Klebsiella species[a]	Pseudomonas cepacia[c]
Enterobacter species[a]	Citrobacter freundii[a]
Serratia marcescens[a]	Corynebacterium (especially
Candida albicans[b]	JK strains)[d]

[a] Frequently associated with contaminated infusate.
[b] Most often associated with TPN; usually along the catheter path, but occasionally as a result of contaminated infusate.
[c] May arise from a water source (e.g., infusate) or may reflect cutaneous colonization.
[d] JK bacteremia occurs almost exclusively in severely immunosuppressed patients who are or have been receiving broad-spectrum antibiotics and who have indwelling intravascular devices.

From Mandell GL, et al (eds): Principles and Practice of Infectious Diseases. New York, Churchill Livingstone, 1990, p 2191, with permission.

12. Where should blood cultures be obtained to document catheter-related bacteremia?

Blood cultures should be drawn from both catheter and peripheral sites. Blood cultures drawn through the catheter are associated with a high false-positive rate for the diagnosis of catheter-related bacteremia. The diagnosis is best made by removal of the catheter with semiquantitative tip culture.

13. What is the treatment of catheter-related infection?

Treatment depends on the stage of infection and the pathogen. As a general rule, if catheter-related bacteremia or septicemia is suspected, the catheter must be removed and replaced if access is needed. Most of the infectious complications are self-limited and resolve after removal of catheter. If empirical antibiotic therapy is needed, vancomycin is the drug of choice while awaiting cultures because of an increased incidence of oxacillin-resistant Staphylococcus.

Coagulase-negative Staphylococcus can be treated in nonimmunosuppressed patients by removal of catheter alone and/or intravenous antibiotics for 3–7 days.

Staphylococcus aureus–associated bacteremia should be treated with removal of catheter and IV antibiotics for 2–3 weeks because of a higher association with endocarditis.

Yeast colonization or infection of catheter can be treated with removal of catheter. The presence of positive blood cultures, persistent fever despite catheter removal, retinal lesions, or immunosuppression mandates a prolonged course of amphotericin B.

14. What are other ways to prevent catheter infection?

Recently reported new techniques that seem to prevent infection:
- **Vitacuff** (a subcutaneous collagen cuff at the catheter entry site impregnated with silver): its use has been associated with a three-fold reduction in colonization and a four-fold reduction in bacteremia. Its drawbacks are cost and the need for specialized training.
- **Chlorhexidine gluconate:** skin decontamination prior to insertion of catheter with greater reduction of infection than use of iodine solutions.
- **PNB ointment** (polymyxin-neomycin-bacitracin): at skin entry site.
- **Specialized teams:** in charge of dressing changes and maintenance.

CONTROVERSIES

15. Should femoral lines be used routinely?
For: Easier technique with no risk of pneumothorax. No randomized study has proved that this location is associated with an increased risk of catheter-related infection.
Against: Close location to urogenital and rectal areas with their associated gram-negative bacteria flora. Greater risk for arterial cannulation with complication of distal embolization.

16. Which site is more at risk for catheter-associated infection: internal jugular or subclavian?
Not clear. Because of different studies in terms of design and patient selection, no recommendation can be made.

17. Do routine guidewire changes every 48–72 hours decrease the incidence of catheter-related infection?
For: Easy technique without risk of pneumothorax or other complications. Anecdotal reports show reduction of risk of infection.
Against: No well-designed study has proved this.

18. Is it necessary to wear mask and sterile gown?
For: Widely recommended by most authorities. Inexpensive.
Against: No randomized study supports this practice.

BIBLIOGRAPHY

1. Armstrong CW, Mayhall CG, Miller KB, et al: Prospective study of catheter replacement and other risk factors for infection of hyperalimentation catheters. J Infect Dis 154:808–815, 1986.
2. Benezra D, Kiehn TE, Gold JW, et al: Prospective study of infections in indwelling central venous catheters using quantitative blood cultures. Am J Med 85:495–498, 1988.
3. Bozzetti F, Terno G, Bonfanti G, et al: Prevention and treatment of central venous catheter sepsis by exchange via guidewire. Ann Surg 198:48–52, 1983.
4. Cercenado E, Rodriguez M, Romero T, et al: A conservative procedure for the diagnosis of catheter-related infections. Arch Intern Med 150:1417–1420, 1990.
5. Collignon PJ, Soni N, Pearson IY, et al: Is semiquantitative culture of central vein catheter tips useful in the diagnosis of catheter-associated bacteremia? J Clin Microbiol 24:532–535, 1986.
6. Cooper GL, Hopkins CC: Rapid diagnosis of intravascular catheter-associated infection by direct Gram staining of catheter segments. N Engl J Med 312:1142–1147, 1985.
7. Corona ML, Peters SG, Narr BJ, et al: Infections related to central venous catheters. Mayo Clin Proc 65:979–986, 1990.
8. Flowers RH, Schwenzer KJ, Kopel RF, et al: Efficacy of an attachable subcutaneous cuff for the prevention of intravascular catheter-related infection. JAMA 261(6):878–883, 1989.
9. Graeve AH, Carpenter CM, Schiller WR: Management of central venous catheters using a wire introducer. Am J Surg 142:752–755, 1981.
10. Gregory JA, Schiller WR: Subclavian catheter changes every third day in high-risk patients. Am Surg 51:534, 1985.
11. Hampton AA, Sheretz RJ: Vascular-access infections in hospitalized patients. Surg Clin North Am 68:57–71, 1988.
12. Henderson DK: Bacteremia due to percutaneous intravascular devices. In Mandell GL, Douglas RG, Bennett JE (eds): Principles and Practice of Infectious Diseases. New York, Churchill Livingstone, 1990, pp 2189–2198.
13. Hilton E, Haslett TM, Borenstein MT, et al: Central catheter infections: Single- versus triple-lumen catheters. Am J Med 84:667–671, 1988.
14. Maki DG: Risk factors for nosocomial infection in the intensive care unit. Arch Intern Med 149:30–35, 1989.
15. Mantese VA, German DS, Kaminski DL, et al: Colonization and sepsis from triple-lumen catheters in critically ill patients. Am J Surg 154:597–600, 1987.
16. Moyer MA, Edwards LD, Farley L: Comparative culture methods on 101 intravenous catheters. Arch Intern Med 143:66–69, 1983.

17. Myers ML, Austin TW, Sibbald WJ: Pulmonary artery catheter infections. Ann Surg 201:237–241, 1985.
18. Norwood S, Ruby A, Civetta J: Catheter-related infections and associated septicemia. Chest 99:968–975, 1991.
19. Pinilla JC, Ross DF, Martin T: Study of the incidence of intravascular catheter infection and associated septicemia in critically ill patients. Crit Care Med 11:21–24, 1983.
20. Senagore A, Waller JD, Bonnell BW, et al: Pulmonary artery catheterization: A prospective study of internal jugular and subclavian approaches. Crit Care Med 15:35–37, 1987.
21. Snyder RH, Archer FJ, Endy T, et al: Catheter infection. Ann Surg 208:651–653, 1988.

43. TOXIC SHOCK SYNDROME

Mary Bessesen, M.D.

1. What is toxic shock syndrome (TSS)?
TSS is a multisystem disorder manifested by high fever, hypotension, and erythroderma.

2. What is the case definition of TSS?
A case of TSS is diagnosed when either three or more of the following criteria are met in the presence of desquamation or five or more in the absence of desquamation:
1. Temperature $> 38.9°$ C
2. Rash: diffuse erythroderma, with subsequent desquamation
3. Systolic blood pressure < 90 mm Hg
4. Multisystem involvement (three or more of the following):
    Gastrointestinal: diarrhea, vomiting
    Muscular: severe myalgias or CPK > 5 times normal
    Mucous membranes: frank hyperemia
    Renal insufficiency in the presence of sterile pyuria
    Hepatitis
    Thrombocytopenia
    Disorientation
5. Negative serology for Rocky Mountain spotted fever, leptospirosis, and measles

3. What risk factors predispose to TSS?
The classic case profile is a young (15–25 years old), menstruating female. However, any staphylococcal infection can predispose to TSS, including surgical wound infections, furuncles, and abscesses. Postpartum cases can occur after vaginal or cesarean delivery. Nasal reconstructive surgery carries an especially high risk of TSS.

4. What are the signs and symptoms of TSS?
The typical presentation is one of high fever, rash, and confusion. There may be a prodrome of myalgias, vomiting, and diarrhea. Patients are listless, but focal neurologic findings are not seen. Examination of patients with menstruation-associated TSS reveals vaginal hyperemia and exudate that yields *Staphylococcus aureus* on culture. In nonmenstrual cases, a careful examination usually reveals a focus of staphylococcal infection. It is important to note that this focus is frequently subtle. The drainage from a wound infection causing TSS may be only serous-appearing, rather than grossly purulent. This is a toxin-mediated disease, and the local appearance is not one of intensive purulence. Drainage of local infections is a key point in management.

5. What are the common laboratory findings?

Leukocytosis with marked left shift, thrombocytopenia, azotemia, sterile pyuria, and elevated transaminases are common but not invariable findings. Blood cultures are usually sterile, as are cerebrospinal fluid (CSF) cultures. Cultures of the local site of infection are usually positive for *S. aureus.*

6. What is the differential diagnosis of TSS?

Streptococcal scarlet fever, measles, leptospirosis, Rocky Mountain spotted fever, Stevens-Johnson syndrome, and Kawasaki's disease can mimic TSS. Multiorgan involvement is usually absent in streptococcal scarlet fever, and the primary focus yields *Streptococcus pyogenes.* In contrast, a toxic-shock-like syndrome associated with group A streptococcal infections has recently been reported. Patients usually have a focus of streptococcal infection, and positive blood cultures are common. Toxin A, which has 50% homology with staphylococcal toxin B, is produced by most isolates. Exclusion of measles, leptospirosis, and Rocky Mountain spotted fever requires both a careful history for potential exposures and serologic testing. Stevens-Johnson syndrome is characterized by target lesions and is commonly associated with antecedent drug use. Kawasaki's disease is characterized by fever and rash without multisystem involvement. It is most commonly seen in children under the age of 6 years, and is associated with thrombocytosis rather than thrombocytopenia.

7. What is the bacterial etiology of TSS?

S. aureus is the etiology. Virtually all isolates from menstruation-associated cases are phage type 1.

8. What bacterial virulence factors are important in TSS?

TSST-1 (toxic shock syndrome toxin 1) is produced by the isolates that cause most cases of menstruation-associated TSS. In cases not associated with menstruation, the majority of staphylococcal isolates produce TSST-1; a substantial minority produce staphylococcal enterotoxin B.

9. What host factors are important in the production of TSS?

The absence of preexisting antibody to TSST-1 is associated with TSS. Antibody to TSST-1 is produced in response to colonization with toxin-producing strains, and rates of seropositivity increase with age. More than 90% of persons over the age of 25 years are seropositive.

10. What is the treatment for TSS?

The primary intervention consists of fluid resuscitation and supportive care. Any focus of staphylococcal infection must be drained. In women, a vaginal examination must be performed as soon as the patient is stabilized, and any foreign bodies (such as tampon or diaphragm) removed. After cultures of the local site and the blood are obtained, an antistaphylococcal penicillin (nafcillin or oxacillin) should be administered intravenously.

11. What are the complications of TSS?

Complications include the adult respiratory distress syndrome, cerebral edema, myocardial dysfunction, and hypocalcemia.

12. What are the sequelae of TSS?

The majority of patients enjoy a full recovery. Occasionally there are persistent cognitive deficits, mild renal failure, electroencephalographic abnormalities, and cyanotic extremities. Telogen effluvium (temporary hair loss) is common.

13. How can TSS be prevented?

Primary prevention involves education of the public either to avoid the use of tampons or to use the least absorbent product consistent with an individual's needs. Recurrent cases can be reduced by antistaphylococcal therapy to eradicate *S. aureus*.

14. What is the incidence of TSS?

The incidence is estimated to be one case per 100,000 women of menstrual age per year.

15. What is the mortality rate of TSS?

The case fatality ratio has diminished from 5.6% to 3.3%.

16. Can TSS recur?

Yes. Because many patients do not produce antibodies against TSST-1, recurrent episodes are seen.

CONTROVERSY

17. Should intravenous immunoglobulin (IVIG) be used in the therapy of severe cases of TSS?

For:

1. Persons with preexisting serum antibody against TSST-1 are at very low risk for TSS, suggesting that antibody may prevent or ameliorate disease.

2. Commercial preparations of IVIG have high titers of antibody to TSST-1. IVIG is well tolerated.

3. Animal studies have shown that IVIG administered prior to challenge with toxin-producing strains of *S. aureus* or TSST-1 prevents TSS in rabbits.

Against:

1. No human studies of IVIG for TSS have been performed. It is dangerous to apply data from animal studies to clinical medicine.

2. The use of IVIG for TSS may blunt the patient's immune response, thereby increasing the risk of TSS recurrence.

3. In the animal studies, IVIG was administered prior to challenge with TSST-1 or *S. aureus*. Administration of IVIG after the syndrome has occurred may not be efficacious.

4. IVIG is very costly.

BIBLIOGRAPHY

1. Bartlett P, Reingold AL, Graham DR, et al: Toxic shock syndrome associated with surgical wound infections. JAMA 247:1448–1450, 1982.
2. Chesney PJ: Clinical aspects and spectrum of TSS: Overview. Rev Infect Dis 11:S1–7, 1989.
3. Jacobson JA, Kasworm EM, Crass BA, Bergdoll MS: Nasal carriage of toxigenic *Staphylococcus aureus* and prevalence of serum antibody to toxic-shock-syndrome toxin 1 in Utah. J Infect Dis 153:356–358, 1986.
4. Reduced incidence of menstrual toxic shock syndrome–United States, 1980–1990. MMWR 39:421–423, 1990.
5. Resnick SD: Toxic shock syndrome: Recent developments in pathogenesis. J Pediatr 116:321–328, 1990.
6. Schlievert PM, Shands KN, Dan BB, et al: Identification and characterization of an exotoxin from *Staphylococcus aureus* associated wiith toxic-shock syndrome. J Infect Dis 143:509–516, 1981.
7. Stevens DL, Tanner MH, Winship J, et al: Severe group A streptococcal infections associated with a toxic shock-like syndrome and scarlet fever toxin A. N Engl J Med 321:1–7, 1989.
8. Todd J, Fishaut M, Kapral F, Welch T: Toxic-shock syndrome associated with phage-group-1 staphylococci. Lancet 2:1116–1118, 1978.
9. Vergeront JM, Stolz SJ, Crass BA, et al: Prevalence of serum antibody to staphylococcal enterotoxin F among Wisconsin residents: Implications for toxic-shock syndrome. J Infect Dis 148:692–698, 1983.

44. AIDS IN THE INTENSIVE CARE UNIT

David M. Guidot, M.D.

1. What is the principal differential diagnosis of diffuse pulmonary infiltrates in a patient with the acquired immunodeficiency syndrome (AIDS)?

The most common cause of diffuse pulmonary infiltrates in a patient with AIDS is *Pneumocystis carinii* pneumonia (PCP), which accounts for greater than 80% of ICU admissions in AIDS patients and remains the most common cause of death in all AIDS patients. Other diagnoses to consider, either as primary etiologies for the infiltrates or as coexistent pathologies with PCP, include cytomegalovirus (CMV) pneumonia, diffuse lymphangitic spread of Kaposi's sarcoma, and mycobacterial disease (most commonly *Mycobacterium avium-intracellulare*). Cardiogenic pulmonary edema should be considered in the patient who has received large volumes of intravenous fluids, particularly if underlying renal and/or cardiac insufficiency is present. The adult respiratory distress syndrome (ARDS) may complicate PCP and may explain persistent infiltrates and hypoxemia in a patient who has received a full course of PCP therapy.

2. What are the available methods for diagnosing PCP and/or other AIDS-related pulmonary disorders in the critically ill patient?

1. **Sputum examination.** In the outpatient setting and/or medical ward, relatively stable patients can be evaluated for the presence of PCP by specialized stains of induced sputum. However, more invasive methods usually must be employed in critically ill patients to ensure the greatest chance that a rapid and accurate diagnosis can be made.

2. **Bronchoalveolar lavage (BAL).** BAL is highly sensitive in diagnosing PCP and may offer evidence for other etiologic agents as well. BAL can be performed in either spontaneously breathing or intubated patients and has greater than 90% sensitivity in diagnosing first presentations of PCP. The sensitivity decreases in patients who have been on PCP prophylaxis and/or have recurrent PCP, in which the parasite burden may be less and thus more difficult to detect by lavage alone. BAL can also detect other agents such as CMV and mycobacteria in pulmonary secretions. However, these agents may reflect colonization and not tissue invasion and therefore must be interpreted with caution when recovered by BAL alone.

3. **Transbronchial biopsy.** Transbronchial biopsy (TBB) does not significantly increase the sensitivity in the diagnosis of first-presentation PCP but can improve PCP detection in recurrent or atypical cases in which BAL is negative. In addition, TBB can detect lymphangitic involvement with Kaposi's sarcoma, provide histologic evidence of CMV infection, and detect tissue granulomata and/or acid-fast bacilli in mycobacterial infection. TBB involves a much greater risk of complications than does BAL alone, including significant hemorrhage and/or pneumothorax, and thus is reserved for special circumstances in the ICU setting.

4. **Open-lung biopsy.** On rare occasions, an open-lung biopsy may be necessary if BAL and/or TBB fails to yield a diagnosis. This was more common in the early years of the epidemic, before the spectrum of AIDS-related pulmonary complications was known and before improved techniques for examining sputum and lavage samples had been developed.

3. What are the treatment modalities for PCP with associated respiratory failure?

Medical treatment of the primary infection consists of essentially either trimethoprim/sulfamethoxazole (TMP/SMX) or pentamidine isethionate. Each is effective in about half of treated patients with PCP. Agents related to TMP/SMX, including trimetrexate and dapsone-trimethoprim, are also available. Other agents used as second-line therapy include dapsone and alpha-difluoromethylornithine (DFMO). The management of respiratory failure, pending successful therapy of the primary infection, is supportive. With severe hypoxia and/or respiratory acidosis, intubation and mechanical ventilation are necessary. Frequently, high concentrations of oxygen and high levels of positive end-expiratory pressure (PEEP) are necessary to maintain adequate tissue oxygenation. Some patients with relatively mild respiratory failure from PCP may be supported with continuous positive airway pressure (CPAP) ventilation. CPAP may also be employed in weaning from mechanical ventilation. Even with aggressive ICU care, outcome depends on successful treatment of the Pneumocystis infection.

4. What are the complications of therapy for severe PCP in the ICU?
Both TMP/SMX and pentamidine isethionate have protean complications. TMP/SMX can cause severe rash, fever, anemia, neutropenia, elevated liver enzymes, and thrombocytopenia. Pentamidine isethionate can cause neutropenia, renal insufficiency, elevated liver enzymes, hyponatremia, hypoglycemia, orthostatic hypotension, and anemia. The efficacy of these agents is largely tempered by their extensive side effects. The complications of the ventilatory support of patients with severe PCP are similar to those in other patients with respiratory failure. Mechanical ventilation, particularly with high levels of PEEP, is associated with impaired cardiac output and barotrauma principally manifested by pneumothorax formation.

5. What are the principal CNS infections associated with AIDS that may affect the mental status of AIDS patients in the ICU?
Cryptococcal meningitis, herpes encephalitis, and brain abscesses from toxoplasmosis are the three most common CNS infections identified in these patients. Primary treatment for cryptococcal meningitis and toxoplasmosis may control these infections. Herpes encephalitis carries an extremely poor prognosis even with treatment.

6. What is the prognosis for patients with PCP and/or other AIDS-related infections who develop respiratory failure and require mechanical ventilation?
The outcome has been universally poor, with most centers reporting mortalities between 80% and 100% in the first 5 years of the epidemic. More recent reports suggest there has been an improvement in outcome, citing mortalities of 30% to 60%. Several published reports suggest that treatment with corticosteroids can improve survival in these patients. However, improved survival cannot be definitively linked to adjunctive use of corticosteroids. Other factors, such as improved care and general health of patients with HIV infection prior to development of PCP and physician selection of younger and previously healthier patients as candidates for aggressive ICU care, may contribute to the apparent improvement in outcome. Early in the epidemic, most patients were mechanically ventilated. As the poor outcome of these patients became apparent, fewer patients were treated with aggressive support. The present selection of a subgroup with a better survival may be influencing present outcomes. Clearly the primary therapies for PCP—TMP/SMX and pentamidine—have not changed, and supportive ventilatory care has not changed significantly in the past 5 years. Thus, despite recent optimistic reports, the prognosis for patients with AIDS who develop respiratory failure associated with PCP and/or CMV appears in general to be poor. Short-term ICU survival has not been translated into any apparent meaningful long-term survival.

7. Does knowledge of the prognosis of respiratory failure associated with PCP affect patients' and/or physicians' decisions regarding intubation and mechanical ventilation?
Surveys conducted by the group at San Francisco General Hospital indicate that early in the course of HIV infection, patients overestimate their chances of survival should they

develop respiratory failure from PCP, and the majority say they would elect to be intubated. However, as the disease progresses and they witness the outcome of friends with AIDS and talk to counselors, they are far less likely to request resuscitation. Physicians who care for significant numbers of AIDS patients are well aware of the grim prognosis in this setting and, when surveyed, indicate they rarely that feel intubation and mechanical ventilation are appropriate for severe PCP. Surveys indicate that physicians with less experience with such patients are much more likely to recommend these measures.

8. Are there any prognostic variables that can predict a subset of patients with respiratory failure who may benefit from mechanical ventilation?
Few studies address this question. However, experienced investigators report that patients who present with their first infection with PCP, particularly those who were in good previous health, may have a better prognosis than patients who are debilitated and/or have recurrent PCP. There do not appear to be any distinct physiologic, radiographic, or prophylactic treatment variables (such as inhaled pentamidine) that can assist the physician in this decision. A San Francisco study, performed retrospectively, determined that a higher serum albumin level predicted a better outcome. This likely reflects better overall health. In that study, the investigators did not find that patient age, previous episodes of PCP, duration of HIV illness or anti-PCP therapy predicted outcome.

9. Do AIDS patients wish to discuss with their physicians issues regarding resuscitation?
A large survey of male AIDS patients in San Francisco revealed that the majority of them had thought a great deal about the limits of care they preferred and wanted to discuss these issues with their physicians. However, at the time of the survey, only a minority of these patients had discussed these issues with their physicians. The finding that most AIDS patients have thought about limits of care and wish to discuss it with their physicians is similar to findings in other surveys of non-AIDS patients with terminal diseases. Although the San Francisco survey may not be generalizable to all AIDS populations, physicians should actively explore these issues with AIDS patients, particularly in the ICU, where the therapeutic options range from comfort care to maximal cardiopulmonary support. Ideally, such discussions should be held prior to the development of significant respiratory distress.

10. What are the risks of HIV transmission to healthcare workers in the ICU?
The primary risk to healthcare workers for HIV infection in the ICU is from needlesticks. Numerous studies place the risk of HIV transmission from a contaminated needlestick to be approximately 0.5% per episode. HIV has been identified in saliva and there have been a few reports of transmission of the virus from human bites. However, there have been many documented human bites in which transmission has not occurred. HIV has also been found in tears and vaginal secretions, but evidence that these secretions could be a source of transmission to healthcare workers is lacking. The HIV virus has not been found in urine or stool, although urine does contain antibodies to HIV. Contact with these secretions likely represents far less risk than does contact with contaminated blood. Thus, the greatest risk for transmission to workers in the ICU is accidental puncture with contaminated needles. Given the uncertainty about HIV transmissibility to healthcare workers, all blood, secretions, and contaminated instruments should be handled appropriately. Universal blood and secretion precautions have been formulated and should be carefully followed with all patients. Particular caution should be exercised in handling all contaminated needles. These should be promptly placed in appropriate containers and *not be recapped.* Recapping needles is a common cause of accidental skin puncture. It is also important to note that the majority of people in this country who are estimated to be infected with HIV have not been tested for antibodies to HIV. Thus, universal precautions should be used in the care of all patients, including those in the ICU.

CONTROVERSY

11. Should patients with respiratory failure from PCP be treated with adjunctive corticosteroids?

For:

1. Several reports from different institutions have shown improved survival in patients treated with corticosteroids compared with historical controls.

2. There is evidence that a significant percentage of AIDS patients have unrecognized adrenal insufficiency and are thus unable to mount the necessary adrenal response to stress.

3. Steroids may limit the interstitial inflammatory response and rapid development of interstitial fibrosis, both of which are pathologic features of patients who die from PCP.

Against:

1. A prospective, randomized controlled study at San Francisco General Hospital failed to support the efficacy of corticosteroids in PCP.

2. Corticosteroids theoretically may impose an additional immunosuppressive effect on these patients, increasing their susceptibility to other infections such as CMV and herpes-viruses.

BIBLIOGRAPHY

1. Consensus Statement on the use of corticosteroids as adjunctive therapy for Pneumocystis pneumonia in the acquired immunodeficiency syndrome. N Engl J Med 323:21:1500–1504, 1990.
2. Devita M, Greenbaum D: The critically ill patient with the acquired immunodeficiency syndrome. In Shoemaker WC, et al (eds): Textbook of Critical Care. Philadelphia, W.B. Saunders, 1989, pp 865–869.
3. El-Sadr W, Simberkoff MS: Survival and prognostic factors in severe *Pneumocystis carinii* pneumonia requiring mechanical ventilation. Am Rev Respir Dis 137:1264–1267, 1988.
4. Gerst P, Fildes J, Rosario P, Schorr J: Risks of human immunodeficiency virus infection to patients and healthcare personnel. Crit Care Med 18:12:1440–1448, 1990.
5. Layon AJ, D'Amico R: Intensive care for patients with acquired immunodeficiency syndrome— Medicine versus ideology. Crit Care Med 18:11:1297–1299, 1990.
6. Luce JM, Wachter RM, Hopewell PC: Intensive care of patients with the acquired immunodeficiency syndrome: Time for a reassessment? Am Rev Respir Dis 137:1261–1263, 1988.
7. MacFadden D, Hyland R, Inouye T, et al: Corticosteroids as adjunctive therapy in treatment of *Pneumocystis carinii* pneumonia in patients with acquired immunodeficiency syndrome. Lancet June 27, 1987, pp 1477–1479.
8. Montaner J, Russel J, Ruedy J, Lawson L: *Pneumocystis carinii* pneumonia in the acquired immunodeficiency syndrome: A potential role for systemic corticosteroids. Chest 95:881–884, 1989.
9. Mottin D, Denis M, Dombret H, et al: Role for steroids in treatment of *Pneumocystis carinii* pneumonia in AIDS. Lancet August 29, 1987, p 519.
10. Rogers PL, Lane HC, Henderson DK: Admission of AIDS patients to a medical intensive care unit: Causes and outcome. Crit Care Med 17:113–117, 1989.
11. Sprung CL, Steinberg A: Acquired immunodeficiency syndrome and critical care. Crit Care Med 18:11:1300–1302, 1990.
12. Steinbrook R, Lo B, Moulton J, et al: Preferences of homosexual men with AIDS for life-sustaining treatment. N Engl J Med 314:7:457–460, 1986.
13. Wachter RM, Cooke M, Hopewell PC, Luce JM: Attitudes of medical residents regarding intensive care for patients with the acquired immunodeficiency syndrome. Arch Intern Med 148:149–152, 1988.
14. Wachter RM, Luce JM, Turner J, et al: Intensive care of patients with the acquired immunodeficiency syndrome. Am Rev Respir Dis 134:891–896, 1986.
15. Wachter R, Russi M, Bloch D, et al: *Pneumocystis carinii* pneumonia and respiratory failure in AIDS. Am Rev Respir Dis 143:251–256, 1991.

VI: Renal Disease

45. HYPERTENSION

Jeffrey Schelling, M.D., and Stuart Linas, M.D.

1. Define the clinical spectrum of severe hypertension.
Severe hypertension can be classified in many ways, but there are three major categories: hypertensive crisis or emergent hypertension, hypertension with end-organ dysfunction (such as angina), and uncontrolled or urgent hypertension.

Hypertensive crisis is the turning point in the course of hypertension when immediate management of elevated blood pressure plays a decisive role in the eventual outcome. Although there are a number of causes of emergent hypertension, the most common etiology is malignant or accelerated hypertension. Accelerated hypertension is severe hypertension (diastolic blood pressure usually > 120 mm Hg) in the setting of retinal hemorrhage and exudates (cotton wool spots). Malignant hypertension is accelerated hypertension with papilledema.

Hypertension with end-organ dysfunction is a form of severe hypertension because blood pressure reduction may be associated with relief of clinical symptoms.

Urgent hypertension is elevated blood pressure in the absence of end-organ dysfunction. Because it is only an abnormal "number," urgent hypertension is not associated with the dire consequences of the other types of severe hypertension.

2. Define the two hemodynamic determinants of blood pressure. Which is the predominant problem in malignant hypertension?
Arterial blood pressure is the product of cardiac output and systemic vascular resistance. Malignant hypertension is caused by increased systemic vascular resistance.

3. What are the most common underlying causes of malignant hypertension? Is an evaluation for secondary hypertension necessary?
Approximately 95% of all patients with hypertension have essential hypertension. However, essential hypertension is the underlying cause in only 50% of malignant hypertension. Because secondary hypertension (e.g., renovascular hypertension, pheochromocytoma) is a precipitant in the remaining 50% of patients with malignant hypertension, an evaluation for secondary hypertension is usually warranted. This is particularly true in whites and in patients either younger than 30 years or older than 60 years.

4. What are the potential complications of untreated and treated malignant hypertension?
Studies from the 1950s and 1960s revealed that the mortality from untreated malignant hypertension was 80–90%. Most of the deaths were due to acute renal failure. With the initiation of prompt antihypertensive therapy and acute dialysis (if necessary), morbidity and mortality have become due primarily to cardiovascular disease (stroke, myocardial infarction, and congestive heart failure).

5. Describe the acute treatment of malignant hypertension.
The acute treatment of choice is intravenous sodium nitroprusside. The initial dose is 0.5 μg/kg/min, and should be increased by 0.5 μg/kg/min every 2–3 minutes until a

diastolic blood pressure less than 110 mm Hg has been attained. Further acute decreases in blood pressure may result in vital organ hypoperfusion, as blood flow autoregulation may be altered to accommodate chronically elevated blood pressure. Other parenteral drugs that are less ideal (but acceptable) for the acute treatment of malignant hypertension include diazoxide, trimethaphan, and labetalol. Blood pressure should be monitored continuously during therapy. If there is concern about the accuracy of sphygmomanometric readings, monitoring should be done with an indwelling arterial catheter.

6. Outline a chronic antihypertensive regimen to follow successful acute treatment of malignant hypertension.

Because malignant hypertension is mediated by increased systemic vascular resistance, it is recommended that chronic therapy include a vasodilator such as hydralazine, pinacidil, or minoxidil. Vasodilators cause reflex tachycardia and sodium retention; therefore, it is usually necessary also to include a beta blocker and a diuretic. In some cases, chronic blood pressure reduction may be achieved with less potent vasodilators, such as angiotensin-converting enzyme (ACE) inhibitors or calcium channel blockers.

7. What is the prognosis following a successfully treated episode of malignant hypertension?

The prognosis is related primarily to the degree of azotemia and the efficacy of acute antihypertensive therapy. In the best circumstances, the 1-year mortality is about 10%.

8. Describe the acute antihypertensive treatment in a patient with a pheochromocytoma.

Hypertension from pheochromocytomas is caused by vascular smooth muscle $alpha_1$ receptor activation, which results in vasoconstriction. Thus, the best acute treatment is intravenous administration of the $alpha_1$-blocker phentolamine. Sodium nitroprusside is also a reasonable choice. Beta blockers should initially be avoided because they cause both unopposed peripheral $alpha_1$ receptor stimulation and decreased cardiac output.

9. Describe the acute medical management of a patient with aortic dissection.

The initial therapeutic aim is to decrease both blood pressure and cardiac contractile force (dp/dt). This has traditionally been best achieved with sodium nitroprusside plus a beta blocker. Trimethaphan or labetalol are also effective in this setting.

10. What is the treatment for cocaine-induced hypertensive crisis?

Cocaine causes hypertension by inhibiting catecholamine reuptake at nerve terminals. Therefore, $alpha_1$ blockade with phentolamine or labetalol is effective. If hypertension is severe, sodium nitroprusside is the drug of choice.

11. Which antihypertensive drugs are associated with hypertensive crisis following abrupt withdrawal?

Clonidine and beta blockers may result in "rebound hypertension" after acute withdrawal. Both need to be tapered over several days to avoid this complication.

CONTROVERSIES

12. Why are clonidine, beta blockers, and diuretics undesirable choices for treatment of malignant hypertension?

Each medication works, at least partly, by reducing cardiac output. While this may result in acute blood pressure reduction, it may also further increase systemic vascular resistance. Therefore, vasodilator therapy is a better choice for malignant hypertension treatment.

13. Prescribe the best antihypertensive regimen for a patient with preeclampsia.
Preeclampsia is hypertension, proteinuria, and edema combined, and it occurs after the 20th week of gestation. The traditional treatments of choice are hydralazine or alpha-methyldopa. If these drugs are ineffective or poorly tolerated, labetalol is a reasonably safe and effective alternative. Medications to be avoided because of potential teratogenesis include sodium nitroprusside, trimethaphan, diazoxide, ACE inhibitors, beta blockers, and calcium channel blockers. Furthermore, the safety of many antihypertensive drugs during pregnancy is unknown. Because preeclampsia and eclampsia may be life-threatening, it may be necessary to prescribe potent antihypertensives (sodium nitroprusside, minoxidil) with uncertain fetal toxicity potential.

BIBLIOGRAPHY

1. Anderson RJ, Reed WG: Current concepts in treatment of hypertensive urgencies. Am Heart J 111:211–219, 1986.
2. Calhoun DA, Oparil S: Treatment of hypertensive crisis. N Engl J Med 323: 1177–1183, 1990.
3. Houston M: Hypertensive emergencies and urgencies: Pathophysiology and clinical aspects. Am Heart J 111:205–210, 1986.
4. McRae RP, Liebson PR: Hypertensive crisis. Med Clin North Am 70:749–767, 1986.
5. Nolan CR, Linas SL: Accelerated and malignant hypertension. In Schrier RW, Gottschalk CW (eds): Diseases of the Kidney. Boston, Little, Brown, 1988, pp 1703–1824.
6. Perez-Grovas H, Herrera-Acosta J: Mechanism and treatment of malignant hypertension. Semin Nephrol 8:147–154, 1988.
7. Silver HM: Acute hypertensive crisis in pregnancy. Med Clin North Am 73:623–638, 1989.
8. Vidt DG: Current concepts in treatment of hypertensive emergencies. Am Heart J 111:220–225, 1986.

46. ACUTE RENAL FAILURE

Joseph Shapiro, M.D.

1. How is acute renal failure (ARF) diagnosed?
ARF is best diagnosed by the observation of a rapid deterioration in renal function, specifically glomerular filtration rate (GFR). GFR is clinically best determined by an estimation of the clearance of creatinine. In many cases, if it is simply assumed that creatinine production is constant, a rising serum level of creatinine demonstrates that the clearance of creatinine has fallen. Until the patient achieves a steady state, the level of renal function cannot be assessed by the serum creatinine concentration. If a patient with previously normal renal function suddenly loses all renal function, serum creatinine will rise by only 1–2 mg/dl per day.

2. What features distinguish acute from chronic renal failure?
When a patient presents some time after the onset of ARF, this distinction may not be that simple. In other words, when the serum creatinine is already extremely high (10 mg/dl or greater), it may not increase much more. As a rule of thumb, chronic renal failure is more likely to be associated with anemia, normal urine output, and small shrunken kidneys on ultrasound examination than is acute renal failure. It has been reported that chronic but not acute renal failure may be associated with an increase in the serum osmolal gap, i.e., the difference between measured and calculated serum osmolality. Most nephrologists would

agree that if kidneys are normal sized on ultrasound examination, a renal biopsy may be warranted.

3. What is the urine output of patients with ARF?
Although oliguria (urine output less than 500 ml/24 hours in adults) implies the presence of ARF, often ARF is associated with normal or even increased urine flow. In the last decade, nonoliguric ARF has come to be recognized as being as common as oliguric ARF. Generally, however, oliguria denotes a worse prognosis in the setting of acute tubular necrosis.

4. What is the clinical classification of ARF?
As for many things in medicine, it is generally better to start off with big categories and zoom in. In ARF, the causes are classified as prerenal, intrarenal or parenchymal, and postrenal or obstructive.

Prerenal azotemia occurs when the renal perfusion pressure falls below the autoregulatory threshold for maintenance of normal GFR. This may occur in states of total body salt and water depletion such as dehydration, in conditions in which total body salt and water is excessive such as heart failure and cirrhosis, or from local lesions that decrease renal perfusion pressure such as renal artery stenosis. Typically such patients have a concentrated urine with relatively low sodium concentration, have relatively benign urinalysis, and can be treated by optimization of hemodynamic parameters. A special case of prerenal azotemia, called the hepatorenal syndrome, however, usually does not respond to such therapy and generally requires liver transplantation to correct the abnormal renal hemodynamics that result from liver failure.

Intrarenal or parenchymal renal failure may be classified as glomerular or tubulointerstitial. Acute glomerulonephritis from a variety of causes may cause ARF. Tubulointerstitial causes of ARF are more common and include acute interstitial nephritis, usually resulting from drug allergy; precipitation of myeloma proteins in the tubular fluid seen with myeloma kidney; and acute tubular necrosis, which is the most common tubulointerstitial form. Parenchymal causes of ARF are generally associated with isotonic urine that is high in sodium concentration and an active urinary sediment that contains clues to the etiology of the renal failure.

Postrenal or obstructive renal failure is a common cause of ARF and may result from either intraluminal or extraluminal obstruction at any site from the beginning of the collecting system to the tip of the urethra. Typically the urine (if elaborated) is isotonic or dilute and relatively high in sodium. Although examination of urine sediment may provide clues to the etiology of obstruction, often it does not.

5. What are the pathophysiologic mechanisms operant in acute tubular necrosis?
It has been known for some time that renal ischemia, toxic injury to the kidney, or a combination of these insults could cause prolonged loss of renal function. Physiologically, decreased GFR must result from an alteration in glomerular hemodynamic factors such as a decrease in the effective surface area or permeability of the glomerulus (Kf), from a decrease in glomerular blood flow, or from an abnormality in tubular integrity, including obstruction of tubular flow by cellular debris or backleak of ultrafiltrate through a porous tubule. In fact, each of these pathogenetic features can be shown to be operant in some experimental models of ARF. The major mechanism by which renal failure is induced may be different from the primary mechanism by which it is maintained. For example, in ischemic ARF, decreases in renal and glomerular blood flow may cause the initial loss of renal function. However, it is the tubular necrosis, with its attendant obstructing debris and backleak of ultrafiltrate, that maintains the low GFR. The tubular mechanisms are usually important in the maintenance of ARF from most causes seen clinically. Therefore, pharmacologic efforts to improve renal blood flow are not, by themselves, generally effective in shortening the duration of ARF.

6. How does one approach the differential diagnosis of ARF?

The approach to the patient with ARF requires a good history and physical exam in concert with judiciously ordered laboratory and imaging tests. The history is extremely important in determining whether antecedent renal ischemia might have occurred, settings for which include surgery, other causes of hypotension, or dehydration. In addition, exposure to nephrotoxic drugs such as aminoglycosides or nonsteroidal anti-inflammatory agents or endogenous substances can be elicited. The physical examination is most useful in establishing the volume status of the patient as well as in obtaining clues of any systemic illness (such as vasculitis) that may present as ARF. Evaluation of the neck veins is essential. Although urinary obstruction may be detected by other means, the finding of suprapubic dullness after voiding is a valuable clue to the presence of bladder outlet obstruction.

7. How does examination of the urine help in the differential diagnosis of ARF?

Laboratory evaluation begins with careful examination of the urine. A concentrated urine points more to prerenal causes, whereas isotonic urine suggests parenchymal or obstructive causes. Typically, the urine sediment of patients with prerenal azotemia demonstrates occasional hyaline casts or finely granular casts. In contrast, the presence of renal tubular epithelial cells and "muddy" granular casts strongly suggests acute tubular necrosis; microhematuria and red blood cell casts suggest glomerulonephritis; and white cell casts containing eosinophils suggest acute interstitial nephritis. As discussed above, benign urine sediment is quite compatible with urinary obstruction.

8. What are the implications of urinary electrolytes in the differential diagnosis of ARF?

The determination of urine electrolyte and creatinine concentrations may be helpful in the differential diagnosis of ARF. When used with serum values, urinary diagnostic indices can be generated. Understanding the concepts behind the interpretation of these indices is easier and better than trying to remember specific numbers. Quite simply, if the tubule is working well in the setting of decreased GFR, tubular reabsorption of sodium and water will be avid, and the relative clearance of sodium to creatine will be low. Conversely, if the tubule is injured and cannot reabsorb sodium well, the relative clearance of sodium to creatine will not be low. Therefore, with prerenal azotemia, the ratio of the clearance of sodium to the clearance of creatine ($\times$ 100), which is also called the fractional excretion of sodium ($FENa = UNa/UCr \times PCr/PNa \times 100$), is typically less than 1.0, whereas with parenchymal or obstructive causes of ARF, the FENa is generally greater than 2.0.

9. What are important exceptions to the rules about urinary diagnostic indices described above?

The FENa test is much less useful when patients are nonoliguric. In this setting, the specificity of a low FENa for prerenal azotemia is markedly diminished. In addition to nonoliguria, several causes of ATN, specifically dye-induced acute tubular necrosis or acute tubular necrosis associated with hemolysis or rhabdomyolysis, may typically be associated with a low FENa. Patients who have prerenal azotemia but have either persistent diuretic effect, chronic tubulointerstitial injury, or bicarbonaturia may have a relatively high FENa. In the last case, the fractional excretion of chloride (FECl), which is calculated in an analogous way, will be appropriately low ($<1\%$). Finally, the early stages of acute renal failure from glomerulonephritis, transplant allograft rejection, or urinary obstruction may be associated with a low FENa.

10. How is ARF prevented?

Acute tubular necrosis often results from a combination of insults and is most likely to occur in particular clinical settings as well as in older patients, so that avoidance and prophylaxis are often possible. Acute tubular necrosis usually occurs following surgery or preexisting dehydration. In these settings, nephrotoxic drugs such as radiocontrast dye, aminoglycosides, amphotericin B, nonsteroidal anti-inflammatory agents, and some cancer chemotherapeutic agents such as cisplatin and methotrexate are far more potent in causing ARF. Optimizing volume status and establishing a relatively high rate of urine flow will minimize the risk of ARF. In specific situations such as administration of radiocontrast dye or cisplatin or in relatively high-risk surgery such as open-heart or biliary tract surgery, mannitol (12.5–25 gm administered as an IV infusion) may be a useful adjunct in preventing ARF.

11. How is established ARF treated?

The key point in treatment is to make an accurate diagnosis. Different causes of ARF require different therapies. Prerenal azotemia is treated by optimizing hemodynamic factors. The approach will obviously differ among patients. In dehydration, simple volume resuscitation will be effective. In congestive heart failure, diuresis, by virtue of resultant decreases in afterload, may improve renal perfusion. Urinary obstruction must be relieved.

Parenchymal ARF is also addressed in a diagnosis-directed manner. Acute glomerulo-nephritis may respond to immunosuppressive medications and/or plasmapheresis. Acute interstitial nephritis usually mandates discontinuation of an offending allergen, usually a drug, and may resolve more quickly with the administration of steroids.

Acute tubular necrosis is best treated, as discussed above, by prevention. Although pharmacologic agents such as calcium channel blockers and atrial natriuretic factor may ameliorate established experimental ARF, these agents are not yet approved for use in the clinical setting. Because nonoliguric acute tubular necrosis has a lower associated mortality and morbidity than oliguric acute tubular necrosis, there is some excitement about the administration of high-dose loop diuretics (1–3 gm/24 hr given as an IV infusion or as repeated boluses) in concert with renal doses of dopamine (1–3 μg/kg/min) to such patients. This therapy, which converts some patients with oliguric acute tubular necrosis to a nonoliguric state, certainly allows for easier management of the patient's volume and nutritional status. Whether this approach actually improves the prognosis is not clear. Optimization of fluid status and avoidance and/or therapy of electrolyte disorders are the mainstays of conservative management of ARF.

12. Which electrolyte disorders accompany ARF?

The most common are hyperkalemia, hypermagnesemia, hyperphosphatemia, hypocalcemia and acidosis.

13. What is the approach to hyperkalemia in patients with ARF?

Hyperkalemia most commonly occurs with oliguric acute tubular necrosis or urinary obstruction. It is truly a medical emergency. A serum potassium over 6.0 mandates an EKG, searching for peaked T waves, diminished P-wave amplitude, or prolonged QRS complex. Any of these findings is an indication for parenteral therapy. The quickest-acting parenteral therapy is the administration of calcium, as either the chloride, gluceptate, or gluconate salts. This therapy does not affect the serum potassium but does antagonize the effects of hyperkalemia on the membrane potential of the heart, and will prevent or reverse the cardiac effects of hyperkalemia. Administration of 1–2 ampules of calcium (4.8–9.6 mEq) will have immediate effects, but these effects persist only as long as the resultant hypercalcemia. Potential adverse effects include possible precipitation of calcium and phosphate in a hyperphosphatemic patient. Generally, this risk is outweighed by the risk of untreated hyperkalemia. Another rapidly effective approach is the administration of insulin. This drives potassium into cells and lowers the serum potassium. In patients who have a normal serum glucose, insulin (10 units IV) is generally administered with dextrose (one ampule of D50W or an infusion of D10W). The effects of insulin last somewhat longer than those of calcium and can be prolonged by a constant infusion of insulin, usually administered with glucose to prevent hypoglycemia. Bicarbonate may also be used to raise arterial pH and to shift potassium into cells. Complications include potentially adverse hemodynamic effects of intravenous bicarbonate and volume expansion from the sodium load of the drug.

Other useful approaches include removal of potassium from the body with potassium-binding resins (Kayexalate), increased urinary excretion with diuretics if possible, and hemodialysis or peritoneal dialysis. These methods of removing potassium from the body take longer to work than parenteral calcium, insulin, and bicarbonate, and therefore must be considered only after the medical emergency is addressed.

14. What abnormalities in calcium, phosphate, and magnesium accompany ARF?

In patients with ARF, phosphate excretion is minimized and hyperphosphatemia generally results. This process is accelerated in conditions in which tissue breakdown with attendant release of phosphate into the extracellular fluid occurs. Increases in serum phosphate concentration cause microprecipitation of calcium and resultant hypocalcemia. Although this is not usually clinically important, occasionally severe hypocalcemia causes tetany, seizures, and cardiac arrhythmias, which are largely preventable by the judicious administration of oral phosphate binders, usually aluminum hydroxide. Rarely, hemo-dialysis with porous membranes must be undertaken to lower the serum phosphate. If the hyperphosphatemia is extremely severe, a low calcium dialysate bath should be used to avoid extensive calcium-phosphate precipitation. Hypermagnesemia generally results in patients with ARF who are receiving magnesium-containing antacids or cathartics. Because the kidney is the usual organ that excretes magnesium, these agents should certainly be avoided in patients with ARF.

15. What abnormalities in acid-base balance accompany ARF?

The kidney is the organ that generally excretes acid generated by metabolism of a typical Western diet; therefore, ARF is often associated with acidosis. Although the degree of metabolic acidosis is generally minor, occasionally other contributing factors such as ongoing lactic acidosis cause severe metabolic acidosis.

Oral sodium bicarbonate may be useful in treating metabolic acidosis associated with ARF if the acidosis is relatively mild. It is not clear, however, whether intravenous sodium bicarbonate, especially if administered as a bolus, should be used. In some cases, either intravenous or oral sodium bicarbonate may be contraindicated by coexisting volume expansion. A growing body of literature suggests that the deleterious hemodynamic effects of intravenous bolus of bicarbonate contraindicate its use. The mechanism of these deleterious hemodynamic effects may involve the generation of CO_2 when bicarbonate is mixed with acidotic blood. This CO_2 can diffuse across cell membranes and potentially produce a paradoxical intracellular acidosis in cardiac and vascular tissue. Hemodialysis against a bicarbonate bath may be used to address acidosis in this setting without causing increases in $PaCO_2$; however, most extremely acidotic patients are hemodynamically unstable to start with, making hemodialysis difficult to perform. The therapeutic approach to severe metabolic acidosis with or without ARF failure is controversial.

16. What is the uremic syndrome?

The uremic syndrome is a symptom complex associated with renal failure. It may occur with chronic and acute renal failure, and involves virtually all organs of the body. Major manifestations are nausea and vomiting, pruritus, bleeding disorder, encephalopathy, and pericarditis. The syndrome generally mandates initiation of nonconservative therapy for ARF such as hemodialysis, peritoneal dialysis or continuous arteriovenous hemofiltration. The pathogenesis of the uremic syndrome is still poorly understood; however, neither urea nor creatinine produces any of the known manifestations of uremia.

17. What are the indications for nonconservative therapy of ARF?

Indications for nonconservative therapy such as dialysis include uremic signs or symptoms, fluid overload and/or electrolyte abnormalities that are refractory to conservative management. It has become the standard of care to provide nonconservative therapy when the BUN exceeds 100 mg/dl or the serum creatinine exceeds 10 mg/dl, especially in the setting of oliguric ATN. These latter guidelines are not absolute and must be interpreted in the light of other clinical features.

18. What are the options for nonconservative therapy of ARF?

The three main options for nonconservative therapy of ARF are hemodialysis, peritoneal dialysis, and continuous arteriovenous hemofiltration (CAVH). There are, of course, variations of each of these modalities. Hemodialysis involves the pumping of blood through an artificial kidney where solutes are removed primarily by dialysis along a concentration gradient and water is removed by ultrafiltration driven by a pressure gradient. Central venous access, anticoagulation, a skilled technician, and expensive equipment are mandatory for this process. Peritoneal dialysis involves the repetitive instillation and removal of fluid into the peritoneal cavity. Solute removal again results primarily by dialysis along a concentration gradient, and fluid removal occurs by ultrafiltration driven by an osmotic pressure gradient. Although this method is less efficient and less rapid than hemodialysis, no central venous access, anticoagulation, skilled technician, or expensive equipment is necessary. Finally, CAVH describes the perfusion of a hemofilter by the patient's own blood pressure. Ultrafiltration of fluid and solute is driven by this hydrostatic pressure gradient. Arterial and venous access are necessary, as is anticoagulation. However, no skilled technician or expensive equipment is necessary to perform this procedure. The advantages and disadvantages of each of these techniques, in general, depend on the expertise in performing them.

BIBLIOGRAPHY

1. Anderson RJ, Gabow PA, Gross PA: Urinary chloride concentration in acute renal failure. Min Elect Metab 10:92–97, 1984.
2. Anderson RJ, Linas SL, Berns AS, et al: Nonoliguric acute renal failure. N Engl J Med 296:1134–1138, 1977.
3. Appel BB: Aminoglycoside nephrotoxicity. Am J Med 159:427–443, 1990.
4. Better OS, Stein JH: Early management of shock and prophylaxis of acute renal failure in traumatic rhabdomyolysis. N Engl J Med 322:825–829, 1990.
5. Burke TJ, Cronin RE, Duchin KL, et al: Ischemia and tubule obstruction during acute renal failure in dogs: Mannitol in protection. Am J Physiol 238:F305–F314, 1980.
6. Burke TJ, Arnold PE, Gordon JA, et al: Protective effect of intrarenal calcium membrane blockers before or after ischemia. J Clin Invest 74:1830–1841, 1984.
7. Cantarovich F, Locatelli A, Fernandez JC, et al: Furosemide in high doses in the treatment of acute renal failure. Postgrad Med J 47:13–17, 1971.
8. Graziani G, Cantaluppi A, Casati S, et al: Dopamine and furosemide in oliguric acute renal failure. Nephron 37:39–42, 1984.
9. Hou SH, Bushinsky DA, Wish JB, et al: Hospital acquired renal insufficiency: A prospective study. Am J Med 74:243–248, 1983.
10. Levinsky NG: Pathophysiology of acute renal failure. N Engl J Med 296:1453–1457, 1977.
11. Maguire WC, Anderson RJ: Continuous arteriovenous hemofiltration in the intensive care unit. J Crit Care 1:54–56, 1986.
12. Miller TR, Anderson RJ, Linas SL, et al: Urinary diagnostic indices in acute renal failure. Ann Intern Med 89:47–50, 1978.
13. Nakamoto M, Shapiro JI, Chan L, Schrier RW: The invitro and invivo protective effect of atriopeptin III in ischemic acute renal failure in the rat. J Clin Invest 80:698–705, 1987.
14. Old CW, Lehrener LM: Prevention of radiocontrast induced acute renal failure with mannitol. Lancet 1:885, 1980.
15. Paller MS: Drug-induced nephropathies. Med Clin North Am 74:909–917, 1990.

16. Schetz M, Lauwers PM, Ferdinande P: Extracorporeal treatment of acute renal failure in the intensive care unit: A critical view. Intens Care Med 15:349–357, 1989.
17. Schrier RW, Conger JD: Acute renal failure: Pathogenesis, diagnosis, and management. In Schrier RW (ed): Renal and Electrolyte Disorders. Boston, Little, Brown, 1986, pp 423–460.
18. Shapiro JI, Anderson RJ: Urinary diagnostic indices in acute renal failure. AKF Nephrol Let 1:13–16, 1984.
19. Shapiro JI, Anderson RJ: Sodium depletion states. In Brenner BM, Stein J (eds): Topics in Nephrology. New York, Churchill Livingstone, 1985, pp 155–192.
20. Shapiro JI, Mathew A, Whalen MA, et al: Different effects of bicarbonate and Carbicarb in normal volunteers. J Crit Care 5:1–4, 1990.
21. Shapiro JI, Whalen M, Chan L: Hemodynamic and hepatic pH responses to bicarbonate and Carbicarb during acidosis. Mag Reson Med 16:403–410, 1990.

47. DIALYSIS

Arlene Chapman, M.D.

1. What is dialysis? What is peritoneal dialysis?

Hemodialysis—the process of separating crystalloids and colloids in solution by the difference of their rates of diffusion through a semipermeable membrane. Crystalloids pass through readily; colloids very slowly or not at all. Hemodialysis is controlled by (1) blood flow rate, (2) permeability of the membrane, (3) duration of dialysis, and (4) transmembrane pressure. Ultrafiltration is also achieved by removing water and solute through convective transport.

Peritoneal dialysis—dialysis through the abdominal wall within the peritoneal cavity. Dialysis occurs across the peritoneal membrane and is affected by thickness or inflammation of the membrane, blood flow to the peritoneal lining, the size of the peritoneal cavity, and the presence of infection.

2. What are absolute and relative indications for acute dialysis?

Absolute indications include life-threatening hypoxia secondary to excess fluid volume; systemic acidemia; hyperkalemia not controlled by conservative measures; drug overdoses that are effectively cleared by dialysis such as lithium, theophylline, and acetaminophen; and confusion, coma, or pericarditis due to uremia. **Relative indications** include acute renal failure with blood urea nitrogen (BUN) increasing to or above 100 mg/dl (this varies depending on the muscle mass of the patient), platelet dysfunction with clinical evidence of bleeding, and fluid overload. Recent evidence suggests that more frequent, efficient dialysis with a lower BUN is generally associated with better renal and patient outcome.

3. What new dialytic techniques are available for critically ill patients?

Continuous arteriovenous hemofiltration (CAVH) is a technique in which convective transport is applied through an extracorporeal circuit that does not use a blood pump. Removal of solutes is accomplished by ultrafiltration and replacement with a balanced electrolyte solution. CAVH can adequately dialyze a patient who is not severely catabolic and is better tolerated by patients with hemodynamic instability than is hemodialysis.

CAVHD is continuous arteriovenous hemodialysis or hemodiafiltration, in which diffusive transport is used with dialysate administered in a single pass countercurrent to blood flow. No blood pump is required and dialysate flow rates are 5% of those used in conventional hemodialysis. Flow is maintained by the patient's arterial pressure. Because high flow rates and high transmembrane pressures are not used, expensive monitoring equipment is not needed. However, continuous supervision, frequent filter replacements, and systemic anticoagulation are necessary.

Both therapies require vascular access (arterial and large venous), anticoagulation, and frequent filter changes (approximately every 24–72 hours). CAVH is best used for large volumes of fluid removal or when therapy requires large fluid volumes (total parenteral nutrition, medications, pressor agents). When the patient requires dialysis as well as fluid removal, CAVHD is more appropriate.

4. What are the indications for acute peritoneal dialysis?
Acute peritoneal dialysis is absolutely indicated in cerebral hemorrhage. Large compartmental shifts and increases in intracerebral pressure occur quickly with hemodialysis, worsening the cerebral hemorrhage. Peritoneal dialysis is also used when anticoagulation is unsafe or when the patient has severe congestive heart failure and marginal systemic blood pressures that do not tolerate hemodialysis. Poor vascular access and absence of a catabolic state are two relative indications for peritoneal dialysis. Patients with undiagnosed intraabdominal disease or recent abdominal surgery should not be considered candidates for peritoneal dialysis. The most frequent complications are infection or peritonitis, ileus and indigestion, shortness of breath from decreased diaphragmatic excursion, and peritoneal leaking from the catheter site.

5. Which ICU patients most often require acute dialysis?
The most common cause of acute renal failure in critical care patients is acute tubular necrosis. The events leading to acute tubular necrosis in the ICU are usually septicemia or cardiovascular surgery. Less common causes include burns, cardiopulmonary arrest, liver failure, rhabdomyolysis, antibiotic nephrotoxicity, and primary renal disease. The relative incidences vary depending on the hospital setting of the ICU. Of all patients with acute renal failure, postoperative patients most often require acute dialysis, whereas nephrotoxin-induced renal failure requires acute dialysis less often.

6. What complications commonly occur during acute dialysis?
The commonest complications are hypotension, bleeding, infection, and encephalopathy. Now that H_2 blockers and Carafate are available, gastrointestinal bleeding occurs less often. In most critical care patients with multiorgan failure (MOF), cardiac arrhythmias during dialysis may occur.

7. What is dialysis disequilibrium syndrome? How is it prevented?
Dialysis disequilibrium syndrome is a variety of symptoms related to the central nervous system that occur during or immediately after hemodialysis. Minor symptoms include nausea, vomiting, dizziness, headache, blurred vision, restlessness, cramping, and tremors. Major symptoms include confusion, psychosis, seizures, and coma. This is most commonly seen during initial dialysis sessions in patients with high BUN concentrations, in the elderly, and in children, and is a diagnosis of exclusion. The cause is most likely related to increases in intracranial or cerebrospinal fluid (CSF) pressure from water accumulation due to unequal urea concentrations in the CSF and plasma compartments.

This syndrome can be avoided by early intervention in acute and chronic renal failure (BUN < 150 ml/dl), starting with brief dialysis sessions with a gradual increase in dialysis time and blood flow rate using a small-surface-area dialyzer. Dialysis disequilibrium can be practically treated by adding osmotically active solutes, including dextrose, fructose, mannitol, sodium chloride, and glycerol, to the plasma compartment during dialysis.

8. What is available to treat dialysis-induced hypotension?

Dialysis-induced hypotension occurs due to vascular instability or circulating volume contraction. In critical care patients, vascular instability results from myocardial dysfunction and poor cardiac output, volume contraction, or endothelial damage and poorly contracting arterial vessels. In patients with central cardiac monitoring, the decreased intravascular volume and vascular instability can be differentiated from central volume overload. In all patients, dry weight estimations should be reassessed with withdrawal or adjustment of antihypertensive medications. In patients with increased pulmonary capillary wedge or right atrial pressures due to myocardial dysfunction, positive inotropic agents such as dobutamine can be used. In patients with diminished peripheral resistance or poorly contracting vessels, agents such as dopamine and norepinephrine (Levophed) can be used to increase peripheral resistance. These patients may also benefit from crystalloid infusion with isotonic saline (Ringer's lacate), in 200–500 ml boluses, colloid infusion albumin in 25-gm doses, mannitol 25% in 50-ml volumes, or blood products in the form of whole blood should the patient's hematocrit warrant transfusion. All patients who suddenly become hypotensive during dialysis treatment when volume removal has not been large should be investigated for changes in cardiac status due to cardiac tamponade, myocardial infarction or cardiac arrhythmia due to hypokalemia, hypomagnesia, or hypocalcemia, as well as bacteremia.

9. How does one dialyze a patient with a bleeding disorder?

Specific dialyzer membranes such as EXVAL are available that remain free of thrombosis when heparin is not used. Low-dose heparin can be used to maintain dialyzer membrane viability with minimal additional risk for bleeding. When early thrombosis is apparent, saline flushing can be used successfully. Standard heparin infusion is 500 units/hr. Target activated bleeding times are usually 9–10 minutes. Heparin infusions can be treated to the minimum bleeding time, done regionally with protamine, or given until evidence of filter thrombosis occurs. Dialysis-induced bleeding can be stopped by discontinuing dialysis and administering protamine or DDAVP intravenously.

10. What are first-use reactions during hemodialysis?

First-use reactions occur in patients when a new dialyzer membrane is used, not just the first time a patient is dialyzed. Symptoms include chest or back pain, diaphoresis, nausea, shortness of breath, hypertension or hypotension, and mental status changes such as confusion. This most often occurs with cuprophane membranes, and is thought to be due to complement activation. Dialyzers are reused today because of improved membrane biocompatibility, which decreases the incidence of first-use reactions and is cost efficient.

11. What is the difference between acetate and bicarbonate dialysates?

Acetate was originally used as the buffering agent in dialysate fluid. However, with the development of more efficient dialyzers, patients with systemic acidemia, liver disease, and severe congestive heart failure developed side effects owing to acetate accumulation, including diaphoresis, headaches, nausea, vomiting, and hypotension. Given that intact liver function is required for conversion of acetate to bicarbonate, almost all ICU patients are dialyzed with a bicarbonate dialysate. Bicarbonate is less stable and more difficult to prepare than acetate, but it is safer for the patient.

12. What determines survival in ICU patients who require dialysis due to acute renal failure?

Acute renal failure carries a high mortality rate (33–81%), and ICU patients who require dialysis have higher mortality rates (64–88%) than patients dialyzed in standard dialysis units. Confounding variables such as pulmonary insufficiency, jaundice, and peritonitis have been shown to affect survival negatively in patients with acute renal failure. Failure to recover renal function is most often associated with adult respiratory distress syndrome, the need for mechanical ventilation, and the need for antibiotics. Patient survival during acute renal failure is unlikely when the need for mechanical ventilation occurs and three or more other organ systems have failed.

13. Are there patients with acute renal failure in intensive care settings who will not benefit from acute dialysis?

Patients requiring mechanical ventilation have been reported to have 82–100% mortality during acute renal failure. Other investigators have found 100% mortality in patients with failure of more than three other organ systems. However, the decision to institute or discontinue dialysis in critically ill patients with a small chance of survival rests with the patient, the family, the primary physician, and the nephrologist. As improvements occur in respiratory care and new dialytic techniques (CAVH, CAVHD) are developed, reevaluation of patient survival with acute renal failure in the ICU may show improvement.

BIBLIOGRAPHY

1. Brezis M, Rosen S, Epstein FM: Acute renal failure. In Brenner B, Rector FC (eds): The Kidney, 3rd ed. Philadelphia, W.B. Saunders, 1986, pp 772–773.
2. Cameron JS: Acute renal failure in the intensive care unit today. Intens Care Med 12:64–70, 1986.
3. Cerra FB, Anthore S: Colloid osmotic pressure fluctuations and the disequilibrium syndrome during hemodialysis. Nephron 13:245–249, 1974.
4. Coggins CM, Fong LST: Acute renal failure associated with antibiotics, anesthetic agents and radioactive agents. In Brenner BM, Lazarus JM (eds): Acute Renal Failure, 4th ed. New York, Churchill Livingstone, 1988, pp 292–352.
5. Conger JD, Anderson RJ: Acute renal failure including cortical necrosis. In Massry SG, Glasscock RJ (eds): Textbook of Nephrology. Baltimore, Williams & Wilkins, 1983, pp 215–232.
6. Eioffi WG, Astrukaga T, Gamelli RL: Probability of surviving postoperative acute renal failure. Ann Surg 200:205–211, 1984.
7. Finn WF: Recovery from acute renal failure. In Brenner BM, Lazarus JM (eds): Acute Renal Failure. Philadelphia, W.B. Saunders, 1983, pp 753–774.
8. Harter HR: Reviews of significant findings from the National Cooperative Dialysis Study and recommendations. Kidney Int 23:5107–5112, 1983.
9. Kjellstrand CM, Bakseth RO, Klinkmann M: Treatment of acute renal failure. In Schrier RW, Gottschalk CW (eds): Diseases of the Kidney, 4th ed. Boston, Little, Brown, 1988, pp 1501–1542.
10. Ruth GS, Briggs JD, Mare JG, et al: Survival from acute renal failure with and without multiple organ dysfunction. Postgrad Med J 56:244–247, 1980.
11. Spiegel DM, Ullian ME, Zerbe GO, Berl T: Determinants of survival and recovery in acute renal failure patients dialyzed in intensive care units. Am J Nephrol 11:44–47, 1991.
12. Voerman HJ, Strack von Schijndel RJ, Thijs LG: Continuous arterial-venous hemodiafiltration in critically ill patients. Crit Care Med 18:911–914, 1990.

---

48. PERITONEAL DIALYSIS

Hildegarde M. Schell, R.N., B.S.N.

---

1. When is peritoneal dialysis (PD) the preferred treatment modality for patients with acute or chronic renal failure?

PD is the preferred renal replacement therapy when hemodialysis is contraindicated secondary to the patient's unstable cardiovascular status or when vascular access is difficult to obtain. Issues such as a patient's refusal of blood transfusions or mobile lifestyle would be indicators for choosing PD as long-term therapy.

2. What are the contraindications for PD?

Acute PD does not adequately remove uremic metabolites from patients in hypercatabolic states. The patient is at risk for an acute hydrothorax if a patent peritoneal-pleural fistula is present. If a patient's history includes multiple abdominal surgeries or previous episodes of peritonitis, there may be scarring and adhesions that prevent an adequate transfer surface area of the peritoneum.

3. What types of catheters are commonly used for PD?

For temporary PD, a rigid cannula made of polyvinyl chloride can be inserted over a stylet. A trochar or peritoneoscope may be used. These cannulas are for single-use only (24–48 hours). They are inserted and removed at the bedside. Rigid cannulas have an increased risk of mechanical complication (organ perforation) and cause discomfort to the patient. A straight or curled silicone rubber catheter with a single Dacron polyester cuff can be placed for acute or long-term use. These can be inserted surgically or at the bedside with a special introducer. The single cuff and double cuff Silastic catheters were developed by Tenchkhoff primarily for chronic PD patients. The cuffs allow subcutaneous tissue ingrowth to stabilize the catheter, provide a barrier to microorganisms, and provide a water seal. These catheters have a radiopaque stripe to allow visualization on x-ray.

4. How soon after catheter placement can PD be initiated?

Dialysis can be initiated with temporary rigid catheters once the exit site is secure and protected with a sterile dressing. The dressing should be assessed frequently for movement or loss of the catheter and for dialysate leakage. Chemstrip glucose will differentiate dialysate fluid from exudate at the exit site. There are various break-in techniques for chronic Silastic catheters. The goals during break-in are to prevent leaks, to maintain a patent catheter, and to minimize intraabdominal pressure by limiting physical activity (bed rest) and discouraging Valsalva maneuvers. One common technique is to use frequent rapid exchanges of small volumes (50–500 cc) of heparinized dialysate for the first 24–48 hours or until the effluent is clear.

5. What are the mechanical complications of PD?

Mild to moderate bleeding, secondary to abdominal trauma, usually occurs during the first 24 hours. A large amount of blood that does not clear with exchanges may indicate vascular injury. **Organ perforation** may occur when using a rigid catheter or during placement of the rigid or Silastic catheter. An increase in urine flow with dialysate infusion may indicate a perforated bladder. Abdominal pain, nausea, vomiting, and watery diarrhea are signs of a perforated bowel. **Poor inflow or outflow** can be the result of a kinked catheter or tubing, an air lock in the tubing, or constipation that inferferes with flow. **Dialysate leakage** around the catheter into the abdominal wall or externally is usually caused by overfilling or inadequate catheter stabilization. **Abdominal pain** can be the result of hot or cold dialysate, the use of hypertonic dialysate, a rapid rate of infusion, or the pressure caused by a malpositioned catheter. Intraperitoneal air can cause **shoulder pain** referred from the diaphragm. Anesthetics (lidocaine 2%, 3–5 cc/L) or parenteral analgesics may be administered for patient comfort.

6. What anatomy and physiology are involved in PD?

The peritoneum acts as the dialyzing membrane. Its size approximates body surface area. The peritoneum obtains its blood supply from the arteries of the abdominal wall and the celiac and mesenteric arteries. Blood returns to circulation via the portal vein and vessels of the abdominal wall. Movement of solutes, drugs, and water across the peritoneal membrane occurs through diffusion, osmosis, and ultrafiltration. Diffusion is influenced by the permeability of the peritoneum as well as the solute's characteristics. Osmosis and ultrafiltration are influenced by the surface area and permeability of the peritoneum as well as by the oncotic, hydrostatic, and osmotic pressure gradients. Dopamine can be used to increase ultrafiltration by increasing hydrostatic pressure. The osmotic pressure gradient is determined by the concentration of dextrose in the dialysate.

7. What is the PD process?

An **exchange** or cycle includes the **infusion, dwell and drainage** of dialysate. Dialysate infuses into the peritoneal cavity by gravity in approximately 5–15 minutes. The height of the dialysate, the tubing length, and intraabdominal pressure may affect the infusion rate. The dwell time allows diffusion and osmosis to take place. Dwell time in acute PD is 10–30 minutes versus 2–6 hours in chronic PD exchanges. Drainage of the dialysate occurs by gravity in approximately 10–30 minutes. Catheter position, length and occlusion of the tubing, intraabdominal pressure, and distance from the abdomen to the drainage bag may affect the rate of drainage. Effluent is another term used for the outflow solution.

8. What are the different techniques of PD therapy?

Acute PD is a therapy option for acute renal failure. A temporary or long-term catheter may be placed for access. In acute PD, dialysate is infused, dwelled for short periods of time (10–30 minutes), and drained completely. Patients with chronic renal failure may choose continuous ambulatory peritoneal dialysis (CAPD) or intermittent peritoneal dialysis (IPD). These techniques require a permanent catheter for access. CAPD involves 4–6 exchanges a day (7 days a week), including a longer 8- to 12-hour dwell during the night. Continuous cyclic peritoneal dialysis (CCPD) involves a cycler machine that automatically allows the infusion, dwell, and drain of 3 or 4 exchanges every 2–3 hours during the night. During the day, one 10- to 12-hour dwell of hypertonic dialysate prevents excessive reabsorption of fluid. IPD also involves a machine that automatically cycles exchanges 10–14 hours, 3 or 4 times per week, and during the night. Between the dialyses, no dialysate is left in the peritoneal cavity.

9. What is the composition of the dialysis solution?

The dialysis solution (dialysate) is composed of electrolytes, a buffer, and dextrose. The electrolytes include sodium 132 mEq/L, chloride 96 mEq/L, potassium none, calcium 3.5 mEq/L, and magnesium 0.5 mEq/L. They are present in the combined forms: sodium chloride, calcium chloride, and magnesium chloride. Sodium lactate is the buffer currently used in the United States. Dextrose is used to generate an osmotic pressure gradient in the peritoneal cavity and to enhance ultrafiltration. Most commonly used dextrose concentrations are 1.5, 2.5, and 4.25% solutions. Dextrose and calcium are absorbed from the dialysate into the systemic circulation.

10. Does the temperature of the dialysate affect dialysis?

Warming the dialysate to approximately 37°–38°C (tepid to touch) enhances solute transport and aids patient comfort. Warm water baths are not recommended because they increase the risk of contamination. Dry heating via a heating pad or a microwave is preferred. Microwave heating does not change the pH or chemistry of the dialysate. Medications should be administered after heating, just prior to infusing the dialysate. The plastic overwrap on the dialysate bag should be left on during the heating process. If the infused dialysate is too cold, the patient may become hypothermic and have subjective complaints. If the infused dialysate is too hot, the patient may have an increase in body temperature, flushing, and abdominal pain. This can also burn and scar the peritoneal membrane, decreasing effective surface area needed for dialysis.

11. Which laboratory values should be monitored during PD?
In acute PD, a rapid drop in creatinine and blood urea nitrogen is not likely. Longer dwell times are needed for more efficient removal of these solutes. Special attention should be paid to the electrolyte values. Hyperkalemia may persist if there is a problem with the PD system. Hypokalemia frequently occurs in acute PD if not monitored and treated by adding potassium chloride (KCl) to the dialysate or by giving supplemental IV or oral KCl. Hypercalcemia is rare but may occur because calcium is systemically absorbed from the dialysate. Magnesium is minimally removed in PD. Glucose monitoring is important because dextrose is absorbed from the dialysate. Serum albumin and transferrin levels help to assess protein loss and nutritional status. A rise in the hematocrit may occur with the initiation of PD secondary to the concentrated red cell mass and decreased plasma volume. The hematocrit eventually returns to the patient's baseline level.

12. How is peritonitis diagnosed?
Patients with peritonitis typically present with cloudy effluent, rebound tenderness, and abdominal pain. Less common signs and symptoms include fever, chills, nausea, and vomiting. Samples of the cloudy effluent should be obtained from the drainage bag with aseptic technique. The effluent should be sent to the laboratory for a cell count, differential, Gram stain, and culture. A normal cell count from uninfected effluent is 0–50 μl with mononuclear cells. A cell count of $\geq 100/\mu l$ with a differential of $>50\%$ neutrophils may indicate an infection. The most common organisms of infectious peritonitis are gram-positive cocci, mainly *Staphylococcus epidermidis* and *Staphylococcus aureus*. Gram-negative rods have been noted in a number of cases. The average peritonitis rate for CAPD is 1.4 episodes/year. A majority of these episodes are related to breaking aseptic technique during bag or line changes.

13. How is infectious peritonitis treated?
Infectious peritonitis has been treated with various protocols of oral (PO), intravenous (IV), and/or intraperitoneal (IP) antimicrobial agents. Oral agents are not commonly used to treat peritonitis. Recent trials with ciprofloxacin have been successful in treating gram-positive and negative organisms. A loading dose of IV vancomycin followed by IP doses has shown excellent activity against gram-positive cocci. Intraperitoneal therapy for a positive Gram stain usually includes a combination of an aminoglycoside with vancomycin until culture results are available. IP therapy for 7–14 days is recommended. Fungal peritonitis may be treated with IP amphotericin B or flucytosine. Early catheter removal is recommended because reports of the efficacy of these agents are inconsistent. Heparin (1 unit/cc) may be added to the dialysate to prevent potential adhesion formation and scarring of the peritoneum.

14. What medications are commonly given intraperitoneally?
IP administration of any medication has an inherent risk of contaminating the system. Aseptic technique is imperative. All injection ports and multiple-dose vials should be disinfected prior to use.
   Heparin in a 1:1 concentration is commonly used in the dialysate for a few days after catheter placement. Heparin inhibits fibrin formation, thereby preventing the catheter from clotting. Heparin is also used during episodes of peritonitis to decrease the risk of adhesion formation. Excessive potassium can be removed in acute PD because the dialysate is potassium free. **Potassium chloride** (2–4 mEq/L) should be added to the dialysate once the serum potassium reaches normal levels. Intravenous or oral supplements should be given if hypokalemia persists. **Insulin** may be required in nondiabetic and diabetic patients secondary to the absorption of dextrose from the dialysate. The dose usually needs to be increased in dialysates containing higher dextrose concentrations. **Antibiotics** are given intraperitoneally when treating peritonitis.

15. Are systemic drugs cleared by peritoneal dialysis?
Systemic drugs that are water soluble, poorly bound to protein and/or have a low molecular weight (<20,000 daltons) are easily transported across the peritoneal membrane. Increased dosages of drugs that are removed by peritoneal dialysis may need to be given. Aminocaproic acid and theophylline are removed by peritoneal dialysis. Digoxin, cimetadine, and phenytoin are not removed in significant amounts. Drugs administered intraperitoneally, such as insulin and antibiotics, may be absorbed systemically. Heparin is poorly absorbed from the dialysate and does not result in systemic anticoagulation.

16. How is hypervolemia managed?
Fluid overload is usually related to inadequate use of high-dextrose-containing (hypertonic) dialysate. Technical complications, including dialysate leaks and catheter malfunctions, are also possible reasons for inadequate dialysis. Clinical signs and symptoms include positive fluid balance, hypertension, weight gain, edema, and shortness of breath. Fluid intake should be limited. The dialysate should be changed to a higher dextrose concentration with shorter dwell times to facilitate fluid removal. Acute renal failure may require rapid exchanges (every half hour) of 1- to 2-liter bags of 4.25% dextrose dialysate. Once fluid overload is corrected, an isotonic dialysate should be used to avoid the complications of excessive fluid removal.

17. What complications are related to increased intraabdominal pressure?
There is a positive relationship between increased intraabdominal pressure and increased dialysate volumes used in peritoneal dialysis. Coughing, Valsalva maneuver, straining, and other activities that increase intraabdominal pressure should be avoided during dialysis. Common complications are hernias (incisional, inguinal, and umbilical) and dialysate leaks. Repair of the hernia is usually indicated. Leaks are manifested by exit site drainage or edema of the genitalia and/or anterior abdominal wall. Decreasing the dialysate volume and dialyzing in the supine position will decrease intraabdominal pressure. Dialysis can be stopped for 24 hours. If the leak persists, removal and replacement of the catheter are indicated. Less common complications are low back pain, gastroesophageal reflux, decreased forced vital capacity, and progressive decrease in left ventricular systolic function in patients on long-term peritoneal dialysis.

18. How is acute hydrothorax clinically manifested?
Acute hydrothorax, which is caused by an acquired or congenital defect in the diaphragm, usually manifests on the right side and may present as a pleural effusion or massive hydro-thorax on chest x-ray. The patient will appear dyspneic and tachypneic. The dialysate will drain poorly, resulting in fluid retention. The fluid from the pleural tap will have similar composition to the dialysate, including a high glucose content (≥ 40 mmol/L). Methylene blue can be added to the dialysate to confirm the diagnosis. Cessation of the PD exchange facilitates resolution of the acute hydrothorax. Pleural effusions should be monitored closely.

19. What are the nutritional considerations for patients on PD?
PD is associated with large protein losses (5–15 gm/day) into the dialysate. Most of the protein loss is albumin, which has a lower molecular weight than other proteins. Amino acids (2–4 gm/day) and water-soluble vitamins are also lost in the dialysate. Glucose (60–80%) from the dialysate is absorbed, especially with the high-dextrose concentrations. Early assessment of nutritional status is imperative. These patients need both an adequate amount of protein to maintain nitrogen balance and supplemental vitamins (folic acid, vitamin B_6, and vitamin C).

20. What is included in the documentation of PD?

Continuous monitoring of the patient's total intake and output is imperative. A dry weight should be obtained after draining the dialysate. The dialysate solution, the volume, and any added medications ordered should be documented (i.e., 2.5% 1,000 cc with 1,000 U heparin IP). The outflow (effluent) volume, color, and consistency need to be noted. The exchange balance (outflow volume–inflow volume) and a cumulative balance monitor dialysis output. The catheter exit site should be assessed for redness, exudate, and tenderness.

BIBLIOGRAPHY

1. Cole GA: Manual of Peritoneal Dialysis: Practical Procedures for Medical and Nursing Staff. Dordrecht, Netherlands, Kluwer Academic Publishers, 1988.
2. Green A: The management of hydrothorax in CAPD. Peritoneal Dialysis International 4:271–279, 1990.
3. Hirszel P, Lasrick M, Maher J: Augmentation of peritoneal mass transport by dopamine. J Lab Clin Med 94:747–754, 1979.
4. Linblad AS: Hematocrit values in the CAPD/CCPD population: A report of the National Registry. Peritoneal Dialysis International 4:275–282, 1990.
5. Nolph KD (ed): Peritoneal Dialysis. Dordrecht, Netherlands, Kluwer Academic Publishers, 1989.
6. Ronco C, Feriani M, Chiaramonte S, et al: Pathophysiology of ultrafiltration in peritoneal dialysis. Peritoneal Dialysis International 2:119–126, 1990.
7. Wadhwa NK, Kenward DH, Kennedy B, et al: Heating of peritoneal dialysis fluid by microwave oven in hospital practice—a method of choice. Peritoneal Dialysis Bulletin 3:187–188, 1983.

49. CONTINUOUS ARTERIOVENOUS HEMOFILTRATION

Connie Glavis, M.S., R.N.

1. What is continuous arteriovenous hemofiltration (CAVH)?

CAVH is an extracorporeal hemofiltration system designed to remove plasma water and toxins from the vascular space. This technique is designed for ultrafiltration without a blood pump.

2. When is CAVH indicated?

CAVH is indicated in an acutely ill, hemodynamically unstable patient in acute renal failure who is either too unstable to tolerate hemodialysis or requires such large volumes for parenteral nutrition and/or drug titration that a mode of therapy that provides slow, continuous fluid removal is necessary.

3. Why is CAVH tolerated by an unstable patient who is unable to tolerate hemodialysis?

CAVH provides a more physiologic process of ultrafiltration similar to that of the glomerulus. Less hemodynamic instability occurs because it is a slow, continuous process compared with the intermittent, episodic nature of hemodialysis. The system is low volume, so there is not significant diversion of cardiac output through the filter. The CAVH filter does not activate the complement system or leukocytes. It permits continuous control of volume.

4. Summarize the advantages and disadvantages of CAVH.

Continuous Arteriovenous Hemofiltration

Advantages

Better tolerated in hemodynamically unstable patients

Allows for removal of large volumes of fluid

Does not require pumps, machines, or continuous monitoring by dialysis nurses

Can be done continuously at bedside in the ICU

Disadvantages

Need for arterial access

Demands *intense* ICU nursing care (can lose 3–900 ml/hr)

Clotting in cartridge leads to decreased efficiency

From Parrillo JE (ed): Current Therapy in Critical Care Medicine, 2nd ed. Philadelphia, B.C. Decker, 1991, p 256, with permission.

5. What pump provides the blood flow within the system?

The pressure gradient between the arterial and venous blood pressures provides flow through the filter. An arterial catheter is connected to tubing that carries blood through the filter and back to the patient via a venous catheter. A semipermeable membrane within the filter allows plasma water or ultrafiltrate to pass through the filter and into a drainage bag.

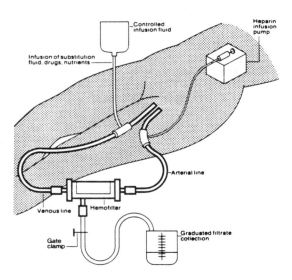

The CAVH system. (From Ossenkoppele GJ, et al: Crit Care Med 13:102–104, 1985, with permission.)

6. How is the ultrafiltrate formed?

Formation of the ultrafiltrate is a function of the net pressure differences across the membrane. The oncotic pressure within the blood space holds plasma water within the blood. However, hydrostatic pressure within the blood forces plasma water across the filter into the collection bag. Negative hydrostatic pressure provided by the weight of the ultra-filtrate column on the filter moves plasma water across the filter. Thus, the transmembrane pressure gradient (TPG) is the difference between the oncotic pressure and hydrostatic pressures within the system. The amount of ultrafiltrate removed is controlled by maintaining an adequate blood pressure and adjusting the height of the drainage bag. However, blood flow through the filter is the primary determinant of ultrafiltrate volume.

7. What factors influence blood flow through the filter?

Blood flow within the filter depends on adequate blood pressure. A mean arterial pressure greater than 65 mm Hg is usually necessary to maintain flow. The pressure gradient between arterial and venous pressures will affect flow. The vascular access must be large enough to allow adequate flow to and from the filter. Blood viscosity influences flow, and a hematocrit less than 45 will allow adequate flow. The tubing connecting the filter to the patient is short with a relatively large internal diameter that will minimize loss of flow within the system. Blood flow may be calculated by:

$$BFR = \frac{(UF\ ml/min)(Hct_v)}{(Hct_v) - (Hct_m)}$$

8. What solutes are in the ultrafiltrate?

Solutes move across the filter via convection. The ultrafiltrate consists of plasma water and solutes less than 60,000 daltons. Proteins and protein-bound substances are not removed from the blood. Solutes are in similar concentrations as in plasma.

9. If solute concentration in the ultrafiltrate is the same as in the plasma, how does clearance occur?

Clearance or reduction of the concentration of solutes in the plasma occurs by removing large volumes of ultrafiltrate and replacing it with fluid. Thus, the clearance obtained with CAVH is primarily due to dilution. The removal of large volumes of plasma water and solutes and simultaneous replacement with a "clean" IV solution reduces uremic toxins. The "coffeepot analogy" provides a concrete example of this concept. Imagine a coffeepot filled with very strong, concentrated coffee. If you empty the pot halfway, the volume of coffee is reduced but the remaining coffee is as strong as it was before. However, if you fill the pot with clean water, the strength or concentration of the coffee is reduced. Similarly, CAVH works most efficiently when large volumes of ultrafiltrate (10 ml/min) are removed from the blood and replaced with clean IV solution. Simply removing small amounts of ultrafiltrate without replacing fluids will not lower uremic toxin blood levels. Creatinine clearance for spontaneous CAVH is approximately 10 ml/min.

10. How can removal of drugs by CAVH be predicted?

Nonprotein-bound drugs may be removed with ultrafiltration. The rate of drug removal depends on the amount of drug in the ultrafiltrate and the rate of ultrafiltrate formation. It may be calculated by:

Concentration in UF × UF rate

or

Steady-state arterial concentration × unbound fraction × UF vol/time

However, because of multiple uncontrollable variables, the actual amount of drug removed may vary from predictions.

11. Is anticoagulation necessary?

As blood passes across the filter, it will clot if coagulation is normal. Patients with coagulopathies may not need additional anticoagulation to maintain the filter. With normal coagulation times, the goal is to anticoagulate the filter with as little systemic anticoagulation as possible. However, it is currently not possible to anticoagulate the filter without some systemic effect. A recommended dose of heparin is 20 u/kg IV bolus just prior to filter connection, followed by a heparin drip connected to the arterial or prefilter side of the filter, titrated to maintain the patient's activated clotting time (ACT) $>$ 100 or the partial thromboplastin time (PTT) 1–1½ times normal. The range of titration is dictated by monitored coagulation times, but is usually 7–10 u/kg. A lower heparin concentration in the drip solution allows greater mixing and better anticoagulation in the filter.

12. What type of vascular access is necessary?
Because the system is run by the patient's blood pressure, large-bore arterial and venous access are required for adequate blood flow. Percutaneous femoral 7-French arterial and venous catheters provide adequate flow. CAVH catheters are available. A Quinton catheter may be placed in the vein to be used for hemodialysis when the patient is more stable. Arterial and venous access must be of similar size in order not to impede flow. If femoral access is not possible, a Scribner shunt may be used. An arteriovenous fistula usually does not provide sufficient arteriovenous pressure gradient to allow adequate flow through the system.

13. How is the filter prepared prior to use?
All filters are cleared with heparinized normal saline. Several filters are available, and each manufacturer has its own recommendations. In general, about 2 liters of heparinized saline (5000 u/L) are run through the filter to clear the blood pathway and the semipermeable membrane of any glycerin and air.

14. What replacement fluid is administered?
The replacement solution is determined according to the patient's metabolic needs. Extremely large volumes of fluid are removed from the patient, which requires close monitoring of electrolytes with appropriate replacement. Alkali replacement can be with bicarbonate, lactate, or acetate. Magnesium, calcium, and bicarbonate must be administered in separate containers to prevent precipitation. Administration of total parenteral nutrition (TPN) is possible because of the unrestricted administration of fluids; in fact, much of the electrolyte control can be maintained with TPN. This technique may eliminate the need for multiple replacement solutions.

15. How is the replacement solution administered?
The filtration replacement fluid (FRF) may be administered to the patient either prefilter or postfilter. Prefilter administration is through the port on the arterial line of the connecting tubing and provides better clearance rates because it dilutes the plasma, drawing urea from the red blood cells into the plasma and then across the filter. However, it requires more fluid administration because much of this fluid will pass into the ultrafiltrate without ever having gone to the patient. Postfilter administration is through the port on the venous connecting tubing and will run directly into the patient. This method of administration requires less fluid and is more cost efficient.

16. What calculations are necessary to determine filtration replacement fluid volumes?
Because several hundred milliliters are removed from the patient per hour, fluid replacement is calculated and administered at least hourly:

$$FRF = (UFR) + \text{all other losses} - \text{(all other fluids given)}$$
$$\pm \text{ desired fluid removal rate.}$$

For example, if 800 cc of ultrafiltrate were removed, total IV fluids administered (excluding FRF for the last hour) were 200 cc, and it was desired to remove a negative balance of 100 cc/hr, the formula would be: FRF = 800 – 200 = 600 – 100 = 500. Therefore, to maintain a negative balance of 100 cc/hr, 500 cc of replacement fluid would be administered over the next hour. Because this 500 cc is being given to make the fluid balance a negative 100 cc for the last hour, it will *not* be included as IV intake for this hour.

17. What are the common complications of CAVH?

Complications are remarkably rare and most can be prevented if the patient is monitored closely. Some complications are filter clotting, access complications, hemorrhage, and filter rupture.

18. How is filter clotting predicted?

Over time, the filter will clot off, the blood flow will be reduced, and ultrafiltration will cease. As blood flow decreases through the filter, certain signs can be noted clinically. Initially, the venous connecting tubing will become cooler than the arterial tubing. Second, the arterial connecting tubing will become cooler. Third, the ultrafiltrate rate will decrease. Finally, separation of the red cells and plasma will be noticed in the connecting tubing. By frequently monitoring the tubing for temperature changes, early clotting can be detected and the filter may be changed without interruption in filtration or loss of access catheters. Depending on blood flow and anticoagulation, filters may last from a few hours to 92 hours.

19. Should the ultrafiltrate be heme tested to detect filter rupture?

Because of blood contact with the filter, the ultrafiltrate will always test heme positive. A heme-positive ultrafiltrate is therefore not indicative of filter rupture. Filter rupture, which is quite rare, may be detected by visibly pink ultrafiltrate. A ruptured filter allows red blood cells to cross the filter and enter the ultrafiltrate. At any sign of blood in the ultrafiltrate, the filter should be changed immediately.

20. Are certain precautions necessary to prevent hemorrhage?

Internal bleeding may be prevented by frequent monitoring of coagulation times and appropriate regulation of heparin. Bleeding from the CAVH circuit can be prevented by ensuring that all connections are securely Luerlocked. The access site and all tubing and connections should be kept uncovered and visible at all times.

21. Is it possible to remove less fluid from the patient?

It is possible to remove small volumes of fluid with the CAVH filter. This technique is referred to as slow continuous ultrafiltration (SCUF). Fluid removal is controlled by raising the drainage bag, thus decreasing the amount of hydrostatic pressure created by the height of the ultrafiltrate column on the filter. A C-clamp may be placed on the ultrafiltrate line to further reduce the amount of ultrafiltrate. This technique removes small volumes and will not provide any clearance of toxins. It may be used in conjunction with hemodialysis but it is not adequate alone as renal replacement therapy.

22. Will suction applied to the ultrafiltrate port provide greater volumes of ultrafiltrate?

Suction may be applied to the ultrafiltrate port on certain filters. In general, suction is not applied to plate filters because of increased risk of filter rupture. Each manufacturer has recommendations for suction but, in general, not more than 200 mm Hg of suction should be applied to the filter. A hazard to the application of suction to the system is loss of the patient's blood pressure as the primary determinant of ultrafiltration rate. If the patient has a hypotensive episode, the suction will continue to draw ultrafiltrate across the filter. Without suction, a hypotensive episode will reduce or eliminate the production of ultrafiltrate.

23. Is better clearance possible when a dialysate solution is added to the system?

Most filters allow the addition of a dialysate solution to the system. The dialysate enters the filter opposite the venous port on the filter and runs countercurrent to the blood flow. It runs across the filter and exits out the ultrafiltrate port. The dialysate provides an osmotic gradient, increasing clearance rates. Continuous arteriovenous hemodialysis (CAVHD) has been demonstrated to have creatinine clearance rates of 20 ml/min. The degree of clearance depends on the rate of dialysate through the filter. It has been demonstrated that a dialysate rate of approximately 1500 cc/hour provides adequate clearance rates. Dialysate solutions that are marketed for peritoneal dialysis are commonly used for CAVHD.

24. Is CAVH or CAVHD more cost-effective than hemodialysis?
No reliable cost analyses have been reported in the literature. However, a breakdown of all charges to an "average" patient on CAVHD for a 24-hour period is nearly equal to the charge for a single hemodialysis treatment. The major cost of CAVH and CAVHD is the large volume fluids used in this treatment.

25. Is CAVH associated with a higher survival rate?
Various mortality rates from uncontrolled studies are reported in the literature; however, the hemodynamically unstable, critically ill patient who typically is a CAVH candidate has a high mortality rate associated with the multisystem organ failure that is present. It is virtually impossible to determine if the institution of CAVH reduces mortality. However, CAVH has been demonstrated to be an effective renal replacement therapy for the critically ill patient who cannot tolerate hemodialysis.

BIBLIOGRAPHY

1. Baldamus CA, Quesshorst E: Outcome for longterm hemofiltration. Kidney Int 28(Suppl 17):S41–S46, 1985.
2. Bartlett RH, Mault JR, Dechert RE, et al: Continuous arteriovenous hemofiltration: Improved survival in surgical acute renal failure? Surgery 100:400–408, 1986.
3. Golper TA, Pullam J, Bennett WM: Removal of therapeutic drugs by CAVH. Arch Intern Med 145:1651–1652, 1985.
4. Kaplan AA, Longnecker RE, Folker VW: CAVH: A report of six months' experience. Ann Intern Med 100:358–367, 1984.
5. Kramer P, Bohler J, Kehr A, et al: Intensive care potential of CAVH. ASAIO Trans 28:28–32, 1982.
6. Kramer P, Kaufhold G, Grone HJ, et al: Management of anuric ICU patients with arteriovenous hemofiltration. Int J Artif Organs 3:225–230, 1980.
7. Kramer P, Wigger W, Rieger J, et al: Arteriovenous hemofiltration: A new and simple method for treatment of overhydrated patients resistant to diuretics. Klin Wochenshr 55:1121–1122, 1977.
8. Lauer A, Alvis R, Avram M: Hemodynamic consequences of CAVH. Am J Kidney Dis 12:110–115, 1988.
9. Lauer A, Scaggi A, Ronco C, et al: CAVH in the critically ill patient: Clinical use and operation characteristics. Ann Intern Med 99:455–460, 1983.
10. Mault JR, Dechert RE, Lees P, et al: CAVH: An effective treatment for surgical acute renal failure. Surgery 101:478–484, 1987.
11. Olbricht C, Muellen C, Schurek HJ, Stolte H: Treatment of acute renal failure by continuous spontaneous hemofiltration. ASAIO Trans 28:33–39, 1982.
12. Ossenkopple GJ, Muelen J, Bronsveld W, Thijs LG: CAVH as an adjunctive therapy for septic shock. Crit Care Med 13:102–104, 1985.
13. Oyama C, Levin N, Magilligan DJ: Pulmonary edema: Reversal by ultrafiltration. J Surg Res 36:191–197, 1984.
14. Paganini EP, Nakamoto S: Continuous slow ultrafiltration in oliguric acute renal failure. ASAIO Trans 26:201–204, 1980.
15. Paganini EP, Suhoza K, Swann S, et al: Continuous renal replacement therapy in patients with acute renal dysfunction undergoing intraaortic balloon pump and/or left ventricular device support. ASAIO trans 32:414–417, 1986.
16. Parillo JE (ed): Current Therapy in Critical Care Medicine, 2nd ed. Philadelphia, B.C. Decker, 1991.
17. Pattison ME, Lee SM, Ogden DA: CAVH: An aggressive approach to the management of acute renal failure. Am J Kid Dis 11:43–47, 1988.
18. Price CA: Continuous renal replacement therapy: The treatment of choice for acute renal failure. ANNA 18:239–244, 1991.

19. Stevens PE, Davies SP, Brown EA, et al: CAVHD in critically ill patients. Lancet, July 16, 1988, pp 150–152.
20. Voerman HJ, Strack von Schijndel RJ, Thijs LG: Continuous arterial-venous hemodiafiltration in critically ill patients. Crit Care Med 18:811–814, 1990.

50. RHABDOMYOLYSIS

Richard Hock, M.D.

1. What is rhabdomyolysis?

Rhabdomyolysis is a clinical and laboratory syndrome resulting from skeletal muscle injury with release of muscle cell contents into the plasma. It may be subtle or massive in presentation; however, muscle necrosis does not necessarily occur. In general, the following substances are released from muscle cells during rhabdomyolysis: creatine phosphokinase (CPK), creatinine, aldolase, lactate dehydrogenase (LDH), glutamine, serum glutamic oxaloacetic transaminase (SGOT), myoglobin, purines and electrolytes, primarily phosphorus and potassium.

2. What are the basic mechanisms in the pathophysiology of rhabdomyolysis?

The occurrence of rhabdomyolysis after exposure to a multitude of apparently unrelated substances or processes can be explained by several basic mechanisms. The predisposing cause may be multifactorial. Inadequate delivery of oxygen and nutrients, excessive energy use, metabolic poisons, potassium depletion, direct muscular toxins, and hypersensitivity reactions have all been implicated as basic mechanisms of muscle injury. On a molecular level, sarcolemmic sodium-potassium-adenosine triphosphate activity is impaired in damaged muscle, thus diminishing the extrusion of sodium from the sarcoplasm and interfering indirectly with the efflux of calcium and water from the cell. As the cytosolic free calcium level increases, activation of neutral proteases occurs, which disrupts myofibrils and induces muscle damage.

3. What is the most common etiologic factor in rhabdomyolysis?

There are more than 50 reported causes of rhabdomyolysis; however, alcohol use, compression injury, and seizures are the main causes, with over half of all cases of rhabdomyolysis having more than one factor identified. Since 1988, numerous case reports have implicated cocaine as a cause of rhabdomyolysis, with up to one-third of cases presenting in acute renal failure usually associated with hypotension, hyperpyrexia, and markedly elevated CPK levels (mean 28,000 units/L).

4. Can a uniform clinical presentation be anticipated in rhabdomyolysis?

The clinical presentation of rhabdomyolysis can be extremely varied. The classic presentation of myalgias, weakness, and dark urine occurs in the minority. Approximately 50% of patients with rhabdomyolysis do not have muscle pain on admission. However, limb swelling or tenderness that occurs after admission in the presence of intravenous fluid therapy may indicate a recent episode of rhabdomyolysis. Because toxins and drugs are the usual factors involved in rhabdomyolysis, other symptoms and findings may predominate, causing rhabdomyolysis to be overlooked.

5. Discuss the numerous laboratory abnormalities associated with rhabdomyolysis.

CPK activity is the most sensitive indicator of muscle damage and may continue to increase several days after admission. Hyperkalemia, hyperuricemia, and hyperphosphatemia occur from the release of cellular contents. Hypocalcemia can occur in up to two-thirds of cases and is generally attributed to the deposition of calcium salts in injured or necrotic muscle, possibly facilitated by the elevated phosphorus level. Both anion gap and nonanion gap metabolic acidosis have been described in rhabdomyolysis, with the former being generated by unidentified organic acid(s) released or produced. The urinalysis in rhabdomyolysis may show proteinuria and hematuria. The orthotoluidine dipstick for heme does not distinguish between myoglobin and hemoglobin. Furthermore, up to 20% of patients with rhabdomyolysis will have a negative dipstick for heme, suggesting there is no myoglobin in the urine.

6. How frequent is acute renal failure, and what are its risk factors for rhabdomyolysis?
The frequency of acute renal failure in rhabdomyolysis is not known and varies in the literature from 10–30%. To date there has not been a prospective trial to identify factors in nontraumatic rhabdomyolysis that may predispose to acute renal failure. In earlier studies by Gabow et al., measurable myoglobinuria and peak CPK level did not predict an increased risk of renal failure. Acute renal failure does develop in 100% of patients suffering from rhabdomyolysis resulting from traumatic crush syndrome if intravenous hydration is withheld the first 12 hours after presentation.

7. What are the mechanisms of nephrotoxicity in rhabdomyolysis?
They are not completely understood. The most commonly suggested theory based on animal studies is a direct nephrotoxic component of myoglobin named ferrihemate, which dissociates from myoglobin at or below pH 5.6. The other determinant of myoglobin toxicity in the kidney is the urine flow rate, with high flow rates rarely associated with renal dysfunction. Other possible mechanisms of renal damage are (1) alterations of renal blood flow by mechanisms that inhibit the vasodilating effect of endothelium-derived relaxation factor (EDRF) in the kidney; (2) tubular obstruction from precipitation of myoglobin, protein, and uric acid crystals; and (3) formation of thrombin in the glomeruli due to disseminated intravascular coagulation. Further evidence for decreased renal perfusion is also provided by the low fractional excretion of sodium (FENa) of less than 1% often seen in myoglobinuric acute renal failure during the oliguric phase.

8. Besides acute renal failure, what are other possible complications of rhabdomyolysis?
    1. As muscles swell in confined spaces, elevated fascial compartment pressures can occur with surprisingly little muscle necrosis, and may not be evident until several days after the initial insult, possibly brought on by aggressive intravenous fluid hydration. This "second-wave phenomenon" is characterized by a rebound elevation in falling CPK levels and other signs of compartment syndrome.
    2. Acute respiratory failure has been reported in rhabdomyolysis and, when primary, is generally associated with rhabdomyolysis of the diaphragm and intercostal muscles, which may make weaning from mechanical ventilation difficult.

9. What should be the initial treatment of rhabdomyolysis?
It is the same as for any serious illness: ensuring an adequate airway, ventilation, and perfusion as well as addressing the underlying process. Excessive exertion from fighting restraints, seizures, or abnormal posturing should be controlled with sedatives or anticonvulsants. If an agitated, combative state persists, one may need to consider mechanical ventilation and pharmacologic paralysis with a nondepolarizing neuromuscular blocking agent. For the patient with hyperthermia, controlling excessive muscular activity is essential, followed by passive cooling techniques. Hypotension, hypoxemia, hypokalemia, and hypophosphatemia should be reversed, because these factors will contribute to ongoing rhabdomyolysis.

10. Should hypocalcemia be treated in rhabdomyolysis?

Although hypocalcemia is common in rhabdomyolysis, even severe hypocalcemia rarely causes symptoms. Treatment of asymptomatic hypocalcemia is discouraged since it may potentially increase deposition of calcium in damaged muscle and further augment rhabdomyolysis.

CONTROVERSY

11. How should acute renal failure be prevented in rhabdomyolysis? Construct a treatment plan.

There is no consensus about how to predict which patients with rhabdomyolysis will proceed to acute renal failure. Substantial animal data suggest that myoglobinuric renal failure is prevented if good urine output is maintained and extremes of aciduria are prevented. Thus, as a direct result of animal studies, coupled with the predominance of acute renal failure in traumatic crush syndrome if timely intravenous hydration is not initiated, it has become standard to treat rhabdomyolysis aggressively with intravenous hydration to maintain a urine output generally greater than 150 cc/hr. In the surgical literature that addresses the crush syndrome, it is now recommended to begin early normal saline intravascular repletion followed by forced mannitol-alkaline diuresis, maintaining urine output greater than 300 cc/hr and urinary pH greater than 6.5 until no evidence of myoglobinuria is present. Loop diuretics are avoided because of the potential disadvantage of acidifying the urine and causing myoglobin precipitation; however, acetazolamide may be used if arterial pH is greater than 7.5, because this agent will correct metabolic alkalosis and increase urinary pH. Despite impressive animal studies, there is still no controlled, prospective trial in humans with nontraumatic rhabdomyolysis to determine whether these interventions are of value in preventing acute renal failure. The key factors are that maintaining good urine flow will prevent acute renal failure in rhabdomyolysis and that mannitol is superior to both normal saline and bicarbonate therapy in achieving this goal.

A possible treatment plan in rhabdomyolysis to help prevent acute renal failure is offered below:

1. Check urinary pH and dipstick for presence of myoglobin (orthotoluidine positive in the absence of red blood cells).

2. If intravascularly volume-deficient, begin normal saline hydration.

3. Once euvolemia is achieved, if myoglobinuria is still present, give 0.5 gm/kg of mannitol to achieve a urine output greater than 150 cc/hr.

4. If severe systemic acidemia and/or aciduria is present, consider giving bicarbonate therapy until urinary pH is greater than 6.5. If metabolic alkalemia results, a dose of acetazolamide can be used (except in the setting of salicylate intoxication).

5. If bicarbonate is used, follow serum electrolytes and calcium every 4–6 hours.

6. In the setting of pulmonary edema, use furosemide instead of mannitol to maintain urinary flow rate.

7. If evidence of compartment syndrome develops and/or if CPK levels continue to rise, search for underlying disease process and strongly consider the addition of mannitol.

BIBLIOGRAPHY

1. Better O, Stein J: Early management of shock and prophylaxis of acute renal failure in traumatic rhabdomyolysis. N Engl J Med 322:825–829, 1990.
2. Corwin H, Schreiber M, Fang L: Low fractional excretion of sodium: Occurrence with hemoglobinuric and myoglobinuric-induced acute renal failure. Arch Intern Med 144:981–982, 1984.

3. Curry SC, Chang D, Connor D: Drug and toxin induced rhabdomyolysis. Ann Emerg Med 18: 1068–1082, 1989.
4. Eneas J, Schoenfeld P, Humphreys M: The effects of infusion of mannitol-sodium bicarbonate on the clinical course of myoglobinuria. Arch Intern Med 139:801–805, 1979.
5. Gabow P, Kaehny W, Kelleher S: The spectrum of rhabdomyolysis. Medicine 61:141–152, 1982.
6. Grossman R, Hamilton R, Morse B, et al: Nontraumatic rhabdomyolysis and acute renal failure. N Engl J Med 291:807–817, 1974.
7. Knochel J: Rhabdomyolysis and myoglobinuria. Semin Nephrol 1:75–86, 1981.
8. Koffler A, Fridler R, Massry S. Acute renal failure due to nontraumatic rhabdomyolysis. Ann Intern Med 85:23–28, 1976.
9. Llach F, Felsenfeld A, Hawssler M. The pathophysiology of altered calcium metabolism in rhabdomyolysis-induced acute renal failure. N Engl J Med 305:117–123, 1981.
10. Morris C, Alexander E, Bruns F, Levinsky N. Restoration and maintenance of glomerular filtration by mannitol during hypoperfusion of the kidney. J Clin Invest 51:155, 1972.
11. Ron D: Prevention of acute renal failure in traumatic rhabdomyolysis. Arch Intern Med 144:277–280, 1984.
12. Roth D: Acute rhabdomyolysis associated with cocaine intoxication. N Engl J Med 319:637–677, 1988.
13. Ward M: Factors predictive of acute renal failure in rhabdomyolysis. Arch Intern Med 148:1553–1557, 1988.
14. Wynne JW, Goslen JB, Ballinger WE, et al: Rhabdomyolysis with cardiac and respiratory involvement. South Med J 70:1125–1128, 1977.
15. Zager R: Studies of mechanisms and protective maneuvers in myoglobinuric acute renal injury. Lab Invest 60:619–629, 1989.

51. HYPOKALEMIA AND HYPERKALEMIA

Alan S. Hanson, M.D., and Stuart Linas, M.D.

1. Why is tight regulation of serum potassium (K) critical?

Because only about 65 mEq of the body's total 3400 mEq of K is extracellular, changes in extracellular fluid (ECF) K, either by compartmental shifts or by net gain or loss, will significantly alter the ratio of extracellular to intracellular K. Because this ratio determines the resting membrane potential, small changes in ECF K can profoundly affect neuro-muscular excitability.

2. What are the manifestations of hypokalemia?

By depressing neuromuscular excitability, hypokalemia leads to muscle weakness, with quadriplegia, hypoventilation, adynamic ileus, and orthostatic hypotension. Severe hypokalemia disrupts cell integrity, leading to rhabdomyolysis. Renal effects include the stimulation of renal ammonia production, which can promote encephalopathy in patients with advanced liver disease. Among the most critical are the cardiac consequences, including atrial and ventricular arrhythmias. The EKG shows S-T segment depression and flattened T waves, which makes for prominent U-waves, such that the Q-T interval appears prolonged.

3. What are the causes of K deficiency?

(1) **Poor intake** is a common cause in elderly, alcoholic, and anorexic patients. (2) **Gastro-intestinal (GI) losses** can be due to either diarrhea, which is rich in K (including cases of villous adenoma and laxative abuse), or to vomiting or nasogastric suction. As gastric fluid K is only 5–10 mEq/L, the major loss in the latter case is via renal K wasting due to

bicarbonaturia from the ensuing metabolic alkalosis. (3) **Renal K loss** can be due to mineralocorticoid excess (e.g., hyperaldosteronism, Cushing's syndrome, or ACTH-producing tumor) or to conditions that secondarily elevate aldosterone (e.g, cirrhosis, congestive heart failure, and nephrotic syndrome), in which K deficiency is usually promoted by diuretics. Bartter's syndrome is a rare cause seen mostly in children. Hyperglycemia leads to K loss by osmotic diuresis. The most common cause of renal K loss is use of diuretics.

4. When does serum K falsely estimate body K?

Intracellular/extracellular K shifting has a profound effect on serum K values. The reciprocal movement of K and H across the cell membrane results in a rise in serum K of approximately 0.6 mEq/L for every drop in pH of 0.1 unit in the case of acidemia, and a fall in serum K of 0.1–0.4 mEq/L for every rise in pH of 0.1 unit in the case of alkalemia. Hormones that drive K into cells include insulin and catecholamines. An example of the importance of acid-base balance and insulin in K homeostasis is in diabetes with ketoacidosis. In this situation, the administration of insulin moves K into cells by both direct and indirect means (correction of acidosis).

5. How can the K deficit be estimated?

It is not possible to predict accurately the total body K deficit based on serum values, but a useful rough estimate can be made as follows: for a 70-kg patient, K = 3 mEq/L implies a 100–200 mEq deficit, and K = 2 mEq/L implies a 300–600 mEq deficit. In patients with acid-base disorders, one must first account for compartmental K shifting, as discussed above, before estimating K replacement.

6. How is hypokalemia treated?

In most cases, potassium chloride (KCl) is used. In metabolic acidosis, replacement with K bicarbonate or equivalent (e.g., K citrate, acetate, or gluconate) is recommended to help alleviate the acidosis. Alcoholics and diabetics out of control often have phosphate deficiency and should receive some of the potassium as K phosphate. Oral replacement is the safest route, and administration of doses of up to 40 mEq multiple times daily is allowed. Delayed-release formulations tend to reduce the GI upset seen with the higher doses.

7. When is intravenous replacement necessary? What are the risks?

When oral administration is not possible, as when the GI tract is nonfunctional, or in life-threatening situations such as severe weakness, respiratory distress, cardiac arrhythmias, or rhabdomyolysis, K must be replaced intravenously. Infusion rates must normally be limited to 10 mEq/hr to prevent the potentially catastrophic effect of a K bolus to the heart. In extreme situations, under cardiac monitoring and frequent serum level checks, infusion rates of up to 30 mEq/hr can be used (see also Controversy below).

8. In what other circumstances is special care in replacement necessary?

- K-depleted patients who are also on digitalis therapy (especially overdose) are prone to serious arrhythmias and must be treated urgently.
- K overload rarely occurs during replacement *except* in the following circumstances: renal failure, use of K-sparing diuretics (spironolactone, amiloride, triamterene), and possibly use of angiotensin-converting enzyme (ACE) inhibitors.
- Significant magnesium deficiency causes renal K wasting and often must be corrected before therapy for hypokalemia can be effective.

9. What is pseudohyperkalemia? What are its causes?

In certain situations, an elevated serum K does not reflect hyperkalemia. Significant K can or from platelets when the platelet count exceeds 1,000,000 mm^3. In these circumstances, a plasma K determination should be obtained. A tight tourniquet, combined with opening and closing of the hand, can artifactually elevate K by as much as 2.7 mEq/L.

10. What are the clinical manifestations of hyperkalemia?

Hyperkalemia results in heart block and asystole. Initially the EKG will show peaked T waves, followed by decreasing amplitude of R waves, prolonged P-R interval, and progressive widening of the QRS complex, until QRS and T blend into a sine-wave pattern. Because cardiac arrest can occur at any point in this progression, hyperkalemia with EKG changes constitutes a medical emergency. Other effects of hyperkalemia include weakness and neuromuscular paralysis (without CNS disturbances) and suppression of renal ammoniagenesis, which may result in a metabolic acidosis.

11. What are the causes of hyperkalemia?

1. **Cellular shifts:** Redistribution of even small amounts out of the large intracellular pool can significantly raise serum K. Causes include acidosis, hyperosmotic state, and insulin deficiency. Certain drugs may contribute, including beta blockers and digitalis.

2. **Increased endogenous K** release due to tumor lysis, rhabdomyolysis, brisk hemolysis, or heavily catabolic states such as severe sepsis may raise serum K, particularly in the setting of renal failure.

3. **Increased exogenous K** sources include oral K replacement, K-rich foods, TPN, salt substitutes, and high-dose K penicillin.

4. **Decreased renal K excretion** is the leading cause, as 90% of K intake is renally excreted under normal circumstances. Despite this, only late in the course of chronic renal failure (GFR < 10 ml/min) is the renal failure the *sole* cause of hyperkalemia. Primary defects in K excretion out of proportion to decrement in GFR are seen in certain diseases: systemic lupus erythematosus, sickle cell disease, obstructive uropathy, and postrenal transplantation. Drugs that impair K excretion include K-sparing diuretics, ACE inhibitors, nonsteroidal drugs, and heparin (the latter by suppression of aldosterone synthesis and secretion). Finally, hypoaldosteronism reduces K excretion, and, in addition to Addison's disease, this includes renal diseases associated with impaired renin production such as diabetes mellitus and chronic interstitial nephritis.

12. What is the treatment of hyperkalemia?

The presence of serum K > 6.5 or of EKG changes or severe weakness mandates emergent therapy. The general approach is to use therapy from each of the following three categories for definitive treatment.

1. **Membrane stabilization:** Calcium raises the cell depolarization threshold and reduces myocardial irritability. One or two ampules of IV calcium chloride results in improvement in EKG changes within seconds, but because K levels are not altered, the beneficial effect lasts only about 30 minutes.

2. **Shift K into cells:** IV insulin (e.g., 10-unit bolus of regular), with glucose administration if necessary to prevent hypoglycemia, begins lowering serum K in about 2–5 minutes and lasts a few hours. Correction of acidosis with IV sodium bicarbonate (e.g., 2 ampules) has a similar duration and time of onset.

3. **Removal of K:** Loop diuretics can sometimes cause enough renal K loss in patients with intact renal function, but usually a GI K-binding resin must be used (e.g., Kayexalate, 30 gm PO or 50 gm by retention enema). The resin is given with a cathartic to remove the K from the gut and prevent development of a solid mass in the bowel. Note that as K is drawn into the gut lumen, sodium is absorbed, giving the patient a net volume load. Acute hemodialysis is effective at K removal and must be used when the GI tract is nonfunctional or when serious fluid overload is already present.

CONTROVERSY

13. Should intravenous K be administered via central venous catheter?

For:

1. K infused via peripheral vein can cause local pain and may result in phlebitis, particularly if the concentration exceeds 40 mEq/L.

2. Extravasation peripherally can result in skin necrosis.

3. Central administration rates of 10–20 mEq/hr have rarely been associated with problems.

Against:

High intracardiac K concentrations can result from direct right atrial K infusion, causing increased danger of arrhythmias.

BIBLIOGRAPHY

1. Androgue HJ, Madias NE: Changes in plasma potassium concentration during acute acid-base disturbances. Am J Med 71:456, 1981.
2. Beigelman PM: Potassium in severe diabetic ketoacidosis. Am J Med 54:419, 1973.
3. Bia MJ, DeFronzo RT: Extrarenal potassium homeostasis. Am J Physiol 240:F257, 1981.
4. DeFronzo RA, Bia MJ, Smith D: Clinical disorders of hyperkalemia. Annu Rev Med 33:521, 1982.
5. Fisch C: Relation of electrolyte disturbances to cardiac arrhythmias. Circulation 47:408, 1973.
6. Gabow PA, Peterson LM: Disorders of potassium metabolism. In Schrier RW (ed): Renal and Electrolyte Disorders, 3rd ed. Boston, Little, Brown, 1986, pp 207–249.
7. Kassirer JP, Harrington JT: Diuretics and potassium metabolism: A reassessment of the need, effectiveness and safety of potassium therapy. Kidney Int 11:505, 1977.
8. Linas SL, Berl T: Clinical diagnosis of abnormal potassium balance. In Seldin DW, Giebisch G (eds): The Regulation of Potassium Balance. New York, Raven Press, 1989.
9. Patrick J: Assessment of body potassium stones. Kidney Int 11:476, 1977.
10. Sterns RH, Cox M, Feig PU: Internal potassium balance and the control of the plasma potassium concentration. Medicine 60:339, 1981.
11. Tannen RL: Relationship of renal ammonia production and potassium homeostasis. Kidney Int 11:453, 1977.

52. HYPONATREMIA AND HYPERNATREMIA

Stuart Senkfor, M.D., and Tomas Berl, M.D.

1. Why is sodium homeostasis critical to volume control and osmolar stability?

Sodium and its corresponding anion represent almost all the osmotically active solutes in the extracellular fluid. As such, its serum concentration closely reflects the tonicity of body fluids. In fact, serum osmolality can be closely calculated by $2 \times [Na^+] + 10$ under normal circumstances (see question #16, formula 1, for pathophysiologic conditions). Slight changes in tonicity are counteracted by thirst regulation, antidiuretic hormone (vasopressin) secretion, and renal concentrating or diluting mechanisms. This preservation of normal osmolality (290 mOsm/L) guarantees cellular integrity by regulating net movement of water across cellular membranes. Abnormalities in sodium concentration primarily reflect changes in total body water. In contrast, alterations in total body sodium cause derangements in extracellular fluid volume. A decrease in total body sodium is associated with hypovolemia, whereas an increment in total body sodium is associated with hypervolemia.

2. Does hyponatremia simply represent a low sodium state?

No. Hyponatremia is defined as a serum sodium concentration of less than 135 mEq/L. However, serum sodium concentration tells very little about total body sodium or volume status. Hyponatremia can occur in low total body sodium (hypovolemic), normal total body sodium (euvolemic), and excess total body sodium (hypervolemic) states. Physical examination will be the major source of volume assessment. Helpful findings include tachycardia, dry mucous membranes, orthostatic hypotension (hypovolemia), edema, extra heart sound (S_3), jugular venous distention, and ascites (hypervolemia).

3. How can hyponatremia develop in a hypovolemic patient?

Hypovolemic hyponatremia represents a decrease in total body sodium in excess of a decrease in total body water. Sodium and water loss can be due to renal and extrarenal sources. For example, renal losses can be due to glycosuria, diuretic use, mineralocorticoid deficiency, and intrinsic renal disease. Extrarenal losses include vomiting, diarrhea, excessive sweating, burns, and third spacing. Hypovolemia leads to hyponatremia by limiting the kidney's ability to excrete water. This happens by both renal and extrarenal mechanisms. Hypovolemia results in a decrease in renal perfusion, a decrement in glomerular filtration rate (GFR), and an increase in proximal tubule reabsorption, all serving to limit water excretion. More important is the effect of hypovolemia to supersede the expected inhibition of vasopressin release by hypotonicity and thereby maintain the secretion of the hormone by a nonosmotic pathway. This limits renal diluting ability, and any water taken in is retained, culminating in hyponatremia. Therefore, hypovolemia results in antidiuretic hormone secretion, decreased renal perfusion, decreased GFR, increased proximal tubular sodium reabsorption, and maximum water reabsorption. The latter occurs despite the presence of hypotonicity due to nonosmotic release of antidiuretic hormone.

4. How does hypervolemic hyponatremia differ from hypovolemic hyponatremia?

Once again, the kidneys are at the center of the problem, due either to intrinsic renal disease or renal compensation secondary to an extrarenal abnormality. Physical examination will reveal edema and no evidence of volume depletion. Intrinsic renal disease with markedly decreased GFR (acute or chronic) prevents the adequate excretion of sodium and water. Intake of sodium in excess of what can be excreted leads to hypervolemia (edema); excessive intake of water leads to hyponatremia. Homeostasis is lost and volume overload (edema), hyponatremia, and edema develop. In contrast, congestive heart failure, hepatic cirrhosis, and nephrotic syndrome limit the ability of an intrinsically normal kidney to excrete excess sodium and water.

5. Is euvolemic hyponatremia, then, due only to an increase in total body water?

Although there may be a slight decrement in total body sodium, the hyponatremia is primarily due to an increase in total body water as a consequence of nonosmolar release of antidiuretic hormone or production of an antidiuretic-hormone-like substance by tumors. The syndrome of inappropriate antidiuretic hormone secretion is a common cause of euvolemic hyponatremia and is associated with malignancies, pulmonary disease, central nervous system disorders, and drugs. The latter category includes hypoglycemic agents, psychotropics, narcotics, and chemotherapeutic agents. Other causes of euvolemic hyponatremia include psychogenic polydipsia, hypothyroidism, adrenal insufficiency, pain, surgery, and anesthesia.

6. Can hyponatremia occur without a change in total body sodium or total body water?

It can occur in two settings. The first is designated as pseudohyponatremia, which is only a laboratory abnormality in patients with severe hyperlipidemia or hyperproteinemia, as these substances occupy an increasingly large volume in which the sodium determination is made. Serum sodium is low in these pathologic states when using a flame photometry method, but normal when using an ion-specific electrode. The second setting occurs when large quantities of osmotically active substances (such as glucose or mannitol) cause hyponatremia but not hypotonicity. In such states, water is drawn out of cells to extracellular space, diluting the plasma solute and equilibrating osmolar differences. Serum sodium will decrease approximately 1.6–1.8 mEq/L for every increase of 100 mg/dl over normal glucose levels. In view of this, the serum sodium should not be interpreted without an accompanying serum glucose and the appropriate correction made if the glucose exceeds 200 mg/dl.

7. Is there a difference between acute and chronic hyponatremia?
Yes, acute hyponatremia is a distinct entity in terms of morbidity and mortality as well as treatment strategies. Acute hyponatremia most commonly occurs in the hospital (as in the postoperative setting), in psychogenic polydipsia, and in elderly women on thiazide diuretics. Chronic hyponatremia is defined as having a duration greater than 48 hours. The great majority of patients who present to physicians or to emergency rooms with hyponatremia should be assumed to have chronic hyponatremia.

8. What are the signs and symptoms of hyponatremia?
Hyponatremia is the most common electrolyte disorder, with a prevalence of about 2.5% in hospitalized patients. Although the majority of patients are asymptomatic, symptoms do develop in patients with a serum sodium of less than 125 mEq/L or in whom the sodium has decreased rapidly. Gastrointestinal complaints of nausea, vomiting, and anorexia occur early, but neuropsychiatric complaints such as lethargy, confusion, agitation, psychosis, seizure, and coma are more common. Clinical symptoms roughly correlate with the amount and rate of decrease in serum sodium.

9. Is there a standard therapy for hyponatremia?
Although controversy exists regarding treatment strategies, there is a consensus that not all hyponatremias are alike. Two major facts that should direct therapy are duration (acute versus chronic) and the presence or absence of neurologic symptoms.

    The dilemma of therapy involves balancing symptoms of cerebral edema versus the treatment risks of a demyelinating syndrome. In patients with acute symptomatic hyponatremia, the risk of delaying treatment and allowing the consequences of cerebral edema to culminate in a seizure and respiratory arrest clearly outweighs any risk of treatment. Hypertonic saline and furosemide (which promotes free water excretion) should be given until symptoms subside. In contrast, the asymptomatic chronic hyponatremia patient in high-risk categories (alcoholism, malnutrition, and liver disease) is at greatest risk for complications of the correction of hyponatremia, namely central pontine myelinolysis. Such patients are best treated with water restriction.

10. What are some helpful guidelines for treatment of hyponatremia?
Both delay of therapy and overly aggressive therapy, especially in high-risk patients (alcoholism, malnutrition, liver disease), place patients at greater risk for treatment complications. Reasonable guidelines include a rate of sodium increase of less than 2 mEq/L/hr, with a maximum increase of 20 mEq/L/day, not to exceed a final goal of 130 mEq/L. In moderately symptomatic patients, this can be accomplished with hypertonic saline, furosemide diuresis, and hourly sodium monitoring.

    In chronic asymptomatic patients, simple free water restriction (i.e., 1000 cc/day) will allow a slow and relatively safe correction of serum sodium. However, this requires patient cooperation, which may be difficult to obtain from outpatients. In selected patients, who are resistant to free water restriction, an antidiuretic hormone antagonist (demeclocycline, 600–1,200 mg/day), or increased urinary solute excretion may be necessary.

The most difficult therapeutic dilemma is posed by patients who have cerebral symptoms and have hyponatremia of unknown duration. Such patients are also at risk of a demyelinating disorder if treated too aggressively, yet the presence of symptoms is reflective of central nervous system dysfunction. These patients should be treated with careful (hourly) monitoring of serum sodium, as hypertonic saline and lasix are given. The rate of increase should not exceed 2 mEq/L/hr and the total increment should not exceed 20 mEq/24 hr, no matter how low the initial sodium.

11. What is central pontine myelinolysis?

Central pontine myelinolysis is a rare neurologic disorder of unclear etiology characterized by symmetric midline demyelination of the central basis pontis. Extrapontine lesions can occur in the basal ganglia, internal capsule, lateral geniculate body, and cortex. Symptoms include motor abnormalities that can progress to flaccid quadriplegia, respiratory paralysis, pseudobulbar palsy, mental status changes, and coma. Central pontine myelinolysis is frequently fatal in 3–5 weeks, but survival with residual deficit is increasingly observed. Magnetic resonance imaging and, to a lesser extent, CT scanning can be used to document the alterations in white matter. Although central pontine myelinolysis can occur in patients without a history of hyponatremia, it is one of the major concerns as a complication of therapy. Risk factors include a change in serum sodium of greater than 20–25 mEq/L in 24 hours, correction of serum sodium to normal or hypernatremic range, symptomatic and coexistent alcoholism, malnutrition, and liver disease.

12. Can hypernatremia also occur in hypovolemic, euvolemic, and hypervolemic states?

Yes, and these categories, based on physical examination, provide a useful framework for understanding and treating patients. Hypovolemic hypernatremia tends to occur in the very young and the very old. It is typically due to extracellular fluid losses and the inability to intake adequate amounts of free water. Febrile illnesses, vomiting, diarrhea, and renal losses are common etiologies.

Euvolemic hypernatremia can also be due to extracellular loss of fluid without adequate access to water or from loss of control of water hemostasis. Diabetes insipidus, either central (inadequate antidiuretic hormone secretion) or nephrogenic (renal insensitivity to antidiuretic hormone), results in the inability to reabsorb filtered water, resulting in systemic hypertonicity but a hypo-osmolar urine.

Hypervolemic hypernatremia, although uncommon, is iatrogenic. For example, sodium bicarbonate injection during cardiac arrest, administration of hypertonic saline, saline abortions, and inappropriately prepared infant formulas are several examples of induced hypernatremia.

13. What are the causes of diabetes insipidus?

Central diabetes insipidus can result from trauma, tumors, strokes, granulomatous disease, and central nervous system infections, but it commonly follows neurosurgical procedures. Nephrogenic diabetes insipidus can occur in acute or chronic renal failure, hypercalcemia, hypokalemia, and sickle cell disease, or it may be drug related (lithium, demeclocycline, and loop diuretics).

14. What are the signs and symptoms of hypernatremia?

In awake and alert patients, thirst is a prominent symptom. Anorexia, nausea, vomiting, altered mental status, agitation, irritability, lethargy, stupor, coma, and neuromuscular hyperactivity are common.

15. What is the best therapy for hypernatremia?

The first priority is circulatory stabilization with normal saline in patients with significant volume depletion. Once hypotension has been corrected, patients can be rehydrated with oral water, intravenous D5W, or even one half normal saline. Water deficit can be calculated (see question 16) and can be corrected at a rate no greater than 2 mEq/L/hr and over 48 hours. In patients with central diabetes insipidus, a synthetic analogue of antidiuretic hormone, namely DDAVP, can be administered, preferably by intranasal route.

16. What are some helpful formulas for assessing sodium abnormalities?

Serum osmolality = $2[Na^+]$ + glucose/18 + BUN/2.8 + ethyl alcohol/4.6

Total body water (TBW) = body weight × 0.6

TBW excess in hyponatremia = TBW $(1 - [$serum $Na^+]/140)$

TBW deficit in hypernatremia = TBW (serum $[Na^+]/140 - 1)$

BIBLIOGRAPHY

1. Anderson RJ: Hospital-associated hyponatremia. Kidney Int 29:1237–1247, 1986.
2. Arieff AI: Hyponatremia associated with permanent brain damage. Adv Intern Med 32:325–344, 1987.
3. Arieff AI: Osmotic failure: Physiology and strategies for treatment. Hosp Pract May 15, 1988, pp 173–194.
4. Ashraf N, et al: Thiazide-induced hyponatremia associated with death or neurologic damage in outpatients. Am J Med 70:1163–1168, 1981.
5. Ayus CJ, et al: Treatment of symptomatic hyponatremia and its relationship to brain damage. N Engl J Med 317:1190–1195, 1987.
5. Berl T: Treating hyponatremia: Damned if we do and damned if we don't. Kidney Int 37:1006–1018, 1990.
7. Brass EP, Thompson WL: Drug-induced electrolyte abnormalities. Drugs 24:207–228, 1982.
8. Clifford B: Hyponatremia and the brain. Am Fam Phys 38:119–124, 1988.
9. Narins RG, Riley L: Polyuria: Simple and mixed disorders. Am J Kidney Dis 17:237–241, 1991.
10. Votey R, et al: Disorders of water metabolism: Hyponatremia and hypernatremia. Emerg Med Clin North Am 7:749–769, 1989.

VII: Gastroenterology

53. ACUTE UPPER GASTROINTESTINAL TRACT HEMORRHAGE

John Schaefer, M.D.

1. What is the initial evaluation for upper gastrointestinal (UGI) hemorrhage?
A brief description of the bleeding episode includes information about hematemesis, melena, bloody stool, weakness, and syncope. Additional useful information is previous bleeding episodes, recent dyspepsia, retching, and use of nonsteroidal anti-inflammatory drugs (NSAIDs) or alcohol. Known concomitant illness and medication should be noted. A survey physical examination should note mental status, vital signs with postural changes, cardiac and pulmonary functions, and signs of hepatic disease or bleeding diathesis. A rectal examination should evaluate the presence of melena, red blood, and stool for occult blood.

2. What are the first steps in management?
Start crystalloid infusion by at least one large-bore intravenous (IV) access. Place a gastric tube of sufficient size to aspirate blood clots (size 24 Fr via nose or 34 Fr via mouth). Send blood for initial chemistries, clotting parameters, counts, and cross match. Expedite admission to the hospital.

3. Who best manages the patient?
Until bleeding stops, the patient is best managed by a combined and coordinated medical-surgical team in an intensive care unit.

4. How should the patient be monitored?
A flow chart should clearly indicate serial vital signs in response to the type and amount of IV fluids and blood products administered. All accumulated blood should be cleared from the stomach by copious gastric lavage. Continued or recurrent bleeding can then be documented by appearance of fresh blood on frequently repeated lavage. Periodic hematocrit values should be noted.

5. What is the value of gastric lavage?
The return of blood confirms a UGI source of hemorrhage. Any therapeutic benefit from gastric lavage is unproved. Properly irrigated, however, the tube offers the best on-line monitor for continued or recurrent hemorrhage and clears the stomach in preparation for early diagnostic endoscopy, radiography, or emergency surgery.

6. When should the patient receive blood transfusions?
Almost all patients presenting in clinical shock (with a blood pressure < 90 mm Hg) will need blood transfusions. Blood should also be given if vital signs remain unstable despite crystalloid infusion or if the hematocrit can be predicted to fall below 30% while bleeding continues. A sufficient number of transfusions should be given so that when bleeding stops, the final, stabilized hematocrit should be no lower than the 27–30% range for most patients.

7. How can cessation of hemorrhage be determined?

It is often difficult to tell exactly when bleeding stops or recurs. Frequent gastric irrigation that remains free of fresh blood is the best early sign of cessation of UGI bleeding. The additional observation of bile-stained gastric returns is also useful in excluding the duodenum as the site of ongoing bleeding. A restful-appearing patient with both stable vital signs and an appropriate elevation of hematocrit in response to blood transfusions is a helpful sign.

8. How can the amount of acute blood loss be clinically assessed?

There may be no detectable cardiovascular changes with acute blood loss up to 500 ml. With blood loss approaching 1,000 ml, patients usually exhibit resting tachycardia, significant postural fall in systolic blood pressure with increased heart rate, and delayed capillary refill, and they are often anxious and somewhat irritable. All findings may clear with IV infusion of crystalloid solution. When acute blood loss exceeds 2,000 ml, patients are in clinical shock and have systolic blood pressure below 90 mm Hg. They appear pale, sweaty, and often mentally confused and will require blood transfusions for stabilization.

In general, stool may become positive for chemical detection of blood with as little as 20 ml upper tract bleeding, melenic in nature with 200 ml or more, and frankly bloody with 1,000 ml or more blood loss.

9. How can serial hematocrit determinations be of value?

The hematocrit level must be interpreted in light of the known time lag for blood volume reconstitution. With acute blood loss and normal hydration, it takes up to 8 hours for one half of the final hematocrit drop to occur and up to 72 hours for final equilibration. With IV fluid administration, these times are shortened. Generally, the hematocrit level rises approximately 3% per unit of blood given in a stable patient.

10. What is the best diagnostic approach for determining sources of hemorrhage?

After a patient has stabilized and acute hemorrhage has stopped as evidenced by gastric aspirate free of blood or only blood tinged, then upper endoscopy provides the most accurate diagnosis. Endoscopy is particularly indicated in high-risk older patients (>60 years), those with suspected liver disease (variceal origin), and those taking mucosal barrier breakers (NSAIDs or alcohol). A young patient with new onset of typical peptic symptoms and a mild bleed could be evaluated with a UGI x-ray examination. The radiologic accuracy for diagnosis of duodenal ulcer, however, is significantly reduced in patients with recurrent ulcer, because the duodenal bulb is often deformed and scarred.

11. What is the short-term prognosis for patients with UGI tract hemorrhage?

Approximately 85% of all acute UGI tract hemorrhage stops spontaneously. Of these, about 75% stop within the first 24 hours, and most within the first few hours of hospitalization. Virtually all patients who stop bleeding without intervention have done so before 48 hours of hospitalization. The overall 10% mortality rate has not changed much in the past three or four decades. This, however, must be viewed in light of the fact that recent series include a higher percentage of older patients with more complex medical problems. Compared with elective surgery, patients requiring emergency surgery have a threefold to fivefold increased mortality rate, especially patients over 60 years of age. The worst prognosis, about 60% mortality, occurs among patients with decompensated liver disease and variceal hemorrhage. Another high-risk category is nonvariceal hemorrhage in patients over age 60 with unstable vital signs, copious fresh blood on gastric aspiration, and bloody stools. These findings, "red from above and red from below," are indicative of a massive ongoing hemorrhage with high mortality.

12. When should emergency surgery be considered?

Multiple factors must be considered, and decisions for each patient must be individualized by combined medical-surgical consultation. Emergency surgery should be considered for patients meeting any of the following criteria.

1. After 5 units of blood in first 24 hours and still bleeding.
2. After 3 units of blood between 24 and 48 hours in hospital and still bleeding.
3. Need for blood transfusion to maintain stability or hematocrit level after 48 hours in hospital.
4. Clinically significant rebleed after 24 hours or more of treatment after cessation of initial bleeding episode.
5. Additional influential factors:
   - Earlier surgery for patients over age 60
   - Point source bleeding (peptic ulcer, Mallory-Weiss tear) makes for a better surgical candidate than one with gastritis or variceal bleed
   - Blood type and units available
   - Associated illness

13. Aside from surgery, what interventional therapy is available?

The role of endoscopic intervention is currently evolving. Esophageal variceal sclerosis and, more recently, variceal banding are effective means of controlling variceal hemorrhage. Many see these as the best initial and even definitive forms of therapy. Others prefer sclerosis as a temporizing procedure in high-surgical-risk patients, followed by elective portal decompression or a selective shunting procedure when and if the operative risk improves. Control of variceal hemorrhage by Sengstaken-Blakemore tube compression together with intravenous vasopressin therapy is also an acceptable form of therapy, but because it does not address the underlying pathogenesis of variceal bleeding, early recurrence of hemorrhage is common. Electrocoagulation and laser therapy for arterial bleeding with peptic ulcers have their advocates as well. Local injection of the ulcer bed with absolute alcohol or vasoconstrictive agents has also been successful in stopping arterial hemorrhage. All of these attempts at endoscopic control of UGI tract hemorrhage depend on the enthusiasm and expertise available at a given institution.

BIBLIOGRAPHY

1. Bornrman PC, Theodorou NA, Shuttleworth RD, et al: Importance of hypovolemic shock and endoscopic signs predicting recurrent hemorrhage from peptic ulceration. Br Med J 291:245, 1985.
2. Fleisher D: Etiology and prevalence of severe persistent upper gastrointestinal bleeding. Gastroenterology 84:538, 1983.
3. Johnson JH, Sones JQ, Long BW, Posey EL: Comparison of heater probe and YAG laser in endoscopic treatment of major bleeding from peptic ulcers. Gastrointest Endosc 31:175, 1983.
4. Morris DL, Hawker PC, Brearley S, et al: Optimal timing of operation for bleeding peptic ulcer. Prospective randomized trial. Br Med J 288:1277, 1984.
5. Paquet KJ, Feussner H: Endoscopic sclerosis and esophageal balloon tamponade in acute variceal hemorrhage from esophagastric varices: A prospective controlled trial. Hepatology 4:580, 1984.
6. Silverstein FE, Gilbert DA, Tedesco FD, et al: The National ASGE survey on upper gastrointestinal bleeding. II. Clinical prognostic factors. Gastrointest Endosc 27–80, 1981.
7. Swan CP, Storey DW, Bown SG, et al: Nature of the bleeding vessel in recurrently bleeding gastric ulcers. Gastroenterology 90:595, 1986.

54. ACUTE PANCREATITIS

John Schaefer, M.D.

1. What are the diagnostic criteria for acute pancreatitis?

The diagnosis is usually made on a constellation of clinical findings, and pathologic confirmation is seldom obtained. The most common presentation is epigastric pain of variable severity, often with radiation to the left upper quadrant and back associated with an elevated serum amylase.

2. What conditions are implicated in the etiology of acute pancreatitis?

Approximately 80% of pancreatitis is associated with alcoholism or biliary tract stones. In about 10% of cases, no precipitating cause can be identified. Other infrequent causes of pancreatitis include hypertriglyceridemia ($>1,500$ mg/dl), trauma including postendoscopic retrograde pancreatography, hypercalcemia, drug use, and viral infections. Postoperative pancreatitis is a particularly severe form of the disease.

3. How do laboratory tests help in diagnosis?

An elevated serum amylase is the most sensitive laboratory test, but it is not altogether specific. Alternative causes of an elevated serum amylase include perforated peptic ulcer, bowel infarction, salivary gland trauma or infection, renal failure, and macroamylasemia. A serum isoamylase assay distinguishes between pancreatic and salivary origin of amylase. A recently introduced semiautomated isoamylase separation process may prove more specific than total amylase for detecting acute pancreatitis. An elevated value for renal excretion of amylase persists longer than an elevated serum amylase and is useful when patients are evaluated four or five days after onset of illness. The test for serum lipase has become more reliable and is more specific for pancreatitis than is total serum amylase.

4. What is macroamylasemia?

Macroamylasemia is a benign biochemical finding of a persistently elevated serum amylase with a normal or reduced renal excretion rate of amylase in the absence of any evidence of renal insufficiency. It results from the binding of amylase to serum proteins. This macromolecular complex is too large for renal glomerular filtration, and thus it accumulates in the serum. Macroamylasemia is not associated with any particular disease state. The main clinical point is to recognize that this cause of elevated serum amylase is not associated with ongoing pancreatic disease.

5. How valuable are plain abdominal radiographs and imaging techniques?

The single most important reason to obtain abdominal films is to help exclude surgical conditions such as perforated viscus or bowel infarction that may simulate acute pancreatitis. Visible gallstones or pancreatic calcifications can be helpful, but together with localized or generalized ileus, they are nonspecific for acute pancreatitis. Both ultrasound and computed tomography are excellent in defining an enlarged, inflamed pancreas and peripancreatic necrosis associated with moderate to severe acute pancreatitis. The pancreas, however, may often appear normal in patients with a mild form of pancreatitis.

6. How can the severity of acute pancreatitis be estimated?

On admission, it is not always possible to predict either the severity or the probable course of acute pancreatitis. Clearly the level of serum amylase does not correlate with the severity of illness. Patients with mild, recurrent pancreatitis, particularly in association with alcoholism, usually have a short, uncomplicated hospitalization and negligible mortality.

Severe pancreatitis is often heralded by cardiopulmonary findings of shock or persistent hypotension, hypoxia, pleural effusion, and pulmonary infiltrates of adult respiratory distress syndrome (ARDS). Variable additional developments of renal insufficiency with oliguria, low serum calcium, falling hematocrit, persisting ileus, overt ascites, and mental confusion portend a mortality rate greater than 80%.

7. What are the treatment and prognosis of acute pancreatitis?

Mild cases subside spontaneously within a few days and require only intravenous hydration and analgesics for pain relief. They show only interstitial edema and inflammation and often subside without permanent damage to the pancreas. Severe pancreatitis is associated with extensive necrotizing and often hemorrhagic tissue destruction. Early in the course, large retroperitoneal and intraperitoneal fluid sequestration develops with resultant hypovolemia, hypotension, hemocentration, and oliguria. Vigorous intravenous fluids in addition to electrolyte, colloid, or blood replacement are required. Many patients die despite the best supportive treatment. Early mortality is often caused by a combination of cardiovascular collapse, ARDS, and renal failure. After the first or second week of illness, pancreatic and retroperitoneal sepsis become an important mortality factor, and patients who survive severe pancreatitis are usually left with some degree of permanently destroyed pancreatic tissue.

8. What is the typical course of alcoholic pancreatitis?

An acute episode of pancreatitis often follows a few days after a patient ends an alcoholic binge. The initial episode of acute alcoholic pancreatitis is usually more severe than any subsequent relapses. Although pathologic confirmation is seldom obtained, the elements of chronic pancreatitis, such as glandular destruction and fibrosis, are usually present at the time of the first clinical attack. The chronic element is thought to represent glandular destruction from a proteinaceous precipitation, of uncertain mechanism, within the small pancreatic ducts. Recurrent painful episodes are common with persistent alcohol abuse and even with abstinence. Punctate pancreatic calcifications and pseudocyst formation are not uncommon. Small pseudocysts identified only by ultrasound or computed tomography may subside spontaneously over time. Pseudocysts larger than 5 cm in diameter that persist or enlarge over 6 weeks require drainage. Cyst drainage is most often accomplished by anastomosis to the stomach or small bowel. In some patients, percutaneous tube drainage can be successful. Continuing destruction of pancreatic tissue may cause clinically important exocrine pancreatic dysfunction with severe fat malabsorption. Less often, patients may also develop secondary diabetes mellitus from islet cell destruction and may benefit from pancreatic enzyme replacement and insulin therapy. Chronic retroperitoneal pain is often a therapeutic dilemma.

9. What are the cardinal features of gallstone pancreatitis?

Acute pancreatitis associated with biliary tract disease occurs from the passage of small gallstones through the common bile duct and ampulla of Vater. It is most often seen in middle-aged and older women. The serum amylase values tend to be markedly elevated (more than fivefold elevation), and the liver-associated biochemical tests are often abnormal. Fever and rigor of cholangitis are sometimes present. An early ultrasound that shows gallstones constitutes useful supportive information. In most patients, the acute episode subsides within a few days of treatment with nasogastric suction, IV fluids, and antibiotics when cholangitis is suspected. If the clinical picture fails to improve, or if it deteriorates, surgical decompression with common bile duct drainage must be performed. For patients at high surgical risk, endoscopic sphincterotomy and stone extraction are acceptable and even preferential alternatives. Patients with biliary-tract-induced pancreatitis seldom develop chronic pancreatitis or pseudocyst formation. If the biliary tract pathology is corrected, recurrences do not take place.

10. What is the role of surgery in acute pancreatitis?

There is no role for surgical intervention in a typical uncomplicated case of acute pancreatitis. There are, however, a number of circumstances when surgery is indicated. Perhaps the most difficult decision concerning the need for surgical exploration occurs when the diagnosis of acute pancreatitis is uncertain and alternative, surgically correctable conditions cannot be excluded with reasonable certainty. When pancreatic abscess is highly suspected or confirmed by guided needle aspiration, the patient needs generous surgical external drainage and perhaps debridement of necrotic retroperitoneal tissue. Common duct drainage (surgically or endoscopically) is necessary when either common duct obstruction, pancreatitis, or cholangitis do not respond to conservative medical therapy. In patients with severe pancreatitis and deteriorating clinical status, placement of multiple abdominal drains and large-volume peritoneal lavage are often advocated. The rationale is to remove and thereby reduce the absorption of accumulated, biologically noxious substances from the peritoneal cavity. This approach is supported by animal experiments and uncontrolled clinical studies. Unfortunately, several randomized studies have not confirmed benefit. Finally, it is prudent to surgically explore the patient with acute pancreatitis caused by penetrating or blunt abdominal trauma when major pancreatic duct fracture is suspected.

BIBLIOGRAPHY

1. Acosta JM, Ledesma CL: Gallstone migration as a cause of acute pancreatitis. N Engl J Med 290:484, 1974.
2. Beger JG, Bittmer R, Buchler M, et al: Hemodynamic data pattern in patients with acute pancreatitis. Gastroenterology 90:74, 1986.
3. Corfield AP, Cooper MJ, Williamson RCN: Acute pancreatitis: A lethal disease of increasing incidence. Gut 26:724, 1985.
4. Frey CF: Classification of pancreatitis: State of the art 1986. Pancreas 1:62, 1986.
5. Kalthoff L, Layer P, Claiw JE, Di Magno EP: The course of alcoholic and non alcoholic chronic pancreatitis. Digest Dis Sci 29:553, 1984.
6. Kelly TR, Wagner DS: Gallstone pancreatitis: A prospective randomized trial of the timing of surgery. Surgery 104:600, 1988.
7. Levitt MD: Diagnosis of acute pancreatitis. Intern Med Specialist 8:99, 1987.
8. Mayer AD, McMahoy MJ, Corfield AP, et al: Controlled clinical trial of peritoneal lavage for treatment of severe acute pancreatitis. N Engl J Med 312:399, 1985.
9. Reber HA. Surgical intervention in necrotizing pancreatitis (editorial). Gastroenterology 91:479, 1986.
10. Singh M, Simsek H: Ethanol and the pancreas: Current status. Gastroenterology 98:1051, 1990.
11. Steinberg WM, Goldstein SS, Davis ND, et al: Diagnostic assays in acute pancreatitis: A study of sensitivity and specificity. Ann Intern Med 102:576, 1985.
12. Warshaw AL, Gongliang J: Improved survival in 45 patients with pancreatic abscess. Ann Surg 202:408, 1985.

55. HEPATITIS AND CIRRHOSIS

Mark W. Bowyer, M.D.

1. What is hepatitis?

Hepatitis refers to any inflammatory process that involves liver parenchyma and may result in anything ranging from mere laboratory abnormalities to a fulminant illness with high mortality. The most common etiologic factor is viral.

2. Which viruses are responsible?

Viral hepatitis may be caused by the A, B, C, D, and E hepatitis virsues; the Epstein-Barr virus; and cytomegalovirus. In general, they tend to cause similar clinical pictures ranging from asymptomatic to a rarely severe illness.

3. What are the characteristics of hepatitis A?

The hepatitis A virus is an enterovirus of the family Picornaviridae, which causes an enterically transmitted disease acquired by ingestion of material that has been fecally contaminated. The virus passes through the stomach, replicates in the lower intestine, is transported to the liver, and begins to replicate in the cytoplasm. Cellular damage occurs as the body's immunologic defenses attempt to kill the virus.

The average incubation period to onset of symptoms is about 32 days but ranges between 3 and 6 weeks. Classically, there is a prodromal phase during which malaise, anorexia, epigastric or right upper quadrant pain, fever, rashes, diarrhea, and constipation are frequent complaints. The disease is usually recognized during the icteric phase, when dark urine and jaundice prompt patients to seek medical attention. Liver tests at this time reveal elevated aminotransferase levels, and the clinical diagnosis can be confirmed by detection of the IgM antibody to the virus.

The severity of the illness is age related. Older adults tend to have worse symptoms than young adults. Most cases of acute hepatitis resolve rapidly over several weeks with complete clinical and biochemical recovery.

4. What are the characteristics of hepatitis B?

The hepatitis B virus (HBV) is the prototype of a new class of viruses, the Hepadnaviridae. Clinical expression of infection with HBV may range from a carrier state to fulminant hepatitis. In classic acute hepatitis B, the incubation period varies from 60 to 180 days. As with hepatitis A, there is a prodromal phase that in hepatitis B is more insidious and more prolonged, with arthritis and urticarial rash as additional symptoms. As in hepatitis A, symptoms tend to improve with the onset of jaundice. During the icteric phase, the bilirubin tends to rise less steeply than in hepatitis A, but it reaches higher levels, and the jaundice lasts longer. There is a slower rise in aminotransferase levels, which peak much later than in hepatitis A.

Unlike hepatitis A, acute hepatitis B may become chronic hepatitis and cirrhosis. Patients may also have an asymptomatic infection and may continue to carry the virus in the blood even in the absence of significant evidence of liver disease (healthy carriers).

HBV infection can be spread via parenteral transmission. Blood is the most effective vehicle for transmission, but the virus is present in other body fluids as well (e.g., saliva and semen). HBV infection is a common problem among intravenous drugs abusers, homosexuals, and the sexual partners of infected patients. Vertical transmission may occur to infants from mothers who experience hepatitis B infection during the last trimester of pregnancy.

5. What laboratory tests are available for hepatitis B? How are they interpreted?

Sensitive immunoassays are available to measure the antigens associated with HBV and the antibodies it induces. The antigenic activity of the virus DNA core is designated HBc (core) Ag. The other surface coat of the virus has distinctive antigenicity and is designated HBsAg. These antigens evoke specific antibodies, and both constitute important immunologic markers of the infection and its course.

During a typical case of acute hepatitis B, HBsAg is first detected in blood during the incubation period as early as 1 week after infection. The HBsAg level begins to decline after the onset of the illness and usually becomes undetectable within 3 months after exposure. The presence of HBsAg in serum indicates a potential for infectivity. Anti-HBc appears in the serum toward the end of the incubation period and persists during the acute illness and for several months to years thereafter. Anti-HBs is detected during convalescence (several weeks to months after disappearance of HBsAg) and persists for a prolonged period. A high titer of anti-HBs confirms immunity to HBV. Persistence of HBsAg is a sign of chronic hepatitis B.

6. What are the characteristics of hepatitis C?
Hepatitis C is the name recently given to this single-stranded RNA virus distantly related to the flavivirus family. The hepatitis C virus is the major cause of posttransfusion, community-acquired, cryptogenic non-A, non-B hepatitis. Until the recent availability of serologic tests, it was responsible for 90–95% of all cases of posttransfusion hepatitis.

The incubation period to rise in aminotransferases is about 6–8 weeks. Symptoms are usually of moderate severity; many cases (40–75%) are asymptomatic. Jaundice is uncommon (10%) and usually mild. There is a high rate of progression to chronic hepatitis and, eventually, cirrhosis. Early identification of infection is difficult. Alanine aminotransferase is more likely to be elevated than aspartate aminotransferase.

7. What are the characteristics of hepatitis D?
Hepatitis D (or delta agent) is an incomplete RNA viral particle similar to plant viruses, which requires the presence of HBV for infection and replication to occur. Infection can occur only in HBsAg carriers exposed to the delta agent or in patients who are simultaneously infected with both HBV and hepatitis D. Acute simultaneous infection with both viruses may be associated with fulminant hepatitis. Chronic infection with hepatitis D is frequently associated with chronic active hepatitis or cirrhosis.

8. What is hepatitis E?
The hepatitis E virus produces a water-borne disease similar to but generally milder than hepatitis A. It has an average incubation period of 40 days and is epidemic in a number of developing countries. Fulminant hepatitis may occur, especially among pregnant women, with mortality of up to 20%.

9. What is fulminant viral hepatitis?
Fulminant hepatitis occurs in about 1% of cases of acute viral hepatitis requiring hospitalization. In fulminant hepatitis, massive hepatocellular necrosis occurs and is felt to be related to an abnormally rapid clearance of the viral antigens. Type B hepatitis accounts for approximately 50% of cases, with hepatitis C about 45% and hepatitis A about 5%. Fulminant hepatitis can also occur with a variety of hepatotoxic drugs and uncommon diseases. The end product is fulminant hepatic failure (FHF). FHF is manifested by signs and symptoms of encephalopathy within 3–8 weeks of the onset of the illness. A profound coagulopathy occurs as a result of massive liver necrosis, and the prothrombin time (PT) is the most sensitive laboratory parameter. If the PT exceeds control by 10 seconds despite vitamin K supplementation, FHF has evolved. Renal failure usually due to volume depletion and cerebral edema is a frequent sequela of FHF.

10. How is fulminant hepatitis treated?
No specific form of treatment other than transplant has proved beneficial in fulminant hepatitis. The goal of current therapy is to sustain life and control hepatic failure over a time period sufficient to allow hepatic regeneration before the patient dies of liver failure. Intense, supportive care is directed at respiratory support, prevention of hypoglycemia, avoiding factors that might worsen encephalopathy, prevention of renal failure, treatment of infections, and treatment of cerebral edema. Transplantation for fulminant hepatitis is controversial; if it is considered, timing is critical because patients who are in stage IV encephalopathy with cerebral edema have a much poorer prognosis with treatment.

11. What is the prognosis for patients with fulminant hepatitis?

The overall survival rate of patients with fulminant hepatitis is 20–25%. Survival correlates best with age of the patient and deepest level of encephalopathy reached. In patients who reach only stage II encephalopathy, over 50% survive. In contrast, the survival rate of those who progress to stage IV encephalopathy is only 20%.

12. What is chronic hepatitis?

Chronic hepatitis is defined as the presence of liver inflammation that persists for more than 6 months. There are two major variants: chronic persistent hepatitis and chronic active hepatitis. Chronic persistent hepatitis is a relapsing, remitting, benign, self-limited condition that is not associated with progressive liver damage and does not lead to liver failure or cirrhosis. Chronic active hepatitis is a vicious disease characterized by progressive destruction of hepatocytes over a span of years with continued erosion of the hepatic functional reserve and eventual development of cirrhosis. It is estimated that about 5–10% of patients with acute hepatitis B and possibly as many as 33% of those with hepatitis C may develop chronic disease.

13. What are some nonviral causes of hepatitis?

Hepatic injury can be induced by a variety of chemical agents, drugs, and metabolic diseases. Drugs associated with chronic hepatitis or cirrhosis include acetominophen, aspirin, chlorpromazine, dantrolene, ethanol, halothane, isoniazid, methyldopa, nitrofurantoin, propylthiouracil, and sulfonamides. Other hepatotoxins include carbon tetrachloride, phosphorus, tetracycline, several chemotherapy agents, *Amanita phalloides* (mushroom toxin), and anabolic steroids. Metabolic diseases such as Wilson's disease, alpha$_1$-antitrypsin deficiency, and certain autoimmune diseases are associated with hepatitis and liver disease.

14. What is cirrhosis?

Cirrhosis is a diffuse process characterized by fibrosis and a conversion of normal liver architecture into structurally abnormal nodules. The architectural disorganization of the liver is irreversible once established, and management is directed at both prevention of further liver cell damage and treatment of the complications.

15. What are the major causes of cirrhosis?

Alcohol is by far and away the most common cause of cirrhosis, accounting for 60–70% of cases. Chronic viral hepatitis, autoimmune hepatitis, primary sclerosing cholangitis, primary biliary cirrhosis, hemochromatosis, Wilson's disease, and idiopathic causes also lead to cirrhosis.

16. What are the major complications of cirrhosis?

Progressive liver cell failure and portal hypertension are sequelae of cirrhosis; they result in four major complications—ascites, spontaneous bacterial peritonitis, hepatic encephalopathy, and upper gastrointestinal bleeding—all of which may lead to admission to an intensive care unit.

17. How is cirrhotic ascites managed?

The initial management of cirrhotic ascites is conservative, emphasizing sodium restriction and bed rest. It is estimated that 10–20% of cirrhotic patients with ascites can be adequately treated this way. Patients who do not respond to these conservative measures require diuretic therapy. Spironolactone is the agent of choice because of its physiologic action, potassium-sparing effects, and relative safety. Combination therapy with spironolactone and furosemide is used in those patients who do not respond to spironolactone. In cases of diuretic-resistant ascites, therapeutic paracentesis should be considered, with possible albumin replacement. In patients truly unresponsive to other therapy, the use of a peritoneovenous shunt should be considered, bearing in mind there is a high rate of complication and no proven prolongation of survival with these devices.

18. How is hepatic encephalopathy best managed?
Treatment of hepatic encephalopathy is focused on reversing any preciptiating factors and reducing the absorption of gut-derived bacterial protein degradation products. If a specific drug is implicated, it should be stopped. Dietary protein intake is reduced, and lactulose is used to lower stool pH and increase bacterial clearance. Gut sterilization with either metronidazole or neomycin may help. Once a precipitating factor has been identified and treated, the recovery rate reaches around 80%.

19. How is upper gastrointestinal tract bleeding associated with cirrhosis managed?
Approximately 70% of bleeding episodes in cirrhosis are due to variceal hemorrhage, but other causes such as gastritis, ulcer and Mallory-Weiss tears should be kept in mind. Initial management is focused on resuscitation with simultaneous attempts to reduce portal venous pressure (e.g., vasopressin). Once the patient has been resuscitated, endoscopy is performed to define the cause of bleeding. If bleeding is due to esophageal varices, injection sclerotherapy becomes the preferred method and has a success rate of around 85% in the arresting of bleeding. An alternative approach is resection of the lower esophagus, which will almost always stop the bleeding but carries with it a high mortality. There is a high risk of rebleeding with both methods of therapy. Shunt surgery has all but been abandoned in the emergency setting. However, it may be beneficial for a small group of patients with well-compensated cirrhosis and troublesome variceal bleeding. This operation has significant mortality and is often accompanied by severe encephalopathy.

20. What is the role of liver transplantation in cirrhosis?
Although the final role of transplantation in patients with cirrhosis has yet to be established, liver transplantation has become a definitive treatment for end-stage cirrhosis. The one-year survival rate following transplant ranges between 50 and 70%, and most such patients survive three years. The use of liver transplantation in patients with alcoholic cirrhosis or cirrhosis due to hepatitis B remains controversial.

BIBLIOGRAPHY

1. Alaniz C: Management of cirrhotic ascites. Clinical Pharm 8:645–654, 1989.
2. Alexander GJM: Immunology of hepatitis B virus infection. Br Med Bull 46:354–367, 1990.
3. Bonino F, Negro F, Brunette MR, Verma G: Hepatitis delta virus infection. Prog Liver Dis 9:485–496, 1990.
4. Carithers RL, Fairman RP: Critical care of patients with severe liver disease. In Shoemaker WC, et al (eds): Testbook of Critical Care, 2nd ed. Philadelphia, W.B. Saunders, 1989, pp 686–697.
5. Choo QL, Weiner AJ, Overby LR, et al: Heptatitis C virus: The major causative agent of viral non-A, non-B hepatitis. Br Med Bull 46:423–441, 1990.
6. Epstein O: Management aspects of cirrhosis. The Practitioner 231:395–401, 1987.
7. Fagan EA, Williams R: Fulminant viral hepatitis. Br Med Bull 46:462–480, 1990.
8. Fattovich G, Brollo L, Giustina A, et al: Natural history and prognsotic factors for chronic hepatitis type B. Gut 32:294–298, 1991.
9. Gust ID, Feinstone SM: Hepatitis A. Prog Liver Dis 9:371–378, 1990.
10. McIntyre N: Clinical presentation of acute viral hepatitis. Br Med Bull 46:533–547, 1990.
11. O'Grady JG, Williams R: Liver transplantation for viral hepatitis. Br Med Bull 46:481–491, 1990.
12. Schade RR, et al: Orthotopic liver transplantation for alcoholic liver disease. Hepatology 11:159–164, 1990.
13. Schiff ER, Reddy KR, Jeffers LJ: Relevant aspects of hepatobiliary disease. In Civetta JM, Taylor RW, Kirby RR (eds): Critical Care. Philadelphia, J.B. Lippincott, 1988, pp 1283–1289.

56. PERITONITIS

Mark W. Bowyer, M.D.

1. What is the peritoneum?

The peritoneum is a highly evolved and specialized organ that functions to maintain the surface integrity of the intraabdominal structures and to provide a smooth, lubricated surface so that the intestines can move freely. The peritoneum is a serous membrane that, if flattened out, would cover an area of 1.7–2.2 square meters. It is composed of a monocellular layer of flattened mesothelial cells that rests on a thin layer of fibroelastic tissue.

2. What is the difference between the parietal and the visceral peritoneum?

The parietal peritoneum is the portion of the peritoneum that lines all of the abdominal cavity, covering the abdominal wall, diaphragm, and pelvis. The visceral peritoneum is the portion of the peritoneum that covers all the intraabdominal viscera and mesenteries and is identical with the visceral serosa.

3. What features are unique to the peritoneum overlying the diaphragm?

The peritoneum overlying the diaphragm is interrupted by intracellular gaps called stomata, which serve as entrances into diaphragmatic lymphatic channels called lacunae. The lacunae ultimately drain into the substernal lymph nodes and then into the thoracic duct. In contrast to the nondiaphragmatic peritoneal surface, which behaves as a passive, semipermeable membrane allowing bidirectional exchange of water and electrolytes, the diaphragmatic stomata are capable of absorbing particulate matter, including bacteria.

4. What is peritonitis?

The term peritonitis refers to a generalized or local inflammation of the peritoneal membrane. Inflammation may be initiated by a variety of etiologic insults with a resultant cascade of events that includes transudation of fluid, edema formation, and vascular congestion of the tissue layer immediately adjacent to the mesothelium. These events in turn lead to secondary endocrine, cardiac, respiratory, renal, and metabolic responses. Classically, peritonitis is a life-threatening process due to bacteria from perforation of or trauma to intraabdominal organs. Other primary and secondary forms of peritonitis occur but are less common.

5. What are the clinical manifestations of classic peritonitis?

Patients appear gravely ill early in the clinical course. Characteristically, they lie quietly, supine, and with knees flexed; they have shallow breathing, because any motion intensifies their abdominal pain. Abdominal pain is almost always the predominant symptom and when fully developed is steady, unrelenting, and burning. The abdomen is distended and tender over the entire extent of the peritoneum involved in the inflammatory process. Rigidity of the abdominal muscles is produced by voluntary guarding followed by spasm as the parietal peritoneum becomes inflamed. As the peritonitis advances, the reflex spasm may become so severe that boardlike abdominal rigidity is produced. Anorexia is almost always present and is frequently accompanied by nausea and vomiting. The patient often complains of chills and feeling feverish. Temperature elevation usually of a spiking nature is common, or, more ominously, hypothermia is present. Tachycardia and diminished pulse reflect hypovolemia early, and hypovolemic shock may occur rapidly as the peritonitis progresses. Increasing tissue demands for oxygen as well as acidosis lead to tachypnea, which is characteristically shallow, as deep respirations intensify the abdominal pain.

6. What is primary peritonitis?

Primary peritonitis is a diffuse bacterial infection of the peritoneal cavity that occurs in the absence of disruption of the gastrointestinal tract. Prior to widespread use of antibiotics, primary peritonitis occurred most commonly in the pediatric population and was caused by *Streptococcus pneumoniae*. Currently, spontaneous bacterial peritonitis occurs in patients with ascites secondary to liver disease and now constitutes the most common type of primary peritonitis. The third type of primary peritonitis is related to continuous ambulatory peritoneal dialysis.

7. How is spontaneous bacterial peritonitis (SBP) diagnosed?

SBP is a frequent and severe complication of cirrhosis. The incidence in cirrhotic patients with ascites ranges from 15–50% with a mortality of more than 50%. Prognosis can be improved by early diagnosis and therefore requires both knowledge of the clinical signs and symptoms of SBP and a high index of suspicion. The onset of symptoms may be insidious, but there is a high prevalence of jaundice, fever, encephalopathy, and abdominal pain or tenderness. About one-third or more of patients with SBP have no symptoms or signs directly referable to the abdomen. In such cases, deterioration of liver function, such as increasing encephalopathy, increasing ascites, or increasing jaundice, must lead to a suspicion of infection. Temporary resistance to diuretics may be an early sign of SBP. In about 10% of cases SBP is silent and is diagnosed by systematic paracentesis. In summary, the clinical spectrum of SBP ranges from a silent subclinical state to a severe and rapidly fatal illness.

The key to the diagnosis of SBP is examination of the ascitic fluid. A Gram-stained smear of centrifuged ascites may provide clues to the causative organism in 22–77% of cases; cultures require 24–72 hours to become positive. The best single predictor of infection is the absolute polymorphonuclear leukocyte (PMN) count. A PMN count $> 500/mm^3$ is highly suggestive of SBP; it should be treated as if it represented SBP, pending culture results. Treatment should be continued regardless of culture results if there are $> 1,000/mm^3$ of PMNs. When the PMN count is ambiguous, use of ascitic fluid pH levels of < 7.35 or ascitic lactate levels > 25 mg/dl may offer additional diagnostic assistance.

8. How is SBP treated?

Successful treatment of SBP requires prompt intravenous antibiotic therapy directed at the likely predominant pathogens. The Gram stain of centrifuged ascites is the most useful test to guide the initial selection of an antimicrobial regimen. If the Gram stain is unrevealing or there is no obvious organism or potential source, treatment should be broad spectrum and empirical. A literature review of 15 series involving 253 cases revealed that gram-negative bacilli accounted for 69% of cases. Of the gram negatives, *Escherichia coli* was the most common (68%), followed by Klebsiella (16%); smaller numbers of patients had Proteus, Pseudomonas, and Serratia. Gram positives were found in 30% of cases, with Streptococcus species accounting for 86%. Anaerobes, including Bacteroides and Clostridium, accounted for 5% of the pathogens. Based on these findings, empirical treatment with ampicillin and an aminoglycoside is recommended. Empirical therapy directed against anaerobes, Pseudomonas, and Staphylococcus is not indicated unless these pathogens are suspected on clinical grounds or by Gram stain. As always, antimicrobial therapy should be adjusted when the results of culture and sensitivity testing become available.

9. How is peritonitis diagnosed in peritoneal dialysis (PD) patients?

The manifestations of peritonitis in this patient group may be vague and include mild abdominal pain, low-grade fever, and mild abdominal tenderness. A definition of peritonitis in this group has been established and includes at least two of the following criteria: (1) the presence of microorganisms on Gram stain or culture of the peritoneal effluent, (2) cloudy fluid with inflammatory cells, and (3) symptoms of peritoneal inflammation. Occasionally the dialysis effluent may be contaminated with microorganisms, but there are no signs of clinical infection. This finding does not constitute peritonitis, and dialysis should be continued without treatment.

10. What is the treatment for peritonitis among PD patients?
Initial therapy involves drainage of residual abdominal fluid and instillation of antibiotics via the dialysis cannula. Tobramycin plus cephalothin are used empirically and adjusted depending on culture and sensitivity data. Therapy is usually continued for 7 days following the last positive culture. Catheters need be removed only when there is a persistently infected exit site or tunnel tract, when there are recurrent episodes of peritonitis caused by the same organism, or when laparotomy is required for fecal peritonitis.

11. What is secondary peritonitis?
Secondary bacterial peritonitis is classic peritonitis defined as peritoneal infection due to perforation of a hollow viscus. It commonly occurs with trauma or with such entities as perforated appendicitis, perforated duodenal ulcer, perforated sigmoid colon due to diverticulitis, volvulus, cancer, strangulation obstruction of the small bowel, and postoperative peritonitis due to anastomotic disruption. The diagnosis is usually a clinical one, and the classic findings of abdominal pain are associated with peritoneal signs, including tenderness, guarding, and increased abdominal wall tone. Leukocytosis with a left shift, free air under the diaphragm, or evidence of ileus support this diagnosis. In patients in whom a history or physical may not be reliable (e.g., head-injured patients, paraplegics, the elderly, or patients on steroids), diagnostic peritoneal lavage may be a useful method of determining the presence of peritonitis requiring surgery.

12. How should secondary peritonitis be managed?
The treatment of secondary peritonitis is primarily operative. The goals of the operative management of peritonitis are to eliminate the source of contamination, reduce the bacterial inoculum, and prevent recurrent or persistent sepsis. Important aspects of the perioperative care are fluid resuscitation and appropriate antibiotic therapy. These infections are almost always polymicrobial and contain a mixture of aerobic and anaerobic bacteria; therefore, antibiotic treatment should be directed against both gram-negative enteric bacteria and *Bacteroides fragilis*.

13. What is tertiary peritonitis?
Secondary peritonitis that cannot be controlled, whether due to impaired host defense mechanisms or overwhelming infection, progresses to persistent diffuse (tertiary) peritonitis. The clinical picture is one of occult sepsis without a well-defined focus of infection. Despite aggressive management, progressive multiple-system organ failure frequently develops, after which, ultimately, death results.

14. How does the peritoneum normally deal with an infection?
The peritoneum deals with an infection in three ways: (1) by direct absorption of bacteria into the lymphatics via the stomata of the diaphragmatic peritoneum; (2) by local destruction of bacteria through phagocytosis by either resident macrophages or polymorphonuclear granulocytes attracted to the peritoneal cavity; and (3) by localization of the infection in the form of an abscess.

15. What are the characteristics of intraperitoneal abscesses?
Intraperitoneal abscesses arise during resolution of generalized peritonitis and most commonly occur in the pelvis or subphrenic areas. These locations are a reflection of the anatomy of the peritoneum, which permits gravity-dependent flow of infected material into these dependent cavities. Clinical symptoms may be vague early on but commonly include

paralytic ileus, anorexia, abdominal distention, recurrent or persistent fever, chills, abdominal pain, and tachycardia. CT scanning and ultrasound have a diagnostic accuracy of greater than 90%. Radionucleotide scans may be useful but have much less specificity.

16. How are intraperitoneal abscesses treated?

Three basic principles of management are (1) drainage of the abscess, (2) use of antibiotics, and (3) general care of the patient's status, that is, correction of nutritional or metabolic derangements. Percutaneous drainage is the treatment of choice for most intraabdominal abscesses and is successful in greater than 85% of cases. Failure of percutaneous drainage requires open surgical drainage.

17. What are the common causes of nonbacterial (aseptic) peritonitis?

Aseptic (chemical) peritonitis develops whenever irritant materials gain entry into the peritoneal cavity. This inflammatory reaction may lead to the general clinical symptoms and physiologic sequelae associated with bacterial peritonitis. Secondary bacterial invasion may then occur even without apparent bacterial contamination. Substances that commonly cause aseptic peritonitis are gastric contents, pancreatic juice, bile, urine, blood, meconium, chyle, mucus, foreign bodies, and barium. Certain drugs may cause peritonitis. Several cases have been reported of patients who developed striking thickening of the visceral peritoneum after prolonged treatment with beta blockers.

18. What is granulomatous peritonitis?

There is a group of diseases characterized by a peritoneal reaction that includes formation of granulomas and is associated with a markedly increased incidence of adhesion formation. Tuberculous peritonitis, Candida peritonitis, amebic peritonitis, and peritonitis secondary to Histoplasma or Strongyloides are examples. These diseases are relatively rare but are on the increase due to the AIDS epidemic. Iatrogenic cause of granulomatous peritonitis is contamination of the peritoneal cavity by glove lubricants or cellulose fibers from disposable gauze pads.

BIBLIOGRAPHY

1. Diethelm AG: The acute abdomen. In Sabiston DC (ed): Textbook for Surgery, 13th ed. Philadelphia, W.B. Saunders, 1986, pp 790–809.
2. Farthmann EH, Schoffel U: Principles and limitations of operative management of intraabdominal infections. World J Surg 14:210–217, 1990.
3. Hallak A: Spontaneous bacterial peritonitis. Am J Gastroenterol 84:345–350, 1989.
4. Hau T: Bacteria, toxins, and the peritoneum. World J Surg 14:167–175, 1990.
5. Hoffman SH: Tropical medicine and the acute abdomen. Emerg Med Clin North Am 7:541–609, 1989.
6. Jung PJ, Merrell RC: Acute abdomen. Gastroenterol Clin North Am 17:227–244, 1988.
7. Maddaus MA, Ahrenholz D, Simmons RL: The biology of peritonitis and implications for treatment. Surg Clin North Am 68:431–443, 1988.
8. Pollock AV: Non-operative antiinfective treatment of intraabdominal infections. World J Surg 14:227–230, 1990.
9. Reins HO: Evaluating the acute abdomen in an ICU patient. In Civetta JM, Taylor RW, Kirby RR (eds): Critical Care. Philadelphia, J.B. Lippincott, 1988, pp 567–576.
10. Rotstein OD, Meakins JL: Diagnostic and therapeutic challenges of intraabdominal infections. World J Surg 14:159–166, 1990.
11. Rotellar C, Black J, Winchester JF, et al: Ten years' experience with continuous ambulatory peritoneal dialysis. Am J Kidney Dis 17:158–164, 1991.
12. Walker AP, Condon RE: Peritonitis and intraabdominal abscesses. In Schwartz SI, Shires GT, Spencer FC (eds): Principles of Surgery, 5th ed. New York, McGraw-Hill, 1989, pp 1459–1489.
13. Wilcox CM, Dismukes WE: Spontaneous bacterial peritonitis: A review of pathogenesis, diagnosis, and treatment. Medicine 66:447–456, 1987.

VIII: Endocrinology

57. DIABETIC KETOACIDOSIS

Philip S. Mehler, M.D.

1. What is diabetic ketoacidosis (DKA)?
DKA is an emergent metabolic complication of diabetes mellitus due to a state of relative or absolute insulin deficiency and a relative or absolute increase in counterregulatory hormones. It is characterized by the triad of acidosis, ketosis, and hyperglycemia.

2. What is the pathophysiologic basis of DKA?
Insulin deficiency is the focal point of this disorder and causes both hyperglycemia and hyperketonemia. Under normal states, insulin ensures the storage of glucose as glucagon in the liver and of free fatty acids as triglycerides in adipose tissue. With a deficiency of insulin, there are both increased hepatic glucose production through increased glycogenolysis and gluconeogenesis and decreased glucose utilization. The result is hyperglycemia.

The hyperketonemia is similarly due to a state of insulin deficiency. As a result of the depressed insulin level and the concomitantly elevated levels of catecholamines and other counterregulatory hormones, there is excess production of free fatty acids from the breakdown of triglycerides. Free fatty acids are converted to ketone bodies in the liver. There is also decreased ketone utilization, which contributes to the hyperketonemia.

3. What other physiologic derangements are present in DKA?
In addition to hyperglycemia and hyperketonemia, there are other fluid and electrolyte disturbances. These are predominantly a result of hyperglycemia, which in turn causes glucosuria and, subsequently, osmotic diuresis with loss of electrolytes and concomitant volume depletion. In the average 70-kg man with established DKA, there is a 3–5 liter saline deficiency, a 300–500 mEq sodium deficiency, and a 150–250 mEq potassium deficiency.

4. What are the common signs and symptoms of DKA?
Hyperglycemia is manifested by polyuria, polydipsia, polyphagia, lassitude, weight loss, and visual difficulties. The mental status ranges from lethargy to deep coma; 20% of patients present in a stuporous state. Nausea, vomiting, and abdominal pain, which are not usually due to definite intraabdominal pathology, frequently complicate the early course of DKA. Acidosis is also responsible for one of the classic signs of DKA: Kussmaul breaths, which are long, deep, and sighing respirations made in an attempt to compensate for the metabolic acidosis by lowering arterial PCO_2. An odor of decaying apples or "Juicy Fruit" gum on the patient's breath, another positive sign of DKA, is due to acetone; the other ketoacids are odorless. Further, the patient with DKA is hypothermic because of the inability of available substrate to generate heat.

5. What is the significance of abdominal pain in DKA?
Abdominal pain is commonly found in DKA. The definite cause is unknown, but gastric distention and stretching of the liver capsule have been offered as possible explanations for the pain, which is present approximately 20% of the time. Generally, the pain resolves

promptly with treatment for DKA, but at the time of the initial evaluation, signs and symptoms indicative of an intraabdominal process should be pursued. Further, if abdominal signs and symptoms persist in spite of adequate treatment, one most definitely should consider underlying intraabdominal processes. This is especially true in patients over the age of 40 with DKA, since abdominal pain is likely to have an underlying cause in this group, such as pyelonephritis or appendicitis. Unexplained abdominal pain is more common in younger patients with severe DKA. The serum amylase is elevated approximately 75% of the time in DKA, but the cause is not known. It is not specific for pancreatitis.

6. What are the usual laboratory findings in DKA?

DKA is characterized by hyperglycemia, acidemia, bicarbonate level less than 15 mEq/L, and ketonemia with positive values defined as greater than a 1:2 dilution. Hyperglycemia need not be impressive. Fifteen percent of patients with DKA have a glucose level less than 300 mg/dl. Also, although the majority of patients with DKA have an anion gap metabolic acidosis, there is a spectrum of different types of metabolic acidosis, ranging from purely anion gap to the nongap hyperchloremic type. The factor that determines which type of acidosis is present is linked with the patient's volume status on admission to the hospital. In addition, patients can present with a mixed acid-base problem, including coexistent metabolic acidosis, alkalosis, and respiratory alkalosis due, for example, to a combination of DKA in a patient who has been vomiting, and is thus volume contracted, and who has severe abdominal pain with resultant hyperventilation.

7. What are the other laboratory abnormalities seen in DKA?

Hyponatremia is seen in more than half of patients with DKA. Usually it is in the form of pseudohyponatremia, which does not mean that the low-sodium concentration is incorrect. Rather, it does not necessarily indicate that there is low-serum osmolality, since hyperglycemia is also present. The usual correction fraction for this is that for each 100 mg/dl increase in the glucose level, the sodium concentration decreases by 2 mEq/L. Hypertriglyceridemia can also cause this phenomenon.

Potassium levels are also frequently abnormal. They can be either elevated or depressed, but all patients are total-body-potassium depleted. However, because of the transcellular shifts of potassium seen with insulin deficiency and acidosis, the initial potassium value can vary. Of substantial importance is the fact that during the course of therapy, the serum potassium level drops precipitously because of insulin therapy, correction of the acidosis, and increased urine output with intravenous fluid repletion. Thus an initially "normal" serum potassium needs to be closely followed and repleted soon thereafter while treatment of the DKA ensues. A low potassium level on admission is an important finding, and potassium should be added to the first liter of fluids.

Lastly, as is the case with potassium, most patients with DKA are hyperphosphatemic on presentation to the hospital due to the effects of metabolic acidosis. Yet most of the patients are total body-phosphorus-depleted, which is further exacerbated by phosphorus moving into cells with treatment of the DKA. In DKA, the nadir is reached 2–3 days after admission to the hospital. However, in controlled studies, routine phosphate replacement has not been shown to be of benefit unless there is documented hypophosphatemia.

8. Is the determination of serum ketone levels helpful in the treatment of patients with DKA?

Serum ketones should be determined once, at the outset, in any patient in whom DKA is suspected. In general, significant ketonemia is not present unless the serum ketones are positive at a dilution of 1:2 or greater. There are three blood ketones: betahydroxybutyrate, acetoacetate, and acetone. In DKA, the ratio of betahydroxybutyrate to acetoacetate is only mildly elevated. However, in some cases of DKA, the great majority of the ketones may exist as betahydroxybutyrate, which is not picked up by the qualitative ketone measurements that detect only acetoacetate. Thus plasma ketones may be "falsely" low or negative. In fact, during successful therapy of DKA, these serum ketones may paradoxically rise or fail to fall, which is a result of decreased production of betahydroxybutyrate due to insulin treatment as well as from the conversion of betahydroxybutyrate (not measured) to acetoacetate (measured) prior to its utilization. Serial ketone levels therefore can be misleading and are not recommended.

9. How is DKA treated?

In order to avoid potential complications, there must be meticulous attention to detail. Insulin, fluids, and potassium supplementation are the cornerstones of therapy. The end point of insulin therapy is correction of acidemia and hyperglycemia. Unless there is severe insulin resistance, rarely will one require insulin doses in excess of 5–10 u/hr. Until the mid-1970s, larger doses of insulin—40–100 u/hr—were used; currently, low-dose insulin therapy (5–10 u/hr) is utilized. After rapid intravenous infusion of 5–10 u/hr of regular insulin, begin an insulin drip at 5–10 u/hr or .1 u/kg/hr, and measure the plasma glucose concentration 1 hour after starting the insulin infusion and at 1–2 hr intervals thereafter. If the glucose concentration is falling at a predictable rate of 75 mg/dl/hr, continue the drip at 5–10 u/hr. If the glucose concentration is unchanged or is slightly decreased, then the patient is insulin resistant, and infusion should be increased to 10–20 u/hr. Do not discontinue the insulin infusion if "hypoglycemia" (blood sugar less than 250 mg/dl) develops. When this glucose level is reached, switch the intravenous flush to one containing glucose, and continue the infusion at the previous rate. Remember that it takes longer to clear the ketoacidosis (10–20 hr) than it does to correct the hypoglycemia (4–8 hr). Also, most diabetologists agree that at least the first 2–3 liters of fluids should be in the form of isotonic saline to correct hypovolemia. Once this has been infused, hemodynamic considerations and attention to the serum sodium concentration should guide the choice of additional fluids.

10. Given that it may be misleading to follow serial ketone measurements during treatment of DKA, what is the best indicator of resolution of DKA?

The most reliable indicator of DKA resolution is the anion gap. Glucose will correct simply as a consequence of fluid repletion and thus cannot be relied on. Urinary ketones tend to remain detectable long after resolution of DKA. Therefore they are also not good predictors of successful treatment. However, when the anion gap returns to normal, ketoacid production has ceased. Once the electrolytes demonstrate a normal anion gap, continue the insulin infusion for a few more hours to ensure that control has been achieved. After that, if the patient can eat, one can return to the patient's previous insulin regimen if known and if satisfactory, and discontinue the insulin infusion.

11. Why do most patients develop a hyperchloremic nongap acidosis after therapy for DKA?

Although there are probably several factors that account for this finding, the most dominant factor is that renal threshold for ketones is quite low. Therefore with volume expansion there is increased excretion of ketones in the urine. These excreted ketones are "bicarbonate equivalents," which limit the availability of substrate to regenerate bicarbonate. Approximately 75% of patients recovering from DKA develop a hyperchloremic metabolic acidosis, which resolves over 48–72 hours. Development of the hyperchloremic metabolic acidosis does not indicate that the insulin infusion has failed.

12. What are the most common precipitants for development of DKA?

In most series, noncompliance with medication and infection are the most common precipitating events. Often, no definable cause is found. Leukocytosis by itself is not a sensitive or specific indicator of infection in DKA because leukocyte counts in the 20,000 range are commonly seen in DKA due to stress and hemoconcentration. Recently it has been shown that an elevated band count (10 or greater) is a sensitive and significant indicator of occult coexisting infection. Total leukocyte count, blood glucose, serum bicarbonate levels, and temperature have little value in predicting covert infection.

13. What are the major complications in DKA?
The mortality rate in DKA is in the 5–10% range. Diabetics rarely die of ketoacidosis itself. Normally, death is attributable to associated medical conditions. Hypothermia and coma are negative prognostic signs. A few complications are potentially associated with the therapy of DKA. The major ones are hypoglycemia, hypokalemia, hypophosphatemia, and cerebral edema. With regard to the latter, if sudden coma develops 12–24 hr after starting therapy, particularly in a younger patient, increased intracranial pressure should be suspected. Most cases of cerebral edema occur in patients whose blood sugar is rapidly reduced to the 250 range. Multiple theories have been advanced to explain this phenomenon; the most plausible one involves unfavorable osmotic gradients that develop during therapy.

CONTROVERSY

14. What is the role of bicarbonate therapy in the treatment of DKA?
There is lack of complete agreement regarding the use of bicarbonate therapy in the treatment of DKA. Those who favor it point to the deleterious side effects that acidosis causes. Those who are against its routine use are concerned with the potential for overshoot alkalosis and the development of paradoxical CNS acidosis. Recently a prospective study was performed to answer this question. Variable doses of sodium bicarbonate based on initial arterial pH (6.9–7.14) were given to patients in the treatment group and were withheld from the control group. Bicarbonate therapy did not significantly affect the outcome of DKA as measured by the time required for plasma glucose levels to reach 250 mg/dl, blood pH to reach 7.3, or bicarbonate levels to reach 15 mEq/L. No beneficial clinical or biochemical effects were noted. It must be remembered, however, that the minimum pH in the study was 6.9, and therefore there currently are no definitive data with regard to bicarbonate use in these patients with more severe DKA. Based on the aforementioned studies, many clinicians believe that bicarbonate should not be used in DKA, at least in those patients with pH of greater than 6.9.

There are, however, those who would argue that when the serum bicarbonate level is less than 5 mEq/L, bicarbonate should be administered. They criticize the aforementioned studies based on the study design and the fact that the patients were given only an average of 120 mEq of bicarbonate, and therefore they caution clinicians to continue considering alkaline therapy for severe DKA. Their argument is predicated on the fact that although more than 90% of ketoacidotic patients treated with only saline and insulin recover, a small fraction of patients dying from ketosis do so because of the deleterious hemodynamic effects of acidemia. These effects include myocardial dysfunction, arrhythmias, and antagonism of the effects of pressor-type compounds.

Those who support such usage argue that paradoxical cerebrospinal fluid acidosis has never been shown to cause clinically important sequelae. Also, concern regarding a decrease in tissue oxygenation through eradication of the beneficial Bohr effect has never been shown to alter in vivo tissue oxygenation in a clinically significant manner.

Ultimately each case of DKA must be evaluated on an individual basis in terms of the use of bicarbonate. A prudent approach may be to use small quantities of bicarbonate therapy if respiratory compensation is at its limit and serum bicarbonate is of the order of 5 mEq or less. In this scenario, any further diminution of the bicarbonate concentration would be associated with a severe decline in serum pH.

BIBLIOGRAPHY

1. Adrogue HJ, Wilson H, Boyd AE: Plasma acid base patterns in diabetic ketoacidosis. N Engl J Med 307:1603–1610, 1982.
2. Boris LR, Murphy MB, Kitabchi AE: Bicarbonate therapy in severe DKA. Ann Intern Med 105:836–840, 1986.
3. Fischer JN, Kitabchi AE: A randomized study of phosphate therapy in the treatment of DKA. J Clin Endocrinol Metab 47:177–180, 1983.
4. Gelfand RA, Matthews DE, Bier DM: Role of counter regulatory hormones in the catabolic response to stress. J Clin Invest 74:2238–2248, 1984.
5. Israel RS: Diabetic ketoacidosis. Emerg Med Clin North Am 7:859–871, 1989.
6. Kiefe C: Bicarbonate therapy in severe DKA. Ann Intern Med 106:635–636, 1986.
7. Kitbachi AE, Murphy MB: Diabetic ketoacidosis and hyperosmolar hyperglycemic nonketotic coma. Med Clin North Am 72:1545–1563, 1988.
8. Oh MS, Banergi MA, Carol HJ: The mechanism of hyperchloremic acidosis during the recovery phase of DKA. Diabetes 30:310–313, 1981.
9. Slovis CM, Mork EG, Bain RP: Diabetic ketoacidosis and infection. Am J Emerg Med 5:1–5, 1987.
10. Vinicor F, Lehrner LM, Carn RC: Hyperamylasemia in DKA: Sources and significance. Ann Intern Med 91:200–204, 1979.
11. Winegrad AI, Kern EFO, Simmons DA: Cerebral edema in DKA. N Engl J Med 312:1184–1185, 1985.

58. HYPEROSMOLAR NONKETOTIC COMA

Philip S. Mehler, M.D.

1. What is hyperosmolar nonketotic coma (HNC)?

This syndrome is classically defined as consisting of a plasma osmolarity greater than 350 mOsm/L, a plasma glucose greater than 600 mg/dl, and lack of ketoacidosis in a diabetic patient with an alteration of the level of consciousness. Currently it is appreciated that this is somewhat of a misnomer, becuase very few patients present with actual coma. Almost 50% of these patients may have a small increase in their anion gap and also mild metabolic acidosis.

2. Why do some diabetics present with diabetic ketoacidosis (DKA) and others with HNC?

The exact answer to this question is unknown. It has been thought that patients with HNC have enough endogenous insulin to suppress the release of free fatty acids but an insufficient amount to facilitate glucose transport and metabolism. However, this is probably not the reason, since it has been shown that insulin levels in both DKA and HNC are essentially identical. Rather, it presumably involves the availability of free fatty acids. Glucagon is one of the major mediators of ketogenesis, and the level of glucagon is significantly lower in HNC than it is in DKA, as are the lipolytic hormones such as growth hormone and cortisol. Therefore, availability of free fatty acids for ketogenesis is also less in HNC compared with DKA. Hyperosmolarity itself may also suppress ketone body formation.

3. How does HNC differ from DKA?

Generally, the average age of patients who present with HNC is much higher than with DKA. Two thirds have no previous history of diabetes in contrast to those with DKA, most of whom have been previously diagnosed as diabetic. Because a portion of HNC patients do not develop ketonemia, they have a much longer duration of symptoms prior to coming to medical attention as opposed to those with DKA, who are usually ill only 2–3 days before coming to the hospital. Because of this prolonged prehospital phase, patients with HNC have a much more severe level of dehydration and a higher degree of hyperglycemia and hyperosmolarity compared with the DKA population. In patients with DKA, there is rarely any significant change in mental status; in patients with HNC, a significant proportion have some degree of stupor. Further, the blood sugar tends to be much higher in hyperosmolar syndrome than in DKA, and acidosis is very mild, if present at all.

4. What is the basic pathophysiology of HNC?

The central causative mechanism involves a hyperglycemia-induced osmotic diuresis. The hyperglycemia emanates from a commonly identified diabetogenic stressor, such as infection, which precipitated the onset of the syndrome. This exhausts insulin reserves by hyperglycemic desensitization of the beta cell as well as induces a state of peripheral resistance to the effects of insulin. The resultant severe hyperglycemia, with average levels greater than 600 mg/dl, causes development of the glycosuric diuresis. This in turn results in hypertonicity and dehydration, because although a substantial amount of sodium is lost through the kidney due to osmotic diuresis, the water loss is greater relative to the extracellular fluid.

Further, osmotically activated glucose is located primarily in the extracellular fluid. When the concentration of glucose rises, water is osmotically drawn from the intracellular fluid until the intracellular fluid and the extracellular osmolarity are equalized. Such intracellular dehydration may be a prominent factor in producing the aforementioned central nervous system dysfunction in these patients. In response to this water shift, the serum sodium concentration falls 1.6 mEq/dl for every 100 mg rise of the serum glucose above 100.

There are additional pathophysiologic aspects to this syndrome. The decrement in intravascular volume impairs renal function and causes the glomerular filtration rate to fall. As this occurs, plasma glucose continues to rise. Additionally, a problem arises with the thirst mechanism in many patients with HNC. It is not mere coincidence that this syndrome is largely restricted to the infirm and neglected institutionalized patient who cannot recognize or respond to the need for water. Thus, the massive osmotic diuresis and its associated changes progress unabated until a change in mental status brings these patients to medical attention.

5. What are the main precipitants of this syndrome?

In contrast to DKA, in which a definable cause for the development of that state is often lacking, approximately one-half of patients with HNC have an associated illness that precipitated the syndrome. Sepsis, myocardial infarction, pancreatitis, gastrointestinal bleeding, hyperalimentation, and medications—including thiazide, steroids, and phenytoin, to name but a few—are the most frequently noted associated culprits. Presumably these stressors cause beta cell insufficiency in concert with peripheral insulin resistance and promote the development of profound hyperglycemia.

6. What are the common clinical manifestations?

The history is punctuated by insidious onset. Symptoms are often present for days to weeks before arrival at the hospital. If a history can be elicited, it is usually notable for complaints of progressive weakness, malaise, and perhaps hints of some possible precipitating events. Physical examination reveals substantial evidence of dehydration with tachycardia, hypotension, cool skin temperature, and decreased skin turgor. In contrast to DKA, there is usually no hypothermia. A depressed cognitive state, ranging from profound stupor to mild clouding of the sensorium, runs the entire gamut of neurologic abnormalities, including Babinski reflexes, seizures, and alterations of strength and sensation. With prompt and proper treatment, all of these neurologic abnormalities dissipate.

7. What are the laboratory findings associated with HNC?

The average serum sodium is 140 mEq/L, with a range of 119–188 being in the medical literature. In contrast to DKA patients, since patients with HNC are usually not profoundly acidotic, initial hyperkalemia is distinctly uncommon. Given the osmotic diuresis, there is generally potassium depletion due to urinary potassium losses. The serum bicarbonate level is usually mildly depressed to a level of 17–19 mEq/L with a small increase in the anion gap that is somewhat of a difficult finding to explain. At one time, it was presumed that this was attributable to an accumulation of lactic acid. However, further research has discounted lactic acid as the organic acid causing an increase in the anion gap. Currently it is not clear why these patients have an increase in the anion gap, but presumably it is due to accumulation of organic acids that remain undefined. Serum glucose usually exceeds 600 mg/dl, with values most commonly in the 1,000 mg/dl range, and serum osmolarity is greater than 320 mOsm/L. A leukocytosis with a white blood cell count of 15,000–20,000 is frequently found, usually due to the effects of dehydration. Similarly, hemoconcentration results in a hematocrit in the 55–60 range.

8. How is HNC treated?

The major aims of therapy for HNC are to reduce hyperosmolarity and restore intravascular volume. Although there is some controversy about what type of intravenous fluids to use, it is clear that a patient in a hyperosmolar state who is profoundly hypotensive and who has orthostatic blood pressure changes should initially receive normal saline at a rapid rate to expand volume. In this instance, volume repletion should take precedence over all other considerations. Even with the use of normal saline, the hypertonic state will also correct, because the isotonic fluid is hypotonic relevant to the patient at that time. Once blood pressure has risen to an acceptable level and urine output is adequate, it is controversial whether to continue with normal saline or switch to a more hypotonic type of fluid.

The rate of correction is also controversial. Most clinicians feel that it should be achieved slowly over 24–48 hrs. The water deficit in this setting can be calculated based on the "true" serum sodium concentration and on the assumption that 60% of the body's weight is water. An example follows: If body weight is 70 kg, this is multiplied by .6 to calculate total body water, which would equal 42 liters. If the "true" serum sodium concentration is 154 mEq/L, the water needed to lower serum sodium to 140 can be calculated as follows:

$$42 \times 154 = 140x$$
$$x = 46.2$$
$$46.2 - 42 = 4.2 \text{ liter deficit}$$

Half of this 4-liter deficit should be replaced over the first 12 hours, and the remaining estimated deficit during the second 12 hours. A rate of 2 mOsm/hr is usually advocated. Faster correction may be associated with deleterious CNS changes, because as extracellular osmolarity is rapidly decreased, an osmotic gradient may develop between the brain and the plasma, which could result in the movement of water into the brain, causing cerebral edema.

9. What is the role of insulin?

Given the fact that these patients have been ill for 1–2 weeks before seeking medical care and are usually severely volume depleted, a large amount of fluid is held in the intravascular space by the osmotic effect of glucose. Early reviews of HNC described many deaths among patients receiving insulin for the treatment of their condition. Presumably death was caused by rapidly progressive shock and hypotension concomitant with the rapid fall in blood glucose levels due to insulin. As insulin is given and glucose moves into cells, fluid follows, markedly compromising the integrity of the intravascular compartment. Further it has been shown that glucose levels will correct substantially with fluid replacement alone. Insulin should be administered only after sufficient volume has been infused to replete intravascular volume. If a continuous infusion of insulin is going to be used, doses of 0.5 u/kg/hr are usually sufficient and are less than used in DKA.

In managing these patients, it is also crucial to search for and treat any underlying illnesses that are commonly found to precipitate HNC, especially infectious diseases.

10. What are the major potential complications of the treatment of HNC?
A number of complications have been reported, one of which is vascular occlusion, which is probably due to the combined effects of hypotension, dehydration, hemoconcentration, and resultant hyperviscosity rather than a discrete, independent coagulopathy unique to HNC. Anticoagulant treatment is not routinely recommended. Aggressive volume repletion should negate the propensity for vascular thrombosis. An additional hematologic complication is disseminated intravascular coagulation. Cerebral edema may develop as HNC is being treated; its cause is somewhat equivocal but may be related to a rapid water shift into the brain if hypotonic fluids are used in the treatment protocol. As will be discussed below, cerebral edema is a rare entity in HNC and the exact mechanism is unclear. A pH-sensitive sodium-acid exchange, which also responds to insulin, may cause a transport of sodium into the cell in exchange for acid, resulting in cell swelling. Adult respiratory distress syndrome and rhabdomyolysis are two other serious complications that have been described in these patients.

CONTROVERSY

11. The major area of controversy in HNC concerns the choice of fluids. Some clinicians prefer hypotonic electrolyte solutions; some prefer isotonic ones. Basically, the argument is as follows: those who advocate isotonic fluids claim that use of hypotonic solutions causes too rapid a fall in extracellular fluid osmolarity. This rapid decrease in turn can cause cerebral edema, because with water loss at the onset of the illness, there is formation of new intracellular particles called idiogenic osmoles. These as yet undefined particles protect brain cell volume. With a rapid fall in extracellular fluid osmolarity, water is osmotically drawn into the brain by the idiogenic osmoles. These osmotically active particles take a finite period of time to return to an osmotically inactive state. This school of thought therefore recommends using isotonic solutions, which are actually hypotonic with regard to the patient's hyperosmolar state.

Those who believe that hypotonic fluids should be used partly justify their contention based on the deleterious potential of administration of excessive sodium as well as chloride, which can result in pulmonary edema. In addition, isotonic solutions do not remain hypotonic compared with the patient's serum, as their serum osmolarity decreases. The possibility of cerebral edema is dismissed as being purely theoretical since it is an extremely rare complication of HNC. Also, if it were a real concern, one would expect it to occur more frequently in nonketotic coma compared with DKA, but clinical experience indicates the exact opposite trend. Since mental status changes seem to correlate with the level of osmolarity, practitioners in the hypotonic camp advocate rapid reduction with a hypotonic fluid such as half-normal saline.

BIBLIOGRAPHY

1. Cahill GF: Hyperglycemic hyperosmolar coma: A syndrome almost unique to the elderly. J Am Geriatr Soc 31:103–105, 1983.
2. Carol P, Matz R: Uncontrolled diabetes mellitus in adults: Experience in treating DKA and hyperosmolar non-ketotic coma with low dose insulin regimen. Diabetes Care 6:579–585, 1983.
3. Kitbachi AE, Murphy MB: Diabetic ketoacidosis and hyperosmolar hyperglycemic non-ketotic coma. Med Clin North Am 72:1545–1563, 1988.
4. McCurdy DK: Hyperosmolar, hyperglycemic, non-ketotic diabetic coma. Med Clin North Am 54:683–699, 1970.

5. Pope DW, Dansky D: Hyperosmolar hyperglycemic non-ketotic coma. Emerg Med Clin North Am 7:849–857, 1989.
6. Rieff AI, Carol H: Non-ketotic hyperosmolar coma with hyperglycemia: Clinical features, pathophysiology, acid base balance, plasma cerebral spinal fluid equilibria and the effects of therapy in 37 cases. Medicine 51:73–94, 1972.
7. Rieff AI, Kleeman CR: Studies on mechanisms of cerebral edema in diabetic coma: Effects of hyperglycemia and rapid lowering of plasma glucose in normal rabbits. J Clin Invest 52:571–583, 1973.
8. Rosenthal NR, Barrett EJ: An assessment of insulin action in hyperosmolar hyperglycemic non-ketotic diabetic patients. J Clin Endocrinol Metab 60:607–610, 1985.
9. Wachtel PJ, Sillman RA, Lamberton P: Predisposing factors for the diabetic hyperosmolar state. Arch Intern Med 147:499–501, 1987.
10. Waldhaus LW, Kleinberger G, Korn A: Severe hyperglycemia: Effects of rehydration on endocrine derangements in blood glucose concentration. Diabetes 28:578–584, 1979.
11. Worthy IG: Hyperosmolar coma treated with intravenous sterile water. Arch Intern Med 146:945–947, 1986.

59. ADRENAL INSUFFICIENCY

Daniel Bessesen, M.D.

1. What structures and hormones control secretion of cortisol?

Cortisol secretion is under the control of a regulatory system called the hypothalamic-pituitary-adrenal (HPA) axis. In response to stimulation from higher brain centers, including the hippocampus, the arcuate and supraoptic nuclei of the hypothalamus secrete a 41-amino-acid compound identified as corticotropin-releasing hormone (CRH) into the portal circulation of the pituitary, where it stimulates the secretion of adrenocorticotropic hormone (ACTH). This peptide hormone enters the systemic circulation, where it stimulates the production and secretion of the glucocorticoid cortisol (and to a lesser extent mineralocorticoids) from the cortex of the adrenal glands. Cortisol or glucocorticoids used as pharmacologic agents then feed back on both the hypothalamus and the pituitary gland to inhibit the production of CRH and ACTH.

2. What is the normal pattern of cortisol secretion in health and under stress?

CRH, ACTH, and cortisol are secreted in a pulsatile manner with diurnal variation in normal individuals. In normals, cortisol is higher in the morning than in the afternoon. With stress, plasma cortisol increases and loses its diurnal variation. The increased cortisol level lasts only as long as the stress. For example, after an operation following significant trauma, one study found baseline cortisol to average 28 μg/dl; if there were no postoperative complications, plasma cortisol and 24-hour urinary cortisol were back to normal within 4 days.

3. What are the clinical signs and symptoms of adrenal insufficiency (AI)?

AI may present with complaints of anorexia, nausea, vomiting, abdominal or flank pain, diarrhea, fever, orthostatic dizziness, fatigue, and weakness. On physical exam, there may be fever (as high as 40°C), orthostatic or frank hypotension, tachycardia, and abdominal tenderness that can mimic an acute abdomen. The hypotension is caused in part by the volume depletion that accompanies electrolyte losses but is also due to a peripheral vasodilation, which occurs because of the lack of the permissive effect that cortisol provides for the vasoconstrictive effects of catecholamines. High-output congestive heart failure has even been reported. If the condition is chronic, hyperpigmentation—in particular, hyperpigmentation of gums, areolae, scars, and skinfolds—may be seen.

4. What are the laboratory abnormalities associated with AI?

The most common abnormality is hyponatremia. Hyperkalemia and hypochloremia may also be seen. Hypoglycemia may be present and may be severe. The complete blood count may show a leukocytosis and eosinophilia, and with volume depletion the hematocrit may be elevated. Occasionally the blood urea nitrogen may be elevated.

5. What is the differential diagnosis of AI?

Inadequate cortisol secretion can result from inadequate secretion from the adrenal glands due to either destruction or supression (primary AI), inadequate secretion of ACTH from the pituitary gland (secondary AI), or inadequate secretion of CRH from the hypothalamus (tertiary AI). Historically, the most common cause of AI was destruction of the adrenal glands by infectious agents like tuberculosis. Today, the most common cause of adrenal gland destruction is an autoimmune process, which may occur in isolation or along with other autoimmune endocrine disorders like hypothyroidism, type one diabetes mellitus, or gonadal failure.

The most common cause of secondary AI is an adenoma of the pituitary gland. This could be associated with a hormone-secreting syndrome such as acromegaly or galactorrhea/amenorrhea (from high prolactin levels), or a mass lesion in the sella (headaches, peripheral visual field defects). More than half of pituitary adenomas are not associated with a hormone-secreting syndrome. In these cases, by the time ACTH secretion is impaired, follicle-stimulation-hormone secretion and luteinizing-hormone secretion have usually been lost and the individual will have signs and symptoms of hypogonadism. Secondary AI may develop quickly in the setting of hemorrhage into a preexisting pituitary adenoma—so-called pituitary apoplexy. This usually presents with an acute onset of nausea, vomiting, and severe headache, and it may be associated with visual field defects or problems with extraocular movements. Pituitary hemorrhage can occur spontaneously in the postpartum setting, where it is referred to as Sheehan's syndrome. This usually occurs after a significant postpartum hemorrhage and should be considered in any woman who shows signs and symptoms of postpartum AI.

Tertiary AI can occur from infiltrative processes within the hypothalamus, such as sarcoidosis, or with tumors, such as craniopharyngiomas, gliomas of the optic chiasm, dysgerminomas, or pinealomas.

a. What about the patient with a history of chronic steroid use?

This individual may not be able to achieve an appropriate adrenal response to a stressful event such as an infection, myocardial infarction, or abdominal catastrophe and therefore may have relative AI in the setting of acute illness. The ability of pharmacologic preparation of steroids to suppress the normal secretion of the adrenal glands is a function of the potency of the preparation, the dose, and the duration of therapy. At a minimum, a dose of 60 mg of prednisone given for 7 days blunts the maximal cortisol response to ACTH in some individuals. At a maximum, those who have taken 40–60 mg of prednisone for 1–2 years may have a blunted response to ACTH for up to 2 years after discontinuation of the steroids. When in doubt about the type, the dose or the duration of previous steroid therapy, it is prudent to cover these patients with stress doses of steroids during an acute illness.

b. What about the patient with AIDS?

Symptoms usually associated with adrenal insufficiency are common among this group, as is histologic adrenalitis. In one series, involvement of the adrenal glands by cytomegalovirus was found in 37 of 74 patients who came to autopsy. However, most of these had focal fibrosis and inflammation and, clinically, were not adrenally insufficient. It probably takes destruction of 85–90% of the adrenal cortex to cause an abnormal response to ACTH. In a prospective evaluation of 40 patients withg AIDS, a blunted adrenal response to ACTH was found in only 3. Ketoconazole is an antifungal that is commonly used in patients with

AIDS. It has an antiglucocorticoid effect and may precipitate or worsen AI. Overall, biochemically significant AI that would benefit from treatment is uncommon in patients with AIDS but should be both tested for when appropriate and considered in a patient with AIDS who has hyponatremia, hyperkalemia, fever, abdominal pain, or orthostatic hypotension.

c. What about the patient with cancer?

The patient with cancer has a relatively high likelihood of having adrenal metastasis, but AI is uncommon.

d. When should the diagnosis of adrenal hemorrhage be considered?

Bilateral adrenal hemorrhage is an unusual cause of acute AI that occurs spontaneously in very ill individuals in the setting of sepsis, of hypotension, and postoperatively. A significant predisposing factor is thrombocytopenia, particularly related to heparin therapy, or a lupus anticoagulant. The patient on coumadin therapy is also at risk. The diagnosis of bilateral adrenal hemorrhage is suggested by enlargement of the adrenals with increased density on CT scan.

6. Diagnostic tests:

a. Should I do any test at all?

Sometimes when the clinician is faced with a severely ill patient and is considering the diagnosis of AI, there is a sense of urgency to give therapy immediately and then "sort out" the diagnosis later. The problem with this approach is that by the time the diagnosis can be established, the therapy may have impaired the clinician's ability to test adequately for AI, or the patient may have been treated unnecessarily with high doses of steroids for some time. For these reasons, some diagnostic test should be done concurrent with the initiation of empirical therapy. The therapy can then be discontinued if the tests later reveal that the HPA axis was normal.

b. Which test to order?

Again, when choosing a test, the clinician may not want to delay therapy and therefore may simply draw a random cortisol before initiating therapy. The rationale is that the patient is "stressed," and therefore this single value will be adequate to rule out AI. The problem with this approach is that often the value not only is not high enough to guarantee adequate adrenal reserve, but also is not low enough to definitively diagnose AI. The best test therefore is a cosyntropin stimulation test. A baseline cortisol is drawn; then 250 μg of cosyntropin is administered intravenously. A second cortisol can be drawn at 60 minutes. If there is an urgent need to give therapy, 10 mg of dexamethasone can be given after the baseline cortisol is drawn, as it will neither interfere with the assay for cortisol nor inhibit the response to cosyntropin.

c. What is an abnormal response?

There are a number of criteria for determining an adequate response to cosyntropin stimulation. These include a doubling of the baseline value, an increment of 10 μg/dl or greater, and a stimulated value greater than 20 μg/dl. The most important of these criteria is a peak value greater than 20 μg/dl.

7. Therapy:

a. Which steroid preparation to use?

The primary differences between different preparations of steroids are potency and degree of mineralocorticoid effect. Dexamethasone is the most potent glucocorticoid and has little mineralocorticoid effect. Methylprednisolone is much less potent than dexamethasone but shares its relative lack of mineralocorticoid action. This is potentially advantageous if sodium retention is to be avoided. Prednisone and prednisolone are intermediate in their potency and mineralocorticoid effects. Hydrocortisone has the most mineralocorticoid effects of the compounds mentioned and for that reason is the drug most often used in the setting of acute AI.

b. What dose to use?

The dosage should be adequate to replace what the normal adrenal gland would produce under the same physiologic stress. It is convenient to remember three levels of dosing: normal replacement, replacement for moderate stress, and replacement in the setting of life-threatening illness. These doses are as follows.

	Unstressed State	Moderate Stress	Life-threatening Stress
Dexamethasone	.75 mg/d	3–6 mg/d	7.5–30 mg/d
Methylprednisolone	4 mg/d	16–32 mg/d	40–80 mg/d
Prednisone	7.5 mg/d	20–40 mg/d	50–100 mg/d
Hydrocortisone	30 mg/d	80–120 mg/d	300 mg/d
Cortisone	37.5 mg/d		

One should become familiar with the dosing of at least two of these preparations and use them for most applications. A common dosing error is to stay with a maximal dose for too long. The normal adrenal secretion of cortisol returns to baseline within several days of severe stress if the acute event resolves.

BIBLIOGRAPHY

1. Brunko MW, Wolfe R: An unusual cause of an acute surgical abdomen. J Emerg Med 6:411–416, 1988.
2. Dahlberg PH, Goellner MH, Pehling GB: Adrenal insufficiency secondary to adrenal hemorrhage. Arch Intern Med 150:905–909, 1990.
3. Dobs AS, Dempsey MA, Ladenson PW, Polk BF: Endocrine disorders in men infected with human immunodeficiency virus. Am J Med 84:611–616, 1988.
4. Dorin RI, Kearns PJ: High output circulatory failure in acute adrenal insufficiency. Crit Care Med 16:296–297, 1988.
5. Harris MJ, Baker RT, McRoberts W, Mohler J: The adrenal response to trauma, operation and cosyntropin stimulation. Surg Gynecol Obstet 179:513–516, 1990.
6. Pulakhandam U, Dincsoy HP: Cytomegaloviral adrenalitis and adrenal insufficiency in AIDS. Am J Clin Pathol 93:651–656, 1990.
7. Sui SC, Kitzman DW, Sheedy PF, Northcutt RC: Adrenal insufficiency from bilateral adrenal hemorrhage. Mayo Clin Proc 65:664–670, 1990.
8. Soto-Hernandez JL, Verghese A, Hall BD, et al: Secondary adrenal insufficiency manifested as an acute febrile illness. South Med J 82:384–385, 1989.

60. THYROID DISEASE IN THE CRITICAL CARE SETTING

Michael T. McDermott, M.D.

1. Which thyroid conditions are most likely to be encountered in patients in a critical care setting?

The euthyroid sick syndrome is, by far, the most common thyroid condition seen in patients who are critically ill from nonthyroidal illnesses, being present to some degree in almost all such patients. Unrelated thyroid disorders such as thyroid nodules, nodular goiters, and treated or untreated hypothyroidism and hyperthyroidism may also be seen. Much less frequent, but far more serious, are the conditions that may actually be causing the critical illness: thyroid storm and myxedema coma.

2. What is the euthyroid sick syndrome?
The euthyroid sick syndrome consists of a group of abnormalities of the serum thyroid hormone profile seen in patients with both acute and chronic nonthyroidal illnesses. It is not a thyroid disorder per se, but rather a result of changes in peripheral thyroid hormone metabolism induced by the primary nonthyroidal illness.

3. What type of thyroid hormone profile is usually seen in patients with the euthyroid sick syndrome?
Patients with mild to moderate nonthyroidal illnesses most commonly have a modestly decreased serum triiodothyronine (T3) level. Patients with more severe nonthyroidal illnesses often have markedly reduced serum T3 levels and also have decreased serum thyroxine (T4) and increased T3 resin uptake (T3RU). The serum thyroid-stimulating hormone (TSH) level generally is either normal or mildly increased. Occasionally, patients with acute medical problems such as hepatitis, myocardial infarction, or an acute psychiatric condition may actually have transient elevations of both the T4 and T3 levels. Despite these changes in serum hormone levels, patients are euthyroid.

4. What causes these thyroid hormone changes in patients with the euthyroid sick syndrome?
Changes in serum thyroid hormone levels occurring in the euthyroid sick syndrome are due to alterations in peripheral thyroid hormone metabolism and transport. All such patients appear to have impaired conversion of T4 to T3 in the peripheral tissues (mainly liver and kidney), where the majority of the body's T3 is normally generated. More severely ill patients also have reduced thyroid hormone binding to normal transport proteins due to decreased hepatic synthesis of thyroxine-binding globulin (TBG) and to the presence of various circulating factors, such as free fatty acids and tumor necrosis factor, which impair T4 and T3 binding to TBG.

5. How can euthyroid sick syndrome be distinguished from hypothyroidism?
In the euthyroid sick syndrome, serum T3 is decreased proportionately more than is T4, the T3RU tends to be high normal or elevated, and the TSH is normal or mildly increased. In hypothyroidism, serum T4 is reduced proportionately more than T3, the T3RU tends to be low normal or low, and the TSH is usually more significantly increased. In hypothyroidism due to hypothalamic or pituitary disease, the TSH may be normal or low. In difficult cases, other tests such as the free T4 and the reverse T3 (RT3) may be helpful. In the euthyroid sick syndrome, free T4 is usually normal and RT3 is increased; in hypothyroidism, the free T4 and RT3 are both decreased.

6. Should patients with the euthyroid sick syndrome be treated with thyroid hormone?
Management of patients with the euthyroid sick syndrome is controversial. The majority of data from animal models and human studies indicate that treatment of euthyroid sick patients with T4 (levothyroxine) or T3 (liothyronine) replacement is not beneficial and may actually increase mortality. Current opinion favors giving no specific thyroid therapy. The disorder tends to resolve with appropriate treatment of and improvement in the primary nonthyroidal illness.

7. Does the euthyroid sick syndrome have any prognostic significance?
Current evidence would indicate that the prognosis for recovery from critical nonthyroidal illness may be fairly well predicted from the severity of the reduction in T3 and T4 levels.

8. Should patients who are being treated for hypothyroidism or hyperthyroidism and who are critically ill for other reasons be continued on therapy for their thyroid condition?
During a critical illness, patients with coincident hypothyroidism should continue to receive thyroid hormone therapy. Adequate amounts of thyroid hormone are believed to be necessary

for normal healing. Levothyroxine should be continued orally in the usual dosage or may be given intravenously at 50–75% of the usual oral dose. Patients with coincident hyperthyroidism should continue to be treated with antithyroid medications because uncontrolled hyperthyroidism would increase the heart rate and predispose to tachyarrhythmias. However, if granulocytopenia is present, antithyroid drugs should be discontinued because granulocytopenia may be caused or aggravated by these medications. Propylthiouracil and methimazole are administered orally, but methimazole may also be given as a suppository in the same dose.

9. What is thyroid storm?

Thyroid storm is a life-threatening condition characterized by an exaggeration of the manifestations of thyrotoxicosis.

10. What causes thyroid storm?

Thyroid storm usually occurs in patients with preexisting hyperthyroidism and one or more superimposed precipitating factors. The most common precipitating events are thyroid surgery (in patients whose underlying thyrotoxicosis has not been previously well controlled with medications), nonthyroid surgery, infection, trauma, and miscellaneous acute events.

11. What are the most common clinical manifestations of thyroid storm?

Patients with thyroid storm clinically present with multiple systemic manifestations. Fever (>102° F) and tachycardia are nearly always present; tachypnea is usually present, but the blood pressure response is variable. Cardiac arrhythmias are common, and congestive heart failure or ischemic heart disease may ensue. Nausea, vomiting, diarrhea, and abdominal pain are frequent features. Central nervous system manifestations include hyperkinesis, psychosis, and coma. A goiter and/or exophthalmos are helpful if found but may not be present or appreciated. Common laboratory abnormalities include anemia, leukocytosis, hyperglycemia, azotemia, hypercalcemia, and elevated liver-associated enzymes.

12. How is the diagnosis of thyroid storm made?

The diagnosis of thyroid storm must be made on the basis of these somewhat nonspecific clinical findings. Serum thyroid hormone levels will be elevated, but waiting for the results of such tests may cause a critical delay in the initiation of effective life-saving therapy. Furthermore, thyroid hormone levels are unable to distinguish patients with thyroid storm from those who may have uncomplicated thyrotoxicosis as a coincident disorder. Some conditions with which thyroid storm may be confused include sepsis, pheochromocytomas, and malignant hyperthermia.

13. How should patients with thyroid storm be treated?

Patients should be treated for thyroid storm as soon as the diagnosis is suspected on clinical grounds. Propylthiouracil—300–400 mg orally or by nasogastric tube—should be given as soon as possible and repeated every 6–8 hours. If the oral or nasogastric route is impossible, methimazole—30–40 mg per rectum—should be given every 6–8 hours. One hour after the antithyroid drugs are first given, 1–2 gm of sodium iodide should be started and administered intravenously over 24 hours, or 5 drops of saturated solution of potassium iodide (SSKI) may be given orally every 6 hours. Dexamethasone—2 mg intravenously every 6 hours—and (if congestive heart failure is absent) propranolol—40–80 mg orally or 1–2 mg intravenously every 6–8 hours—are also recommended. If these measures are unsuccessful, reserpine, guanethidine, or plasma exchange should be considered. Supportive therapy with oxygen and intravenous fluids is crucial. Antipyretics should be administered and external cooling undertaken if the temperature exceeds 105° F. Many experts have also recommended administering phenobarbital, glucose, and B vitamins. Precipitating factors must also be treated appropriately.

14. What is the prognosis for patients with thyroid storm?
When thyroid storm was first described, the acute mortality rate was nearly 100%. Today the prognosis is significantly improved when aggressive therapy, as described above, is initiated early; however, the mortality rate continues to be approximately 20%.

15. What is myxedema coma?
Myxedema coma is a life-threatening condition characterized by an exaggeration of the manifestations of hypothyroidism.

16. What causes myxedema coma to occur?
Myxedema coma usually occurs in elderly patients with underlying hypothyroidism and one or more superimposed precipitating factors. Important precipitating events include prolonged cold exposure, infection, trauma, surgery, myocardial infarction, congestive heart failure, pulmonary embolism, stroke, respiratory failure, gastrointestinal bleeding, and administration of a variety of drugs, particularly those that have a depressive effect on the central nervous system.

17. What are the most common clinical manifestations of myxedema coma?
Patients with myxedema coma present with numerous systemic manifestations. Moderate to severe hypothermia, bradycardia, and hypoventilation are common; the blood pressure, while generally reduced, is more variable. Pericardial, pleural, and peritoneal effusions are often found. An ileus is present in about two-thirds of patients, and acute urinary retention may also be seen. Central nervous system manifestations include seizures, stupor, and coma; deep tendon reflexes are either absent or exhibit a delayed relaxation phase. Typical hypothyroid changes of the skin and hair may be apparent. A goiter, though frequently absent, is a helpful finding; a thyroidectomy scar may also be an important clue. Laboratory abnormalities include anemia, hyponatremia, hypoglycemia, and elevated serum cholesterol and creatine phosphokinase levels. Arterial blood gases usually reveal carbon dioxide retention and hypoxemia. The electrocardiogram often shows sinus bradycardia, various types and degrees of heart block, low voltage, and T-wave flattening.

18. How is the diagnosis of myxedema coma made?
The diagnosis of myxedema coma must be made on clinical grounds based on the findings described above. Serum thyroid hormone levels are reduced, and TSH is elevated (if there is primary thyroid failure). However, the delay involved in waiting for these test results unnecessarily postpones the initiation of effective therapy in this critical condition.

19. How should patients with myxedema coma be treated?
Treatment for myxedema coma should be initiated as soon as the diagnosis is suspected on clinical grounds. Thyroid hormone replacement is the cornerstone of therapy. Levothyroxine (T4) 0.5 mg should be given intravenously followed by 0.025–0.05 mg each day until the patient is awake; then oral replacement of 0.05–0.1 mg per day should be given. Controversy exists over whether liothyronine (T3) in doses of 0.01–0.025 mg intravenously every 8–12 hours may be preferable, because T3 is more metabolically active than T4; there are currently no convincing data available to settle this question. Hydrocortisone, 75 mg intravenously every 6 hours, is also recommended, since transient or permanent adrenal insufficiency may also be present. Circulation and ventilation must be supported while thyroid hormone levels are being restored. The hypothermic patient should be rewarmed slowly by being covered with a blanket or, when the condition is severe, by central rewarming. Underlying or complicating conditions, such as infection, vascular events, heart failure, hyponatremia, hypoglycemia, and anemia, should be treated appropriately as well.

20. What is the prognosis for patients with myxedema coma?

Myxedema coma originally had a mortality rate of 100%. Today the outlook is much improved for appropriately treated patients, though the mortality rate in recent studies has varied from 0% to 45%.

BIBLIOGRAPHY

1. Brent GA, Hershman JM: Thyroxine therapy in patients with severe nonthyroidal illnesses and low serum thyroxine concentration. J Clin Endocrinol Metab 63:1–8. 1986.
2. Brooks MH, Waldstein SS: Free thyroxine concentrations in thyroid storm. Ann Intern Med 93:694–697, 1980.
3. Chopra IJ, Hershman JM, Pardridge WM, Nicoloff JT. Thyroid function in nonthyroidal illnesses. Ann Intern Med 98:946–957, 1983.
4. Fried JC, LoPresti JS, Micon M, et al: Serum triiodothyronine values: Prognostic indicators of acute mortality due to *Pneumocystis carinii* pneumonia associated with the acquired immunodeficiency syndrome. Arch Intern Med 150:406–409, 1990.
5. Hoffenberg R: Thyroid emergencies. Clin Endocrinol Metab 9:503–512, 1980.
6. Ingbar SH. Management of emergencies: Thyrotoxic storm. N Engl J Med 274:1252–1254, 1966.
7. Kaplan MM, Larsen PR, Crantz FR, et al: Prevalence of abnormal thyroid function test results in patients with acute medical illnesses. Am J Med 72:9–16, 1982.
8. Mackin JF, Canary JJ, Pittman CS: Current concepts: Thyroid storm and its management. N Engl J Med 291:1396–1398, 1974.
9. Menendez CE, Rivlin RS. Thyrotoxic crisis and myxedema coma. Med Clin North Am 57:1463–1470, 1973.
10. Morley JE, Slag MF, Elson MK, Shafer RB: The interpretation of thyroid function tests in hospitalized patients. JAMA 249:2377–2379, 1983.
11. Royce PC: Severely impaired consciousness in myxedema—a review. Am J Med Sci 261:46–50, 1971.
12. Sanders V: Neurologic manifestation of myxedema. N Engl J Med 266:547–552, 1962.
13. Simons RJ, Simon JM, Demers LM, Santen RJ: Thyroid dysfunction in elderly hospitalized patients: Effect of age and severity of illness. Arch Intern Med 150:1249–1253, 1990.
14. Slag MF, Morley JE, Elson MK, et al: Hypothyroxinemia in critically ill patients as a predictor of high mortality. JAMA 245:43–45, 1981.
15. Utiger RD: Decreased extrathyroidal triiodothyronine production in nonthyroidal illness: Benefit or harm? Am J Med 69:807–810, 1980.
16. Wehmann RE, Gregerman RI, Burns WH, et al: Suppression of thyrotropin in the low-thyroxine state of severe nonthyroidal illness. N Engl J Med 312:546–552, 1985.

61. HYPERCALCEMIA

Fred D. Hofeldt, M.D.

1. What is hypercalcemia?

The usual range of calcium measurement when performed as part of a multiphasic screening panel is 8.5–10.5 mg/dl (2.1–2.6 mmol/L). However, when calcium is determined by specific ethylenediaminetetraacetic acid (EDTA) titration method or atomic absorption spectroscopy, values of greater than 10.2 mg/dl are abnormal in women and 10.5 mg/dl in men. An ionized calcium measurement is available in many laboratories, and normal values vary from 4.5 to 5.3 mg/dl (1.1–1.3 mmol/L). Hypercalcemia is defined as a calcium that is elevated outside the normal range on at least three occasions. Serum calcium values between 10.6 and 10.9 mg/dl are often misleading and may not lead to detection of clinically significant disease, whereas values greater than 11.0 mg/dl are almost always indicative of disease.

2. What conditions can falsely elevate a serum calcium level?

- Hyperproteinemic states as may occur during excessive venous stasis during blood collection.
- Hyperalbuminemic states.
- Hypergammaglobulinemia or paraproteinemia states as occur with multiple myeloma.

3. What level of the serum calcium defines a hypercalcemic crisis?

Patients may manifest their symptoms quite variably to any elevated serum calcium level. However, a serum calcium in excess of 14 mg/dl should be considered a critical value and that patient treated under intensive monitoring.

4. How do we correct the serum calcium level for a low serum albumin?

As a rule, approximately 45% of the measured serum calcium is protein bound; 55% is diffusible. The protein-bound fraction is greatest for albumin compared to globulin. For a serum calcium of 10 mg/dl, approximately 0.8 mg/dl will be protein bound to globulin, and 3.7 mg/dl protein bound to albumin. For a low albumin state, the correction is that 1 gram of albumin will bind 0.8 mg of calcium.

For example: If the measured serum calcium is 7.6 mg/dl and albumin is 2.4 gm/dl, what is the corrected calcium? (Assume a normal serum albumin is 4.0 gm/dl.)

$$
\begin{array}{rl}
 & 4.0 \quad \text{normal level} \\
- & \underline{2.4} \quad \text{patient value} \\
 & 1.6 \quad \text{difference} \\
\times & \underline{0.8} \quad \text{amount calcium bound per gram of albumin} \\
 & 1.28 \quad \text{add this to measured calcium to adjust for low albumin state} \\
+ & \underline{7.6} \\
 & 8.88 \quad \text{mg/dl equals corrected calcium value}
\end{array}
$$

Hence the calcium is adjusted into the normal range and is appropriately low for the level of hypoalbuminemia.

5. How do we evaluate hypercalcemia when the serum albumin or total protein is elevated?

$$
\text{corrected serum calcium} = \dfrac{\text{measured serum calcium}}{0.6 + \dfrac{\text{total serum proteins}}{19.4}}
$$

6. What are the signs and symptoms of hypercalcemia?

They are frequently nonspecific but include irritability, weakness, fatigue, anorexia, nausea, vomiting, constipation, photophobia, and polyuria. Severe hypercalcemia may be associated with CNS and cardiac depression with progressive stupor, coma, and shock. Hypercalcemia is associated with a shortening of the Q-T interval, a prolonged P-R interval, and T-wave changes on EKG. The hypercalcemic patient may manifest nephrolithiasis or nephrocalcinosis. Many patients undergoing preventive care evaluations may be incidentally discovered to have a high serum calcium on routine chemistry panel.

7. What is the differential diagnosis of hypercalcemia?

After substantiating that hypercalcemia is a valid condition (by the measurement of at least two other serum calcium measurements) and noting that hyperproteinemia is not present, the clinician may consider primarily the existence of malignancies or hyperparathyroidism. The tumors include either solid tumors such as breast, lung, head and neck, renal, and prostate or hematologic malignancies such a myeloma, lymphoma, and leukemia. The other major consideration is hyperparathyroidism, which may exist with multiple endocrine adenomatosis type I or type II. The other endocrine conditions that can cause hypercalcemia are hyperthyroidism, hypoadrenalism, vitamin D intoxication, and Paget's disease, particularly when associated with immobilization. Certain drugs may be associated with hypercalcemia and include vitamin A intoxication, administration of thiazides and lithium, and the milk-alkali syndrome from the ingestion of absorbable calcium-containing antacids. Other causes include a variety of granulomatous diseases such as sarcoidosis, tuberculosis, and histoplasmosis. Hypercalcemia can also be associated with rheumatoid arthritis, especially during immobilization. Hypercalcemia can be noted in the patients after renal transplant, in the diuretic phase of acute renal failure, and as a condition called benign familial hypocalciuric hypercalcemia.

8. What are the most common causes of hypercalcemia?

Of the many above causes of hypercalcemia, the most common are malignancy in 45% of patients and hyperparathyroidism in another 45%. The large differential diagnosis includes the other 10% of the causes of hypercalcemia. Hence, from a practical approach, the evaluation of hypercalcemic disorders can be broken into two groups of parathyroid-hormone-mediated and parathyroid-hormone-nonmediated hypercalcemia.

9. What effects does parathyroid hormone (PTH) have on renal function?

PTH has many actions on the renal proximal tubule. It causes increased renal loss of phosphate with phosphate wasting, aminoaciduria, and increased tubular reabsorption of calcium; however, because the filtered load of calcium is high and the normal tubule reabsoprtion capacity of calcium is approximately $95 \pm 2\%$, patients with hyperparathyroidism may experience mild hypercalciuria. Hyperparathyroidism also causes a type II renal tubular acidosis, which manifests as a hyperchloremic metabolic acidosis. Parathyroid hormone also stimulates renal gluconeogenesis. Parathyroid hormone acts as a trophic factor for renal 1α hydroxylase regulation and generation of 1,25-dihydroxyvitamin D from its precursor 25-hydroxyvitamin D.

10. What laboratory features suggest that hypercalcemia is PTH-mediated?

Hypophosphatemia is seen in only 40–60% of patients with hyperparathyroidism, and its presentation varies considerably depending on dietary phosphate intake. A chloride greater than 104 mmol/L suggests hyperparathyroidism, as does a serum bicarbonate in the mildly acidotic range. A chloride/phosphate ratio of greater than 33 suggests hyperparathyroidism. An elevated 1,25-dihydroxyvitamin D level may be seen. An elevated PTH level is diagnostic. Today's generation of IRMA (immunoradiometric) and immunochemiluminometric PTH assays are highly specific for the patient with primary hyperparathyroidism and in most cases enable differentiation between patients with non-PTH-mediated hypercalcemia, particularly those with malignancies.

11. Are localization procedures helpful in hyperparathyroidism?

Preoperative localization procedures add little to the initial evaluation of the patient with hyperparathyroidism. The localization procedures lack both sensitivity and specificity in predicting the presence of the adenoma and are expensive. The best localization procedure is an experienced surgeon who in most all cases removes the adenoma or identifies parathyroid hyperplasia.

12. What percent of patients will have parathyroid adenoma?

Approximately 80–90% of patients with primary hyperparathyroidism will have a single parathyroid adenoma. Ten to 15% may have parathyroid hyperplasia. Less than 1% may have parathyroid carcinoma.

13. Does a 24-hour urine calcium measurement help in evaluating a hypercalcemic patient?
Yes. Before establishing the diagnosis of hyperparathyroidism, it is important that benign familial hypocalciuric hypercalcemia be eliminated from consideration. This familial autosomal dominant condition frequently affects family members with nonspecific symptoms, which may suggest a clinically significant disorder. However, when they are evaluated, they have a calcium/creatinine excretion of less than 0.01. These patients may have enlarged parathyroid glands due to increases in the amount of fat within the parathyroid glands. Parathyroidectomy does not cure the hypercalcemia.

The calcium/creatinine ratio (calcium/cr) is calculated as follows.

$$\frac{Calcium\ urine\ \times\ Cr\ plasma}{Creatinine\ urine} = Ca\ plasma*$$

*is total calcium
A value $> .01$ is seen in other hypercalcemic disorders.
A value $< .01$ is seen in benign familial hypocalciuric hypercalcemia.

14. What is the mechanism for hypercalcemia in malignancy?
The malignant tumor may be primarily invasive in bone, which may locally activate bone reabsorption or the tumor may be in a distal site from bone and resorption is stimulated by humoral substances that activate the osteoclast directly or indirectly.

15. What are the known humoral factors that can produce hypercalcemia?
Tumors may produce cytokines (osteoclastic-activating factor) to include interleukin-1, tumor necrosis, and colony-stimulating factor or other humoral substances such as prostaglandins of the E series, 1,25-dihydroxyvitamin D, transforming growth factors (TGF alpha and TGF beta), and the more recently described PTH-like or PTH-related peptide.

16. What is the significance of PTH-related peptide?
PTH-related peptide (PTHrP) was recently extracted and identified by complementary DNA probes to be produced by certain malignancies. PTHrP has been identified from squamous cell carcinoma, small-cell and anaplastic lung carcinoma, melanoma, and renal and breast carcinoma. The peptide is a larger molecular species than PTH, but its homology to the PTH molecule allows it to imitate some of the actions of the parathyroid hormone, particularly activation of bone resorption, phosphate renal wasting, and generation of renal cyclic adenosine monophosphate. Most often, the Cl/PO_4 ratio is < 33 in these malignancies.

17. What therapy is available for the hypercalcemic patient?
   A. Urgent Therapy
      1. Saline
         a. generally safe with 200–300 cc/hr but may need over 10 liters/day with careful monitoring. Use NS:D5W alternate 4:1 ratio with 20 mEq KCl/bottle (can follow urinary K+, Na+, and volume in order to document losses)
         b. may need 15 mg magnesium/hr
      2. Saline plus furosemide
         a. with aggressive management 80–100 mg furosemide intravensouly q 1–2 hrs and replace urinary electrolytes (*NEJM* 283:836, 1970)
         b. less urgent management 40 mg furosemide q 4–6 hr
         c. before using furosemide, be sure patient is adequately hydrated
      3. Calcitonin
         a. 4–8 IU/kg subcutaneously q 6–12 hr

4. Calcitonin plus glucocorticoids
   a. 4–8 MRC units/kg q 6–12 hr
   b. prednisone 40–60 mg/day
5. Intravenous diphosphonates (Didronel, 7.5 mg/kg, with 3 liters of saline over 24 hr and repeated daily for 3 days).
6. Gallium nitrate (avoid use if creatinine > 2.5 mg/dl); give 100–200 mg/m² of body surface in 1,000 cc NS over 24 hours daily for 5 days.
7. Intravenous phosphate
   a. given as 1,000 mg elemental phosphate (0.16 mM/kg) over 8–12 hr during each 24-hour period (caution: can cause hypotension)
   b. avoid use if serum phosphate elevated
8. Dialysis
9. Intravenous EDTA
   a. avoid use because it forms insoluble calcium compounds that damage kidney
B. Chronic therapy (adjunct therapy in addition to treatment of primary cause)
   1. Mobilization
   2. Oral phosphates
      a. 1,000–2,000 mg elemental phosphate (K-Phos, 3 tablets three times daily)
      b. avoid use if elevated serum phosphate
   3. Mithramycin (may also be used in semiacute situations)
      a. 25 μg/kg in 50 cc D5W given as infusion over 3 hr
   4. Glucocorticoids
      a. prednisone 50–60 mg/day
   5. Diphosphonates
      a. oral Didronel 5–20 mg/kg/day
   6. Aspirin or indomethacin (? usefulness) (*NEJM* 293:1278–1282, 1975)

18. (a) What is the treatment of choice for a patient with a serum calcium of 13 mg/dl and minimal symptoms? (b) What if the serum calcium is 19 mg/dl?

(a) Start saline to reexpand intravascular volume, then add furosemide to promote calciuretic diuresis. Other therapies that may need to be added include calcitonin, steroids, and mithramycin. If the hypercalcemia is unresponsive, IV administration of etidronate with saline or gallium nitrate may be helpful.

(b) Saline and furosemide are also first-line therapy for the patient with a calcium of 19 mg/dl. However, in this more critical situation, the next therapies to consider in order to rapidly lower the calcium would be IV diphosphonates, gallium nitrate, or phosphate if the patient does not have hyperphosphatemia. In emergent situations, dialysis is the treatment of choice.

19. What types of therapy can be used in the long-term management of the patient with hypercalcemia?

(1) Treatment of the primary disease causing the hypercalcemia, (2) encouragement of mobilization of the patient, and (3) oral phosphate administration of 1,000–2,000 mg of elemental phosphate, which may be useful if the serum phosphate is not elevated. Other treatments include oral steroids, oral etidronate, and repeated courses of mithramycin.

BIBLIOGRAPHY

1. Abbasi AA, Chemplavil JK, Farah S, et al: Hypercalcemia in active pulmonary tuberculosis. Ann Intern Med 90:324, 1979.
2. Blind E, Schmidt-Gayk H, Scharla S, et al: Two-site assay of intact parathyroid hormone in the investigation of primary hyperparathyroidism and other disorders of calcium metabolism compared with a midregion assay. J Clin Endocrinol Metab 67:353, 1988.

3. Broadus AE, Mangin M, Ikeda K, et al: Humoral hypercalcemia of cancer: Identification of a novel parathyroid hormone-like peptide. N Engl J Med 319:556, 1988.
4. Danks JA, Ebeling PR, Hayman J, et al: Parathyroid hormone-related protein: Immunohisto-chemical localization in cancers and in normal skin. J Bone Miner Res 4:273, 1989.
5. Henderson JE, Shustik C, Kremer R, et al: Circulating concentrations of parathyroid hormone-like peptide in malignancy and in hyperparathyroidism. J Bone Miner Res 5:105, 1990.
6. Lufkin EG, Kao PC, Heath H: Parathyroid hormone radioimmunoassays in the differential diagnosis of hypercalcemia due to primary hyperparathyroidism or malignancy. Ann Intern Med 160:559, 1987.
7. Marx SJ, Stock JL, Attie MF, Downs RW JR, et al: Familial hypocalciuric hypercalcemia: Recognition among patients referred after unsuccessful parathyroid exploration. Ann Intern Med 92:351, 1980.
8. Mundy GR: The hypercalcemia of malignancy. Kidney Int 31:142, 1987.
9. Mundy GR, Ibbotson KJ, D'Souza SM: Tumor products and the hypercalcemia of malignancy. J Clin Invest 76:391, 1985.
10. Purnell DC, van Heerden JA: Management of symptomatic hypercalcemia and hypocalcemia. World J Surg 6:702, 1982.
11. Ralston SH, Gallacher SJ, Patel U, et al: Cancer-associated hypercalcemia: Morbidity and mortality. Ann Intern Med 112:499, 1990.
12. Warrell RP Jr, Israel R, Frisone M, et al: Gallium nitrate for acute treatment of cancer-related hypercalcemia. Ann Intern Med 108:669–674, 1988.

IX: Hematology/Oncology

62. BLOOD PRODUCTS AND COAGULATION

Mark W. Bowyer, M.D.

1. What is measured by the partial thromboplastin time (PTT)?
The PTT assesses activities of the intrinsic pathway of the coagulation cascade. The intrinsic pathway includes factors XII, XI, IX, and VIII. A prolonged PTT with a normal prothrombin time (PT) suggests an inherited defect in coagulation.

2. What is the most common inherited factor deficiency?
Hemophilia A, a factor VIII deficiency, accounts for approximately 75%; factor IX deficiency (hemophilia B) accounts for about 20%.

3. What is measured by the PT?
The PT uniquely assesses the factor VII and therefore the extrinsic pathway of the coagulation cascade. It is prolonged in patients with liver disease.

4. What does heparin do?
Heparin is a synthetic anticoagulant, which markedly accelerates the effects of antithrombin III, a naturally occurring anticoagulant that neutralizes several activated clotting factors. The biologic half-life of heparin is less than 1 hour, so that its effects are reversible in 3–4 hours if an infusion is stopped. Heparin increases the PTT > PT.

5. What does coumadin (warfarin) do?
The major pharmacologic effect of coumadin is antagonism of vitamin K and therefore interference with the hepatic synthesis of vitamin K-dependent clotting factors (II, VII, IX, and X). Coumadin increases the PT > PTT.

6. What is the optimal hematocrit in critically ill patients?
Though controversial, it has been shown that optimal survival in critically ill patients is associated with a hematocrit of around 33%. In humans, oxygen delivery is constant to hematocrits as low as 22%. When the hematocrit is < 10%, arterial lactate levels rise, and mortality is about 70%.

7. What are the indications for the transfusion of blood?
Tissue hypoxia and a hemoglobin of less than 7 (hematocrit < 21) are the only two absolute indications for blood transfusion. Additional factors that must be considered are age of the patient, cause of the anemia, chronicity of the anemia, hemodynamic status, and presence of coexisting cardiac, pulmonary, or vascular disease.

8. How is blood preserved?
Banked blood contains CAPD—citrate, adenine, phosphate, and dextrose—and is stored at 4–7° Celsius to prevent bacterial growth.

9. How long can banked blood be stored?
The refrigerated storage life of blood collected in CAPD is 5 weeks. At the end of this period, about 70–80% of red blood cells are still viable, white blood cells and platelets are nonviable, and the clotting factors have very low levels of activity.

10. What are packed red blood cells?
Packed red blood cells (PRBCs) are made by removing two thirds of the plasma from a unit of whole blood, leaving 200–300 ml of volume. PRBCs are used primarily to restore oxygen-carrying capacity. PRBCs have less anticoagulant than whole blood and cause less volume expansion.

11. How much will one unit of PRBC raise hematocrit?
One unit of transfused PRBCs will raise hematocrit on the average of 3 points.

12. What is fresh frozen plasma (FFP)?
FFP is created when the plasma portion is removed from a unit of whole blood and then frozen. FFP contains factor V, factor VIII, and prothrombin, as well as antithrombin III, protein C, and protein S.

13. What are the indications for giving FFP?
1. Treatment of dilutional coagulopathy in a massively transfused patient.
2. Correction of warfarin anticoagulation (one unit of FFP will decrease the PT by 2 seconds).
3. Treatment of congenital or acquired coagulation factor deficiencies.
4. Treatment of antithrombin III deficiency.

14. What is cryoprecipitate?
Cryoprecipitate is formed when the plasma that is separated from whole blood is rapidly frozen, then allowed to rewarm. Cryoprecipitate contains most of the factor VIII and fibrinogen of the original unit of blood. Cryoprecipitate also contains factor IX, factor VIIIa, and von Willebrand's factor.

15. What are the indications for giving cryoprecipitate?
(1) Hemophilia A (factor VIII deficiency), (2) von Willebrand's disease, (3) hypofibrino-genemic states, and (4) bleeding from thrombolytic therapy.

In most circumstances, except for those listed above, it is preferable to give FFP, as it contains more of the essential clotting factors.

16. What is a hemolytic transfusion reaction?
Hemolytic transfusion reactions occur when ABO or Rh mismatched blood is given. It may occur with as little as 10 cc of blood infused and causes a fulminant, disseminated intravascular coagulation (DIC) with a resultant mortality of about 35%.

17. What are the classic findings in hemolytic transfusion reaction?
Chills, fever, flank or back pain, occipital headache, hypotension, oliguria, and hemoglobinuria.

18. How is a hemolytic transfusion reaction treated?
The most important treatment is to stop the transfusion. The patient is then given mannitol, intravenous fluids, heparin, bicarbonate, inotropes if required, platelets, cryoprecipitate, and ICU support. This treatment is directed toward the DIC that occurs.

19. What are the risks of transmission of transfusion-related disease?
The risk of contracting human immunovirus from a unit of blood is currently about 1 in 40,000. The risk of contracting serum hepatitis is now approximately 1 in 1,000, with the advent of hepatitis C (non-A, non-B) testing. Other rare diseases that may be transmitted by blood include cytomegalovirus, malaria, brucellosis, toxoplasmosis, and the Epstein-Barr virus.

20. What techniques are available to decrease the need for donor blood transfusion?
    Preoperative hemodilution: Blood is withdrawn before surgery, normovolemia is maintained with fluids and after surgery, and the saved blood is reinfused.
    Preoperative autologous blood donation: Patients may donate up to six units of their own blood over the 6 weeks prior to a planned surgery.
    Intraoperative autotransfusion: Blood lost by the patient during surgery is collected, washed, and reinfused.

BIBLIOGRAPHY

1. Anderson BV: Current autologous practices. Transfusion 28:394, 1988.
2. Bove JR: Transfusion associated with hepatitis and AIDS: What is the risk? N Engl J Med 317:242, 1987.
3. Capon SM, Sacher RA: Hemolytic transfusion reactions: A review. J Intens Care Med 4:100, 1989.
4. Coffin CM: Current issues in transfusion therapy: Indications for use of blood components. Postgrad Med 81:343, 1987.
5. Czer LS, Shoemaker WC: Optimal hematocrit value in critically ill postoperative patients. Surg Gynecol Obstet 147:363, 1978.
6. Kruskall MS, Mintz PD, Bergin JJ, et al: Transfusion therapy in emergency medicine. Ann Emerg Med 17:327, 1988.
7. Lisander B: Preoperative haemodilution. Acta Anaesthesiol Scand 32 (Suppl 89):63, 1988.
8. Morduchowicz G, Pitlik SD, Huminer D, et al: Transfusion reactions due to bacterial contamination of blood and blood products. Rev Infect Dis 13:307–314, 1991.
9. NIH Consensus Development Conference Summary: Fresh frozen plasma: Indications and risks. Transfus Med Rev 1:201, 1987.
10. NIH Consensus Development Summary: Perioperative red blood cell transfusion. JAMA 260:2700, 1988.
11. NIH: Transfusion alert: Indications for the use of red blood cells, platelets, and fresh frozen plasma. Publication of the Department of Health and Human Services, Spring 1989.
12. Tarnover A, Clark D: Blood component therapy: New guidelines for avoiding complications. Postgrad Med 86:48, 1989.

63. THROMBOCYTOPENIA AND PLATELETS

Mark W. Bowyer, M.D.

1. How is thrombocytopenia defined?
A platelet count of less than 100,000 per cubic millimeter is generally considered to constitute thrombocytopenia.

2. What are the mechanisms of thrombocytopenia?
A low platelet count may result from one mechanism or a combination of mechanisms. These include abnormal platelet production, disordered platelet distribution, and increased rate of destruction.

3. What disorders lead to abnormal platelet production?

Reduced thrombopoiesis may result from injury to the bone marrow from drugs, chemicals, radiation, or infection. Congenital or acquired marrow failure, marrow invasion from carcinoma, leukemia, lymphoma, or fibrosis and lack of marrow stimulation, as in congenital thrombopoietin deficiency, may all lead to decreased platelet production. Defective maturation of platelets may occur with vitamin B_{12} or folic acid deficiencies or as the consequence of a hereditary disorder such as Wiskott-Aldrich syndrome.

4. What factors may lead to disordered platelet distribution?

Splenomegaly may lead to sequestration of platelets with resultant thrombocytopenia. In normal individuals, about 30% of the circulatory platelets are present in the spleen, whereas in massive splenomegaly, up to 80% of the circulating platelets may be there. This thrombocytopenia is rarely severe enough to produce hemorrhage. Splenectomy restores the platelet count to normal but is rarely needed.

5. What conditions are associated with accelerated destruction of platelets?

The most common causes of accelerated platelet destruction are antibody-mediated platelet injury, increased platelet utilization as in disseminated intravascular coagulation, and severe blood loss with multiple transfusions.

6. What are some of the conditions associated with antibody-mediated thrombocytopenia?

Antibody-mediated thrombocytopenia may be due to autoantibodies as in idiopathic thrombocytopenic purpura, systemic lupus erythematosus, and chronic lymphocytic leukemia, and in association with autoimmune hemolytic anemia. Alloantibodies following transfusions or as a result of fetal-maternal incompatibility also produce thrombocytopenia. Antibodies associated with the administration of certain drugs, such as heparin, quinidine, quinine, and sulfamides, may produce thrombocytopenia. Finally, thrombocytopenia is being seen with increasing frequency as an autoimmune phenomenon associated with AIDS.

7. What is idiopathic thrombocytopenic purpura (ITP)?

ITP is a prototypic example of an autoimmune process. In ITP, IgG antibodies directed against specific platelet antigens are responsible for platelet destruction. Acute ITP is usually self-limited, with life-threatening bleeding occurring only rarely.

8. What is the treatment of chronic ITP?

The initial therapy for ITP consists of corticosteroids. If the platelet count does not rise substantially within 2–4 weeks, splenectomy is usually the next step. Splenectomy produces prolonged remission in 80–90%. Those who fail splenectomy may benefit from vincristine, anabolic steroids, or gamma globulin.

9. What are the characteristics of heparin-induced thrombocytopenia?

Given the almost ubiquitous use of heparin in the intensive care setting, heparin-induced thrombocytopenia merits special attention. The incidence of heparin-induced thrombocytopenia is reported to be around 5%. The mechanism is uncertain but is probably immunologic, and a heparin-dependent platelet-aggregating factor can be found in the serum of many patients. Thrombocytopenia usually occurs 6–12 days after the initiation of heparin therapy or may occur immediately after repeated exposure to the drug. Only minimal amounts of heparin, such as that used for flushing indwelling venous lines, may be necessary. Platelet counts should be made regularly in all patients receiving heparin, and the drug discontinued if the count falls significantly.

10. Does sepsis contribute to thrombocytopenia?

Thrombocytopenia, sometimes profound, commonly is associated with septicemia. An immunologic mechanism has been implicated by studies showing increased amounts of IgG directed against platelets in septic patients. Successful treatment of the septicemia cures the thrombocytopenia.

11. What laboratory test measures platelet function?

The bleeding time is a sensitive measurement of platelet function.

12. What are some causes of platelet dysfunction in the ICU setting?

Many of the drugs utilized in the intensive care unit can cause platelet dysfunction. These include many of the antibiotics, nitrates, local anesthetics, alpha- and beta-blockers, xanthines, diuretics, and dextran. Uremia, which is commonly seen in the ICU, is another important cause of platelet dysfunction. The "toxin" responsible for defect is not well defined, but it appears to be related to impaired platelet–von Willebrand factor interactions.

13. How are platelet dysfunction disorders managed?

All unnecessary drugs should be viewed as suspect and discontinued in patients who have evidence of platelet dysfunction. Platelet transfusion may be necessary in some instances. The primary therapy for uremia-associated platelet dysfunction is dialysis. However, cryoprecipitate, 1-desamino-8-D-arginine vasopressin (DDAVP), and conjugated estrogens have been used with good results.

14. How does aspirin affect platelet function?

Aspirin irreversibly inhibits platelet cyclo-oxygenase, resulting in a function defect that lasts the duration of the platelet's life span (8–9 days). A single aspirin results in a platelet hemostatic defect that remains in 50% of the circulating platelets 5 days after its ingestion.

15. What platelet count is necessary?

A normal platelet count ranges from 150,000 to 400,000/microliter. Experience from patients with leukemias has shown that those with a platelet count greater than 50,000 are unlikely to bleed excessively, even with surgery or trauma. In patients with a count between 5,000 and 50,000, the risk of bleeding depends on the clinical circumstance. When the platelet count is less than 5,000, vascular integrity is disrupted, and spontaneous bleeding is likely to occur.

16. What are the indications for platelet transfusion?

Platelets are transfused prophylactically in patients with a count between 5,000 and 20,000 and in patients with a count of less than 50,000 who need an invasive procedure. Therapeutic uses of platelets include use in patients with a platelet count of less than 50,000 who are actively bleeding and in patients who are bleeding from a functional defect (bleeding time two times normal).

17. How much does a one-unit transfusion of platelets increase the count?

A one-unit transfusion of platelets increases the platelet count by 5,000–10,000.

BIBLIOGRAPHY

1. Becker PS, Miller VT: Heparin-induced thrombocytopenia. Stroke 20:1449–1459, 1989.
2. Belluci S. Autoimmune thrombocytopenias. Balliere's Clin Haematol 2:695–718, 1989.
3. Brannan DP, Guthrie TH: Idiopathic thrombocytopenic purpura in adults. South Med J 81:75–80, 1988.
4. Farmer JC, Parker RI: Coagulation disorders. In Civetta JM, Taylor RW, Kirby RR (eds): Critical Care. Philadelphia, J.B. Lippincott, 1988, pp 1469–1480.

5. Glassman AB: Thrombocytopenia: Proposed mechanisms and treatment in human immunodeficiency virus infection. Ann Clin Lab Sci 19:319–322, 1989.
6. Hardesty RM: Disorders of platelet secretion. Balliere's Clin Haematol 2:673–694, 1989.
7. Miller ML: Heparin-induced thrombocytopenia. Cleve Clin J Med 56:483–490, 1989.
8. Murphy WG, Kelton JG: Idiosyncratic drug-induced thrombocytopenia. Curr Stud Hematol Blood Transf 54:71–88, 1988.
9. Sears DA: Hematologic diseases requiring critical care. In Civetta JM, Taylor RW, Kirby RR (eds): Critical Care. Philadelphia, J.B. Lippincott, 1988, pp 1503–1515.
10. Slichter SJ: Platelet transfusion therapy. Hematol Oncol Clin North Am 4:291–311, 1990.
11. Vermylen J, Blockmans D: Acquired disorders of platelet function. Balliere's Clin Haematol 2:729–748, 1989.

64. DISSEMINATED INTRAVASCULAR COAGULATION

Madeline White, M.D.

1. What is disseminated intravascular coagulation (DIC)?
DIC is not a disease entity in itself but a dynamic condition incorporating clotting activation, thrombin generation, consumption of coagulation factors, deposition of fibrin, and, in turn, fibrinolysis. Both excess thrombin and plasmin can be produced; therefore, both thrombosis and bleeding can be seen simultaneously.

2. What are the various forms of DIC?
It can be acute and fulminant, such as in amniotic fluid embolism and meningococcemia, or chronic, subtle, and asymptomatic, as in some cases of disseminated malignancy and collagen vascular disease. The consumption can occur systemically throughout the entire vascular system, or it can be localized as in hemangiomas, aortic aneurysms, and renal allograft rejection.

3. What characterizes acute and chronic DIC?
In acute DIC, thromboplastic material (endogenous or exogenous) is released suddenly into the vascular system. The balancing mechanisms of coagulation inhibitors and of the fibrinolytic system are overwhelmed. Thrombosis occurs, and coagulation factors are consumed. Major bleeding ensues, and microvascular thromboses cause tissue ischemia and dysfunction.

In chronic DIC, the coagulation activation is met by increased factor and platelet production and increased activity of the fibrolytic system. It is a compensated state, and its presentations are quite variable. Mild bleeding may occur, as may macrovascular thromboses (deep venous thrombosis, arterial emboli), but microvascular thromboses and resulting organ damage are unusual. If nonbacterial thrombotic endocarditis develops, systemic embolization and infarction will be seen. At the other extreme, chronic DIC may present with laboratory abnormalities only.

4. In critical care, which conditions are associated with acute DIC?
Any condition that produces damage or disruption of vascular endothelium or that releases damaged or necrotic tissue into the bloodstream can be the trigger for DIC. Classically, obstetrical complications, sepsis, injuries (especially brain and crush injuries), shock, hypoxia, burns, vasculitis, transfusion reactions, anaphylaxis, immune complex diseases, and treatment of malignancies such as acute promyelocytic leukemia are among the 100 or so causes of acute DIC.

5. What are some of the common causes of chronic DIC?

Malignancies—especially disseminated prostate cancer, mucin-producing adenocarcinomas, and the leukemias like promyelocytic leukemia—can be associated with chronic DIC. Vascular disorders such as giant hemangiomas, aortic aneurysms, and valvular heart disease can produce local consumption with systemic signs. Some obstetrical complications, such as eclampsia and retained dead fetus syndrome, can have a chronic picture. Other associated conditions include acute myocardial infarction, peripheral vascular disease, paroxysmal nocturnal hemoglobinuria, polycythemia vera, myeloid metaplasia, autoimmune diseases, glomerulonephritis, sarcoidosis, amyloidosis, diabetes, hyperlipoproteinemias, and liver disease. At any time, the balance may shift and an acute picture emerge.

6. What are the clinical signs of acute and chronic DIC?

In acute DIC, when microvascular thrombi predominate, skin, kidneys, and lungs are major targets, but brain, gastrointestinal tract, liver, heart, and pancreas are commonly affected. Acral cyanosis, delerium, coma, oliguria, azotemia, hypoxia, dyspnea, and ulceration reflect the tissue ischemia. Damage continues as skin necrosis, gangrene, cerebral infarction, renal cortical necrosis, and pulmonary and bowel infarction develop. If bleeding predominates, petechiae and ecchymoses will appear, and puncture sites ooze. Genitourinary, pulmonary, gastrointestinal, and intracranial hemorrhage can follow.

In chronic DIC, the bleeding may be milder, with oozing of mucous membranes and puncture sites as well as petechiae and ecchymoses. Venous thrombi with pulmonary emboli as well as arterial emboli can be a feature. As stated above, chronic DIC may be silent clinically and disturb lab values only.

7. What lab values indicate DIC in the acute and chronic forms?

In acute DIC, there are prolongation of prothrombin time (PT), activated partial thromboplastin time (APTT), and thrombin time; fall of platelets and fibrogen; and elevation of fibrin/fibrinogen degradation products (FDPs). In the chronic or compensated form, a more variable pattern is seen. Changes similar to acute DIC but less severe can be present. In many cases, however, PT and APTT can be normal or "supernormal" due to the presence of activated factors affecting the in vitro tests. Fibrinogen can be normal or elevated as an acute phase reactant. Platelets can be normal or just slightly depressed. FDP should be elevated in just about all cases. There are numerous other specialized coagulation tests that become abnormal with DIC but are not commonly available.

8. What clues are present in the peripheral smear for DIC?

Features of a DIC smear are red cell fragments (schistocytes), polychromatophilia, leukocytosis with a left shift, and thrombocytopenia. Schistocytes are present in almost all chronic DIC (90%), less so in acute DIC (50%). The other features vary with conditions underlying the DIC.

9. What conditions can alter the findings of DIC?

Because the liver is the main producer of coagulation factors, impairment of its synthetic function can confuse the diagnostic picture of DIC and hamper recovery from consumption. Poor reticuloendothelial clearance of FDPs can allow elevated levels beyond the active generation time and cause platelet dynsfunction and prolonged thrombin times. Fibrinogen, as an acute phase reactant, can be normal or elevated, and only by comparing levels over time can consumption be documented.

10. What is the treatment of of DIC?

In both acute and chronic DIC, initial therapy is directed toward the triggering event. Hemodynamic support is critical in acute fulminant DIC. More specific tools, depending on the cause of DIC, include evacuation of the uterus, antibiotics, and antineoplastic therapy. If the inciting event cannot be reversed, or, if reversed, a prolonged recovery time is expected, therapy may be needed for the DIC process itself to prevent further thromboses and exsanguination. Most authors urge stopping the consumption process with intravenous or subcutaneous heparin before replacing specific coagulation components (fresh frozen plasma, cryoprecipitate, platelets). If bleeding continues after consumption is controlled and hemostatic factors are replaced to satisfactory levels, a few consider antifibrinolytic therapy with epsilon-aminocaproic acid. Its use is hazardous, since blocking fibrinolysis may accelerate microvascular clotting.

In chronic DIC, hemorrhage is not usually life threatening, but thrombosis may be a serious complication. After attention to the triggering event, anticoagulation may or may not be appropriate. Subcutaneous heparin, oral anticoagulants, and antiplatelet agents (aspirin, dipyridamole) have had variable success. Component therapy is rarely needed.

11. How is the efficacy of DIC therapy evaluated?

The clinical situation and the lab parameters should stabilize or improve. FDP should fall, and fibrinogen levels should rise in 3–6 hours if liver function is adequate. Improvement in platelets, PT, and APTT may vary with replacement efforts and with the endogenous production rates of the various elements. Thrombotic and bleeding phenomena should gradually cease.

Here is how Feinstein[6] handles heparin therapy:
1. Initiate heparin at 7.5 U/kg/hr IV.
2. One or 2 hours later give platelets to reach a count of 50,000 (one pack should increase count by 5,000–10,000), and give cryoprecipitate to reach a fibrinogen of 150 (one unit should increase fibrinogen by 5–10 mg/dl).
3. Measure platelet and fibrinogen levels 30–60 minutes posttransfusion.
4. Repeat determinations every 6–12 hours.
5. If adequate counts and levels cannot be attained or counts and levels fall, increase heparin by 2.5 U/kg/hr.
6. Repeat sequence of evaluation.

Bick[2] offers an alternative approach. Faced with continued significant bleeding or clotting 4 hours after aggressive therapy for the inciting event, he starts subcutaneous heparin (80 U/kg every 4–6 hrs). In 3–4 hours, he looks for increased fibrinogen, falling FDPs, and slow or rapid correction of other lab abnormalities. Cessation of problematic bleeding or clotting should follow.

CONTROVERSIES

12. Is heparin really indicated in DIC?

There are a few objective studies. Most authors agree that termination of the inciting event is the most desirable approach. This is most effective in obstetric complications, when evacuation of the uterus, hemodynamic support, and component therapy as needed can be successful. The numerous other causes of DIC are more difficult to control, and heparin may be used to blunt the consequences of ongoing DIC. Some believe that heparin is indicated in amniotic fluid embolism, severe transfusion reactions, macrovascular thromboses, prevention of DIC with treatment of promyelocytic leukemia, retained fetus syndrome, purpura fulminans, septic abortion, heat stroke, and septicemia. Others feel that it is of no help in sepsis, shock, or obstetric complications. Its use in patients with renal or hepatic failure, extensive vascular damage, severe thrombocytopenia, or hypofibrinogenemia is hazardous. Most authors stress that, if heparin is administered, careful monitoring of its efficacy, as outlined above, is the key to responsible therapy.

13. What dose of heparin is effective?

Full-dose heparin is used for embolic events and major vessel occlusion. The dose necessary to control microvascular thromboses and to stop consumption remains controversial. Some recommend full-dose heparin; others feel that low-dose heparin (500 units/hr intravenously or 80 units/kg every 4–6 hr s.c.) may suffice to prevent new thromboses at the microvascular level.[2,6] The dose of heparin can be increased if necessary to achieve therapeutic efficacy, and there is less risk of hemorrhage with the lower dosing levels. Intravenous heparin allows better moment-to-moment control than subcutaneous heparin. Whatever method is chosen, the clinical situation, fibrinogen, and FDP levels along with platelet counts should be monitored for stabilization or improvement.

14. What other tests can aid in diagnosis of DIC?

In the DIC process, fibrin is generated, then lysed by plasmin. FDP levels are felt to be the most sensitive test for the combined result of thrombin and plasmin activation. FDP measures the products of both fibrinogen and fibrin degradation. The D-Dimer test detects elevated levels of fragments of cross-linked fibrin. It specifically shows that thrombin has been produced, causing the cross-linking of fibrin clot via activated factor XIII and that fibrinolysis has occurred via plasmin action. It is a confirmatory test for interpreting elevated FDP and is specific for fibrin degradation.

BIBLIOGRAPHY

1. Baker WF: Clinical aspects of disseminated intravascular coagulation: A clinician's point of view. Semin Thromb Hemost 15:1–57, 1989.
2. Bick RL: Disseminated intravascular coagulation and related syndromes: A clinical review. Semin Thromb Hemost 14:294–338, 1988.
3. Carr JM, McKinney M, McDonoagh J: Diagnosis of disseminated intravascular coagulation. Am J Clin Pathol 91:280–287, 1989.
4. Carr ME: Disseminated intravascular coagulation: Pathogenesis, diagnosis and therapy. J Emerg Med 5:311–322, 1987.
5. Cembrowski GS, Griffin JH, Mosher DF: Diagnostic efficacy of six plasma proteins in evaluating consumptive coagulopathies. Arch Intern Med 146:1997–2002, 1989.
6. Feinstein DI: Treatment of disseminated intravascular coagulation. Semin Thromb Hemost 14:351–362, 1988.
7. Fruchtman S, Aledort LM: Disseminated intravascular coagulation. J Am Coll Cardiol 8:159B–167B, 1986.
8. Ratnoff OD: Hemostatic emergencies in malignancy. Semin Oncol 16:561–571, 1989.
9. Williams WJ, Beutler E, Erslev AJ (eds): Hematology, 4th ed. New York, McGraw-Hill, Inc., 1990.

65. SICKLE CELL DISEASE

Kathryn Hassell, M.D.

1. What is sickle cell disease?

The term "sickle cell disease" refers to a group of inherited hemoglobinopathies in which abnormal beta-hemoglobin chains are produced as a result of a single amino acid substitution. Hemoglobin S is produced when valine is substituted for glutamic acid in the sixth position of the beta chain; hemoglobin C is produced when lysine is substituted in the sixth position. Patients can carry one hemoglobin S gene (AS) and have sickle cell trait; this is not associated with significant disease except for concentrating defects in the kidney, occasional hematuria, and, less commonly, papillary necrosis.

Patients who have two hemoglobin S genes (SS) have sickle cell anemia. This is characterized by hemolytic anemia, with a baseline elevated reticulocyte count and indirect bilirubin, as well as episodic painful ischemic events due to sickling of the red blood cells, with occlusion of small blood vessels by the deformed cells.

Patients who have one hemoglobin S gene and one hemoglobin C gene have Hgb SC disease. Clinically, this is usually associated with milder anemia and fewer painful episodes than sickle cell anema.

Patients who have one gene for hemoglobin S and a gene mutation for beta-thalassemia have S-β^+ thalassemia disease. This form of sickle cell disease is usually less severe, with mild anemia and relatively few painful episodes compared with sickle cell anemia.

When sickle cells are exposed to extreme conditions, such as hypoxia or osmotic changes (e.g., dehydration), the sickle hemoglobin can polymerize, and the red cell assumes a sickled shape, which occludes small vessels and can cause acute and chronic organ damage.

2. How is sickle cell disease diagnosed?
Sickle cell hemoglobins can be detected by hemoglobin electrophoresis. Due to the differences in charges, hemoglobin S and hemoglobin C migrate differently from normal hemoglobin A. Use of a "sickle cell prep," which detects the presence of hemoglobin S, cannot distinguish between sickle cell trait (AS), sickle cell anemia (SS), Hgb SC disease, or S-β^+ thalassemia, because it does not quantitate the amount of sickle hemoglobin present.

3. What evaluation should be done for a patient presenting with a painful sickle cell crisis?
A painful crisis, characterized in many patients by diffuse pain in the back, abdomen, or extremities, is often brought on by a precipitating event, which must be corrected and/or reversed to prevent further sickling. Extremes of temperature and heavy physical exertion often predispose to crises; dehydration can occur easily with poor oral intake or excessive fluid losses due to the renal concentrating defect induced by chronic ischemia to the renal medulla. Infections are frequently present and can precipitate a painful crisis. Despite thorough evaluation, however, the precipitating event of some crises cannot be determined.

Evaluation should include careful history-taking and a thorough physical examination with attention to possible sites of infection. Laboratory studies should include a complete blood count, with a reticulocyte count, to be sure the patient is producing red blood cells in response to the increased destruction of sickled cells. Cultures of urine, sputum, and blood should be done, especially in the setting of fever. A chest x-ray is useful if hypoxia is present, there is a history of pulmonary disease, or there are pulmonary signs or symptoms.

4. What infections are common in sickle cell disease?
Because patients with sickle cell anemia (SS) have generally infarcted their spleen by age 3 or 4, they are susceptible to encapsulated organisms, including *Hemophilus influenzae, Streptococcus pneumoniae,* and *Neisseria meningitidis.* Pyelonephritis is also common, is often associated with bacteremia, and predisposes to sickling with subsequent papillary necrosis. Osteomyelitis can also develop and is most commonly caused by Staphylococcus, though there is an increased incidence of Salmonella osteomyelitis in sickle cell patients compared with other patients.

5. How are painful sickle cell crises treated?
The usual approach to painful crisis includes intravenous fluids to attain and maintain adequate hydration. Supplemental oxygen by nasal cannula is given to reverse any hypoxia that may precipitate sickling. Parenteral analgesics, usually meperidine (Demerol) or morphine sulfate, are given intravenously on a fixed schedule (not p.r.n.) until the pain has subsided enough to use oral analgesics. Evidence of infection (positive urinalysis

or cultures) is treated appropriately, and in the setting of fever, "empirical" intravenous antibiotics may be necessary.

6. What is acute chest syndrome?

Acute chest syndrome develops in the setting of an acute painful crisis and is characterized by chest pain, fever, increasing hypoxia, and, in many cases, development of bilateral pulmonary infiltrates on chest x-ray. It may occur in the setting of pneumonia but is probably pathophysiologically distinct and represents infarction of lung tissue due to sickled cells. Heparin is not an effective therapy. Treatment usually involves a red blood cell exchange transfusion (see below) to remove sickled blood and arrest the process. Because it is often difficult to differentiate between worsening pneumonia and acute chest syndrome, intravenous antibiotics are also given.

Arterial hypoxia syndrome, a rare complication of severe painful vaso-occlusive crises (often in patients with Hgb SC disease), is characterized by bone pain, fever, dyspnea, hypoxia, and confusion, with or without renal failure and disseminated intravascular coagulation (DIC). This is felt to be due to fat emboli from infarcted, liquefied bone marrow.

7. What is aplastic crisis?

Aplastic crisis is characterized by a rapid fall in hemoglobin associated with few or no reticulocytes and indicating a failure of the bone marrow to respond to increased cell turnover. Folate deficiency can occur in the setting of chronic hemolytic anemia if the patient does not take supplemental folate, and this may precipitate an aplastic crisis. Parvovirus (B19) has been associated with bone marrow suppression and subsequent aplastic crisis; other viral infections or severe bacterial infections may also suppress the bone marrow. Treatment of aplastic crisis becomes necessary when the hematocrit becomes dangerously low. Packed red blood cells are given to support an adequate hematocrit until bone marrow suppression is resolved, folate is repleted, and the reticulocyte count improves.

8. What is splenic sequestration?

Splenic sequestration does not occur in adults with hemoglobin SS because they have infracted their spleen by age 3 or 4. In Hgb SC disease or S-β^+ thalassemia, however, the disease is relatively mild and splenic function can be preserved into adulthood. Splenic sequestration is characterized by rapid, painful enlargement of the spleen, with rapid falls in hemoglobin and occasionally platelets due to sickling and sudden intravascular pooling of blood in the spleen. In adults, the sequestration is often relatively mild, with only a 1–2 gm/dl drop in hemoglobin; transfusion is rarely required for support. Very rarely, the spleen may become so massive and/or necrotic as to require splenectomy.

9. What cerebrovascular complications can occur with sickle cell disease?

Stroke may affect as many as 6–12% of patients with sickle cell anemia in childhood or young adulthood. In children, strokes tend to be thrombotic in nature, while adults tend to have hemorrhagic strokes. These strokes are usually due to large-vessel disease, and abnormal vessels can be seen on angiogram or magnetic resonance imaging in some cases. Acute management involves red blood cell exchange transfusion to remove sickling red blood cells and enhance oxygen-carrying capacity. Simple blood transfusions are not recommended because blood viscosity may be increased with increased hematocrit if sickled cells are not removed. Hyperventilation should be avoided, and anticonvulsants are sometimes needed, since seizures can occur during acute infarction.

10. What other acute complications may develop with sickle cell disease?

Intrahepatic sickling can occur, with rapid rises in liver enzymes, a fall in hemoglobin due to sequestration in the liver, and, in severe cases, an extreme rise in conjugated bilirubin and prothrombin time, indicating acute liver failure. Acute renal failure, in the absence of sepsis or other systemic illness, is relatively uncommon. Priapism can occur with or without systemic painful crisis. Gallstones are very common due to chronic hyperbilirubinemia and may cause acute cholecystitis or common bile duct obstruction. Acute myocardial infarction is not more common in patients with sickle cell disease than in the general population; however, pulmonary hypertension due to recurrent pulmonary infarction by sickled cells may be more common.

11. What are the surgical risks for patients with sickle cell disease?

Patients with sickle cell anemia who undergo general anesthesia may be at increased risk for development of acute painful crisis and acute chest syndrome. Studies are under way to determine if preoperative simple transfusion or exchange transfusion can decrease this risk; all major operations should be preceded by some form of transfusion to reduce the percentage of Hgb S and to increase oxygen-carrying capacity. Patients should be carefully monitored for hypoxia, with a minimum of 50% oxygen in combination with the anesthetic agent, to avoid precipitation of red cell sickling. Adequate hydration should be carefully maintained.

12. What is the role of acute transfusion in sickle cell disease?

Packed red blood cell transfusions are indicated in the setting of severe anemia with hemodynamic instability or severe hypoxia. The final hematocrit after transfusion should not exceed 25% because blood viscosity may increase at hematocrits higher than this. If life-threatening events such as acute stroke, acute liver failure, acute chest syndrome, acute priapism, or arterial hypoxia syndrome develop, red blood cell exchange transfusion should be performed. In this procedure, blood is removed in 70–90 mg/kg aliquots through an arterial or venous line, with replacement with whole blood or "reconstituted" packed red blood cells. Alternatively, an apheresis instrument can be used in an automated exchange procedure through a double-lumen dialysis catheter.

In all cases of transfusion, an effort should be made to match transfused units to minor antigens on the patient's red blood cells (minor antigen match), as sickle cell patients otherwise tend to rapidly develop multiple alloantibodies, making future cross-matching difficult.

CONTROVERSIES

13. What is the role of continuing blood transfusions chronically in sickle cell patients who have had a stroke?

Currently, chronic, monthly blood transfusions are recommended for patients who have had a stroke. The emergent exchange transfusion done acutely essentially eliminates the patient's own sickle cells; chronic transfusions can suppress the bone marrow, prevent reaccumulation of sickle cells, and theoretically reduce the risk for recurrent stroke. However, some studies have shown that strokes can recur despite transfusions; in other patients, discontinuation of chronic transfusion has not led to recurrent stroke. Further studies are under way.

14. What is the role of hydroxyurea (Hydrea) in the treatment of sickle cell disease?

In some patients with sickle cell disease, there is persistent production of hemoglobin F (fetal hemoglobin), with a corresponding decrease in the percentage of hemoglobin S. Such patients have been observed to have a milder form of sickle cell disease. It was noted that hydroxyurea could increase the production of hemoglobin F, and a number of studies have shown this could be achieved in sickle cell patients. Thus far, however, no studies have shown that this increase in hemoglobin F has consistently made a difference in the clinical severity of these patients' disease; such studies are under way.

15. Is pulse oximetry reliable in sickle cell patients?
Noninvasive assessment of oxygen saturation can be done using a pulse oximeter, with good correlation to measured saturation by arterial blood gas. It has recently been noted, however, that pulse oximetry may be off by as much as ±4% compared with measured oxygen saturation by blood gas, especially in patients with hemoglobins of less than 11 gm/dl. If there is doubt about hypoxia, an arterial blood gas is indicated.

BIBLIOGRAPHY

1. Allon M: Renal abnormalities in sickle cell disease. Arch Intern Med 150:501, 1990.
2. Baum KF, Dunn DT, Maude GH, Sergeant GR: The painful crisis of homozygous sickle cell disease: A study of the risk factors. Arch Intern Med 47:1231, 1987.
3. Castro O, Finke-Castro H, Coats D: Improved method for automated red cell exchange in sickle cell disease. J Clin Apheresis 3:93, 1986.
4. Charache S, Lubin B, Reid CD: Management and therapy of sickle cell disease. NIH Publication No. 89-2117, 1989.
5. Deneberg BS, Criner G, Jones R, Spann J: Cardiac function in sickle cell anemia. Am J Cardiol 51:1674, 1985.
6. Gibson J: Anesthesia for sickle cell disease and other hemoglobinopathies. Semin Anesthesiol 6:27, 1987.
7. Gilliland DG, Bridges KR: Management strategies for acute sickle cell crises: Recognizing painful crisis, aplastic crisis, sickle lung syndrome. J Crit Illness, 1988, p 25.
8. Ponez M, Kane E, Gill F: Acute chest syndrome in sickle cell disease: Etiology and clinical correlates. J Pediatr 107:861, 1985.
9. Prohovnik I, Pavlakis SG, Pionelli S, et al: Cerebral hyperemia, stroke and transfusion in sickle cell disease. Neurology 34:344, 1989.
10. Shubert TT: Hepatobiliary system in sickle cell disease. Gastroenterology 90:2013, 1986.

66. ONCOLOGIC EMERGENCIES

Susan L. Kelley, M.D.

1. What are the causes of superior vena cava (SVC) syndrome?
1. Malignant intrathoracic tumors: Extrinsic compression of the SVC by mediastinal malignancy accounts for 80–95% of the cases of SVC syndrome. Primary lung cancer (generally small cell or squamous cell carcinoma) or lymphomas constitute the most common histologies of tumor involved. Other malignancies that may cause SVC compression include thymic tumors, breast cancer, testicular cancer, and metastatic disease from carcinoma of unknown primary site.
2. Mediastinal fibroses/chronic mediastinitis.
3. Thrombosis, primary or secondary to instrumentation or indwelling catheters.
4. Granulomatous disease of mediastinal lymph nodes.
5. Idiopathic causes.

2. What are the clinical manifestations of SVC syndrome?
Symptoms commonly consist of swelling of the face, trunk, and/or upper extremities; dyspnea; dysphagia; chest pain; and cough. Some patients complain of neurologic symptoms such as dizziness, vision changes, or syncope. Physical findings include facial edema, plethora, distended neck veins, and distention of the superficial veins of the chest wall and

anterior abdominal wall. Signs of airway obstruction or increased intracranial pressure such as tachypnea, stridor, lethargy, or papilledema require prompt initiation of treatment.

3. How is the diagnosis of SVC syndrome made?

It is based on the clinical manifestations, although chest x-ray findings support the diagnosis in 80% of cases. Tissue diagnosis of malignancy must be confirmed before definitive therapy is initiated. Diagnosis may be obtained via sputum cytology, lymph node biopsy, bronchoscopy, bone marrow biopsy, or, if necessary, thoracotomy.

4. What is the treatment for SVC syndrome?

Mediastinal irradiation is the therapy for most cases of SVC syndrome due to malignancy. Greater than 75% of patients respond within 3 weeks. Chemotherapy should be the initial mode of treatment in patients with SVC syndrome due to small cell carcinoma of the lung or lymphoma. The right upper extremity must be avoided for intravenous drug administration due to the increased risk of thrombosis and phlebitis. The role of anticoagulation in treatment of SVC syndrome is controversial. Initial improvement is usually observed within 3–5 days.

5. What is the tumor lysis syndrome?

Hyperphosphatemia, hyperkalemia, hyperuricemia, and hypocalcemia can ocur 1–5 days after significant malignant cell lysis from chemotherapy. In severe cases, acute renal failure, cardiac arrhythmias, or convulsions may ensue.

6. What are the risk factors for tumor lysis syndrome?

The major risk factor is a large tumor burden with a rapidly proliferating tumor that is highly responsive to chemotherapy. These malignancies include non-Hodgkin's lymphoma, acute lymphoblastic leukemia, chronic myelogenous leukemia in blast crisis, and Burkett's lymphoma. Other predisposing factors are dehydration, obstructive uropathy, renal insufficiency, and an increased lactate dehydrogenase or uric acid prior to initiation of chemotherapy.

Tumor lysis syndrome can be minimized using vigorous intravenous hydration to maintain high urine volumes. Alkalinization of the urine with intravenous sodium bicarbonate and administration of allopurinol before chemotherapy is initiated decrease the risk of urate nephropathy. Frequent monitoring of blood urea nitrogen, creatinine, uric acid, calcium, phosphate, and potassium levels is required to detect metabolic aberrations.

7. What are the symptoms of hyperleukocytosis?

Hyperleukocytosis syndrome results from leukocyte sequestration within the capillaries of patients with severe leukocytosis (a white blood cell (WBC) count $> 100,000/\mu l$). Organs most commonly affected include the lungs and brain, and thus the presenting manifestations may include tachypnea, dyspnea, hypoxia, mental status changes, and signs of increased intracranial pressure or intracerebral hemorrhage. Patients may also present with abdominal pain, priapism, and symptoms of vascular insufficiency. Although the syndrome may occur with any type of leukemia, the leukocytosis associated with chronic lymphocytic leukemia results in fewer symptoms because the lymphocytes are smaller, more deformable, and less likely to lodge in the microvasculature.

8. How should hyperleukocytosis syndrome be treated?

Immediate therapy for severe symptomatic hyperleukocytosis consists of leukapheresis, which can achieve transient lowering of the WBC count by 20–50%. Definitive chemotherapy of the underlying leukemia can then be initiated. Supportive care such as oxygen and treatment for elevated intracranial presure or bleeding must also be administered.

9. What is hyperviscosity syndrome? How is it treated?
Resistance to blood flow (viscosity) is due to the presence of the formed elements of blood (primarily red blood cells) and the plasma proteins. Hyperviscosity syndrome occurs primarily in patients with tumors producing immunoglobulins, most notably immunoglobulin M. Serum hyperviscosity has also been described in autoimmune diseases that lead to the formation of circulating immune complexes.

The signs and symptoms of hyperviscosity syndrome are due to occlusive changes in small blood vessels, especially those in the brain and peripheral nervous system, eyes, kidneys, and distal extremities. Bleeding may occur; epistaxis is common. The diagnosis is based on clinical findings and may be confirmed by measurement of elevated serum or whole blood viscosity. However, the threshold of elevated viscosity at which clinical symptoms occur is variable.

Manifestations of hyperviscosity syndrome respond transiently to plasmapheresis, which reduces viscosity through decreased immunoglobulin concentration. Definitive treatment of the underlying disease, including chemotherapy, appropriate for the condition causing the syndrome, should be started promptly.

10. What are the predisposing factors for infection in cancer patients?
Patients with cancer are "compromised hosts" at risk for infection due to the underlying malignancy and as a result of anticancer therapy. Risk factors for infection include defects in cellular and humoral immunity, disruption of mucosal and skin integrity, tumor-related obstruction, granulocytopenia, and iatrogenic procedures. The patient's endogenous flora is the major source of infection.

11. How should the febrile, neutropenic patient be evaluated?
The problem of fever without an apparent source must be addressed promptly in a patient with a neutrophil count of less than $500/\mu l$. A careful history and physical exam should include evaluation of all potential mucosal and epithelial portals of entry. The sinuses, oral cavity, and perirectal areas are important sources of infection in neutropenic patients. Any indwelling venous catheters should be inspected and palpated. The laboratory evaluation should include Gram stain and cultures of blood, urine, sputum, throat, stool, and other available fluids. Lumbar puncture should be performed if CNS infection is suspected. Chest x-rays should always be obtained along with radiologic evaluation of the paranasal sinuses, abdomen, and other sites as clinically indicated.

12. What is the treatment for fever in the neutropenic patient?
After cultures have been obtained, empirical broad-spectrum antibiotic coverage should be initiated promptly. The specific empirical therapy to initiate remains controversial, but most studies support the use of an aminoglycoside in combination with an extended spectrum penicillin so that coverage for gram-negative and gram-positive flora is accomplished. Antibacterial therapy should not be discontinued until the neutrophil count is adequate, even though the fever may resolve and all cultures may be negative. In one study, 40% of afebrile patients with persistent neutropenia required reinstitution of antibiotics within 3 days of stopping initial therapy. In patients with positive cultures, therapy should be continued for 10–14 days or until the neutrophil count is greater than $500/\mu l$, whichever is longer. Special considerations include therapy for staphylococcal, viral, and fungal infections. There is currently no role for granulocyte transfusions in treatment of neutropenic, febrile patients.

13. What is acute graft-versus-host disease (GVHD)?
The bone marrow infused during an allogeneic transplant also contains immunocompetent T cells removed from their "self" environment and transferred into a foreign, "nonself" recipient. If the donor is histoincompatible and the recipient is unable to destroy the donor lymphoid cells, acute GVHD results. Acute GVHD develops most frequently in the setting of bone marrow transplantation, since large numbers of lymphoid cells are transferred, but

GVHD is also observed after solid organ transplants. Acute GVHD may develop within days of marrow transplantation but generally does not occur until after early bone marrow engraftment. The target organs of acute GVHD are the skin, gastrointestinal tract, liver, and lymphatic organs. An increased risk of developing acute GVHD is associated with the degree of histoincompatibility between donor and recipient, patient and donor age and gender, prior transfusion history, and infections before transplant. The reported incidence of GVHD is 40–50% in many studies. It is the primary cause of death in 20–30% of allogeneic bone marrow transplant recipients. The overall prognosis after bone marrow transplantation is significantly influenced by the occurrence of acute GVHD. Mortality from infectious complications is increased in patients who develop acute GVHD because GVHD is accompanied by profound immunodeficiency. Other causes of increased mortality include hepatic failure, bowel perforation, and intestinal hemorrhage.

14. How is acute GVHD treated?

The primary goal is to prevent acute GVHD. Various immunosuppressive drugs have been used both alone and in combination to prevent GVHD. Cyclosporine A and methotrexate have been used most commonly, but the optimal therapy to prevent acute GVHD has not yet been determined. Once acute GVHD develops, the management of patients must include both specific therapy directed toward immunologic control and supportive care measures to protect the patient from life-threatening infections. Strict isolation in a controlled environment is critical, as are measures to minimize entry of pathogens through skin and mucosal portals. Prophylactic antimicrobial therapy is necessary to prevent specific opportunistic infections; empirical, broad-spectrum antibiotic and antifungal therapy should be initiated if the clinical course suggests acute infection. All blood products must be irradiated to destroy alloreactive lymphocytes and should be serologically screened in order to minimize exposure to infectious agents or to cells capable of initiating a new GVHD reaction.

BIBLIOGRAPHY

1. Adelstein DJ, Hines JD, Carter SG, et al: Thromboembolic events in patients with malignant superior vena cava syndrome and the role of anticoagulation. Cancer 62:2258–2262, 1988.
2. Bjornson B: Hyperleukocytic and hyperviscosity syndromes. In Heffernan J, Witzburg RA, Cohen AS (eds): Clinical Problems in Acute Care Medicine. Philadelphia, W.B. Saunders, 1989, p 266.
3. Bloch KJ, Maki DG: Hyperviscosity syndromes associated with immunoglobulin abnormalities. Semin Hematol 10:113, 1973.
3a. Bustamante CI, Wade JC: Herpes simplex virus infections in the immunocompromised cancer patient. J Clin Oncol 9:1903–1915, 1991.
4. Cohen LF, Balow JE, Magrath IT, et al: Acute tumor lysis syndrome: A review of 37 patients with Burkitt's lymphoma. Am J Med 68:486–491, 1980.
5. Deeg HJ, Cottler-Fox M: Clinical spectrum and pathophysiology of acute graft-vs.-host disease. In Burakoff SJ, Deeg HJ, Ferrara J, Atkinson K (eds): Graft-vs.-Host Disease. New York, Marcel Dekker, 1990, p 311.
6. Gerson SL, Lazarus HM: Hematopoietic emergencies. Semin Oncol 16:532–542, 1989.
7. Helms SR, Carlson MD: Cardiovascular emergencies. Semin Oncol 16:463–470, 1989.
8. Henslee-Downey PJ: Treatment of acute graft-vs.-host disease. In Burakoff SJ, Deeg HJ, Ferarra J, Atkinson K (eds): Graft-vs.-Host Disease. New York, Marcel Dekker, 1990, p 457.
9. Lazarus HM, Creger KJ, Gerson SL: Infectious emergencies in oncology patients. Semin Oncol 16:543–560, 1989.
10. McGrath MA, Penny R: Paraproteinemia: Blood hyperviscosity and clinical manifestations. J Clin Invest 58:1155, 1976.
11. Pizzo PA, Robichaud KJ, Gill FA, et al: Duration of empiric antibiotic therapy in granulocytopenic cancer patients. Am J Med 67:194–200, 1979.
12. Silverman P, Distelhorst C: Metabolic emergencies in clinical oncology. Semin Oncol 16:504–515, 1989.
13. Strauss RG, Connett JE, Gale RP, et al: A controlled trial of prophylactic granulocyte transfusion during initial induction therapy for acute myelogenous leukemia. N Engl J Med 305:597–603, 1981.

X: Neurology

67. COMA

Brian J. Kelly, M.D.

1. Define coma.
Coma is a condition in which the patient appears asleep but is incapable of responding either to external stimuli or inner needs. A patient in coma is unable to interact appropriately with the environment.

2. Which anatomic structures must be malfunctioning to produce coma?
Coma can be produced only by bilateral cerebral hemispheric dysfunction or by injury to the reticular activating system (RAS).

3. What can we deduce about the etiology of coma by understanding its anatomy?
Dysfunction of the RAS and/or cerebral hemispheres can be produced by structural or metabolic lesions. A structural lesion would have to be huge to affect both cerebral hemispheres and produce coma. Structural lesions of the RAS are usually associated with focal neurologic signs because of its anatomic location in the brain stem, adjacent to multiple cranial nerves and ascending and descending tracts. Therefore, in the absence of focal neurologic signs, coma is usually the result of a global toxic or metabolic suppression of the cerebral hemispheres and/or the RAS.

4. What are the initial steps in managing a patient with coma?
First, Airway Breathing, and Circulation (ABCs) should be addressed. Oxygen should be administered via face mask, and, if the patient does not have a secure airway, intubation should be performed. Empirical therapy for reversible causes of coma such as Wernicke's encephalopathy and narcotic overdose should be initiated with thiamine and naloxone. A bedside blood glucose determination should be performed; if hypoglycemia is present, D50W should then be administered.

5. How do you diagnostically approach a comatose patient?
It is important to have a systematic approach to coma. The patient's history as obtained from relatives, friends, or paramedics may reveal an obvious cause such as drug or alcohol overdose, sepsis, or abnormalities of glucose metabolism. Assessment of the vital signs may suggest an infectious etiology or a respiratory disorder. A thorough general examination should be performed with specific attention to possible foci of infection in the ears, mouth, skin (decubiti or needle tracts), lungs, heart, and abdomen. The fingers, fundi, and mucous membranes should be inspected for signs of emboli, and the neck should be assessed for nuchal rigidity. A rectal examiantion should be done to assess the stool for blood. While it is impossible to do a full neurologic exam on a comatose patient, one can usually ascertain if focal findings are present. The pupillary and corneal reflexes can be tested easily, and the fundi should be visualized. The oculovestibular reflex and gag should be tested. Motor withdrawal from a painful stimulus, deep tendon reflexes, and plantar reflexes should be assessed; they should be symmetrical.

6. Match the following clinical signs with the cause of coma with which it is associated:

1. Purpuric rash	A. Basilar skull fracture
2. Battle sign	B. Atropine poisoning
3. Bilateral, large, fixed pupils	C. Meningitis
4. Unilateral, large, fixed pupil	D. Third-nerve palsy suggesting
5. Nuchal rigidity	temporal lobe herniation
6. Gynecomastia, spider angiomas	E. Anoxic encephalopathy
7. Bilateral pinpoint pupils	F. Locked-in syndrome
8. Unilateral chemosis and proptosis	G. Chronic liver disease
9. Myoclonus	H. Narcotic overdose
10. Quadriplegia, loss of lower cranial	I. Meningococcemia
nerve function, but retained	J. Diabetic ketoacidosis
vertical eye movements	

1. I; 2. A; 3. B; 4. D; 5. C; 6. G; 7. H; 8. J; 9. E; and 10. F

7. How does the finding of a new focal abnormality on neurologic examination affect the management of a comatose patient?
Focal neurologic abnormalities generally indicate intrinsic structural CNS pathology such as a tumor, abscess, or infarct, although severe metabolic derangements such as hypoglycemia may present with such findings. Imaging with CT or MRI should be considered mandatory early in the management of such patients.

8. Does a nonfocal neurologic exam in a comatose patient exclude a mass as the cause of coma?
No, although most cases of coma with a nonfocal neurologic exam are due to toxic-metabolic causes, bilateral subdural hematomas, subarachnoid hemorrhages, and frontal lobe masses may not show any gross focal abnormalities on neurologic testing.

9. What initial laboratory evaluations should be performed in coma of uncertain etiology?
A drug screen and alcohol level, complete blood count, serum electrolytes, calcium, phosphate, magnesium, creatinine, blood urea nitrogen, and liver and thyroid function tests should be ordered. An arterial blood gas analysis is mandatory, and cultures of blood, urine, and sputum should be obtained if infection is likely. A CT scan of the head should be performed if an etiology is not obvious or if focal signs are present on neurologic exam. A lumbar puncture should be performed if a primary CNS infection is likely, but only after the presence of a CNS mass has been excluded.

10. What is the approach to the comatose trauma patient?
Although the general approach is similar, the likelihood of a structural cause of coma is high in these patients. The ABCs need to be attended to first, but one should assume a cervical spine injury is present until this has been excluded by visualization of all seven cervical vertebrae. The patient's coma may be secondary to a hypotensive hemorrhage, hypoxia, drug or alcohol ingestion, or a primary CNS mass such as an epidural or subdural hematoma. If the patient has focal signs on exam or evidence of a third-nerve palsy, immediate neurosurgical consultation is indicated. If an obvious cause of coma is not evident, early neuroimaging with a CT scan is indicated.

11. What are the common causes of coma in the ICU?
Most cases of coma in a medical-surgical (nontrauma) ICU are toxic-metabolic in nature and are often multifactorial. Sepsis, hypotension, hypoxia, hypothermia, acid-base disorders, glucose, electrolyte abnormalities, and the side effects of medications are common causes. Hepatic and uremic failure often contribute to coma. Primary CNS infections such as

meningitis or encephalitis are less common but need to be considered in the appropriate setting. If a severe coagulopathy is present, intracranial hemorrhage and subdural hematomas should be excluded. Focal signs on exam suggest a structural lesion such as a CNS infarction, tumor, or abscess and should be evaluated with a CT or MRI scan. If no obvious cause for coma is apparent, an EEG to exclude nonconvulsive status epilepticus is indicated.

BIBLIOGRAPHY

1. Adams RD, Victor M: Principles of Neurology, 2nd ed. New York, McGraw-Hill, 1981.
2. Alguire PC: Rapid evaluation of comatose patients. Postgrad Med 87:223–228, 1990.
3. Kleeman CR: Metabolic coma. Kidney Int 36:1142–1158, 1989.
4. Plum F, Posner J: The Diagnosis of Stupor and Coma, 3rd ed. Philadelphia, F.A. Davis, 1980.

68. BRAIN DEATH

Dorre Nicholau, M.D.

1. What is brain death?
Historically both lawmakers and physicians defined death as the cessation of heart and lung function. The first attempt to legally define brain death as an alternative to the conventional definition was in 1968 when the Harvard criteria were published. Although the basic guidelines set forth by the Harvard criteria are still valid today, several modifications have been adopted. These include the recognition of persistent spinal reflexes in brain death and more stringent guidelines for the determination of apnea. The most recent guidelines for the determination of brain death are established in "The Report of the Medical Consultants on the Diagnosis of Death to the President's Commission for the Study of Ethical Problems in Medicine, Biomedical, and Behavioral Research," published in 1981. This report is endorsed by the American Medical Association, the American Bar Association, and the National Conference of Commissioners on Uniform State Laws. This document introduces the Uniform Determination of Death Act. Under this act, death is defined as: "1. The irreversible cessation of circulatory and respiratory functions, or 2. The irreversible cessation of all functions of the entire brain, including the brainstem."

2. What are the current guidelines for the determination of brain death?
1. **The cessation of cerebral function.** This requires clinical evidence of a state of deep coma. The patient must be unreceptive and unresponsive to noxious stimuli. True decerebrate or decorticate posturing is not consistent with the diagnosis of death, although peripheral spinal cord reflexes may persist.
2. **The cessation of brainstem function.** This requires the lack of brainstem reflexes, together with the persistence of apnea despite adequate stimulus to breathe ($pCO_2 > 60$). If brainstem reflexes cannot be clinically evaluated with certainty, further confirmatory tests are recommended.
3. **Demonstration of irreversibility.** This requires that the cause of coma is established and is sufficient to account for the loss of brain function. The possibility of recovery of any brain function must be excluded. Finally, the cessation of all brain function must persist for an appropriate period of observation and/or trial of therapy. In the absence of confirmatory tests, the patient should be observed continuously in an intensive care setting for a period of 12 hours. If anoxic brain damage is suspected, observation for 24 hours is recommended.

The absence of cerebral blood flow as measured by radiologic techniques is the only measure of cerebral function that does not require additional clinical observation and laboratory evaluation to confirm the diagnosis of brain death.

3. When can a patient be declared brain dead?

In a concise review, Pitts (1984) distilled the current criteria for brain death into three requirements:

1. The cause of brain injury must be known. The cause of brain injury can be determined clinically through careful history and physical exam in the case of obvious severe head trauma and/or prolonged cardiac arrest. In general, however, diagnostic imaging studies are used to produce convincing evidence of brain damage. CT, MRI, and, in rare cases, cerebral angiography are performed to confirm the cause of brain injury.

2. Metabolic and toxic CNS depression must be excluded. Reversible causes of apparent brain death must be ruled out. These include pharmacologic agents such as barbiturates, benzodiazepines, and neuromuscular blockade; endogenous metabolic disorders such as severe hepatic encephalopathy, hyperosmolar coma, hyponatremia, and uremia; severe systemic hypotension, with a concomitant decrease in cerebral blood flow; and hypothermia. Loss of thermoregulation is often associated with brain death. Normothermia must be restored prior to the determination of brain death.

3. There must be no demonstrable brain function. The diagnosis of brain death requires that there be no evidence of brain function. The patient must be unresponsive without spontaneous movement or response to pain. The possibility of neuromuscular blockade by pharmacologic agents must be ruled out by history and/or the application of a peripheral nerve stimulator.

4. How is the cessation of brainstem function demonstrated?

The absence of brainstem function is demonstrated by the **absence** of brainstem reflexes and the **presence** of apnea. Tendon reflexes are often preserved. Tests for brainstem reflexes are as follows:

1. **Pupillary response to light:** the pupils in brain death are classically described as "fixed and dilated" (5–6 mm in size), without response to light. Factors that may influence pupillary size in critically ill or comatose patients are:

Small, reactive: metabolic or sedative drugs. Glutethimide (Doriden) and scopolamine are the only two seditive drugs that cause dilated pupils.

Unilateral fixed, dilated: Cranial nerve (CN) III palsy (transtentorial herniation with compression of CNIII)

Fixed, midposition: midbrain pathology

Pinpoint: pontine pathology vs. opiates (pontomedullary lesions interrupt sympathetic pathways, leaving CNIII, the parasympathetic pathway, intact and unopposed)

2. **Doll's eyes**, or oculocephalic reflex: tests midbrain and pontine function. In a comatose patient with an intact brainstem, the eyes will lag behind when the head is turned suddenly to one side. This lag in eye movement will not be present in brainstem injury. The oculocephalic reflex is never present in conscious patients.

3. **Cold calorics**, or the oculovestibular reflex: also tests pontine function. This reflex generally persists after the oculocephalic reflex has disappeared, so it is important in patients who lack an oculocephalic response. The test is done by introducing iced water into the external auditory canal of one ear. A normal reflex results in nystagmus, with the slow component toward the side of the stimulation and the fast component to the opposite side of stimulation. The brainstem and cortex are responsible for slow and fast movements, respectively. Cortical injury, producing coma, results in the slow deviation of the eyes without the fast component. Brainstem injury produces a deeper coma and the absence of all eye movements.

4. **Medullary function.** Lack of medullary function is demonstrated by the absence of the cough and gag reflexes, but the most reliable marker of medullary death is cessation of spontaneous respirations as demonstrated by the performance of an apnea test.

5. How is an apnea test performed?

To demonstrate apnea, one must provide the injured brainstem with an adequate stimulus to breathe. In the apnea test, the arterial tension of carbon dioxide provides the stimulus.

The minimum level of pCO_2 required to demonstrate apnea in the severely injured or "dead" brain is a matter of debate in the literature, but minimum levels of 44–60 mm Hg have been recommended.

Guidelines for Apnea Testing

1. Ventilate with 100% O_2 for at least 5 min to produce a normal pCO_2 (37–40 mm Hg) and hyperoxia prior to disconnection from the ventilator.
2. After disconnection from mechanical ventilation, maintain 100% O_2 flow to endotracheal tube by T-piece.
3. Continue apnea for 5–10 min or until hypoxia or ventricular arrhythmias result.
4. Follow pCO_2 by arterial blood gas measurements to document a final pCO_2 of >60 mm Hg.

Adapted from Pitts LH: Determination of brain death. West J Med 140:628–631, 1984.

6. Are spinal reflexes absent in brain death?

No. Current guidelines recognize the persistence of spinal reflexes in brain death; approximately 75% of patients with documented brain death exhibit some spinal reflex.

7. What is the role of the EEG in the diagnosis of brain death?

The EEG is not required to determine brain death. It can be used as a confirmatory test in cases in which the history is questionable and/or the clinical exam is not adequate. However, the following may result in an isoelectric EEG that is indistinguishable from brain death. When one or more of these factors are present, further confirmatory tests that measure cerebral blood flow should be conducted.

Hypothermia produces a transient, reversible electroencephalographic silence (ECS). Therefore, a rectal temperature of at least 32.2° C (90° F) is required prior to the determination of brain death by EEG.

Cardiovascular shock may result in reversible ECS. In this case, loss of electrical activity is secondary to the decreased cerebral perfusion pressure resulting from systemic hypotension (cerebral perfusion pressure = mean arterial presure – intracranial pressure). Electrical activity may be restored by increasing systemic blood pressure. Therefore, a systemic blood pressure of at least 80 mm Hg is a prerequisite to the diagnosis of brain death by EEG.

Barbiturate coma or toxic levels of other CNS depressant drugs (methaqualone, diazepam, meprobamate, trichlorethylene) may also result in ECS, and therefore the possibility of drug overdose must be ruled out by careful history and/or appropriate toxicology screen if the EEG is to reliably diagnose brain death. Most CNS depressant drugs would not produce the clinical criteria necessary for the diagnosis of brain death because of their effect on pupil size (most produce small pupils). Exceptions include scopolamine and glutethimide, which produce large pupils.

Deep anesthesia

8. Is there a role for brainstem evoked potentials (BSEP) in the diagnosis of brain death?

In brain death, the brainstem auditory and short-latency evoked responses are abnormal or absent. The observation that all BSEP components after wave I or II are absent in brain death but preserved in toxic and metabolic disorders suggests that BSEPs may be useful in evaluating patients in whom coma of toxic etiology is suspected (in particular, barbiturate coma is known to produce an isoelectric EEG).

9. What additional tests are available to confirm brain death?
Confirmatory tests of brain death measure blood flow and are more specific than the EEG.

Contrast angiography. This invasive technique requires catheterization of the aorta via the femoral or axillary arteries. A definitive test requires the visualization of both the carotid and vertebrobasilar systems. Carotid angiography alone does not visualize the brainstem and posterior fossa, and therefore is inadequate for diagnosing brain death. A positive test is one in which "no flow" is identified within the cranial vault. Typically, the dye column tapers symmetrically with nonfilling of the cervical carotids (pseudo occlusion) or an abrupt block at the cranial base. This is in marked contrast to the bilateral filling of the external carotid system. The vertebral vessels disappear at the atlantooccipital junction. Occasionally, the basilar artery can be seen against the clivis. There is no visualization of the venous phase.

Radionucleotide cerebral imaging. This noninvasive, simple, and safe method of measuring cerebral blood flow may be used in lieu of invasive contrast arteriography. Portable gamma cameras allow bedside exams to be completed in 15 minutes. The test requires IV bolus of sodium pertechnetate technetium 99 m (15–21 mCi/adult) followed by anterior images recorded every 3 seconds for a total of 60 seconds. Counts attributable to the external carotid system are eliminated by subtraction techniques or a tourniquet placed around the forehead to eliminate scalp flow. With normal cerebral blood flow, sequential images show activity over the common carotid arteries—anterior and middle cerebral arteries—capillaries—sagittal sinus—internal jugular bilaterally. Occasionally, the scalp veins drain into the sagittal sinus, resulting in minimal late sagittal sinus activity in the absence of identifiable arterial activity.

10. What are the cardiac manifestations of brain death?
Despite aggressive cardiovascular support, patients determined to be brain dead progress to cardiovascular collapse within 1 week. In fact, most die within the first 2 days after the diagnosis of brain death. The EKG changes associated with the initial stage of brain death include widening of the terminal QRS complex (Osborn waves), prolongation of the QT segment, and nonspecific ST changes.

More advanced stages of brain death are marked by bradycardia, followed by conduction abnormalities, including atrioventricular block and interventricular conduction delays. Atrial fibrillation is relatively common in the terminal stages of brain death, with atrial activity often continuing after the cessation of ventricular complexes.

11. Is it possible to predict which comatose patients will progress to brain death?
It is not possible to determine with confidence which comatose patients will progress to brain death, even though several studies have identified the clinical parameters associated with a poor neurologic outcome. The best predictor of neurologic outcome is the level of brainstem function observed within the first 24 hours after presentation. The lack of pupillary response to light on initial exam is a very poor prognostic sign. By 72 hours after cerebral insult, the motor response to pain increases in predictive value, with absent or posturing response to pain excluding the possibility of independent neurologic recovery.

BIBLIOGRAPHY

1. Barber J, et al: Guidelines for the determination of death. JAMA 246:2184–2186, 1981.
2. Beecher HK: A definition of irreversible coma. JAMA 205:85–89, 1968.
3. Chatrian G: Electrophysiologic evaluation of brain death: A critical appraisal. In Aminoff MJ: Electrodiagnosis in Clinical Neurology. New York, Churchill Livingstone, 1986, pp 669–736.
4. Cooper M, Stirit J: Monitoring. In Sperry R, Stirt J, Stone D: Manual of Neuroanesthesia. Toronto, B.C. Decker, 1989, pp 67–90.
5. Goldie WP, et al: Brainstem auditory and short latency somatosensory evoked responses in brain death. Neurology 31:248–246, 1981.

6. Quaknine GE: Bedside procedures in the diagnosis of brain death. Resuscitation 4:159–177, 1975.
7. Pitts LH: Determination of brain death. West J Med 140:628–631, 1984.
8. Pitts LH, Caronna J: Apnea testing in the diagnosis of brain death (letter to the editor). J Neurosurg 57:433, 1982.
9. Pitts LH, et al: Brain death, apneic diffusion oxygenation and organ transplant. J Trauma 18:180–183, 1978.
10. Ropper AH, Kennedy S, Russell L: Apnea testing in the diagnosis of brain death. J Neurosurg 55:942–946, 1981.
11. Schafer J, Caronna J: Duration of apnea needed to confirm brain death. Neurology 28:661–666, 1978.
12. Schwartz J, et al: Radionucleotide cerebral imaging confirming brain death. JAMA 249:246–247, 1983.
13. Thompson A, Sussmane J: Bretylium intoxication resembling clinical brain death. Crit Care Med 17:194–195, 1989.
14. Tsai SH, et al: Cerebral radionucleotide angiography: Its application in the diagnosis of brain death. JAMA 248:591–592, 1982.
15. Walker A: Cerebral Death. Baltimore, Urban and Schwartzenberg, 1985.

69. STATUS EPILEPTICUS

Brian J. Kelly, M.D.

1. How is status epilepticus defined?

The World Health Organization defines status epilepticus (SE) as "a condition characterized by an epileptic seizure that is sufficiently prolonged or repeated at sufficiently brief intervals so as to produce an unvarying and enduring epileptic condition." Although no time frame is stated here, traditionally the term SE is applied to any seizure that lasts more than 30 minutes.

2. What are the different types of SE? How do they present?

SE is best divided into three categories: convulsive status epilepticus (CSE), nonconvulsive status epilepticus (NCSE), and continuous partial seizures. Although only CSE is life threatening, all forms of status may result in serious disability.

CSE is the best known and most serious type of SE. In this condition, recurrent, generalized tonic-clonic motor seizures occur without the patient's regaining consciousness between seizures. The motor movements may not be symmetrical, and they may have a lateral predominance or even be focal. It is a medical emergency requiring immediate measures to terminate the seizures.

There are two types of NCSE. These are partial complex SE and petit mal SE. Partial complex SE is a condition in which the patient has continued alteration of consciousness lasting more than 30 minutes due to abnormal cortical electrical activity. Generalized tonic-clonic motor activity is absent, but stereotypical movements such as lip smacking, chewing, or picking at one's clothes may occur. The patient may be misdiagnosed as intoxicated or as having a psychiatric disorder.

Petit mal SE is often difficult to distinguish from partial complex SE, except with electroencephalographic (EEG) recordings. Patients appear lethargic but may be able to answer simple questions slowly. Eye blinking may be present, but automatisms are less common than in partial complex SE.

Continuous partial seizures are merely persistent focal motor seizures that last longer than 30 minutes and do not impair consciousness.

3. What are the most common causes of CSE?

Cessation of antiepileptic drugs, withdrawal from alcohol, drug overdose, and cerebrovascular disease are the most common causes of CSE. Other causes include metabolic disorders, cardiac arrest, central nervous system (CNS) neoplasms, trauma, encephalitis, meningitis, and CNS abscess. In about 15% of patients, no etiology for CSE can be found.

4. Why is there urgency in treating CSE?

Experimental data strongly suggest that permanent cell damage occurs in several cortical and subcortical locations after 60 minutes of convulsive status. Additionally, clinical studies have shown that the longer CSE continues, the more difficult it is to control, and the greater the incidence of neurologic sequelae. Status lasting longer than 60 minutes may also result in a number of secondary metabolic disturbances such as lactic acidosis, hypoglycemia, myolysis, myoglobinuria and renal failure, shock, and severe cardiopulmonary failure. These facts underscore the need to have a predetermined plan of action that will control SE in less than 60 minutes.

5. What are the most important initial steps when faced with a patient with CSE?

As always, the ABCs (*A*irway, *B*reathing, and *C*irculation) must be attended to immediately. Supplemental oxygen should be applied and a secure intravenous (IV) line should be started. If an adequate airway and ventilation are not present, an endotracheal tube should be inserted, and ventilation should be assisted. A 0.9% sodium chloride solution should be the initial IV fluid infused, since it can be used to treat hypotension should it occur and is compatible with IV phenytoin (Dilantin).

6. Which tests should be ordered immediately for a patient presenting with CSE?

A complete blood count, anticonvulsant levels, serum electrolytes, glucose, serum osmolarity, blood urea nitrogen, creatinine, calcium, magnesium, and phosphate levels, a drug screen, the alcohol level, and arterial blood gas analysis should be ordered immediately.

7. Once the ABCs have been accomplished, what are the next steps in managing a patient in CSE?

The following approach is intended only as a guideline. Individual circumstances may dictate different therapies.

Although seizures must persist for 30 minutes to be classified as SE, one should not wait until 30 minutes have passed before initiating therapy. If a seizure persists for more than 3 minutes, IV antiepileptic medications should be prepared for injection. If the seizure has not stopped by the time the medication is ready for injection (which usually takes 4–5 minutes), treatment should be started.

Once the IV line is established, thiamine 50 mg IV, followed by 50 cc of 50% dextrose solution should be administered if bedside blood glucose testing demonstrated hypoglycemia. A benzodiazepine (diazapam 0.10–0.15 mg/kg or lorazepam 0.10 mg/kg should be given at a rate no faster than 2 mg/min). Simultaneously, a loading dose of phenytoin (18 mg/kg given at a rate no faster than 50 mg/min) should be infused. A loading dose of phenytoin alone will stop CSE in approximately 80% of cases, but because the effects of the full dose do not occur for 20–30 minutes, many physicians give the benzodiazepine simultaneously because of its more rapid onset of activity.

If seizures persist after the phenytoin infusion has finished, phenobarbital should be given. A loading dose of 15–20 mg/kg is recommended, given at a rate no faster than 100 mg/min until the full dose is given or the seizures stop. Tracheal intubation, if not already secured, is indicated at this time since the cardiorespiratory depressant effects of phenobarbital and the benzodiazepines are additive.

By the time the phenobarbital infusion is complete, at least 30–40 minutes have elapsed. Remember, the goal is to have controlled the seizures before 60 minutes have elapsed. At this point, several options present themselves. If general anesthesia is available, it may be instituted with halothane and neuromuscular blockade to control the seizures. If general anesthesia is not available, an additional dose of 7 mg/kg of phenytoin may be given, again at a rate no faster than 50 mg/min. Alternatively, 50–100 mg of lidocaine IV push may be given. If the lidocaine stops the seizures, a maintenance lidocaine drip should be started at 1–2 mg/min. If these steps are unsuccessful, a barbiturate coma with an agent such as pentobarbital should be administered, or general anesthesia should be instituted, and a neurologist who is an expert on SE should be consulted.

8. What factors should be taken into account when determining which neuromuscular blockers (NMBs) should be administered to a patient with CSE if these agents are necessary?
NMBs all cause profound muscle weakness, but they vary greatly in their duration of action. If continuous EEG recording is not being performed, a short-acting agent should be employed, because it is impossible to ascertain if seizure activity is continuing in the face of neuromuscular blockade. If a long-acting agent is employed without EEG recording, unrecognized SE could continue for hours until the effects of the NMBs wear off.

9. What are the side effects of administering phenytoin too rapidly?
Hypotension can occur if phenytoin is given at a rate faster than 50 mg/min. Additionally, rapid IV administration may result in cardiac dysrhythmias and ventricular standstill.

10. What is the major advantage of phenytoin in treating CSE?
In addition to being highly effective, phenytoin is not a CNS depressant like the benzodiazepines and the barbiturates. Therefore, it is easier to assess the patient's neurologic status after the seizures have stopped.

11. After the seizures are controlled, what are appropriate subsequent management steps?
Once the seizures are controlled, it is important to establish the etiology of the SE. Although discontinuation of anticonvulsant medication is the most frequent cause of SE in patients with a known history of seizures, often SE is multifactorial in etiology. Therefore in all patients it is necessary to rule out metabolic, infectious, and new CNS pathology. Culture of the blood, urine, sputum, and spinal fluid and their analysis are usually indicated. Imaging with CT or MRI should be performed and should generally precede lumbar puncture if focal signs are present on neurologic exam or if there is a suspicion of a significant intracranial mass. Empirical antibiotics should be started immediately if an infectious etiology is suspected, and maintenance doses of anticonvulsants administered and adjusted based on serum levels.

12. Does a fever or a cerebrospinal fluid (CSF) pleocytosis always indicate an infectious etiology in a patient with CSE?
Most patients with SE exhibit an increase in body temperature, which in rare cases may go to extremes (up to 107° F) even in the absence of an infectious etiology. Additionally, a peripheral blood and mild CSF pleocytosis may occur in these patients. While fever and blood and CSF pleocytosis may be the result of CSE, it is imperative that one not attribute these findings to the effect of repeated seizures until all other possibilities have been excluded. Generally, it is better to empirically cover for infectious etiologies until all cultures are negative than to undertreat a serious infection.

BIBLIOGRAPHY

1. Aminoff MJ, Simon RP. Status epilepticus: Causes, clinical features and consequences in 98 patients. Am J Med 69:657–666, 1980.

2. Crawford TO, Mitchell WG, Snodgrass SR: Lorazepam in childhood status epilepticus and serial seizures: Effectiveness and tachyphylaxis. Neurology 37:190–195, 1987.
3. Delgado-Escueta AV, Wasterlain C, Treiman DM, Porter RJ: Management of status epilepticus. N Engl J Med 306:1337–1340, 1983.
4. Leppik IE: Status epilepticus. Neurol Clin 4:633–643, 1986.
5. Uthman BM, Wilder BJ: Emergency management of seizures: An overview. Epilepsia 30(Suppl 2): S33–S37, 1989.

70. CEREBRAL ANEURYSMS

Dorre Nicholau, M.D.

1. What is the incidence of subarachnoid hemorrhage from ruptured intracranial aneurysms?
The incidence of subarachnoid hemorrhage from intracerebral aneurysms is estimated to be 15–20 per 100,000 population.

2. What is the incidence of asymptomatic intracranial aneurysms?
Incidental cerebral aneurysms are found at autopsy anywhere from 1.6 to 4.7% of the time. Less than one fifth of all intracranial aneurysms result in rupture.

3. Who is most at risk for intracerebral aneurysm rupture?
Women aged 50–60 incur the greatest risk. Sixty percent of cerebral aneurysms occur in females. Size of the aneurysm is also important. Aneurysms >3 mm in diameter are thought to be at risk for rupture. Larger aneurysms are more likely to rupture than smaller aneurysms. An estimated 2% of aneurysms <5 mm in diameter result in rupture; >40% of aneurysms between 6 and 10 mm in diameter are known to result in rupture. The mean size of aneurysms at rupture has been reported to be from 7.5 mm (at angiography) to 8.5 mm (at autopsy).

4. What risk factors are associated with the development of intracerebral aneurysms?
The most widely accepted risk factors include age (40–60), hypertension, sex (female > male), and genetic factors.

5. What are the major etiologies of cerebral aneurysms?
In a majority of cases, no inciting event or genetic predisposition can be identified.

Genetic: Approximately 6.7% of all cerebral aneurysms run in families. These typically present earlier than nonfamilial aneurysms. The known hereditary syndromes such as Ehlers-Danlos syndrome and polycystic kidney disease account for most but not all of these familial aneurysms. Approximately 16% of patients with polycystic kidney disease develop intracerebral aneurysms.

Mycotic: One to 5% of the intracerebral aneurysms are secondary to septic embolization from valvular vegetations in patients suffering from bacterial endocarditis. These aneurysms typically appear approximately 4–5 weeks after an acute embolic event. They are typically found in the distal middle cerebral artery circulation. Streptococcus is the most common pathogen.

Traumatic: While true traumatic aneurysms are rare, false aneurysms are somewhat more common. False aneurysms result from the complete disruption of the vessel wall with resulting clot formation. Traumatic aneurysms are usually found in association with skull fractures.

6. What are the systemic effects associated with acute aneurysm rupture?

Systemic hypertension and bradycardia result from the initial acute elevation in intracranial pressure. Altered mental status or loss of consciousness may result in aspiration of gastric contents and the development of aspiration pneumonitis. Finally, intracerebral catastrophe is associated with gastrointestinal bleeding.

7. What are the signs and symptoms of intracerebral aneurysmal rupture?

Most signs and symptoms of cerebral aneurysm rupture are the result of blood within the subarachnoid space. Common signs such as headache, photophobia, fever, and nuchal rigidity are all the consequence of blood-induced meningeal irritation. In addition, the presence of blood in the subarachnoid space may obstruct interventricular flow and/or reabsorption of cerebrospinal fluid (CSF) by the choroid villi, resulting in hydrocephalus.

Sudden severe headache is the most common complaint among patients presenting with aneurysm rupture. Nausea and vomiting may accompany the headache, especially when intracranial pressure is elevated. Increased intracranial pressure may be the result of mass effect secondary to hematoma formation, cerebral edema, or hydrocephalus.

Focal neurologic deficits are sometimes evident at the time of presentation. One of the most common is a third-nerve palsy resulting from the rupture of a carotid-posterior-communicating-artery aneurysm. Though focal signs may result from nerve compression by a localized hematoma and/or a more general increase in intracranial pressure, they are often the result of ischemia due to cerebral vasospasm.

Signs and Symptoms of Subarachnoid Hemorrhage

SYMPTOMS OF SUBARACHNOID HEMORRHAGE	SIGNS OF SUBARACHNOID HEMORRHAGE
Sudden, severe headache	Neck stiffness
Nausea and vomiting	Brudzinski's, Kernig's sign
Dizziness	Fever
Vertigo	Hypertension
Fatigue	Blurred vision
Diplopia	Oculomotor paralysis
Photophobia	Hemiparesis
	Confusion and/or agitation
	Coma

From Smith R, Miller J: Pathophysiology and clinical evaluation of subarachnoid hemorrhage. In Youmans JR (ed): Neurological Surgery, 3rd ed. Philadelphia, W.B. Saunders, 1990, with permission.

8. What is a sentinel bleed? Why is it significant?

A sentinel bleed is an initial minor bleed or "leak" from a cerebral aneurysm. It is considered a minor bleed because although it results in a severe headache, it usually does not result in focal signs or altered consciousness. As a consequence, it may go unrecognized or be misdiagnosed (as a migraine headache, for instance). It is important to recognize these bleeds because they often serve as warning signs of subsequent catastrophic events. Proper recognition and care may affect mortality. The mortality rate from ruptured aneurysms identified by sentinel bleeds is reported to be lower than that from aneurysmal bleeds that are not preceded by warning leaks (28.9% vs. 43.2%).

9. How is the diagnosis of subarachnoid hemorrhage (SAH) made?

The presence of red blood cells in the CSF is diagnostic of a subarachnoid hemorrhage. In general, >100 RBC/mm^2 is considered significant. The presence of xanthochromia distinguishes SAH from traumatic lumbar puncture. Acutely, the absence of red blood cells in the CSF does not rule out the possibility of SAH, as 6–12 hours may pass before red cells released in the cranium are found in the lumbar space. Erythrocytes should be evident in the CSF up to 2 weeks after SAH. In practice, the diagnosis of SAH is made by radiologic imaging and CSF analysis. Patients in whom intracranial hemorrhage is suspected should undergo CT scan of the head before lumbar puncture to rule out the possibility of significant mass effect. If increased intracranial pressure is present, the performance of a lumbar puncture could result in transtentorial herniation.

When red blood cells are present in CSF, the possibility of a bloody, "traumatic tap" must be ruled out. Traumatic taps are evident by clearing the fluid with the serial collection of a number of tubes, the lack of xanthochromia after centrifugation, and the presence of leukocytes in proportion to that in the peripheral smear (approximately 2 WBC/1,000 erythrocytes).

10. What factors are associated with poor prognosis after rupture of a cerebral aneurysm?
The degree of meningeal irritation, level of consciousness, and presence of focal motor neurologic deficits can be used to identify patients who are at increased risk of perioperative death. Under these criteria, patients are grouped into five grades.

Classic Presentation and Prognosis for Ruptured Cerebral Aneurysm

GRADE	CRITERIA	ESTIMATED PERIOPER-ATIVE MORTALITY (%)
I	Asymptomatic or minimal headache and slight nuchal rigidity	0–5
II	Moderate to severe headache, no nuchal rigidity other than cranial nerve palsy	2–10
III	Drowsiness, confusion, or mild focal deficit	10–15
IV	Stupor, moderate to severe hemiparesis, possible early decerebrate rigidity and vegetative disturbances	60–70
V	Deep coma, decerebrate rigidity, moribund appearance	70–100

Adapted from Peerless SJ.[11] Grades according to Hunt and Hess.[6]

11. What are the major complications of ruptured intracranial aneurysms?
Vasospasm, hyponatremia, hydrocephalus, aseptic meningitis, vascular occlusions, and recurrent hemorrhage.

12. Which complications are the most significant?
Clinically apparent vasospasm complicates cerebral aneurysm rupture 33% of the time. It produces cerebral ischemia and may result in devastating consequences unrelated to the initial bleed. The incidence of vasospasm typically peaks by days 5–9 after rupture. As many as 20% of focal neurologic deficits resulting from vasospasm may be permanent. Recurrent intracranial hemorrhage occurs in a significant number of patients after aneurysm rupture. The risk of rebleeding is related to the length of conservative management (7% at 1 week, up to 30% at 8 weeks). Rebleeding is associated with an increased risk of death when compared with initial bleeds.

13. What is the etiology of cerebral vasospasm?
The etiology of cerebral vasospasm is unclear, but the incidence and severity are related to the presence of blood in the CSF. Clinically, the amount of blood in the subarachnoid cisterns on CT scan correlates with the degree of vasospasm found at angiography.

14. How is vasospasm diagnosed?

Vasospasm may be diagnosed radiographically by angiography or clinically by the appearance of neurologic deficits. Radiographic narrowing of vessels is apparent by day 4 and peaks by day 7 posthemorrhage. The clinical diagnosis of vasospasm is based on the slow (over hours) progression of neurologic deficits 4–7 days after hemorrhage, once other etiologies, such as rebleeding, have been excluded. Vasospasm is present on angiography in approximately 70% of patients after SAH. Only 20–30% of radiographically apparent vasospasm is clinically significant.

15. What is the treatment of cerebral vasospasm?

To treat cerebral vasospasm, one must attempt to prevent or reverse arterial spasm, while at the same time minimize the ischemia that results from the spasm. The mainstay of treatment includes:

1. Calcium channel blockers to relax vascular smooth muscle.
2. Arterial hypertension to maximize cerebral perfusion pressure.
3. Fluid loading with subsequent hypervolemia and hemodilution to optimize the flow characteristics of blood within the narrowed vessels.
4. Recently, removal of blood from the CSF has been advocated as a treatment of vasospasm. This can be done surgically (at the time of craniotomy) or medically, with the injection of fibrinolytic substances into the CSF. Streptokinase and tissue-plasminogen activator (t-PA) have been used for this purpose.

16. What is nimodipine? How does it work?

Nimodipine is the calcium channel blocker of choice for the treatment of cerebral vasospasm. It works by blocking the influx of calcium across cell membranes and theoretically works to relax vascular smooth muscle. To date there is no in vivo angiographic evidence that nimodipine actually works to reverse cerebral vasospasm. An alternative theory of action suggests that the drug functions to decrease calcium entry into damaged cerebral neurons and thereby reduces neuronal damage. Several clinical trials have shown nimodipine to be effective in reducing the incidence of permanent neurologic damage and death resulting from vasospasm.

Nimodipine is highly lipid soluble and rapidly crosses the blood-brain barrier. Therapeutic doses of nimodipine produce a minimal effect on systemic vessels. When used in recommended doses, it rarely results in systemic hypotension (15%). Bradycardia, headache, and nausea can occur.

17. What is the optimal time from hemorrhage to surgical repair of cerebral aneurysms?

The timing of aneurysm surgery is controversial: there is risk of exacerbating cerebral vasospasm and ischemia with early surgery, but also risk of rebleeding if surgery is delayed. Theoretical advantages of early surgery (0–3 days) include: (1) prevention of rebleeding; (2) mechanical removal of blood from the subarachnoid space, with a resulting decrease in vasospasm; (3) aggressive pursuit of the medical management of vasospasm, deliberate hypertension, and volume expansion without increasing the risk of rebleeding; (4) decrease in medical complications associated with prolonged bed rest; and (5) decrease in patient and family anxiety while awaiting surgery.

Advantages of delayed surgery (>10 days) include: (1) resolution of cerebral vasospasm and return of cerebral autoregulation. Advocates of delayed surgery argue that vasospasm and loss of cerebral autoregulation may reduce the cerebral reserve necessary to perform uncomplicated cerebral surgery and that vasospasm-induced, decreased cerebral blood flow may not be clinically apparent at the time of operation. (2) Decreased cerebral edema results in better operating conditions, and (3) the increased time to surgery allows for stabilization of the patient's general medical condition. Delayed surgery represents the accepted dogma, but recent clinical trials from university centers indicate that early surgery may indeed decrease the overall management of mortality in these patients.

18. Describe the operative repair of cerebral aneurysms.

Several different surgical methods are used to repair cerebral aneurysms:

   1. **Clipping:** The most effective of all the surgical techniques, clipping involves the dissection of the neck of the aneurysmal sac and the placement of a removable spring clip at the origin of the neck from the feeder vessel.

   2. **Trapping:** This technique involves permanently occluding the vessel proximally and distally to the aneurysm and relies on the presence of adequate collateral blood flow to the affected area.

   3. **Proximal ligation:** This technique involves ligation of the feeder artery to reduce blood flow through the aneurysm. The subsequent decrease in flow and transmural pressure results in thrombosis and/or obliteration of the aneurysmal sac. As with trapping, this technique is restricted to specific cases in which collateral blood flow is sufficient to prevent subsequent ischemic damage.

   4. **Wrapping:** Reinforcement of the aneurysmal wall with synthetic material (Gelfoam, etc.) prevents further enlargement of the sac.

19. What nonoperative alternative treatments are available?

At selected centers, cerebral aneurysms may be treated in the interventional radiology suite. The technique is called endovascular balloon occlusion. It involves the placement of a detachable microballoon into the aneurysmal sac. This is typically done by puncture of the femoral artery with a balloon-tipped catheter, which is then directed into the aneurysmal sac by fluoroscopic guidance. Once in the aneurysmal sac, the balloon is inflated with a permanently solidifying agent and then detached from the catheter. This technique successfully occludes the aneurysm while at the same time preserving flow within the parent vessel. The technique may also be used in aneurysms that lack a defined neck. In this case, the balloon is inflated to occlude the feeding vessel. It requires a preliminary test occlusion to demonstrate that occlusion of the feeding vessel will not result in neurologic deficit.

BIBLIOGRAPHY

   1. Allen GS, et al: Cerebral arterial spasm—a controlled trial of nimodipine in patients with subarachnoid hemorrhage N Engl J Med 308:619–624, 1983.
   2. Awad I, Carter P, et al: Clinical vasospasm after subarachnoid hemorrhage: Response to hypervolemic hemodilution and arterial hypertension. Stroke 18:365–372, 1987.
   3. Disney L, Weir B, Petruk K: Effect on management mortality of a deliberate policy of early operation on supratentorial aneurysms. Neurosurgery 20:695–701, 1987.
   4. Espinosa F, Weir B, Noseworthy T: Nonoperative treatment of subarachnoid hemorrhage. In Youmans JR (ed): Neurological Surgery, 3rd ed. Philadelphia, W.B. Saunders, 1990, pp 1661–1668.
   5. Higashida R, et al: Endovascular treatment of intracranial aneurysms with a new silicone microballoon device: Technical considerations and indications for therapy. Radiology 174:687–691, 1990.
   6. Hunt W, Hess R: Surgical risk as related to time of intervention in the repair of intracranial aneurysms. J Neurosurg 28:14–20, 1968.
   7. Kassell NF, et al: Cerebral vasospasm following aneurysmal subarachnoid hemorrhage. Stroke 16:562–572, 1985.
   8. Kassell NF, Boarini DJ: Patients with ruptured aneurysm: Pre- and postoperative management. In Wilkins RH, Rengachary SS (eds): Neurosurgery. New York, McGraw-Hill, 1985, pp 1367–1371.
   9. Mee E, et al: Controlled study of Nimodipine in aneurysm patients treated early after subarachnoid hemorrhage. Neurosurgery 22:484–490, 1988.
  10. Newell D, et al: Angioplasty for the treatment of symptomatic vasospasm following subarachnoid hemorrhage. J Neurosurg 71:654–659, 1989.

11. Peerless SJ: Intracranial aneurysms. In Newfield P, Cottrell J: Handbook of Neuroanesthesia, 1983, pp 173–183.
12. Smith R, Miller J: Pathophysiology and clinical evaluation of subarachnoid hemorrhage. In Youmans JR (eds): Neurological Surgery, 3rd ed. Philadelphia, W.B. Saunders, 1990, pp 1644–1660.
13. Weir B: Intracranial aneurysms and subarachnoid hemorrhage: An overview. In Wilkins RH, Rengachary SS: Neurosurgery. New York, McGraw-Hill, 1985, pp 1308–1329.

71. CEREBRAL VASCULAR ACCIDENTS

Dorre Nicholau, M.D.

1. What is the normal value for cerebral blood flow?

In an adult, cerebral blood flow is approximately 50 ml/100 gr of brain tissue/min. This represents 15% of the normal cardiac output. When cerebral blood flow decreases to <23 ml/100 gm/min, neurologic dysfunction occurs. Short periods of ischemia result in reversible deficits.

2. What are the major risk factors for thrombotic cerebral infarction?

Major risk factors are related to the development of atherosclerotic disease. They include hypertension, smoking, obesity, diabetes mellitus, congestive heart failure, coronary artery disease, and hyperlipidemia. Hypertension is by far the most significant risk factor. Among all ages and both sexes, the presence of hypertension increases the risk of stroke threefold. This increased risk is proportional to the degree of both systolic and and diastolic hypertension. Increased diastolic blood pressure is associated with at least 70% of strokes. The incidence of cerebral infarction increases with age and is 1.3 times higher in males than females.

3. What are the major risk factors for embolic cerebral infarction?

Embolic cerebral events are usually of cardiac origin. Major risk factors include myocardial infarction (MI) with mural thrombus; cardiac arrhythmia, especially atrial fibrillation; bacterial endocarditis; and structural valvular abnormalities such as mitral stenosis. MI is a major risk factor. Approximately 5% of patients presenting with acute MI exhibit clinical evidence of stroke. At autopsy, systemic emboli are present in approximately 50% of patients who die from MI. Atrial fibirllation alone, without evidence of rheumatic heart disease, increases the risk of stroke by approximately fivefold. Elderly patients incur the greatest risk from atrial fibrillation, as the proportion of strokes due to this arrhythmia increases with age. Atheroscleroses of the aorta and carotid arteries are also risk factors.

4. Does drug abuse predispose patients to stroke?

Recently drug abuse has emerged as a significant risk factor leading to stroke in young patients. Four percent of strokes occur in patients under the age of 35. A recent case-controlled retrospective study showed drug abuse to be the most frequently identified potential risk factor among stroke patients in this young age group.

5. Describe the blood supply to the brain.

Four arteries carry blood to the brain. They are the two internal carotid arteries anteriorly and the two vertebral arteries posteriorly. The anterior circulation is fed by the carotid arteries bilaterally. The internal carotid arteries arise from the common carotid arteries. The left common carotid artery is a branch of the left subclavian artery; the right carotid artery arises from the right brachiocephalic trunk. Each common carotid artery bifurcates at the angle of the jaw, into external and internal branches. The internal carotid arteries supply the optic nerves, the retina, and the majority of the cerebral hemispheres (the frontal, parietal, and anterior temporal lobes).

Branches of the internal carotid artery include: (1) ophthalmic artery, (2) posterior communicating artery, (3) anterior choroidal artery, (4) anterior cerebral artery, and (5) middle cerebral artery.

The posterior circulation is fed by two vertebral arteries. The right and left vertebral arteries arise from the subclavian arteries bilaterally and enter the posterior fossa through the foramen magnum. They give rise to the posterior inferior cerebellar artery and the anterior and posterior spinal arteries before merging to form the basilar artery at the level of the pontomedullary junction. The vertebral-basilar system supplies the cervical cord, brain stem, cerebral cortex, and, in most cases, the occipital lobes.

The posterior cerebral artery (PCA) supplies the occipital lobes. In a vast majority of patients (70%), this artery originates from the bifurcation of the basilar artery. In 95% of cases, one or both PCAs arise from the basilar artery, whereas in the remaining 5% the posterior cerebral arteries arise from the internal carotid artery bilaterally.

Branches of the basilar artery include: (1) pontine artery, (2) labyrinthine artery to the middle ear, (3) superior cerebellar artery, and (4) posterior cerebral artery.

6. Describe the circle of Willis.

The vertebral-basilar system is joined to the carotid system by an anastomotic ring. The anterior and posterior communicating arteries link the anterior/posterior and the left/right hemispheric circulations. Four arteries compose the circle: posterior communicating artery, posterior cerebral artery, anterior communicating artery, and anterior cerebral artery bilaterally.

7. Describe the clinical presentation of the major vascular deficiencies.

The neurologic presentation of patients suffering an ischemic cerebral vascular insult depends on the location and size of the infarct. Carotid artery infarction results in unilateral symptoms; vertebral-basilar system infarction usually results in bilateral symptoms.

Carotid artery occlusion results in contralateral hemiplegia, hemihypesthesia, homonymous hemianopia, agnosia, and, if the dominant hemisphere is affected, global aphasia. A minority (15%) of patients exhibit an ipsilateral Horner's syndrome. Often the substantial size of the infarct results in marked cerebral edema, and the patient may present in an obtunded or comatose state. Most carotid artery occlusions are thrombotic. Transient ischemic episodes precede major carotid occlusion approximately 50% of the time.

Total occlusion of the middle cerebral artery results in a clinical picture similar to that described for carotid artery occlusion. However, the resulting motor dysfunction affects the face and upper extremity but typically spares the leg. Branch occlusions result in fewer deficits. Because the mass of tissue damage may be significantly less, mental status may not be as severely depressed. Most middle cerebral artery occlusions are embolic.

Basilar artery occlusion results in bilateral cranial nerve palsies and quadriparesis. If the infarction includes the midbrain reticular activating system, the patient presents in coma. It is possible, however, for the high midbrain and reticular activating system to be spared, while motor pathways are affected. This complete loss of motor function in an awake patient is commonly referred to as the locked-in syndrome.

Unilateral vertebral artery occlusion results in ischemia of the lateral medulla. Ischemia of the spinothalamic tract results in ipsilateral ataxia, facial hypesthesia, and contralateral loss of pain and temperature below the face. Loss of function of the ninth and tenth cranial nerves results in dysphagia and hoarseness. Loss of the ipsilateral sympathetic tract results in Horner's syndrome. Finally, loss of cerebellar fibers results in ipsilateral ataxia. This clinical picture reflects ischemia in the distribution of the posterior inferior cerebellar artery and is commonly referred to as lateral medullary syndrome or Wallenberg's syndrome.

8. Describe basilar artery syndrome.

The vertebral basilar system supplies the contents of the posterior fossa and the visual cortex. Hence, the syndrome usually refers to transient cerebellar and brain stem symptoms, including cranial nerve abnormalities. Bilateral motor and/or sensory deficits may accompany vertigo, dysarthria, ataxia, and diplopia.

9. What is subclavian steal syndrome?

This syndrome refers to the symptoms of vertebral basilar insufficiency when they are provoked by arm exercise. It reflects the diversion of blood (or "steal") from the vertebral artery to the brachial artery. When the vasodilation that accompanies exercise is coupled with a proximal subclavian or innominate artery stenosis, blood may flow retrograde through the vertebral artery to fill the dilated vascular pool in the arm. This syndrome is confirmed when symptoms are associated with a decreased blood pressure in one arm and an ipsilateral supraclavicular bruit. It is more common on the left than on the right.

10. What is a TIA?

A transient ischemic attack (TIA) is a reversible ischemic episode that does not result in infarction or permanent deficit. The attacks occur suddenly and last by definition less than 24 hours; the majority of attacks last less than 15 minutes. Between attacks, patient's neurologic function returns to normal.

Carotid TIAs are associated with carotid atheromatous disease. Ischemia in the carotid distribution results in deficits in the ipsilateral visual field or contralateral sensorimotor function. Visual and hemispheric symptoms typically do not occur simultaneously.

Amaurosis fugax refers to the transient ipsilateral monocular blindness resulting from a TIA. Transient hemispheric attacks refer to ischemia in the region of the middle cerebral artery with focal motor and sensory deficits in the contralateral arm and hand.

Approximately one-third of patients who suffer from a TIA will suffer a major storke within 4 years.

11. What is a RIND?

RIND is a reversible ischemic neurologic disability lasting more than 24 hours but less than 3 weeks.

12. What is a completed stroke?

A completed stroke refers to permanent disability resulting from an ischemic event.

13. What is a lacunar infarct?

The term lacuna is Latin for a small pit or hollow cavity. Cerebral lacunes refer to multiple small infarcts resulting from occlusion of the small penetrating branches (50–150 microns in diameter) of the major cerebral vessels. The infarcted brain tissue then softens and decays, leaving small cavities, 1–3 mm in diameter, which are evident at autopsy. Lacunes produce a variety of sensory and motor symptoms depending on their location. Multiple lacunes may result in loss of intellectual capacity with impairment of recent memory. In some cases, severe dementia may result. Lacunar infarction is usually associated with chronic hypertension.

14. Describe hypertensive encephalopathy.

This term refers to encephalopathy that is preceded by a rapid rise in blood pressure. One theory suggests that the rapid rise in blood pressure is accompanied by loss of cerebral autoregulation, producing areas of focal vasospasm and ischemia together with areas of cerebral vasodilation and increased flow. Cerebral edema often ensues, but is not always present. Hypertensive encephalopathy typically occurs in patients with disorders that produce baseline hypertension. Etiologies are related to age and include: (1) acute glomerulonephritis: children and adolescents, (2) chronic glomerulonephritis: young adults, (3) eclampsia: childbearing females, and (4) malignant hypertension: patients > 30–40 years of age. Symptoms are usually generalized and include headache, nausea, vomiting, confusion, obtundation, or, in severe cases, coma. Focal disturbances, including aphasia, focal or generalized seizures, and hemiparesis, may also occur. The only consistent sign is systemic arterial hypertension. Papilledema and/or hypertensive retinopathy may be present but neither is necessary to make a diagnosis.

15. What is a watershed infarct?
A watershed infarct refers to an area of cerebral ischemia resulting from decreased perfusion pressure. In the case of watershed infarcts, decreased blood flow is usually due to systemic hypotension. Watershed infarcts typically occur bilaterally in boundary zones between major vascular beds such as the middle cerebral artery and the posterior cerebral artery.

16. What is the significance of carotid artery stenosis?
Carotid stenosis may result in cerebral ischemia, presenting as TIAs or in more severe cases, stroke. One third of patients who suffer from a TIA show clinical signs of extracranial carotid disease. In these cases, ischemia is most often the result of atherosclerotic microembolism rather than distal infarction secondary to stenosis.

17. What portion of cerebral vascular accidents reflects extracranial versus intracranial pathology?
The distribution of vascular pathology leading to stroke varies among racial groups. Blacks and Asians are more likely to exhibit intracranial pathology; whites more often exhibit extracranial lesions.

18. Discuss the treatment of acute ischemic stroke.
Therapeutic approaches include hypervolemic hemodilution, calcium channel blockade, heparin anticoagulation, and fibrinolytic therapy.

Hemodilution has proved to be a well-tolerated, effective intervention in the treatment of ischemic stroke. Hematocrit is a major determinant of whole blood viscosity, and clinical studies have demonstrated a correlation between hematocrit and the size of cerebral infarcts, the higher hematocrits generally producing the largest defects. By lowering blood viscosity, it is theoretically possible to increase collateral blood flow to the peri-infarct region and thus limit the size of the subsequent cerebral infarction. This technique relies on hypervolemic hemodilution to lower blood viscosity. By venesection and infusions of dextran and crystalloid, the hematocrit is lowered to a target value of 30–35%, a value thought to maximize both viscosity characteristics and oxygen-carrying capacity of blood. Several studies have shown that hemodilution is effective in improving early neurologic outcome from ischemic stroke. It does not alter mortality.

Calcium channel blockade is a promising experimental approach to the treatment of acute ischemic stroke. Its use in this setting is based on the knowledge that cerebral ischemia produces an intracellular shift of free calcium, which correlates with subsequent cell death. The evolution of acute stroke results in an area of ischemic yet viable cells within the hypoperfused periphery of the injury, called the ischemic penumbra. Early effective antagonism of calcium influx into the cells in this region may prevent their destruction and preserve neurologic function.

Nimodipine is a highly lipid, soluble calcium channel blocker that rapidly crosses the blood-brain barrier. A review of five multicenter, double-blind, placebo-controlled trials of the use of nimodipine in acute ischemic sroke showed improvement in both neurologic outcome and mortality in treated patients compared with matched controls. In the over 800 patients studied, nimodipine reduced the death rate from 12.3% among controls to 7.9% among treated patients. Benefit from nimodipine is most evident in patients who suffer moderate to severe stroke, are older than 65 years of age, and are treated within 12 hours of the onset of symptoms.

Although widely accepted as treatment for acute ischemic stroke for over 30 years, heparin anticoagulation therapy remains controversial in the 1990s. A number of clinical studies have not consistently demonstrated benefit from heparinization in the treatment of acute ischemic stroke. A recent, large retrospective review of heparin treatment of progressive stroke failed to show a relationship between stroke progression and/or hemorrhagic complications and heparin dose, mean PTT or PTT ratio.

Thrombolytic therapy for acute ischemic thrombotic and embolic stroke is under clinical investigation at a number of centers in the United States and Germany. The use of thrombolytic agents in these settings must weigh the potential benefit of recanalization of thrombosed arteries against the risk of hemorrhagic transformation. A preliminary report in December 1990 of 71 patients with angiographically demonstrated cerebral arterial occlusion showed that, while angiographic responders fared better with respect to early recovery of hand and language function than nonresponders, hemorrhagic transformation occurred in 27% of patients treated with recombinant tissue plasminogen activator. Though hemorrhagic transformation is for the most part a benign process, cerebral hemorrhage preceded death in 3 study patients. These studies are ongoing, and the risk-benefit ratio of this treatment, though promising, has yet to be determined.

BIBLIOGRAPHY

1. Adams R, Victor M: Cerebrovascular disease. In Principles of Neurology, 4th ed. New York, McGraw-Hill, 1989, pp 617–691.
2. Bannister R: Disorders of the cerebral circulation. In Brain's Clinical Neurology, 6th ed. London, Oxford University Press, 1985, p 285.
3. Barnett HJ: Cerebral ischemia and infarction. In Wyngaarden J, Smith L (eds): Cecil Textbook of Medicine. Philadelphia, W.B. Saunders, 1988, pp 2162–2163.
4. Dunbabin DW, Sandercock PAG: Preventing stroke by modification of risk factors. Stroke 21:36–39, 1990.
5. Gelmers HJ, Hennerici M: Effect of nimodipine on acute ischemic stroke, pooled results from five randomized trials. Stroke 21(Suppl IV):81–84, 1990.
6. Kaku D, Lowenstein D: Emergence of recreational drug use as a major risk factor for stroke in young adults. Ann Intern Med 113:821–827, 1990.
7. Koller M, Haenny P, Hess K, et al: Adjusted hypervolemic hemodilution in acute ischemic stroke. Stroke 21:1429–1434, 1990.
8. Rowland LP: Merritt's Textbook of Neurology, 8th ed. Philadelphia, Lea and Febiger, 1989.
9. Slivka A, Levy D: Natural history of progressive ischemic stroke in a population treated with heparin. Stroke 21:1657–1662, 1990.
10. Strand T, Asplund K, Eriksson S, et al: A randomized trial of hemodilution therapy in acute ischemic stroke. Stroke 15:980–989, 1984.
11. Wolf P: An overview of the epidemiology of stroke. Stroke 21(Suppl II):4–6, 1990.
12. Zoppo G, and the rt-PA Acute Stroke Study Group: An open, multicenter trial of recombinant tissue plasminogen activator in acute stroke: A progress report. Stroke 21(Suppl IV):174–175, 1990.

72. LANDRY-GUILLAIN-BARRÉ SYNDROME

Brian J. Kelly, M.D.

1. What is the Landry-Guillain-Barré syndrome?

Landry-Guillain-Barré syndrome (LGBS) is an acute or subacute polyradiculoneuropathy that affects all ages and is thought to have an autoimmune cause.

2. Are there any factors that predispose a person to LGBS?

Although cause and effect have never been proved, approximately 50% of LGBS patients will have suffered a recent respiratory or gastrointestinal infection. An additional 15% will have had a recent vaccination. Of all the vaccinations studied, only the 1976–77 swine flu vaccine showed a statistically significant, increased incidence of LGBS, possibly secondary to contamination of the vaccine with the P2-myelin protein from the chick embryos that the vaccine was made from.

3. What is the pathology of LGBS? How does it explain the typical clinical features of LGBS?

The primary pathologic process in LGBS is segmental demyelination of the peripheral nerves due to an autoimmune process that is both humorally and cell mediated. Since the primary process is a loss of myelin, the peripheral nerves that are most heavily myelinated (i.e., motor and joint-position sensory nerves) are more severely affected than unmyelinated or lightly myelinated nerves (i.e., nerves that mediate pain and temperature sensation).

4. What are the typical features of LGBS?

The initial symptoms of LGBS are usually paresthesias in the distal extremities and pain or stiffness in the proximal limbs followed quickly by progressive weakness of the limbs, trunk, and cranial muscles. The weakness is fairly symmetrical, most frequently begins in the legs, and spreads in an ascending fashion, although other patterns of disease progression have been described. Patients lose their reflexes early in the course of the disease. Respiratory function is often compromised due to involvement of the phrenic and intercostal nerves. Cranial nerve deficits occur and may affect speech or swallowing. Vibratory sensation and proprioception are usually severely impaired, whereas pinprick and temperature sensation are often normal.

5. What is the differential diagnosis of subacutely evolving motor weakness?

Causes of Subacute Motor Weakness

Toxins (hexacarbon, lead, thallium, or organophosphate intoxication)	Myasthenia gravis
	Periodic paralysis
Poliomyelitis	Tick paralysis
Botulism	Diphtheritic polyneuropathy
Porphyria	Saxitoxin poisoning

6. How is the diagnosis of LGBS confirmed?

The diagnosis is made on clinical grounds and is supported by nerve conduction studies and electromyography that show evidence of a demyelinating polyneuropathy early in the course of the disease. Spinal fluid analysis typically shows increased protein without a prominent inflammatory cellular response. This rise in protein, however, may not occur until 7–14 days into the illness. Other entities listed in the table above should be excluded by clinical exam and ancillary tests.

7. What is the typical clinical time course for LGBS?

LGBS usually follows a predictable triphasic course:

1. There is an initial period of deterioration in strength lasting 1–3 weeks from the onset of the first symptom to the point of maximum deficit.

2. A plateau phase then lasts several days to 2 weeks, during which there is little change in the neurologic exam.

3. The recovery phase then begins due to remyelination of the damaged nerves. This typically lasts a few weeks to months but in cases of severe nerve damage can be much longer.

8. What are the mortality and morbidity from LGBS?

The mortality rate from LGBS is 2–5%, and virtually all deaths are due to secondary complications from prolonged hospitalization. Major causes of these complications are: (1) sepsis secondary to pulmonary and urinary infections, (2) pulmonary emboli, (3) delayed treatment of respiratory failure, and (4) dysautonomias. These complications can be minimized by excellent medical and nursing care in the intensive care unit (ICU).

9. Which patients with LGBS require ICU observation?

Any patient with significant respiratory muscle or bulbar muscle weakness should be transferred to the ICU for observation. Similarly, patients who show evidence of significant autonomic dysfunction or rapidly progressive generalized weakness should be followed closely in the ICU.

10. What percentage of LGBS patients require respiratory support with a mechanical ventilator?

Between 10 and 23% of patients with LGBS eventially require mechanical ventilation.

11. What is the best way to follow respiratory function in a patient with a neuromuscular disease such as LGBS?

Frequent bedside pulmonary function testing of vital capacity and maximum inspiratory and expiratory pressures is the best method of assessing and following respiratory function. Arterial blood gas determinations frequently remain normal until respiratory failure is severe, and such measurements therefore lead to a false sense of security regarding respiratory status.

12. When should patients with LGBS be intubated?

This issue is controversial, and several factors need to be taken into account. The respiratory failure that patients suffer is due to a combination of respiratory muscle insufficiency leading to hypercapnic respiratory failure plus pneumonia secondary to an inability to adequately cough or protect their airway.

The following are general guidelines for intubation. A patient should be intubated:

1. when the vital capacity becomes less than 15 cc/kg of body weight,

2. when the maximum inspiratory pressure is less than $-30/cm\ H_2O$,

3. when patients have such severe bulbar weakness that they cannot handle secretions or protect their airway, or

4. when patients can no longer maintain normal PCO_2 and pH on arterial blood gas determinations (often a very late sign).

The rapidity of disease progression should also be considered. The more rapidly evolving the motor weakness, the more aggressive the clinician should be regarding early intubation.

13. If a neuromuscular blocker is needed to facilitate intubation, which one should be used?

The safety of succinylcholine in the acute phase of LGBS has not been established. The use of succinylcholine in the chronic phase of LGBS has been associated with hyperkalemia-induced cardiac arrest due to the massive release of potassium from denervated muscle cells. Therefore, a nondepolarizing muscle relaxant such as vecuronium or atracurium should be used whenever possible.

14. Which LGBS patients experience dysautonomias?
Autonomic nervous system dysfunction is usually present if the disease is severe enough to require mechanical ventilation. Dysautonomias can result from any combination of excessive or insufficient sympathetic and parasympathetic activity. Additionally, a wide variety of arrhythmias can occur in these patients and can be a major cause of mortality. Treatment of dysautonomias consists of hydration of the patient and other supportive measures such as avoiding sudden changes in position and using stool softeners to prevent straining-induced vagal stimulation. If drugs are necessary to treat dysautonomias or arrhythmias, small doses of short-acting, titratable agents are recommended.

15. Are there any effective treatments for the neurologic injury associated with LGBS?
Yes. Plasmapheresis has been shown to hasten recovery and decrease the ICU and hospital lengths of stay among patients with severe LGBS when it is initiated within 7 days of onset of symptoms.

16. What is the prognosis in acute LGBS?
Most patients experience excellent recovery in muscle function with time, often returning to normal. A small percentage are left with various degrees of weakness that will persist.

17. Are there any special ICU issues unique to LGBS?
In addition to the obvious need for meticulous pulmonary and nutritional support, special care should be taken to avoid pressure palsies of the arms and the legs. Additionally, LGBS patients are usually completely alert yet often cannot communicate because of intubation and paralysis. They require tremendous emotional support and judicious use of anxiolytics.

BIBLIOGRAPHY

1. Ashbury AK: Diagnostic considerations of Guillain-Barré syndrome. Ann Neurol 9(Suppl):1–5, 1981.
2. Feldman JM: Cardiac arrest after succinylcholine administration in a pregnant patient recovered from Guillain-Barré syndrome. Anesthesiology 72:942–944, 1990.
3. The Guillain-Barré Study Group: Plasmapheresis and acute Guillain-Barré syndrome. Neurology 35:1096–1103, 1985.
4. Koski CL: Guillain-Barré syndrome. Neurol Clin 2:355–366, 1984.
5. Prineas JW: Pathology of the Guillain-Barré syndrome. Ann Neurol 9(Suppl):6–19, 1981.

73. MYASTHENIA GRAVIS

Brian J. Kelly, M.D.

1. What is myasthenia gravis?
Myasthenia gravis (MG) is an autoimmune disorder of neuromuscular transmission manifested by weakness and fatigability of voluntary skeletal muscle. It occurs in two forms: ocular MG, in which the weakness is confined to the extraocular muscles, and the more common, generalized form, in which any skeletal muscle can be involved.

2. What are the ages of peak incidence of MG?

There are two peak ages of incidence of MG depending on gender. For women, the peak incidence is in the third decade; before the age of 30 there is a 4:1 female-male incidence. For men, the peak incidence is in the fifth and sixth decades; at that age, the female-male incidence ratio is approximately 1:1. The incidence of thymoma (a tumor often associated with MG) is much higher in older males with MG than in younger females with MG.

3. What are the usual clinical features of MG?

Weakness, which fluctuates with time and has a predilection for the extraocular and bulbar muscle, is highly suggestive of MG.

4. What is the pathophysiology of MG?

Antibodies to the postsynaptic membrane of the neuromuscular junction result in a marked decrease in the number of functional acetylcholine receptors at this structure. This results in faulty neuromuscular transmission because the acetylcholine released by the presynaptic terminals cannot successfully depolarize the postsynaptic membrane.

5. What other conditions are associated with MG?

Disorders of the thymus are common in patients with MG. Approximately 60% of myasthenics have thymic hyperplasia; 10–15% harbor a thymoma. A variety of autoimmune disorders are associated with MG, including thyroid disorders, pernicious anemia, Addison's disease, diabetes mellitus, lupus erythematosus, rheumatoid arthritis, and polymyositis.

6. How is the diagnosis of MG confirmed?

Clinical findings of fluctuating weakness with a predilection for the extraocular and bulbar muscles strongly suggest the diagnosis. A marked improvement in signs or symptoms following administration of a short-acting acetylcholinesterase inhibitor such as edrophonium (Tensilon) or a decremental response in the size of the compound motor action potential after repetitive electrical stimulation of a motor nerve can confirm the diagnosis. Additionally, serum antibodies to the acetylcholine receptor can be detected in approximately 90% of patients with generalized MG.

7. How is MG differentiated from the Lambert-Eaton myasthenic syndrome (LEMS)?

Although MG and LEMS strongly resemble each other clinically, LEMS does not involve extraocular muscles, so ptosis and diplopia, which are very common with MG, do not occur. Also, by EMG testing, repetitive stimulation of the nerve in MG shows a progressive decline in each muscle contraction, documenting the fatigability with repetitive stimulation. With LEMS, there is actually a paradoxical increase, rather than decrease, in successive muscle contractions when the nerve is repetitively stimulated. This is due to a progressive increase in the amount of acetylcholine released presynaptically by the stimulated nerve.

8. What is the most serious complication of MG?

Fatal respiratory failure can result from severe involvement of the respiratory muscles. Respiratory failure can also result from pulmonary aspiration due to trouble in swallowing and protecting the upper airway secondary to bulbar weakness.

9. What is the best way to assess respiratory function in patients with MG?

As with other neuromuscular diseases, findings of hypoxia, hypercapnia, and acidosis on arterial blood gas analysis may not occur until respiratory failure is profound. Although the findings of a rapid, shallow breathing pattern and the presence of abdominal paradox on physical exam may suggest respiratory failure, frequent assessment of maximum inspiratory and expiratory pressures and vital capacity is the best way to quantitate and follow respiratory function.

10. Does MG affect the autonomic nervous system?

No. The antibodies in MG are directed at the nicotinic acetylcholine receptors on skeletal muscles and not the muscarinic or nicotinic acetylcholine receptors found in the autonomic nervous system.

11. Which two conditions can cause rapidly progressive weakness and respiratory failure in a patient with MG?

Myasthenic crisis, a severe life-threatening worsening of MG, must be differentiated from cholinergic crisis, in which an overdose of acetylcholinesterase inhibitors results in profound weakness due to continuous depolarization of the postsynaptic membrane, which in turn results in a depolarizing type of neuromuscular blockade. Generally, cholinergic crisis causes other symptoms of excessive muscarinic receptor stimulation such as excessive salivation, cramps, diarrhea, and blurred vision. There is also a history of a marked increase in pyridostigmine use. A small dose of edrophonium often differentiates the two conditions, as it usually causes significant improvement in myasthenic crisis but worsens cholinergic crisis. This test should be performed only when emergency airway management is available, because it can cause severe respiratory failure in patients with cholinergic crisis.

12. What are the mainstays of therapy for MG?

Long-acting acetylcholinesterase inhibitors such as pyridostigmine (Mestinon) usually significantly improve neuromuscular function in patients with MG. Other therapies include steroids and occasionally long-term immunosuppressants. Thymectomy is often beneficial and should be seriously considered in patients with generalized MG. Thymectomy results in clinical improvement in about 80% of myasthenics in the absence of invasive thymoma. Plasmapheresis is often used in patients with severe exacerbations and can be an effective temporizing measure. Its expense usually precludes its routine use as a long-term therapy.

13. What is the relative potency of pyridostigmine (Mestinon) given intravenously compared to orally?

Intravenous (IV) pyridostigmine is approximately 30 times more potent than oral pyridostigmine. For dosing purposes, 30 mg of oral pyridostigmine is equivalent to 1 mg of IV pyridostigmine.

14. What conditions or agents can exacerbate MG?

Infection from any source, fever, and surgical or emotional stresses can worsen MG. Aminoglycoside and polymyxin antibiotics, beta blockers, quinidine and procainamide, and several antidepressants and anticonvulsants have been found to worsen MG. Steroids (which are often used to treat MG) can result in a transient worsening of MG in the first few days of therapy, possibly by adversely affecting the balance of various T-lymphocyte subgroups.

15. How should a patient in myasthenic crisis be treated?

When a patient with MG has significant problems with the vital functions of respiration and/or swallowing, he or she should be moved to the ICU. When vital capacity begins to fall to about 15 cc/kg of body weight, or when the patient cannot handle secretions, he or she should be intubated and placed on a mechanical ventilator. The goal then is to restore the patient to independent breathing as soon as possible with the following measures:

1. Initially rest the patient as much as possible. Let the ventilator assume the work of breathing during the 48 hours after intubation. We routinely use continuous mandatory ventilation (CMV), although other modes of ventilation are acceptable.

2. Vigorously treat underlying infections and fevers with appropriate antibiotics and antipyretics. Scrupulous attention to pulmonary toilet and pulmonary embolus prophylaxis is essential.

3. Stop all anticholinesterase medications for 48–72 hours. This drug holiday often restores responsiveness to these medications later.

4. Begin steroids and/or plasmapheresis soon after intubation to hasten neuromuscular recovery.

5. After the patient has recovered from the myasthenic crisis, plans for an eventual thymectomy should be seriously considered.

16. What factors should be considered perioperatively in a myasthenic patient undergoing thymectomy?

The most important goal is to optimize respiratory muscle function preoperatively. Plasmapheresis and steroids are often used to accomplish this. It is advisable to reduce the dose of pyridostigmine as much as possible preoperatively, but not at the expense of compromising respiratory function. The advantage of having a reduced dose of pyridostigmine preoperatively is that after thymectomy, the patient may be overly sensitive to pyridostigmine, and cholinergic crisis may result. If the patient was taking steroids preoperatively, stress doses of steroids should be given perioperatively. Extubation should not be done until all the effects of the inhalational agents used for anesthesia have fully dissipated and it is clear that respiratory function is adequate. It is better to be conservative in the decision to extubate the patient. After extubation, respiratory function should be followed closely, and the patient observed for signs of fatigue.

BIBLIOGRAPHY

1. Adams SL, Mathews J, Grammer LC: Drugs that may exacerbate myasthenia gravis. Ann Emerg Med 13:532–538, 1984.
2. Engel AG: Myasthenia gravis and myasthenic syndromes. Ann Neurol 16:519–534, 1984.
3. Fenichel GM: Myasthenia gravis. Pediatr Ann 18:432–438, 1989.
4. Galdi AP: Diagnosis and Management of Muscle Disease. New York, SP Medical and Scientific Books, 1984, pp 54–72.
5. Rowland LP: Controversies about the treatment of myasthenia gravis. J Neurol Neurosurg Psychiatry 43:659–694, 1980.
6. Seybold ME: Myasthenia gravis: A clinical and basic science review. JAMA 250:2516–2521, 1983.
7. Weschler AS, Olanow CW: Myasthenia gravis. Surg Clin North Am 60:931–945, 1980.

74. DELIRIUM TREMENS

Brian J. Kelly, M.D.

1. What is delirium tremens?

Delirium tremens is the most severe form of alcohol withdrawal and is characterized by profound confusion, tremor, agitation, vivid delusions, and hallucinations, as well as by a dramatic increase in the activity of the sympathetic nervous system as evidenced by fever, tachycardia, sweating, and dilated pupils. Delirium tremens is a consequence of the abrupt withdrawal from alcohol in the chronic alcoholic who has developed tolerance to alcohol.

2. What are the causes of mortality in fatal cases of delirium tremens?

Fortunately, with proper early recognition and ICU care, the mortality for delirium tremens is presently low. In the past, fatalities were secondary to severe hyperthermia associated with coma and cardiovascular collapse. Often, but not universally, a secondary illness such as infection, pulmonary embolus, or cardiac arrhythmia has been a contributing factor.

3. What other drug withdrawal syndromes can mimic delirium tremens?

Withdrawal from barbiturates and sedative-hypnotic drugs can cause a syndrome identical to alcoholic delirium tremens. Because the serum half-life of these drugs is often several days, the withdrawal syndrome may not develop until many days after the drugs are discontinued.

4. What other disorders can mimic delirium tremens?

Delirium from any cause can mimic delirium tremens, and the list of causes of delirium is extensive. Medications, including cimetidine, digoxin, steroids, antihypertensives, and psychoactive drugs, may cause delirium. Structural neurological lesions such as subdural hematomas, subarachnoid hemorrhage, and brain contusions can cause delirium. A variety of metabolic and endocrine disorders such as hypoxia, hyponatremia, hypoglycemia, uremia, thyroid disorders, hypercalcemia, shock, liver failure, and severe hypertension can lead to delirium. CNS infections such as encephalitis or meningitis as well as severe non-CNS febrile illness can cause a delirious state. Various collagen vascular disorders and acute porphyria can cause delirium. Rarely, nonconvulsive status epilepticus can cause delirium.

5. How is delirium tremens recognized and treated?

The key to treating delirium tremens lies in recognizing and treating early signs of alcohol withdrawal before delirium tremens occurs. Delirium tremens may occur in hospitalized patients in whom alcohol abuse was unrecognized several days into their stay and should always be considered in the differential diagnosis of delirium in this setting.

Signs of alcohol withdrawal develop several hours after a significant fall in blood alcohol levels and usually initially consist of mild tachycardia and hypertension, irritability, mild tremor, and low-grade fever. A moderately high blood alcohol level does not exclude early withdrawal, as chronic heavy drinkers can be legally intoxicated after a binge and still be withdrawing as the blood alcohol level drops. As withdrawal progresses, auditory hallucinations and seizures may occur, usually in the first 48 hours after cessation of drinking. Patients who have seizures often go on to have full-blown delirium tremens after the seizures subside. Delirium tremens is characterized by profound confusion, vivid hallucinations (usually visual), and severe signs of autonomic hyperactivity.

Treatment consists of administering sedative-hypnotic agents in the *early* stages of the withdrawal syndrome. It is much easier to prevent delirium tremens than to treat it. The benzodiazepines (diazepam) are frequently used for this purpose, and, when titrated properly, few patients will go on to develop delirium tremens. In mild withdrawal, the purpose of these drugs is to ensure rest and sleep.

6. How should a patient with full-blown delirium tremens be managed?

The approach to treating delirium tremens is similar to that for delirium in general. It is important to keep in mind that drug intoxications, as well as neurologic and infectious illnesses, are often associated with chronic alcohol use and may coexist with or mimic delirium tremens.

The first step is to assess the patient's airway and ventilation to ensure that an adequate airway is present. Hemodynamic status is then evaluated with particular attention to volume status. Patients with delirium tremens are often fluid deficient. Hyperthermia should be aggressively treated.

Oxygen should be administered and an intravenous line started. Immediate laboratory tests include arterial blood gas, electrolytes, serum glucose and calcium, CBC and drug screen. The patient should be placed on a cardiac monitor, and thiamine and D50W should be administered, in that order. If hypoventilation and somnolence are present and may be due to narcotic overdose, naloxone should be administered. Caution should be used in giving naloxone to an agitated patient since it may worsen delirium in opioid-dependent patients who are delirious from another cause and may cause seizures in patients who chronically use meperidine.

The next step is to gain control of the patient so that proper evaluation and therapy can proceed. If physical restraint is necessary, adequate personnel is essential for patient and staff safety. If chemical restraint is required, it is best accomplished with benzodiazepines. Diazepam in starting doses of 5 mg every 5 minutes until sedation usually allows safe titration of dose. Care must be taken in patients with COPD because the major side effect of diazepam is respiratory compromise. Because of the risk of respiratory and hemodynamic problems, sedation should be carried out in an ER or an ICU. Phenothiazines are contra-indicated in delirious patients because they have been associated with severe hyperthermia, seizures, and hypotension. Haloperidol has been used in treating delirium because of its minimal effect on blood pressure and respiration, but has not received FDA approval for intravenous use. Its use also is associated with a small risk of severe hyperthermia and seizures, and its use in the delirious patient is still controversial.

Once the patient is stabilized and sedated, proper diagnostic evaluation and therapy can proceed. The history is often crucial in directing the evaluation and may point to an obvious etiology. If a neurologic cause of delirium is suspected, a CT scan may be indicated and, if normal, should be followed by a lumbar puncture. Most metabolic and endocrinologic causes of delirium are suggested by findings on physical examination or initial laboratory evaluation. Non-CNS infectious diseases can cause delirium and should be excluded by appropriate cultures.

7. What further work-up should be performed if the initial evaluation fails to demonstrate an etiology for a patient's delirium?

If the initial history, physical examination, and laboratory evaluations fail to demonstrate a cause for delirium, neurologic consultation should be considered. Encephalitis and nonconvulsive status epilepticus, as well as a variety of collagen vascular diseases, need to be excluded. Chronic exposure to certain heavy metals and toxins can cause delirium as can porphyria. Degenerative conditions of the brain such as Alzheimer's disease may be associated with episodes of delirium. Although psychiatric disorders may mimic delirium, it is much better to exclude treatable medical conditions first and delay psychiatric therapy than to attribute an organic disorder to a psychiatric disease.

BIBLIOGRAPHY

1. Adams RD, Victor M: Principles of Neurology, 2nd ed. New York, McGraw-Hill, 1981.
2. Chick J: Delirium tremens. Br Med J 298:3–4, 1989.
3. Cushman P: Delirium tremens: Update on an old disorder. Postgrad Med 82:117–122, 1987.
4. Delaney KA, Goldfrank L: Delirium: Assessment and management in the critical care environment. Prob Crit Care 1:78–94, 1987.
5. Plum F, Posner JB: The Diagnosis of Stupor and Coma, 3rd ed. Philadelphia, F.A. Davis, 1980.
6. Romach MK, Sellers EM: Management of the alcohol withdrawal syndrome. Annu Rev Med 42:323–340, 1991.
7. Shoemaker WC, et al (eds): Textbook of Critical Care, 2nd ed. Philadelphia, W.B. Saunders, 1989.

75. SPINAL CORD COMPRESSION

Lynn M. Schnapp, M.D.

1. What is usually the earliest symptom of a mass in the epidural space?
Back pain is almost always present from weeks to months before other neurologic signs. It is the first symptom in about 90% of patients with epidural compression.

2. What are the causes of spinal cord compression?
Metastatic tumors (most common), epidural abscesses, hematomas, and acute midline herniated discs.

3. What are the most common primary tumors responsible for epidural metastases?
In order of decreasing frequency: breast, lung, prostate, kidney, lymphoma, myeloma, melanoma, and gastrointestinal tumors.

4. What is the role of the history in the evaluation of the patient with back pain?
The clinician needs to get a careful history regarding the presence of an underlying malignancy, suggestive of epidural metastasis; or an infectious process, suggestive of an abscess.

The site and character of back pain can be quite helpful in localizing the site of pathology. Local pain often indicates irritation of the nerve ending at the site of injury, and referred pain is felt distant from the site of pathology, but not in the distribution of the nerve; the mechanism is unclear. Radicular pain is due to compression of the spinal root and results in pain felt in the distribution of the affected nerve root. Radicular pain is often positional.

5. What should one look for on physical exam?
In addition to the general physical exam to find evidence of underlying systemic illness, a careful neurologic exam is imperative. Tenderness over the site of vertebral compression can often be elicited. Attention to sensory losses, abnormal deep tendon reflexes, and motor weakness is key. Paraplegia or bowel or bladder dysfunction is a late finding and often irreversible.

6. What is Lhermitte's sign?
The production of parathesias that radiate to arms, legs, and buttocks induced by neck flexion is called Lhermitte's sign. It implies either intrinsic or extrinsic spinal cord pathology.

7. What about the patient with back pain who has a completely normal neurologic evaluation and normal spine films?
In a number of studies, no patient who had a normal neurologic exam and normal spine films had an epidural tumor.

8. How do tumors cause spinal cord compression?
Generally, there are two modes. Solid tumors (e.g., breast and lung) metastasize to bone and then involve the epidural space by extension from the vertebral body. Approximately 15% of epidural metastases arise from extension through the intervertebral foramen. This mode is more commonly seen with hematologic malignancies (e.g., lymphoma).

9. What is the value of plain films to evaluate possible cord compression?
Because epidural compression is due to extension of tumor from the vertebral bodies, in the majority of patients, plain x-rays often show vertebral metastasis at the level of spinal compression. If myelopathy is present, over 80% of patients will have abnormal x-rays.

10. What is the role of bone scan?
Although bone scans are quite sensitive, their predictive value is low because they cannot distinguish tumors from inflammatory or degenerative processes.

11. What is the role of magnetic resonance imaging (MRI)?
MRI is extremely valuable at detecting lesions involving the marrow or spinal cord canal. In the future, MRI may replace myelography as the procedure of choice.

12. What is the treatment of epidural metastases?
If the diagnosis is uncertain (i.e., tumor vs. abscess), then surgery may be both diagnostic and therapeutic. Surgical options include decompressive laminectomy or vertebral body resection.

Steroids are useful in emergency treatment of spinal cord compression by acutely decreasing the edema in the spinal cord. Dexamethasone, 100 mg intravenously, is given, followed by 100 mg/day in divided doses and then tapered within 2–3 days.

Radiation therapy is considered the mainstay of therapy for most patients with epidural metastases. If patients were ambulatory prior to initiation of treatment, then the majority remain ambulatory. However, if paralysis is already present, then less than half will regain neurologic function, hence the need for accurate and rapid diagnosis and treatment.

Chemotherapy has been used in selected patients with sensitive tumors (e.g., lymphomas).

13. What is an epidural abscess? How does it originate?
An epidural abscess is a collection of pus between the dura and overlying bone. It can arise via hematogenous spread from a distant focus of infection such as a skin infection, urinary tract infection, pneumonia, or dental abscess, or from extension from a contiguous process such as vertebral osteomyelitis, psoas abscess, skin decubiti, or wound. The most common organism is *Staphylococcus aureus*, followed by *Mycobacterium tuberculosis*. Gram-negative rods and anaerobes are also seen, particularly in immunocompromised patients and intravenous drug abusers.

14. What are the signs and symptoms of an epidural abscess?
An epidural abscess should be considered in the febrile patient with a backache and localized spinal tenderness. The neurologic symptoms depend on the location and are similar to those of a tumor. Leukocytosis is often present.

15. How is the diagnosis made?
The work-up is similar to that for the patient with malignancy (computerized tomography scan, myelogram), except that special care must be taken to avoid lumbar puncture at the site of a suspected abscess. Progression is often rapid, with paralysis occurring within 24 hours. Therefore, rapid diagnosis and treatment are essential.

16. What is the treatment?
Appropriate antibiotic treatment should be started at once (antistaphylococcal drugs and, in select settings, gram-negative coverage). Length of therapy varies from 3–4 weeks for isolated bacterial abscess to 18–24 months for *M. tuberculosis*. Surgical decompression and drainage are indicated in any bacterial abscess, with the possible exception of *M. tuberculosis*, which may respond to antibiotic therapy alone.

BIBLIOGRAPHY

1. Baker A, Ojemann R, Swartz M, Richardson E: Spinal epidural abscess. N Engl J Med 293:463, 1975.

2. Benson C, Harris A: Acute neurologic infections. Med Clin North Am 70:987, 1986.
3. Patchell R, Posner J: Neurologic complications of systemic cancer. Neurol Clin 3:729, 1985.
4. Posner J: Back pain and epidural spinal cord decompression. Med Clin North Am 71:185, 1987.
5. Rodichok L, Harper G, Ruckdeschel J, et al: Early diagnosis of spinal epidural metastases. Am J Med 70:1181, 1981.

76. HEAD TRAUMA

Dorre Nicholau, M.D.

1. Where does head trauma rank as a cause of death in the United States?

Head trauma ranks second to stroke as a cause of death from neurologic disorders. It is one of the leading causes of death among young Americans aged 1 to 45.

2. What are the leading causes of head trauma?

Motor vehicle accidents 49%; falls 28%; all others 23%.

3. What is the mortality rate associated with severe head trauma?

Most studies report a mortality rate of 30–50% in severe head trauma.

4. What factors are important in predicting outcome from severe head injury?

Factors associated with poor neurologic outcome are
- Intracranial hematoma
- Increasing age
- Abnormal motor response
- Impaired or absent pupillary response to light on initial exam.
- Early systemic insults: hypotension, hypercarbia, and/or hypoxemia.

5. What is the Glasgow coma scale? Why is it important?

Developed in 1974 by the neurosurgical department at the University of Glasgow, the scale was an attempt to standardize the assessment of the depth and duration of impaired consciousness and coma, particularly in the setting of trauma. The scale is based upon eye opening, verbal responses, and motor responses. Of these, motor response is the most sensitive and correlates best with neurologic outcome. A score of 15 is possible in a completely awake and oriented patient. A score of <8 indicates significant brain injury and the possible need for airway protection.

Eye opening		Motor response	
Spontaneous	4		
To speech	3	Motor response	
To pain	2	Obeys commands	6
None	1	Localizes pain	5
Best verbal response		Withdraws from pain	4
Oriented	5	Flexes to pain	3
Confused	4	Extends to pain	2
Inappropriate	3	None	1
Incomprehensible	2		
None	1		

6. What is the significance of primary versus secondary head injury?

Primary injury is direct disruption of brain tissue at the moment of impact. Primary injury may result in contusion, hemorrhage, and/or laceration. Primary injuries account for approximately 50% of the deaths associated with head injuries. There is no treatment for the sudden mechanical disruption of brain tissue.

Secondary brain injury refers to delayed insults, both systemic and intracranial, which can be attributed to initial traumatic injury. Delayed intracranial complications include intracranial hematomas (subdural, epidural, and parenchymal), as well as generalized cerebral edema that results in elevated intracranial pressure. Secondary systemic complications are most often seen in multiple trauma patients. When systemic complications occur, they are associated with a marked increase in mortality. In one series, the presence of hypotension and hypoxemia in head-injured patients increased their mortality rate from 24% to 53%.

7. What percentage of head trauma patients suffer additional traumatic injury?

An estimated 50% have at least one other injury: 29% chest injury, 17% abdominal injury, and 6% spinal cord injury. These patients are at risk for secondary systemic complications.

8. What are the essentials of management of head-injured patients?

1. Management and protection of the airway.
2. Controlled ventilation to maintain normal or low pCO_2.
3. Appropriate triage to early surgery (<4 hr postinjury).
4. Maintenance of cerebral blood flow.
5. Treatment of elevated intracranial pressure.
6. Evaluation and treatment of secondary systemic disorders:
   Gastrointestinal bleeding
   Disseminated intravascular coagulopathy
   Neurogenic pulmonary edema
   Endocrine abnormalities (diabetes insipidus, syndrome of inappropriate antidiuretic hormone)
   Hypotension secondary to hemorrhagic or spinal shock
   Hypoxemia secondary to chest trauma or aspiration

9. What are the important considerations when intubating patients with head trauma?

1. Associated cervical spine fractures occur in 5–10% of head-injured patients. This often depends on the mechanism of injury (motor vehicle accidents, fall > gunshot wound). Care should be taken to avoid hyperextension of the neck at the time of intubation. Awake intubation, axial traction, and/or cricothyrotomy are appropriate options in head-injured patients.

2. These patients are considered to have "full stomachs" and should undergo awake intubation or rapid sequence induction to avoid possible aspiration of stomach contents.

3. Patients with associated traumatic injuries are often hypovolemic, and care should be taken when administering induction drugs to avoid hypotension.

4. Care should also be taken to avoid coughing and straining on the endotracheal tube, as this results in a marked increase in intracranial pressure (ICP).

5. Associated maxillofacial and neck injuries should be noted, as they may increase the difficulty of intubation.

6. Nasal intubations are contraindicated in patients with basilar skull and/or Le Fort fractures.

10. What clues suggest the presence of a basilar skull fracture?

Basilar skull fractures result in hemotympanum, ecchymosis over the mastoid area (Battle's sign), and/or periorbital ecchymosis (raccoon's eyes).

11. What percentage of adult head-injured patients develop intracranial hematoma?
Forty percent of head-injured patients develop intracranial hematoma as a result of the head injury. Of these, an estimated 40% are intracerebral, 20% are subdural, and another 20% are epidural.

12. Why is this significant?
Immediate surgical intervention is imperative if these patients are to survive. In a review of 82 severely head injured patients with significant intracranial hemorrhage (>5 mm midline shift or hemorrhagic contusion >2 cm on CT scan), early surgical evacuation was shown to have a remarkable impact on survival. Those taken to operation less than four hours after injury suffered a 30% mortality rate; those taken to operation more than four hours after injury had a 90% mortality.

13. How does head trauma affect intracranial pressure?
Head trauma increases intracranial pressure. The cranial vault encloses a fixed space, which is occupied by three constituents: brain parenchyma 86%, blood 4%, and cerebrospinal fluid (CSF) 10%. To maintain normal intracerebral pressure, a change in the volume in any one of these constituents must result in a compensatory change in one or both of the remaining two. In head trauma, an increase in mass due to cerebral edema or hematoma must be accompanied by a decrease in blood and/or CSF volume in order to maintain normal intracranial pressure. Physiologic compensatory mechanisms include the displacement and absorption of CSF together with spontaneous hyperventilation (in awake patients), which decreases cerebral blood flow. Unfortunately, these mechanisms are rapidly exhausted, resulting in a rapid rise in ICP. This is demonstrated by the intracranial compliance curve shown below. This pressure-volume curve demonstrates a "critical" volume (the knee in the curve), above which compensatory mechanisms are not effective in the noncompliant cranium.

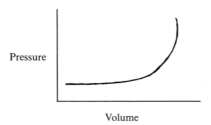

Pressure

Volume

14. What are the mechanisms by which head injury elevates intracranial pressure?
Increased mass secondary to intracranial hematoma formation.
Increased brain tissue secondary to diffuse or localized edema.
Increased blood volume secondary to loss of autoregulation.
Increased CSF volume secondary to obstruction to flow by edema or clot formation.

15. What is the significance of elevated intracranial pressure?
The elevation of ICP without an equivalent rise in systemic mean arterial pressure (MAP) results in a decrease in the cerebral perfusion pressure (CPP) and the risk of brain ischemia.

$$CPP = MAP - ICP$$

Ideally, an arterial line should be placed at the time of ICP monitor placement. This allows accurate moment-to-moment measurement of the systemic MAP and calculation of CPP. The calculation of CPP requires that both transducers be placed at the level of the external auditory canal. A normal ICP is <10 mm Hg. An elevation in ICP >20 in a resting patient for more than a few minutes is associated with a significant increase in mortality. An ICP >40 mm Hg is considered life threatening. A normal CPP is approximately 100 mm Hg. A cerebral perfusion pressure >60 mm Hg is considered to be adequate to prevent further brain ischemia.

16. How is ICP monitored?
The three commonly used methods to monitor ICP are the intraventricular catheter, the subarachnoid screw, and the epidural transducer. See reference 15 for detailed descriptions of each method.

17. Describe the pattern of ICP waves.
C waves are small rhythmic oscillations in pressure that occur at a frequency of 4–8/min. They are associated with ICP measurements of 0–20 mm Hg and are considered normal.

B waves are high-frequency oscillations, 0.5–2/min, which result in pressures between 0 and 50 mm Hg. Though they are not always pathologic, they often progress to A waves.

A waves are periods of extremely elevated ICP, 50–100 mm Hg, which last 5–20 minutes. They are usually superimposed on an elevated baseline and rapidly progress to plateau waves. They are associated with a marked decrease in CPP and are considered life threatening.

18. Which patients should be monitored for increased ICP?
A review of 207 head-injured patients by Narayan in 1982 suggested that two groups of patients should be routinely monitored: (1) those with abnormal CT scans on admission; and (2) those with normal CT scans who demonstrate two or more of the following adverse features on admission: (a) systolic blood pressure <90 mm Hg, (b) age >40, and (c) unilateral or bilateral motor posturing.

Patients who are not routinely monitored should have repeat head CT scans at 12–24 hours. This study showed that 96% of patients with normal CT scans and fewer than two adverse features had normal ICP throughout their ICU course, whereas 53–63% of patients with abnormal CT scans developed elevated ICP.

19. What is the treatment for elevated ICP?
1. Elevation of the head of the bed to >30 degrees to enhance venous drainage.
2. Hyperventilation to a PCO_2 of 25–30 mm Hg.
3. Mannitol, 1 gm/kg emergently, then dose every 1–3 hours to maintain serum Osm 295–305.
4. Furosemide, 0.5 mg/kg, may be used to further dehydrate patients and reduce CSF production.
5. Drainage of CSF from ventriculostomy catheter (most effective in obstructive hydrocephalus, least effective in diffuse edema with narrowed ventricles).
6. Surgical decompression to remove hematoma or necrotic injured brain.
7. Attention to head positioning to avoid jugular venous compression and obstruction to the cranial venous outflow tract.
8. Barbiturates (useful in refractory cases).
9. Seizure prophylaxis to prevent the increase in ICP associated with seizures.

If ICP is unresponsive to therapy, a head CT scan should be done to rule out acute hematoma or hydrocephalus formation.

20. How does hyperventilation decrease ICP?
Hyperventilation decreases ICP by producing cerebral vasoconstriction and a resultant decrease in cerebral blood flow (CBF). A PCO_2 of 20–80 mm Hg gives a relatively linear relationship between PCO_2 and CBF.

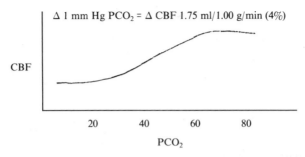

Δ 1 mm Hg PCO_2 = Δ CBF 1.75 ml/1.00 g/min (4%)

CBF

20   40   60   80

PCO_2

This effect is mediated through acute alterations in cerebral interstitial fluid pH, and therefore it generally becomes less effective after 48–72 hours.

21. How does mannitol decrease ICP?

Brain tissue has a slightly greater osmolarity than blood, with a gradient of approximately 3 mOsm/L maintained by the blood-brain barrier. Mannitol is an osmotically active agent that reverses this osmotic gradient and shifts water from the brain to the blood. An increase in blood osmolarity by 10 mOsm/L removes 100–150 ml of water from the brain.

Hyperosmolar treatment of elevated ICP increases the normal serum Osm of 290 to 300–315 mOsm/L. An Osm <300 is ineffective; >315 results in renal and neurologic dysfunction.

22. What is the role of barbiturates in the treatment of increased ICP?

Barbiturates result in a decrease in the cerebral metabolic rate and a decrease in cerebral blood flow, and theoretically they should work to lower ICP. However, this topic is controversial.

23. Is there a role for steroids in the treatment of head injury?

No. Steroids have been shown to increase the incidence of severe pulmonary infections while offering no significant benefit to head-injured patients.

24. What is the effect of PEEP on head-injured patients?

PEEP, or positive end-expiratory pressure, increases intrathoracic pressure. This results in both a decrease in venous outflow from the cranial vault and a decrease in venous return to the heart. The result is an increase in ICP, a decrease in cardiac output (hypotension), and a subsequent decrease in CPP. The effect of a given increment of PEEP is unpredictable, though levels <10 cm H_2O probably do not result in significant hemodynamic alterations.

25. Should dextrose-containing solutions be avoided in head trauma patients?

Infusion of dextrose-containing solutions, especially 5% dextrose and water, is contraindicated in the acute treatment of the neurotrauma patient. Sugar and water pass freely into the brain cell. Once in the cell, the sugar is metabolized, leaving free water behind and causing the cell to swell and cerebral edema to ensue. A number of animal studies show that glucose infusion during cerebral ischemia worsens neurologic outcome. This adverse effect occurs even when the serum glucose level is maintained within the normal range. Normal saline with an osmolarity of 308 mOsm/L is the preferred crystalloid for use in head trauma patients. Plasmalyte, with an osmolarity of 294 mOsm/L, is essentially iso-osmolar with plasma, while lactated Ringer's solution is slightly hypo-osmolar (273 mOsm/L).

BIBLIOGRAPHY

1. Braakman R, Schouten HJA, Blaauw-van Dishoeck M, et al: Megadose steroids in severe head injury: Results of a prospective double-blind clinical trial. J Neurosurg 58:326–330, 1983.
2. Becker D, Miller JD, Ward JD, et al: The outcome from severe head injury with early diagnosis and intensive management. J Neurosurg 47:491–502, 1977.
3. Duffy K, Becker D: State of the art management of severe closed head injury. J Critical Care Med 3:291–302, 1988.
4. Eisenberg H, Frankowski R, Constant C, et al: High dose barbiturate control of elevated intracranial pressure in patients with head injury. J Neurosurg 69:15–23, 1988.
5. Gunnar W, et al: Head injury and hemorrhagic shock: Studies of the blood-brain barrier and intracranial pressure after resuscitation with normal saline solution, 35 saline solution, and dextran 40. Surgery 103:398–407, 1988.
6. Heffner J, Sahn S: Controlled hyperventilation in patients with intracranial hypertension. Arch Intern Med 143:765–769, 1983.
7. Jennett B, Teasdale G, Braakman R, et al: Prognosis of patients with severe head injury. Neurosurgery 4:283–288, 1979.
8. Kalsbeek W, McLaurin R: The national head and spinal cord injury survey: Major findings. J Neurosurg 53:s19–s31, 1980.
9. Marshall L, Smith R, Shapiro H: The outcome with aggressive treatment in severe head injuries. I. The significance of intracranial pressure monitoring. J Neurosurg 50:20–25, 1979.
10. Lanier W, Stangland K, Scheithauer BW, et al: The effects of dextrose infusion and head position on neurologic outcome after complete cerebral ischemia in primates: Examination of a model. Anesthesiology 66:39–48, 1987.
11. Miller J, Becker D, Ward J, et al: Significance of intracranial hypertension in severe head injury. J Neurosurg 47:503–516, 1977.
12. Miller J, Butterworth J, Gudeman S, et al: Further experience in the management of severe head injury. J Neurosurg 54:289–299, 1981.
13. Narayan R, Kishore P, Becker DP, et al: Intracranial pressure: To monitor or not to monitor? J Neurosurg 56:650–659, 1982.
14. Seelig J, Becker D, Miller JD, et al: Traumatic acute subdural hematoma: Major mortality reduction in comatose patients treated within four hours. N Engl J Med 304:1511–1517, 1981.
15. Sokoll M: Monitoring intracranial pressure. In Blitt C: Monitoring in Anesthesia and Critical Care Medicine. New York, Churchill Livingstone, 1985, pp 413–425.
16. Cooper C, Stirt J: Monitoring. In Sperry R, Stirt J, Stone D: Manual of Neuroanesthesia. Philadelphia, B.C. Decker, 1989.

XI: Pharmacology

77. DIURETICS

Lynn M. Schnapp, M.D.

1. What are the indications for use of diuretics?
Traditionally, diuretics have been used for the treatment of hypertension and conditions characterized by volume overload, including congestive heart failure, nephrotic syndrome, and cirrhosis with ascites.

2. Where are the major sites of action of the different diuretic groups?

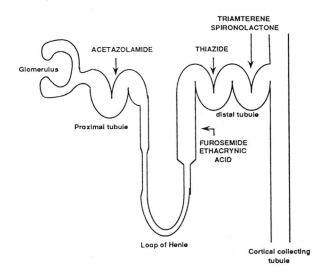

3. Name the classes of diuretics and give examples of each.

Classes of Diuretics and Examples

DIURETIC CLASS	EXAMPLES	
	Generic Name	Brand Name
Thiazides	Hydrochlorothiazide	
	Metolazone	Zaroxolyn
Loop diuretics	Furosemide	Lasix
	Ethacrynic acid	Edecrin
	Bumetanide	Bumex
Potassium-sparing diuretics	Spironolactone	Alactone
	Triamterene	
	Amiloride	Midamor
Carbonic anyhydrase inhibitors	Acetazolamide	Dimox

4. What common metabolic abnormalities are associated with diuretics?

Metabolic Abnormalities with Diuretics

	THIAZIDES	LOOP DIURETICS	CARBONIC ANHYDRASE INHIBITORS	POTASSIUM-SPARING DIURETICS
Hypovolemia	↓↓	↓↓↓	↓	↓
Serum sodium	↓↓	↓↓	↓	↓↓
Serum potassium	↓↓↓	↓↓	↓↓	↑↑
Serum magnesium	↓↓	↓↓	↑	↑
Serum calcium	↑↑	↓	↓	±
Acid-base disturbance	Alkalosis	Alkalosis	Acidosis	Acidosis
Hyperuricemia	↑↑	↑↑	±	±
Carbohydrate intolerance	↑↑	±/↑	±	±
Hyperlipidemia	↑↑	±/↑	±	±

5. A patient is being treated for hypertension with thiazides. Measurement of serum creatinine shows an increase from 1.0 to 1.6 over 6 months. What are the possible mechanisms?

Prerenal azotemia must be considered in any patient being treated with diuretics. Thiazides can cause hypersensitivity interstitial nephritis, which may be accompanied by fever, rash, and eosinophilia. The nephritis is reversible upon discontinuation of the drug. Finally, hypertension iteself can cause renal insufficiency.

6. Should thiazides be used in patients with renal insufficiency?

Thiazides are generally ineffective once the glomerular filtration rate falls below 35 ml/min. Thus, another class of diuretics should be used (e.g., furosemide).

7. What is the role of diuretics in the treatment of acute renal failure?

Traditionally, loop diuretics have been administered during the first 24 hours of development of oliguric renal failure to convert it to nonoliguric renal failure. However, there are scant data in support of this approach.

8. What is the role of furosemide in hypercalcemia?

Loop diuretics decrease reabsorption of sodium and calcium at the loop of Henle, leading to increased excretion of both in the urine. Thus, furosemide is often used in conjunction with fluids containing sodium chloride to treat hypercalcemia.

9. A patient with a history of congestive heart failure on a stable dose of furosemide is admitted for an acute attack of gout and is started on indomethacin. Soon thereafter, the patient experiences an exacerbation of congestive heart failure. What is a possible explanation?

Part of the effect of loop diuretics lies in a prostaglandin-induced increase in renal blood flow. Treatment with nonsteroidal anti-inflammatory drugs can decrease the diuretic effect of furosemide. In the above case, the patient was effectively "seeing" less furosemide because of the administration of indomethacin.

10. Which diuretic may be appropriate in a patient who is volume overloaded and who has concurrent metabolic alkalosis?

Carbonic anhydrase inhibitors (e.g., acetazolamide) induce a sodium bicarbonate diuresis by inhibiting sodium bicarbonate absorption in the proximal tubule. Thus they may be useful in the patient who requires diuresis when the use of thiazides or loop diuretics would worsen preexisting alkalosis. Overall, however, carbonic anhydrase inhibitors are very weak diuretics and have limited use.

11. Which diuretic is often used for first-line therapy of ascites?
Spironolactone, a potassium-sparing diuretic, is particularly useful for the management of ascites when sodium restriction has failed. The usual dose is 100–400 mg/day in divided doses. An occasional patient will require the addition of furosemide.

12. Are potassium-sparing diuretics appropriate single-agent therapy for congestive heart failure?
No. In general, they are not very efficacious when used as monotherapy. They are sometimes used in combination therapy of hypertension to avoid the potassium-depleting effects of the other diuretics.

BIBLIOGRAPHY

1. Frohlich E: Initial therapy for hypertension. Hosp Pract, May 15, 1987, p 89.
2. Jacobson H: Diuretics: Mechanisms of action and use. Hosp Pract, Dec 15, 1987, p 107.
3. Jaeschke R, Guyatt G: Medical therapy for chronic congestive heart failure. Ann Intern Med 110:758, 1989.
4. Levine S: Diuretics. Med Clin North Am 73:271, 1989.

78. INOTROPIC AND VASOPRESSOR DRUGS

Thomas J. Stelzner, M.D.

1. What are the indications for the use of inotropic and vasopressor drugs?
Inotropes and vasopressors are typically used when there is evidence of inadequate perfusion of vital tissues occurring during the course of various pathologic conditions: distributive shock due to sepsis, anaphylaxis, or spinal cord injury; cardiogenic shock due to myocardial infarction, cardiac injury, or valvular dysfunction; and extracardiac obstructive shock resulting from massive pulmonary emboli, pericardial tamponade, constrictive pericarditis, severe pulmonary vascular disease, or, rarely, coarctation of the aorta. Evidence of inadequate perfusion may be overt, as in cardiavascular collapse, or it may be more subtle, indicative of regional maldistribution of organ blood flow with failure to perfuse and maintain individual organ function. Vasoactive drugs may be indicated either to restore overall cardiovascular status or to improve perfusion to various regional vascular beds.

2. What pressors and inotropic drugs are available? What are their mechanisms of action?
A variety of drugs are available, which act primarily by stimulating adrenergic receptors. Alpha-adrenergic agonists mediate peripheral vasoconstriction, beta-1 adrenergic agonists augment cardiac output and heart rate and induce peripheral vasodilation, beta-2 agonists induce bronchodilation, and dopaminergic agonists induce dilation of the renal and mesenteric circulations. Some vasoactive drugs work by directly activating adrenergic receptors; others work at least in part through the indirect release of endogenous intraneuronal stores of catecholamines. This distinction may be important in a few specific clinical situations and should be kept in mind when selecting a vasoactive drug or in gauging the efficacy of a drug in a particular clinical situation (to be discussed).

Epinephrine is a direct-acting, naturally occurring alpha, beta-1, and beta-2 agonist with some differential activity at the various receptors based on dose. At doses of 1–2 μg/min, epinephrine is primarily a beta agonist and would be expected to cause vasodilation and increased stroke volume and heart rate. At 2–10 μg/min, it has both beta and alpha effects, although beta effects again predominate, and at doses >10 μg/min, alpha agonist effects predominate and cause vasoconstriction.

Norepinephrine is a direct-acting, naturally occurring alpha agonist with some beta-1 and virtually no beta-2 activity. It has inotropic effects at doses of 1–2 μg/min and at higher doses is the most potent and dependable vasoconstricting agent available. It also is a venoconstrictor and can increase venous return.

Dobutamine is a direct-acting, synthetic beta-1 agonist, also with beta-2 agonist activity, which acts primarily as an inotrope rather than as a vasopressor due to its lack of alpha agonist activity. It causes less tachycardia than isoproterenol, epinephrine, or dopamine and also may decrease both systemic and pulmonary vascular resistance.

Dopamine is another synthetic drug with both direct and indirect agonist activity at alpha, beta-1, and dopaminergic receptors. It has well-characterized differential activity at these receptor subtypes based on dose, which dictates its dose-dependent functional effects. At 0.5–2 μg/kg/min, dopamine activates dopaminergic receptors. This induces regional vasodilation of the renal and mesenteric circulation leading to increases in renal and gut blood flow. Coexisting therapy with haloperidol or phenothiazines may blunt this dopaminergic effect. At 2–5 μg/kg/min, dopamine activates both dopaminergic as well as beta-1 receptors. At 5–10 μg/kg/min, it is primarily a beta-1 agonist. At doses above 10 μg/kg/min, dopamine also activates alpha receptors. Above 20 μg/kg/min, the alpha effect is the predominant effect of dopamine. Due to its indirect activity, dopamine may have an unpredictable response in patients receiving monoamine oxidase (MAO) inhibitors, tricyclic antidepressants, or cocaine, and it should either not be used or be used with caution in these patients due to possible induction of a hyperadrenergic state. Dopamine also can inhibit insulin secretion and may contribute to hyperglycemia in some patients.

Metaraminol is a synthetic, direct alpha agonist that also has a substantial indirect mechanism of action. It is also taken up by nerve terminals and may serve as a false neurotransmitter. This may partially explain the tendency of patients to develop tolerance or tachyphylaxis to this drug over time. It is less dependable as a vasoconstrictor than either norepinephrine or phenylephrine and is no longer widely used.

Phenylephrine is a synthetic, direct-acting alpha agonist with virtually no beta agonist activity. As such it has less potential to induce arrhythmias or increase myocardial oxygen demand than drugs with beta agonist activity.

Two other inotropic agents are available that do not activate adrenergic receptors. **Amrinone** is a drug that inhibits the enzyme phosphodiesterase, thereby increasing cyclic adenosine monophosphate (cAMP) and smooth muscle cells. The result of this is marked augmentation of stroke volume with little increase in heart rate as well as peripheral vasodilation. This drug is most useful in patients with a severe cardiogenic hypoperfusion state. **Glucagon** is a polypeptide hormone that binds to nonadrenergic surface receptors and activates adenylate cyclase, thereby increasing cAMP. Glucagon appears to be most useful in treating hypoperfusion states induced by or complicated by beta adrenergic blockade.

3. What pharmacologic principles must be considered when choosing or judging the efficacy of a particular vasoactive substance?

Because most of these drugs work via activation of adrenergic receptors, the number of receptors in an individual patient obviously affects the performance of the drug. Adrenergic receptors tend to be up-regulated following chronic adrenergic blockade and tend to be down-regulated in states of adrenergic excess or with chronic beta-adrenergic treatment as in the patient with airflow limitation due to asthma or emphysema. Furthermore, since some of these drugs work by indirectly releasing endogenous intraneuronal stores of catecholamines, the state of these intraneuronal stores also is important. The coexisting use of drugs such a tricyclic antidepressants or cocaine that inhibit the reuptake of norepinephrine at nerve terminals or of drugs that cause accumulations of norepinephrine at nerve terminals (MAO inhibitors) will obviously affect the performance of indirectly acting vasoactive substances. Receptor affinity and efficacy also are important considerations in judging response to a vasoactive drug. Elderly subjects, for example, have increased norepinephrine release with stress, which suggests possible decreased adrenoreceptor function with age. Hypoxia and acidosis are both known to decrease adrenergic receptor affinity, while vascular sensitivity to norepinephrine is increased in the presence of jaundice and hyperlipidemia. Thus a variety of exogenous and endogenous factors may act to either increase or decrease the expected response to a given vasoactive drug and should always be considered in the selection of these compounds.

4. What drugs should be chosen for a given clinical situation, and over what concentrations should they be used?

Vasoactive drugs should be used after careful consideration of the particular hemodynamic state present in each individual patient and only after intravascular volume status has been restored to an adequate level. Once intravascular volume has been restored (pulmonary capillary wedge pressure 12–18 cm H_2O) but perfusion is still judged to be inadequate, the selection of appropriate pharmacologic support should be based on the ability of the drug to correct or augment the hemodynamic deficit present. If the problem is felt to be inadequate cardiac output, the drug chosen should have prominent activity at beta-1 receptors and little effect at alpha receptors that increase afterload and further reduce stroke volume. If the perfusion deficit is due to marked reductions in peripheral vascular resistance, then a drug that increases resistance (an alpha agonist) should be used. The hemodynamic picture is often more complex than those presented above, or other special considerations such as oliguria, underlying ischemic heart disease, or arrhythmias may exist and further complicate the decision-making process.

In general, **epinephrine** is useful in patients with severe reductions in cardiac output in whom the arrhythmogenicity and marked augmentation in heart rate and myocardial oxygen consumption that occur with this drug are not limiting factors. Epinephrine is the drug of choice for anaphylactic shock, due to its activity at beta-1 and beta-2 receptors, and it can also be used in cases of refractory septic shock, due to its ability to activate both beta and alpha receptors at high dose. The usual dosage range is 2–20 $\mu g/min$.

Dopamine is also useful in hypoperfusion due to reduced cardiac output, and it causes less of an increase in myocardial oxygen consumption than epinephrine does. It is particularly useful in patients in whom the reduced output is accompanied by marked regional decreases in renal blood flow, due to its unique ability to activate dopaminergic receptors at low doses. It is also useful in cases of reduced systemic vascular resistance but may be less reliable than norepinephrine. Dopamine tends to cause more tachycardia than dobutamine and unlike dobutamine usually increases rather than decreases pulmonary artery and pulmonary capillary wedge pressures. This effect may be important in the patient with high baseline wedge pressures in whom further increases may precipitate pulmonary edema. Dopamine has differential dose-dependent effects at the dopaminergic, beta, and alpha receptors described above and is used in concentrations of 0.5–20 $\mu g/kg/min$. If dopamine fails to restore mean arterial pressure at 20 $\mu g/kg/min$, norepinephrine should be used.

Norepinephrine is used to restore overall cardiovascular status in cases of reduced systemic vascular resistance and should be the drug of choice when a direct-acting adrenergic agonist is needed (tricyclic overdose, cocaine overdose). Due to the excessive vasoconstriction often noted with this agent, this drug works best with dopamine at low dose in order to preserve renal and mesenteric blood flow. Norepinephrine is used at doses of 1–24 $\mu g/min$.

Dobutamine should be used when reduced cardiac output is considered the cause of the perfusion deficit, and it should not be considered the sole therapy if the decrease in output is accompanied by a significant decrease in mean arterial pressure. This is because dobutamine may cause further reductions in both preload and afterload and further reduce mean arterial pressure. However if both mean arterial pressure and intravascular filling are near normal, a recent study suggests that dobutamine may be more effective than dopamine in enhancing forward flow and in distributing the flow to improve tissue oxygenation. Dobutamine is used at a dose of 2–20 μg/kg/min.

Phenylephrine is used to increase systemic vascular resistance in patients who cannot tolerate any further myocardial stimulation (arrhythmias, angina). It should be given initially at 100–180 μg/min and then at 30–60 μg/min.

5. What parameters should be followed to assess the adequacy of response to a particular vasoactive substance?

The general guidelines to determine the adequacy of success in treatment of shock states include maintenance of mean arterial pressure >60 mm Hg with evidence of adequate regional blood flow to various vital organs. The means of assessing the adequacy of regional tissue perfusion, however, are not ideal, and the best parameters to follow continue to be debated. However, clinical evidence of adequate regional perfusion is always available, and the level of sensorium, urine output, and skin color and termperature are good crude estimates of regional blood flow to brain, kidney, and skin, respectively. Some investigators advocate the use of overall estimates of oxygen transport to assess tissue perfusion. Shoemaker and coworkers use vasoactive drugs along with fluids and blood products to maintain a cardiac index >4.5 L/min/m^2, oxygen delivery >600 ml/min/m^2, and oxygen consumption >170 ml/min/m^2 during the first 2–3 days postoperatively in critically ill surgical patients and have demonstrated improved survival if these parameters can be achieved. Finally, blood lactate levels also serve as an overall marker of tissue hypoxia or underperfusion. A decrease in blood lactate with treatment is a crude marker of improvement in regional blood flow to underperfused vascular beds. A failure to decrease or an increase in lactate levels with adequate blood pressure suggests that regional tissue hypoxia is ongoing and that further attempts to augment oxygen delivery or redistribute blood flow should be attempted.

6. What are the complications of these drugs?

The major adverse effects are related to excessive alpha-or beta-adrenergic stimulation. Although vasoconstriction may be needed to increase mean arterial pressure above a critical level, further vasoconstriction may worsen regional blood flow and cause further tissue hypoxia. The minimum dose of vasopressor (alpha agonist) that brings mean arterial pressure above 60 mm Hg should be used, and excessive vasocontriction should be avoided. Unopposed vasoconstriction is also a potential problem with local extravasation of vasopressors. Peripheral infiltration of intravenous-fluid-containing vasopressors can produce local tissue gangrene if unrecognized or left untreated. Central venous access should be used to deliver vasopressors whenever possible. If peripehral tissue infiltration with a vasopressor does occur, the area should be infiltrated with 5–10 mg of phentolamine (alpha blocker) diluted in 10 cc normal saline to counter the alpha-mediated vasoconstriction. Constriction of pulmonary vessels may cause ventilation perfusion mismatch and actually worsen oxygenation and oxygen delivery. Blood gases should be monitored frequently when beginning therapy with vasoactive drugs, and measures to correct worsening hypoxemia embarked upon so that oxygen delivery is not impaired. The other major complications to be watched for when using vasopressors and inotropes are cardiac in origin. These drugs have the potential to induce a variety of lethal arrhythmias and to markedly increase myocardial oxygen demand. In the patient with limited coronary perfusion, such an increase in oxygen demand can induce cardiac ischemia or infarction.

BIBLIOGRAPHY

1. Fenwick JC, Dodek PM, Ronco JJ, et al: Increased concentrations of plasma lactate predict pathologic dependence of oxygen consumption on oxygen delivery in patients with adult respiratory distress syndrome. J Crit Care 5:81–86, 1990.
2. Hesselvik JF, Brodin B: Low dose norepinephrine in patients with septic shock and oliguria: Effects on afterload, urine flow, and oxygen transport. Crit Care Med 17:179–180, 1989.
3. Higgins TL, Chernow B: Pharmacotherapy of circulatory shock. Dis Month, June 1987, pp 313–361.
4. King EG, Chin WDN: Shock: An overview of pathophysiology and general treatment goals. Crit Care Clin 1:547–561, 1985.
5. Larach DR, Kofke WA: Cardiovascular drugs. In Kofke WA, Levy JH (eds): Postoperative Critical Care Procedures of the Massachusetts General Hospital. Boston, Little, Brown, 1986, pp 464–522.
6. Lollgren H, Drexler H: Use of inotropes in the critical care setting. Crit Care Med 18:S56–S60, 1990.
7. Parrillo JE: Septic shock in humans: Clinical evaluation, pathogenesis, and therapeutic approach. In Shoemaker WC, et al: Textbook of Critical Care. Philadelphia, W.B. Saunders, 1989, pp 1006–1024.
8. Peters JI, Utset OM: Vasopressors in shock management: Choosing and using wisely. J Crit Illness 4:62–68, 1989.
9. Schaer GL, Fink MP, Parillo JE: Norepinephrine alone versus norepinephrine plus low-dose dopamine: Enhanced renal blood flow with combination pressor therapy. Crit Care Med 13:492–496, 1985.
10. Shoemaker WC, Appel PL, Kram HB: Oxygen transport measurements to evaluate tissue perfusion and titrate therapy: Dobutamine and dopamine effects. Crit Care Med 19:672–688, 1991.
11. Shoemaker WC, Kram HB, Appel PL: Therapy of shock based on pathophysiology, monitoring, and outcome prediction. Crit Care Med 18:S19–S25, 1990.
12. Sibbald WJ, Calvin JE, Holliday RL, Driedger AA: Concepts in the pharmacologic and non-pharmacologic support of cardiovascular function in critically ill surgical patients. Surg Clin North Am 63:455–482, 1983.
13. Tuchschmidt J, Oblitas D, Fried JC: Oxygen consumption in sepsis and septic shock. Crit Care Med 19:664–671, 1991.
14. Vernon DD, Banner W, Garrett JS, Dean JM: Efficacy of dopamine and norepinephrine for treatment of hemodynamic compromise in amitriptyline intoxication. Crit Care Med 19:544–549, 1991.
15. Zaloga GP, Delacey W, Holmboe E, Chernow B: Glucagon reversal of hypotension in a case of anaphylactoid shock. Ann Intern Med 105:65–66, 1986.

79. DIGOXIN

Lynn M. Schnapp, M.D.

1. What is thought to be the mechanism of action of digoxin?
Inhibition of the Na^+-K^+ ATPase enzyme.

2. What are the indications for digoxin?
The two major indications are (1) as a positive inotrope in congestive heart failure and (2) to control cardiac arrhythmias.

3. Is digoxin indicated for all patients with congestive heart failure?
Patients who have evidence of a dilated, failing heart and impaired systolic function (as evidenced by an S_3 on physical exam) seem to benefit from digoxin use. Digoxin is not indicated when congestive heart failure is due to diastolic dysfunction.

4. What is the role of digoxin in atrial fibrillation?
Digoxin is used to control ventricular response. It does not convert atrial fibrillation to normal sinus rhythm, but it does slow conduction through the atrioventricular node.

5. How can digoxin be administered?
It can be given orally, with peak effect seen at 2–6 hours, or intravenously, with peak effect at 1–4 hours. Although it can also be given intramuscularly, this is not recommended because of severe pain.

6. What dosage of digoxin should be used?
The general maintenance dose is 0.125–0.50 mg/day (single dose). A steady state is achieved within 6–8 days. Alternatively, one can first give a loading dose of digoxin (1 mg digoxin orally or intravenously for a 70-kg patient to achieve a plasma level of ≅2 ng/ml) prior to maintenance dose to hasten achievement of steady state.

Digoxin Dosage

	ORAL	INTRAVENOUS
Loading dose	0.5–1.5 mg	0.5–1.5 mg
Maintenance dose	0.125–0.5 mg/day	
Time to onset	0.5–2 hr	5–30 min
Time to peak effect	2–6 hr	1–4 hr
Elimination	Renal	Renal
Bioavailability	60–80%	100%

7. Does digoxin have a role in the management of cardiogenic shock?
Unless cardiogenic shock is accompanied by atrial fibrillation or flutter, digoxin has no role.

8. What digoxin level should one aim for?
Toxic level is >2.0 ng/ml. However, there is a great deal of variability between toxic and nontoxic levels among patients. Patients can be digoxin toxic with serum levels <2.0 ng/ml, especially in the face of electrolyte disorders, hypoxemia, or acid-base imbalances.

9. What is the effect of renal failure on digoxin levels?
Because digoxin is eliminated renally, a decrease in the glomerular filtration rate results in prolonged elimination. Thus digoxin needs to be used judiciously in patients with renal insufficiency, and the levels must be monitored closely.

10. How do other drugs affect digoxin levels?
Certain cardiac medications, including verapamil, quinidine, and amiodarone, increase digoxin levels. Drugs that affect electrolyte levels (e.g., diuretics, amphotericin) can have an indirect effect, since hypokalemia, hypomagnesemia, and hypercalcemia can predispose patients to digoxin toxicity even in the presence of "therapeutic" levels. Certain drugs (antacids, cholestyramine) can interfere with gastrointestinal absorption and cause low serum levels.

11. What are the symptoms of digoxin toxicity?
Digoxin toxicity occurs in 5–15% of hospitalized patients on digoxin. Common side effects include gastrointestinal complaints (nausea, vomiting, anorexia), neurologic effects (visual side effects, including alterations in color perception, confusion), and cardiac arrhythmias. The arrhythmias are the most important and can manifest themselves in a variety of ways,

including atrial tachycardia with block, junctional tachycardia, premature ventricular beats, sinus arrest, and atrioventricular block. Irreversible ventricular tachycardia or fibrillation can be seen with digoxin overdose.

12. How is digoxin toxicity treated?

Conservative measures include potassium repletion, suppressive antiarrhythmic therapy (e.g., lidocaine), and discontinuation of digoxin. Temporary transvenous pacing can be used to treat sinus arrest of sinoatrial or atrioventricular block. Digoxin-binding antibodies (Digibind) are available and effective for life-threatening toxicities (ventricular arrhythmias or high-grade atrioventricular block). Each 40-mg vial of Digibind neutralizes 0.6 mg of digoxin stored in the body. An estimate of total body stores can be made from a serum level or estimated digoxin ingestion. Improvement is usually within half an hour of administration. Serum digoxin levels can increase up to twentyfold after administration of Digibind. This increase is due to antibody-bound digoxin, which is pharmacologically inactive. Therefore, serum digoxin levels do not constitute a useful parameter to follow after antibody administration.

13. Should digoxin be used in patients with Wolff-Parkinson-White syndrome?

No. Digoxin may enhance conduction through accessory pathways and cause an extremely rapid ventricular response. Thus digoxin is contraindicated in patients with accessory pathways unless previously proven effective by electrophysiologic studies.

BIBLIOGRAPHY

1. Antman E, Smith T: Current concepts in the use of digitalis. Adv Intern Med 34:425, 1989.
2. Fisch C, Knoebel S: Digitalis cardiotoxicity. J Am Coll Cardiol 5:91, 1985.
3. Haber E: Antibodies and digitalis: The modern revolution in the use of an ancient drug. J Am Coll Cardiol 5:111, 1985.
4. Lewis R: Digitalis: A drug that refuses to die. Crit Care Med 18:S5, 1990.
5. Smith T: Digitalis: Mechanisms of action and clinical use. N Engl J Med 318:358, 1988.
6. Wenger T, Butler V, Haber E, Smith T: Treatment of 63 severely digitalis-toxic patients with digoxin-specific fragments. J Am Coll Cardiol 5:118, 1985.

XII: Surgery

80. BURNS

Mark W. Bowyer, M.D.

1. What is the epidemiology of burn injury?
Over 2 million burns requiring medical attention occur each year in the United States. Of this number, 50,000 persons require hospitalization for an average of 2 months and 14,000 will die. The highest peak incidence occurs in children less than 5 years of age, with the vast majority of burns in this group being secondary to scalds. In adults, most burns are occupationally related. Fires in the home are responsible for only 5% of burn injuries but 50% of burn deaths, mostly due to smoke inhalation.

2. What amount of thermal energy is required to cause cell injury?
The degree of cell injury caused by thermal injury is determined by the temperature and duration of heat exposure. Heat sources less than 45°C (113°F) cause no burn even with prolonged exposure. As temperature increases above this level, the duration of exposure causing tissue damage decreases, such that exposure to water at 54°C (129.2°F) for 30 seconds will cause a partial-thickness burn.

3. How is the depth of a burn injury determined?
Traditionally burn depth has been classified by degrees of injury. **First-degree burns** involve only the outer epidermis layer and are characterized by erythema and mild discomfort. **Second-degree burns** are those in which the entire epidermis and variable portion of the dermis are destroyed. A superficial second-degree burn is heat destruction of the upper third of the dermis. Injury to microvessels perfusing the area leads to leakage of large amounts of plasma into the interstitium with resultant blister formation. Superficial second-degree burns are extremely painful because of exposed sensory nerve endings; healing occurs in 7–14 days with minimal scarring. Deep second-degree burns extend well into the dermal layer with few viable epidermal cells remaining. Reepithelialization is extremely slow and may require months, with dense scarring of very thin skin. Fluid losses and metabolic effects of deep second-degree burns are basically the same as third-degree burns. Full-thickness or **third-degree burns** involve destruction of the entire epidermis and dermis, leaving no residual epidermal cells to repopulate. This wound will not reepithelialize and will therefore require skin grafting.

4. What are the priorities in the initial management of burns?
The burning process must be stopped, followed by the standard ABCs of CPR (see p. 1). Patients require assessment for other injuries that may be life threatening. Intravenous access should be obtained and fluid resuscitation initiated based on the extent and depth of the burn. If applicable, tetanus immunization should be administered. A Foley catheter should be placed and baseline laboratory tests should be done.

5. What are the indications for admission to an ICU or burn center?
Patients with burns who should be admitted to an ICU or burn center include:
- Adults with ≥ 25% body surface area (BSA) burn
- Children with ≥ 20% BSA burn

- Full-thickness burns $\geq$ 10% BSA
- High-voltage electrical injury
- Burns of face, hands, feet, ears, or perineum
- Inhalation injury or associated trauma
- Other medical conditions that increase medical risk (diabetes, extremes of age, or cardiovascular disease)

6. How is the extent of burn injury estimated?

Rapid approximation of the BSA burned in adults may be done using the "rule of nines." This rule divides the skin surface into areas of 9% of the total surface. The area of the patient's palm is approximately 1% and is also useful in estimating percent body surface area burn. Upon admission to a burn unit, more accurate assessment of total body surface area can be determined by using age-related charts designed by Lund and Browder. Careful evaluation of the percent of total body burn is useful for prognostic implications, determination of need for specialized burn care, and as a guide for fluid resuscitation.

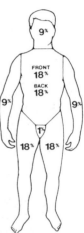

7. What are the systemic consequences of burn injury?

The systemic response to burn injury involves all organ systems with a biphasic pattern of early hypofunction and later hyperfunction characterizing the multisystem response to any injury. As with any major injury, the body increases secretion of catecholamines, cortisol, glucagon, renin-angiotensin, antidiuretic hormone, and aldosterone. The consequence is a tendency toward retention of sodium and water and excretion of potassium by the kidney. Profound hypermetabolism occurs following the burn, with an increase in the metabolic rate and oxygen consumption, which remain elevated until the wound is covered. The evaporative water loss from the wound may reach 300 ml/m^2/hr, which markedly increases heat loss. Additionally, immunologic abnormalities in burn patients may predispose them to infection.

8. What type of fluid therapy should be used in burn resuscitation?

Adequate volume resuscitation is critical to the survival of the victim of a major body burn. Opinions vary regarding the optimal timing and composition of fluids in burn resuscitation. Despite what appear to be radically different approaches, satisfactory results have been obtained with several different formulas. This speaks to the fact that these formulas are merely guidelines and that individual therapy should be tailored to optimize urine output and electrolyte status.

Two of the most popular burn resuscitation formulas are the Parkland and the modified Brooke. The Parkland formula uses lactated Ringer's solution, which is given in a volume of 4 ml/kg/% burn over 24 hours. One-half of this amount is given in the first 8 hours and the second half over the next 16 hours. The modified Brooke formula uses 2 ml/kg/% burn in the first 24 hours. Both formulas use colloids after the first 24 hours and glucose in water as necessary to maintain urine output.

9. What factors should raise suspicion of an inhalation injury?

Inhalation injuries are increased in patients with burns with impaired mental status (alcohol or drugs), in trauma patients, and in those whose burns were from petroleum products or were sustained in a closed space. Inflammation of the oropharyngeal mucosa, facial burns or singed nasal hair, hoarseness, stridor, wheezing and rales and carbonaceous sputum production are all warning signs of possible inhalation injury. Bronchoscopy, xenon-133 perfusion lung scan, and serial arterial blood gas determinations may help in the diagnosis.

10. How are inhalation injuries treated?
Inhalation injuries should be aggressively treated with early intubation prior to airway occlusion from edema. Warm humidified oxygen, pulmonary toilet, treatment of broncho-spasm, and therapeutic bronchoscopy are the cornerstones of treatment. Carbon monoxide intoxication, if present, is treated with 100% oxygen, and the use of hyperbaric oxygen should be considered.

11. What are the principles of burn wound care?
Care of the burn wound can be divided into three separate stages: (1) the presurgical stage, during which the primary goal is to decrease the incidence of burn wound infection with topical antibacterial agents; (2) the surgical phase, during which the wounds are excised of all necrotic material and covered either with autologous skin grafts or with some form of temporary biologic dressing or biosynthetic skin substitute; and (3) the time period after the wound is covered when the primary goal is to prevent wound contracture and scarring in order to preserve or restore function.

12. What topical antimicrobial agens are used in burn wound care?
In the United States, three topical agents are currently used primarily for the coverage of massive burn wound injuries: mafenide acetate (Sulfamylon), silver sulfadiazine (Silvadene), and 0.5% silver nitrate solution. **Mafenide acetate** has a broad spectrum of antibacterial activity and is able to penetrate deeply into the burn eschar. The two most serious side effects are development of metabolis acidosis and severe pain following application. **Silver sulfadiazine** has a broad but more limited antibacterial spectrum and has less eschar penetration than does mafenide acetate. This agent is more widely used because it is not painful when applied. The most serious side effect is a transient leukopenia, which develops 24–72 hours post-burn. **Silver nitrate 0.5% solution** has a broad spectrum of antibacterial activity, absence of hypersensitivity reactions, and painless application. Disadvantages include electrolyte abnormalities, rapid inactivation by precipitation, failure to penetrate eschar, and black staining.

13. Why is it important to prevent burn wound infection?
The mortality associated with generalized burn wound invasion, particularly when systemic dissemination has occurred, is nearly 100%. Invasive burn wound infection necessitates alteration of local wound care and institution of systemic therapy. All tissues involved in the septic process should be excised as soon as the patient can tolerate general anesthesia.

14. How are burn wound infections diagnosed?
Histologic examination of a burn wound biopsy (500-mg sample) is the only definitive means of differentiating the colonization of nonviable tissue from the invasion of viable tissue. Burn wound infection may be suggested from changes in the wound. Local signs of burn wound infection include focal, dark brown, black, or violaceous discoloration; conversion of partical-thickness injury to full-thickness necrosis; unexpected rapid separation of eschar; green pigment in subcutaneous fat; edema and discoloration of unburned skin at the wound margins; and hemorrhagic discoloration of the subeschar tissue.

15. When should escharotomy be done?
Patients who have circumferential burns of an extremity or torso will develop significant edema under the unyielding eschar that will lead to compromised blood flow and, if on the

chest, inhibit chest wall expansion and thus impair ventilation. Escharatomy, with incision through the eschar down to viable fat from proximal to distal margin of the burn, should be performed. Restoration of pulses should be confirmed prior to completion of the procedure.

16. What are the nutritional requirements of the burn patient?
There is marked hypermetabolism and increased catabolism of lean body mass in the burn patient. Nutritional management is aimed at supplying total caloric and nitrogen needs to spare the body tissue mass as much as possible. Total caloric requirments can be calculated by 25 kcal × body weight (kg) + 40 kcal × % burn. Of the total calories, 20–25% should be protein and vitamins and minerals supplied at 2–3 times the recommended daily allowance for normal individuals. The preferred route is via the intestinal tract, with parenteral nutrition being reserved only for those unable to tolerate enteral feeds.

17. What are the major complications associated with major burn injuries?
Gastrointestinal complications include Curling's ulcer, ileus, acalculous cholecystitis, and superior mesenteric artery syndrome. Burn wound infection has been previously discussed, but other sources of infection such as suppurative thrombophlebitis often occur.

18. How should chemical burns be managed?
The solution to pollution is dilution. Cutaneous injury from caustic chemicals can continue as long as the chemical remains; therefore, copious irrigation is essential to lessen the depth of injury. Once the agent has been removed, burn care is identical to care for thermal injuries.

19. How do electrical burns differ from other burns?
Electrical burns are usually caused by contact with high voltage and have entrance and exit wounds. Arrhythmias, especially ventricular fibrillation, are common. Associated fractures are common from falls or current-induced muscle contractions. Vascular and muscle damage may occur with need for fasciotomy and/or amputation. Renal failure secondary to myoglobin and hemoglobin may occur and must be prevented with hydration and alkalinization of the urine. Neurologic damage, including spinal cord deficits and cataract formation, may also occur.

BIBLIOGRAPHY

1. Demling RH. Management of the burn patient. In Shoemaker WC, et al (eds): Textbook of Critical Care, 2nd ed. Philadelphia, W.B. Saunders, 1989, pp 1301–1315.
2. Demling RH: Fluid replacement in burned patients. Surg Clin North Am 67:15–30, 1987.
3. Iteimbach DM: Early burn excision and grafting. Surg Clin North Am 67:93–107, 1987.
4. Herndon DN, Curreri PW, Abston S, et al: Treatment of burns. Curr Prob Surg 24:344–397, 1987.
5. Herndon DN, Langner F, Thompson P, et al: Pulmonary injury in burned patients. Surg Clin North Am 67:31–46, 1987.
6. Monafo WW, Freedman B: Topical therapy for burns. Surg Clin North Am 67:133–145, 1987.
7. Mozingo DW, Smith AA, McManus WF, et al: Chemical burns. J Trauma 28:642–647, 1988.
8. Pasulka PS, Wachtel TL: Nutritional considerations for the burned patient. Surg Clin North Am 67:109–131, 1987.
9. Pruitt BA, Goodwin CW: Thermal injuries. In Davis JH (ed): Clinical Surgery. St. Louis, C.V. Mosby, 1987, pp 2822–2903.
10. Sykes RA, Mani MM, Hiebert JM: Chemical burns: Retrospective review. J Burn Care Rehab 7:343–347, 1986.
11. Waymack JP, Pruitt BA: Burn wound care. Adv Surg 23:261–290, 1990.
12. Wionicki JL, Sato RM, Baxter CR: Current concepts in burn care. Ann Plast Surg 16:242–249, 1986.

81. THE ACUTE ABDOMEN

Christina Finlayson, M.D., and Charles M. Abernathy, M.D.

1. What is an acute abdomen?
The term "acute abdomen" refers to the sudden or gradual onset of abdominal pain that persists over several hours. A "surgical abdomen" implies the additional presence of signs of peritoneal inflammation.

2. What types of stimulation cause abdominal pain?
The visceral organs receive afferent innervation from the parasympathetic and sympathetic nerves. As such, direct injury to the visceral organs such as cutting, crushing, or burning, causes very little in the way of pain sensation. Spasm of hollow organs, distention, and chemical irritation of the peritoneum are perceived as abdominal pain. The abdominal wall and diaphragm receive somatic innervation. Direct injury to those structures from cutting, crushing, or burning will be perceived as painful.

3. What is referred pain?
Diaphragmatic irritation is often perceived by the patient as shoulder and neck pain. Cholecystitis is often perceived as scapular pain, obstruction of the ureter as testicular pain, etc. This is because innervation of visceral organs is along nerve pathways that enter the spinal cord at levels often remote from the site of injury or irritation. Therefore, pain may be perceived in areas distant to the involved structure.

4. How do you evaluate the complaint of abdominal pain?
Whether the patient presents with abdominal pain or develops symptoms after being admitted for another condition, the initial evaluation should be the same. A thorough history is essential and includes location and time of onset of pain, any change in location or severity of pain, and description of quality of the pain (i.e., sharp, stabbing, dull, aching, or burning). Associated symptoms such as vomiting, anorexia, change in bowel habits, urinary complaints, or gynecologic symptoms should be elicited. Blood in vomit or stool or a history of melena is useful.

The physical examination should begin with a careful observation of the shape and contour of the abdomen. A gentle hand in the evaluation of a tender abdomen cannot be overemphasized if patient confidence is to be maintained. Auscultation of all quadrants for presence of bowel sounds and their pitch should be performed before manual palpation. Palpation begins in the least tender area of the abdomen and progresses to the most tender. Peritoneal signs, when present, can be elicited by gentle percussion or by minimal intrusion of the abdominal wall followed by release of pressure. Deep palpation to produce rebound is usually unnecessary and creates discomfort by itself.

5. Which confirmatory tests are helpful in diagnosis?
If history and physical examination reveal a surgical abdomen with little doubt of the diagnosis, radiographic examination is often unnecessary and may lead to delay in resuscitation and therapy. When, however, a surgical emergency is not present and the diagnosis is unclear, selective use of imaging techniques can be valuable. When bowel obstruction or perforation is suspected, abdominal x-rays can show dilation of the small or large intestine, air-fluid levels, or free air within the abdominal cavity. Ultrasound is helpful when aortic or biliary tract disease is suspected. It can accurately identify gallstones, can often evaluate the size of the ducts and pancreas, and has been used in evaluating potential appendicitis. Other modalities that are helpful in evaluation of intraabdominal pathology are CT scan, contrast studies, and nuclear medicine imaging. Angiography is rarely used except when mesenteric arterial occlusion is suspected.

6. What is the role of diagnostic peritoneal lavage (DPL) in evaluation of the patient with the acute abdomen?

DPL is a well-known tool in the evaluation of blunt and penetrating abdominal trauma. Its role in nontraumatic abdominal disease is less well recognized. Patients with suspected peritonitis that is difficult to verify because of an unreliable history or an equivocal physical examination are candidates for DPL. This category of patients includes those with altered mental status, with other medical problems that could account for symptoms (such as pneumonia with gram-negative bacteremia and a potential source that is not intraabdominal), and with septic shock of unknown etiology.

7. Is the differential diagnosis of abdominal pain in the ICU different from that in the ER?

The specific illness that causes abdominal pain in the ER is also seen in the ICU. Because the patient population in the ICU has been shifting to a more elderly base, the differential is weighted toward conditions seen in the aged patient.

8. How are aortic aneurysms diagnosed?

There are two kinds of aortic aneurysms: thoracic and abdominal. Thoracic aneurysms are described as dissecting, where a false lumen is created and blood flow courses in the media of the vessel. This dissection can extend below the diaphragm and even reach the iliac and femoral vessels. Abdominal aneurysms are a dilatation of the vessel wall and become symptomatic when they rupture or "leak." An anterior rupture penetrates freely into the peritoneal cavity and is usually rapidly fatal. Posterior ruptures are contained in the retroperitoneal tissues and patients are more likely to present to the hospital with the complaint of abdominal and back pain. Four radiographic techniques are helpful in diagnosing aortic disruption: (1) Plain radiographs of the abdomen, both AP and lateral, will often show the calcific rim of an abdominal aneurysm. They do not, however, give any indication if the vessel is leaking. A thoracic aneurysm is not dilated and may or may not have associated calcifications; therefore, it will not be identified on plain radiograph. (2) Ultrasound of the abdomen will identify an abdominal aneurysm, but also does not identify evidence of leak. (3) CT scan will demonstrate both thoracic and abdominal aneurysms and can show evidence of dissection or leak. (4) The gold standard for thoracic aneurysm is aortography, which will demonstrate the aneurysm and identify the entrance point of the dissection.

9. What are potential causes of and treatment for small bowel obstruction?

Bowel obstruction can be functional or mechanical. **Functional obstruction** implies an absence or dysfunction of peristalsis without an occlusion of the bowel lumen. This can be caused by early sepsis, the postoperative state, electrolyte abnormalities, or narcotics. These can be treated by nasogastric decompression and correction of the underlying abnormality. **Mechanical causes** of small bowel obstruction include postoperative adhesions, hernias, tumors, intussusception, gallstones, bezoars, etc. These are also treated initially with nasogastric decompression. The decision to treat surgically is often difficult, but guidelines for operative intervention include progression of pain after decompression, failure to improve with decompression, tachycardia, fever, and elevation in white count. A surgeon should be involved early when a small bowel obstruction is suspected.

10. What is Ogilvie's syndrome?

Ogilvie's syndrome, or pseudo-obstruction of the colon, is marked by massive dilation of the colon without mechanical obstruction. It is seen most commonly in elderly, debilitated patients, those from nursing homes, and patients who have undergone orthopedic surgery. If dilation exceeds 9–12 cm, there is a risk of perforation of the cecum. Treatment begins with colonoscopic or rectal tube decompression of the colon. If this is unsuccessful, surgical decompression with cecostomy may be required.

11. What does the constellation of "abnormal pain out of proportion to physical findings" connote?

This symptom pattern is identified in mesenteric ischemia. Acute occlusion of the superior mesenteric artery is usually due to cardiac embolus. It is the most susceptible of the mesenteric vessels because of its large caliber and straight-line takeoff from the aorta. Other causes of ischemia include thrombosis of mesenteric vessels and low flow due to inadequate cardiac output. Early surgical intervention is imperative if the vessels are occluded. Mortality approaches 90%.

12. Name some nonsurgical causes of acute abdominal pain?

Numerous medical conditions that can cause abdominal pain and even mimic a "surgical abdomen" need to be identified early to avoid a needless laparotomy. These conditions commonly include pneumonia, sickle cell anemia, primary peritonitis, infectious gastroenteritis, leukemia, poisoning, pancreatitis, inflammatory bowel disease without perforation, hepatitis, and pelvic inflammatory disease.

BIBLIOGRAPHY

1. Diethelm AG: The acute abdomen. In Sabiston DC (ed): Textbook of Surgery, 13th ed. Philadelphia, W.B. Saunders, 1986.
2. Dodson TF: Evaluation of the acute abdomen in the intensive care unit. In Rippe JM, et al (eds): Intensive Care Medicine. Boston, Little, Brown, 1985.
3. Richardson JD, Flint LM, Polk HC: Peritoneal lavage: A useful diagnostic adjunct for peritonitis. Surgery 94:826, 1983.
4. Sallarides T, Hopkins W, Doolas A: Abdominal emergencies. Med Clin North Am 70:1093, 1986.
5. Steinheber FU: Medical conditions mimicking the acute surgical abdomen. Med Clin North Am 57:1559, 1973.

82. DIAGNOSTIC PERITONEAL LAVAGE

Diane M. Hartman, M.D., and Ernest E. Moore, M.D.

1. What is diagnostic periitoneal lavage (DPL)?

DPL is a procedure that was developed by H. D. Root and associates in 1965 for the evaluation of patients with acute blunt abdominal trauma. DPL replaced the four-quadrant peritoneal tap that was popular at that time. The unique feature of DPL, in addition to aspirating the peritoneal cavity, is the introduction of fluid that is recovered and analyzed for cellular and other particular content.

2. What are the clinical situations in which DPL may be valuable?

DPL became the gold standard for evaluation of blunt abdominal trauma in the early 1970s. In the late 1970s, studies from Brooklyn, Dallas, and Denver expanded the role of DPL to penetrating wounds, particularly stab wounds to the anterior abdomen and lower chest. More recently DPL has been applied in the diagnosis of acute peritonitis and staging of acute pancreatitis, with generally favorable results.

3. What techniques are available to introduce the DPL catheter into the peritoneum?

Conceptually there are three approaches: open, semi-open, and closed techniques. **The open technique** consists of an incision through the abdominal wall, placing the catheter into the peritoneal cavity under direct vision. **The semi-open technique** limits the incision to the skin with a small nick in the fascia, with the catheter and trocar in place, and then advanced across the peritoneum. **The closed technique** is placement of the catheter with trocar in place through the abdominal wall. A more recent variant of this procedure uses a wire guide to facilitate more controlled tunneling of the catheter.

4. What are the advantages and disadvantages of these techniques?

The open technique is considered the standard because it is the most secure route into the peritoneal cavity and is the only safe procedure in patients with previous abdominal surgery, pelvic fracture, or pregnancy. The disadvantages of the open approach include its technical challenge, additional time, and added risk of wound infection. The closed technique of DPL is the quickest and perhaps easiest to perform. The major disadvantage is the blind nature with its inherent risk of injuring underlying abdominal viscera. This risk, however, can be minimized by using the wire guide technique. Currently the semi-open technique is the most widely used because it is a compromise between the open and closed procedures.

5. Must DPL be performed in the operating room?

DPL can be performed readily in the ER, ICU, or ward. The procedure is performed with local anesthesia, generally 1% lidocaine. The entrance site to the abdominal wall must be prepared and draped in the usual sterile fashion.

6. What are the complications of DPL?

In the non-obese patient who has not had a previous abdominal operation or infection, the technical complications are less than 0.5%, with an additional 1% risk of infection. Naturally, the mechanical constraints of obesity or intestinal adhesions increase these risks. Patients with underlying portal hypertension or other coagulation disorders have an increased risk of bleeding.

7. Can DPL be performed in patients with previous abdominal surgery?

With preexistent laparotomy, DPL must be performed with the open technique. If done carefully, this approach is safe, but extensive adhesions may compartmentalize the peritoneal cavity and render the lavage falsely negative.

8. Can DPL be performed in pregnant patients?

The open technique is mandatory in gravid patients. The catheter entrance site chosen is at the top of the fundus of the uterus, and, accordingly, in later pregnancy the catheter entrance site is in the supraumbilical region. While a theoretical concern, DPL has not been associated with induction of labor.

9. What is the sensitivity for intraperitoneal bleeding?

The false-negative rate is less than 1%. The test is extremely useful in blunt trauma because the predominant intraperitoneal injuries are to the spleen and liver. The major limitations of DPL are in the identification of diaphragmatic rupture or perforation of hollow viscera, including the gastrointestinal tract and bladder. The incidence of false-negative studies based on red blood cell analysis with isolated small perforations to these structures is substantial because such lesions tend to bleed minimally.

10. What criteria of bleeding are considered significant following blunt abdominal trauma?

Aspiration of greater than 10 ml of free blood is considered an indication for laparotomy. If the aspirate is not positive, the lavage is done with 1 liter of warm saline (or 15 ml/kg in children), and the effluent analyzed in the laboratory. A red cell count exceeding 100,000/ml^3 is considered positive.

11. What additional indices are considered significant for DPL in blunt abdominal trauma?
Initial aspiration of enteric contents warrants prompt laparotomy. The utility of biochemical markers in the lavage effluent, however, is controversial. A white blood cell count exceeding $400/ml^3$ has been considered significant, but several recent series have shown that this leukocytosis frequently occurs without associated visceral injury. The current standard is to repeat the DPL in 4 hours and operate if the white blood count remains elevated. Additional lavage markers of some value include the amylase and alkaline phosphatase levels, but the threshold for laparotomy remains ill-defined.

12. Has the emergence of contrast-enhanced CT scanning eliminated the need for DPL in the evaluation of blunt abdominal trauma?
DPL and abdominal CT scanning should be considered complementary rather than competitive diagnostic tests (see Controversies). DPL is still the most rapid and reliable means of excluding intraperitoneal hemorrhage in the multisystem-injured patient.

13. Is DPL useful in the evaluation of penetrating abdominal wounds?
In many centers DPL has become the mainstay for evaluating stab wounds to the anterior abdomen. These patients are generally difficult to assess because of intoxication and pain emanating from the abdominal wall stab wound. Stab wounds to the anterior abdomen generally penetrate the peritoneum in approximately two-thirds of patients, of whom about half will incur significant visceral injury. Thus, only one of four patients with a stab wound to the anterior abdomen will require laparotomy. Local wound exploration and DPL provide a safe, quick, and cost effective means of triaging these patients. Interestingly, the DPL criteria for abdominal exploration in stab wounds are similar to those for blunt abdominal trauma. The major difference is the much higher rate of isolated hollow visceral injury following a stab wound; i.e., approximately 2–5% of patients with a negative DPL will have perforation of the small bowel, stomach, or rarely, the colon. For that reason, all patients undergoing DPL for stab wounds must be observed in the hospital for at least 24 hours, and laparotomy performed promptly for any signs of peritoneal irritation.

14. Are the criteria for operation different when DPL is used to evaluate the possibility of abdominal injury via a lower chest wound?
Because small injuries to the diaphragm often bleed minimally, the threshold for laparotomy is reduced in the evaluation of lower chest stab wounds. In fact, a red blood cell count exceeding $5,000/mm^3$ is considered positive. The logic is that red cell contamination cannot be ascribed to the DPL technique and, therefore, must represent intraabdominal injury.

15. Is DPL useful in the evaluation of abominal gunshot wounds?
Gunshot wounds of the abdomen pose a much greater threat than stab wounds. The incidence of significant visceral damage when the missile penetrates the peritoneum approximates 95%. Therefore, it is routine policy to perform laparotomy when the missile appears to have entered the peritoneal cavity. However, in a select group of patients in whom a low-energy missile appears to remain extraperitoneal, DPL may be used as an adjunctive test to avoid laparotomy. In such cases, the red blood cell threshold for laparotomy is $5,000/mm^3$; the rationale is similar to that applied to penetrating wounds to the lower chest.

16. Does DPL have any value in the evaluation of the patient with potential intraabdominal infection?
Several groups have advocated use of DPL in the evaluation of critically ill patients in the ICU with potential intraperitoneal sepsis. The most useful lavage marker appears to be the leukocyte count; i.e., a white blood count exceeding $500/mm^3$ is specific for intraperitoneal inflammation. Nonperforated inflammatory lesions of the peritoneal cavity may not

manifest changes in the lavage fluid. To enhance the sensitivity for abdominal infection, other groups have suggested measurement for endotoxin, lactate, or a variety of enzymes. These reports are promising but inconclusive. Several authors have advocated DPL for the staging of acute pancreatitis, but precise markers remain to be established. Some groups suggest the relative levels of amylase and lipase compared to serum are prognostic; others suggest that blood tinged lavage or ascitic fluid implies pancreatic necrosis.

CONTROVERSY

17. Is DPL or double-contrast CT scanning better in the evaluation of blunt abdominal trauma?

For DPL: DPL is a rapid, safe, and highly sensitive test for intraperitoneal blood. The procedure can be performed during the initial evaluation of the injured patient while other resuscitative maneuvers are ongoing. Thus, DPL is an extremely valuable triage tool in the multisystem-injured patient who remains in shock.

Against DPL: Paradoxically, the major downfall of DPL is that it is too sensitive for intraperitoneal blood and does not indicate the source of bleeding. In the past 5 years, there has been growing enthusiasm for nonoperative management of solid organ injuries, particularly the spleen. DPL may be falsely positive in as many as 15% of patients with major pelvic fracture because of red blood cell diapedesis. DPL does not sample the retroperitoneum; therefore, injuries to the pancreas, duodenum, urinary tract, and major vascular structures may be missed.

For CT scanning: CT scanning affords the opportunity to manage solid organ injuries nonoperatively. This capability is particularly valuable in children, in whom more than two-thirds of splenic injuries can be treated nonoperatively.

Against CT scanning: Accuracy of abdominal CT scanning varies tremendously with patient preparation, scanner, generation, and expertise of the radiologist. Moreover, the logistics of removing a critically injured patient from the ER is less than optimal. Finally, there are risks associated with oral contrast material (aspiration) as well as with intravenous contrast material. Finally, CT scanning is a relatively expensive diagnostic test.

BIBLIOGRAPHY

1. Alyono D, Morrow CE, Perry JF: Reappraisal of diagnostic peritoneal lavage criteria for operation in penetrating and blunt trauma. Surgery 92:751–757, 1982.
2. Cue JI, Miller FB, Cryer HM, et al: A prospective, randomized comparison between open and closed peritoneal lavage technique. J Trauma 30:880–883, 1990.
3. Feliciano DV, Bitondo CG, Steed G, et al: Five hundred open taps or lavages in patients with abdominal stab wounds. Am J Surg 148:772–777, 1984.
4. Jacobs DG, Angus L, Rodriguez A, Militello PR: Peritoneal lavage white count: A reassessment. J Trauma 30:607–612, 1990.
5. Marx JA, Moore EE, Bar-Or D: Peritoneal lavage in penetrating injuries of the small bowel and colon: Value of enzyme determinations. Ann Emerg Med 12:68–70, 1983.
6. Moore EE, Marx JA: Penetrating abdominal wounds: Rationale for exploratory laparotomy. JAMA 253:2705–2711, 1985.
7. Moore JB, Moore EE, Markovchick VJ, Rosen R: Diagnostic peritoneal lavage for abdominal trauma: Superiority of the open technique at the infraumbilical ring. J Trauma 21:570–572, 1981.
8. Moore JB, Moore EE, Thompson JS: Abdominal injuries associated with penetrating trauma in the lower chest. Am J Surg 140:724–730, 1980.
9. Richardson JD, Flint LM, Polk HC: Peritoneal lavage: A useful diagnostic adjunct for peritonitis. Surgery 94:826–829, 1982.
10. Root HD, Hauser CW, McKinley CR, et al: Diagnostic peritoneal lavage. Surgery 57:633–637, 1965.
11. Thompson JS, Moore EE, Van Duzer-Moore S, et al: The evolution of abdominal stab wound management. J Trauma 20:478–484, 1980.

83. WOUND INFECTION AND DEHISCENCE

Charles Abernathy, M.D., and Thomas Rehring, M.D.

1. What are the signs and symptoms of a wound infection?
Local signs include warmth, erythema, pain, and a palpable mass (calor, rubor, dolor, tumor). Systemic signs include increased core temperature, and chills or rigors thought to be secondary to exogenous pyrogens.

2. Which wounds are likely to become infected?
Wounds are divided into clean, clean-contaminated, and contaminated wounds. The overall rate of wound infection is approximately 3%. Acceptable rates of infection for clean wounds (e.g., herniorrhaphy) is less than 2%, for clean-contaminated wounds (e.g., colorectal) less than 3%, and contaminated wounds (gross contamination) less than 6 %.

3. What are the common infecting organisms?
Most clean wound infections are from the skin flora of patients or surgeons (e.g., staphylococci, streptococci). In clean-contaminated and dirty wounds, the organisms are obviously from whatever the source of the contamination was, i.e., the colon, the stomach, etc.

4. What are the risk factors for a wound infection?
Type of operation (i.e., contaminated wounds), local factors (blood supply, foreign bodies, dead space, hematoma), and systemic factors: age (very young or very old), obesity, malnutrition, immunosuppression, cancer, diabetes, liver failure, steroids, and alcohol abuse.

5. When are prophylactic antibiotics indicated?
Prophylactic antibiotics should be used any time foreign material (such as vascular grafts or orthopedic hardward) is used in surgery. The use of antibiotics in multiple trauma is also well established. Less well established is use in biliary tract surgery. Clean elective surgeries such as breast biopsies and inguinal hernias have been addressed by randomized prospective study which indicated that patients receiving prophylactic antibiotics had 48% fewer postoperative infections.

6. Should all patients with penetrating wounds receive prophylactic antibiotics?
Yes. All require coverage of both aerobic and anaerobic bacteria. Length of treatment is determined by which organs are involved. Terminal ileum or colon injuries require the greatest length of treatment (usually 5–10 days).

7. When do wound infections typically manifest?
Frequently, in abdominal wounds the wound infection is undetected until days 3–7 when the erythema and induration of the wound become apparent.

8. What should be done with a red, indurated abdominal incision?
Individual surgeons vary as to whether they take all of the skin suture and subcutaneous sutures out and open the entire wound or remove a limited portion of the skin sutures (and subcutaneous sutures, if present). Anaerobic and aerobic cultures should be obtained, followed by local wound care and appropriate antibiotics.

9. What is the care for a wound that is being allowed to close secondarily?
Necrotic tissue is an ideal bacterial growth medium. Indeed, bacterial overgrowth inhibits epithelialization and healing. Local wound care is therefore critical. Although povidone-iodine

(Betadine) has been shown to be cytotoxic, application of dilute Betadine dressings for 24 hours to a grossly contaminated wound may be advantageous. Routine care involves irrigating the wound with half-strength hydrogen peroxide, and sterile wet to dry normal saline dressing changes two to three times daily to aid in debridement of necrotic material and wound healing.

10. What is the most worrisome diagnosis in a patient 12 hours postoperatively with a temperature of 39° C, an erythematous wound with bullae, and a serosanguinous discharge? What is the treatment?

Necrotizing fasciitis. Treatment includes broad-spectrum intravenous antibiotics, wide debridement, and the consideration of hyperbaric oxygen therapy. In a recent series, the mortality of necrotizing fasciitis approached 30%.

11. What are the risk factors for a wound dehiscence?

Local factors include surgical technique, hemorrhage, and infection. At risk are elderly, debilitated, malnourished, obese patients. Patients on systemic steroids, with diabetes, or with any process that increases intraabdominal pressure are at increased risk. It has been claimed that horizontal incisions have a lower incidence of dehiscence compared with vertical incisions. A recent large-scale retrospective study has largely refuted this theory, however.

12. Which signs herald wound dehiscences?

Serosanguinous discharge from a wound greater than 24 hours postoperatively must *always* be considered as wound dehiscence until proved otherwise.

13. What is the difference between wound dehiscence and evisceration?

Dehiscence means that the abdominal fascia is not intact. It is diagnosed by placing a gloved finger into the wound and feeling the separation of the fascia. Evisceration is protrusion of abdominal contents (usually small bowel) through a wound. Both are basically managed in the same way.

14. How do you manage evisceration? Dehiscence?

If the surgeon is unsure of the diagnosis, the wound may be gently explored with a sterile glove, noting the integrity of the fascia and the contents of the wound cavity. In evisceration, the exposed bowels should be wrapped in sterile, saline-soaked towels and the patient returned to the operating room for closure as soon as possible. In general, dehiscences should also be closed operatively, although in certain difficult, extenuating circumstances (chronic intraabdominal sepsis), dehiscences can be left open, simply accepting the fact that there will be a ventral hernia and allowing the chronic intraabdominal sepsis to drain through the open dehiscence.

BIBLIOGRAPHY

1. Gentry, et al: Perioperative antibiotic therapy for penetrating injuries to the abdomen. Ann Surg 200(5):561–566, 1984.
2. Greenburg, et al: Wound dehiscence. Arch Surg 114:143–146, 1979.
3. Moore FA, et al: Presumptive antibiotics for penetrating abdominal wounds. Surg Gynecol Obstet 169:99–103, 1989.
4. Oreseovich MR, et al: Duration of preventative antibiotic administration for penetrating abdominal trauma. Arch Surg 117:200–205, 1982.
5. Platt, et al: Preoperative antibiotic prophylaxis for herniorrhaphy and breast surgery. N Engl J Med 322:153–160, 1990.

84. ARTERIAL EMBOLI

Thomas A. Whitehill, M.D.

1. What is an arterial embolus?

An embolus is a blood clot that is formed in, or gains access to, the vascular system in one location and is then carried to another site by blood flow where it produces obstruction.

2. What are the usual etiologies of acute arterial emboli?

Cardiac: The heart is by far the predominant source of arterial emboli, cited as the site of origin in 80–90% of cases in all reported series. The type of heart disease responsible for the embolus has shifted from rheumatic to atherosclerotic origin, with coronary vascular disease currently implicated in 60–70% of the cases. Atrial fibrillation is the leading nidus (65–75%), followed by acute myocardial infarction with left ventricular (LV) thrombus (5%) and LV aneurysm (5%); lesser causes include prosthetic valves, dilated cardiomyopathy, and intracardiac tumors.

Noncardiac: Only 5–10% of emboli originate from extracardiac sources. Etiologies include diseased large vessels (aneurysms/plaques), vessel injury secondary to invasive diagnostic/therapeutic maneuvers, intravascular devices, malignant noncardiac tumor emboli, and paradoxical emboli.

3. Where are the common sites that emboli lodge?

Overall, 20% of emboli enter the carotid/vertebral circulations, 10% involve visceral vessels, and 70–80% involve axial/limb vessels. The lower-extremity vessels are involved five times more frequently than those of the upper extremities. Sites of embolic occlusion are most often related to major vessel bifurcations because vessel diameters change most abruptly at these branch points. Embolic obstruction also occurs at points of stenosis. In all series, the common femoral bifurcation is the most frequent site of embolic occlusion, usually noted in 35–50% of series. Taken together, the femoral and popliteal arteries are involved more than twice as often as the aorta and iliac vessels; i.e., only a thrombus of considerable size will have any effect at the aortic or iliac bifurcation unless the vessel is narrowed by preexistent occlusive disease.

4. What is the significance of spontaneous atheroembolism?

Atheroembolism is a generic term for arterial embolization of small thrombus or debris derived from degeneration and ulceration of proximal atherosclerotic plaques. Because of the small size of this embolic debris, the affected arteries are typically capillaries, arterioles, and digital arteries. The clinical manifestations of atheroembolic disease in the carotid circulation are transient ischemic attacks or stroke. Microembolic phenomena of the legs, feet, or toes are often described as livedo reticularis and "blue-toe" syndrome.

5. What is a paradoxical embolus?

A paradoxical embolus originates in the venous circulation and passes into the arterial circulation through an intracardiac shunt. The pathophysiology of a paradoxical embolus involves elevation of right heart pressures either on a chronic or an acute basis with concomitant development of a right-to-left shunt through which emboli can pass. A patent foramen ovale is responsible in most cases. The most common source of the right-sided emboli is a thrombus formed in the lower extremity deep venous system or the pelvic veins. The recurrent nature of paradoxical emboli, leading to involvement of multiple arterial sites, emphasizes the importance of expeditious diagnosis and treatment. In a patient with concomitant acute arterial ischemia and deep venous thrombosis or pulmonary emboli, the diagnosis of paradoxical embolus is probable, and institution of heparin anticoagulation should begin immediately.

6. Name the five "Ps" of acute arterial ischemia. What is the significance of each?
Pulselessness, pain, pallor, paresthesias, and paralysis.

Pulselessness. Sudden loss of a previously known pulse is the hallmark of an embolic occlusion. Recognition of this sign is obviously more difficult if the prior pulse state of the limb is unknown or abnormal due to associated arteriosclerotic occlusive disease.

Pain. Characteristically, pain is described as a severe and steady ache involving major muscle groups below the level of obstruction which worsens at locations increasingly distal to the point of obstruction. In 10–20% of patients, sensory disturbances such as numbness or paresthesias predominate and may mask primary complaints of pain.

Pallor. Initially the limb distal to the occlusion is white and waxy and is often termed cadaveric; subsequently, blotchy mottled areas of cyanosis may appear with eventual blistering and the deeper discoloration typical of early gangrene.

Paresthesias. Advanced ischemia is characterized by diminished to absent motor and sensory function, reflecting ischemia of both muscles and nerves distal to the arterial occlusion. The extent of anesthesia and motor paralysis of a limb is a good index of the degree of tissue anoxia and correlates well with the ultimate prognosis. Sensitivity to two-point discrimination or light touch is often the best guide to viability; its absence demands immediate intervention.

Paralysis. This is a similarly grave sign, indicating a combination of severe neural and skeletal muscle ischemia without reversibility (i.e., impending gangrene). When rigor appears, with its woody hardness associated with involuntary muscle contraction, irreversible ischemia has most likely developed. Although the limb may still be salvaged by surgical intervention, ultimate function is often permanently compromised, and the metabolic effects of revascularization may be profound and sometimes lethal (See question #11.) Determination of the site of occlusion is often possible by careful physical examination. In addition to the site of pulselessness, a point of temperature demarcation (poikilothermia) can usually be noted approximately "one joint" distal to the point of obstruction.

7. What is the differential diagnosis of an ischemic limb?
Acute arterial thrombosis. Sudden in-situ thrombosis may occur in a vessel with preexistent atheromatous occlusive disease. (See question #8.)

Aortic dissection. Acute dissections may cause sudden limb or organ ischemia with abrupt loss of pulses and other signs of acute ischemia. However, it can usually be differentiated from embolic occlusion by the presence of hypertension and chest/intrascapular back pain radiating downward.

Phlegmasia cerulea dolens. This is due to massive iliofemoral deep venous thrombosis and may present with a suddenly painful leg. It is initially differentiated by the sudden acute swelling of the limb that is always present at the onset, an atypical presentation for acute arterial occlusion.

Neurologic disorder. In some patients, neurologic manifestations of acute limb ischemia may predominate and cause confusion with primary neurologic disorders (most commonly with limb numbness). Care must be taken to avoid initial confusion with acute neurologic problems, leading to time-consuming and misdirected therapeutic efforts.

Low output states. The peripheral manifestations of hypovolemia and diminished cardiac output, particularly in a patient with longstanding absent distal pulses, may be confused with acute limb ischemia due to emboli. Recognition of a primary disease state (e.g., sepsis, acute myocardial infarction, pulmonary embolus, acute intraabdominal catastrophe) is requisite for differentiation.

8. How can embolus be distinguished from thrombus historically and clinically?

Patients with an embolus typically have sudden onset of symptoms and a recognizable source for an embolus, most often cardiac disease with atrial fibrillation. As many as 30% of patients with an embolus will have had a prior embolic episode. In contrast, a history of claudication or known pulse deficit is usually absent in the patient with an embolus, with no evidence of occlusive disease present in the contralateral limb on physical exam. The level of temperature change is often quite sharply demarcated in embolic occlusion in contrast to the patient with preexistent occlusive disease and better developed collaterals. Differentiation is of significance in planning treatment. Whereas embolectomy is often successful and the surgical procedure usually limited, attempts at thrombectomy for thrombosis will often fail and sometimes aggravate ischemia, requiring major arterial reconstruction on an emergency basis in a poorly prepared patient. For these reasons, most vascular surgeons prefer to manage acute arterial thrombosis nonoperatively in its initial stages, if feasible.

9. What is the role of two-dimensional echocardiography and angiography in the diagnosis of arterial emboli?

Two-dimensional echocardiography is a sensitive and specific technique used to detect mural thrombus. Diagnostic criteria for an LV thrombus include a mass of echoes in the LV cavity, a dyskinetic underlying myocardium, usual apical location, and a variable echocardiographic texture different from that of underlying myocardium. Left atrial cavity thrombi are detected in up to 75% of patients but rarely when present in the left atrial appendage.

Angiography can be helpful in distinguishing embolic from thrombotic occlusion. In the patient with an embolus, a sharp cutoff, sometimes with an upside-down meniscus in an otherwise normal vessel, is seen (minimal atherosclerotic changes are seen in the patient). In acute embolic occlusion, the distal outflow tract is often not visualized and little useful information is gained. In contrast, patients with acute thrombosis have more obvious and diffuse atheromatous changes and better developed collaterals, with an irregular tapering end point at the site of vascular occlusion. However, the use of angiography to aid in surgical planning is still controversial. The additional time taken for angiography can prolong ischemia and increase the possibility of a poor outcome. Careful clinical judgment is of paramount importance in such management decisions.

10. When should heparin be given during the course of management?

Intravenous heparinization to a partial thromboplastin time of 2.5–3.0 times normal should be begun as soon as the diagnosis of acute arterial ischemia is made in order to prevent clot propagation and to stabilize the patient long enough to allow consideration of diagnostic possibilities and, most importantly, to permit evaluation and initial treatment of the cardiac abnormalities present in the great percentage of patients with embolic disease.

11. What are the potential metabolic complications of reperfusion of an ischemic limb following embolectomy or clot dissolution?

Acidosis, hyperkalemia, renal failure secondary to myoglobinuria, and pulmonary insufficiency secondary to washout of platelet aggregates and thrombotic debris in the venous effluent of the revascularized limb can result. Appropriate expectant management of these metabolic complications by the perioperative team depends largely upon anticipation of their possible occurrence.

12. What is the compartment syndrome? How is it best detected?

Following revascularization, reperfusion of an ischemic limb may bring about significant tissue swelling, leading to compartmental compression, especially in the anterior calf compartment. Concomitant venous thrombosis may exacerbate the situation. Such compartmental swelling may lead to ischemic neurologic compromise or impairment of distal blood flow manifested by a changing neurologic examination or decreased signs of distal perfusion. Although some authorities have advocated the use of increased compartmental pressure measurments (>20–40 mm Hg) as an objective indicator of the need for compartment release by fasciotomy, most surgeons have found them difficult to interpret and of uncertain reliability. Decisions regarding fasciotomy are based upon individual preferences, prior clinical experience, and a changing physical examination.

13. What are the expected outcomes for a patient with acute arterial embolus and extremity ischemia?
The advent of the Fogarty balloon embolectomy catheter has simplified surgical management and improved the results of operative intervention. Currently, limb salvage may be achieved in 85–95% of patients with peripheral emboli who undergo surgical embolectomy. Mortality rates in the range of 10–20% accompany this. Prompt operative intervention is the single most important determinant of success and survival. Factors that continue to exert a negative influence are severity of underlying cardiac problems, increasing incidence of concomitant peripheral atherosclerotic occlusive disease, and systemic metabolic complications associated with increasingly aggressive attempts at late limb salvage.

CONTROVERSIES

14. Is there a role for nonoperative treatment of patients with documented arterial emboli?
Noting the persistently high mortality and rate of limb loss associated with emergency surgical treatment of acute ischemia, Blaisdell and associates first advocated avoidance of an initial surgical approach and reliance on primary treatment with high-dose anticoagulation therapy alone. In their view, the systemic consequences of revascularization in the high-risk patient typically presenting with acute ischemia were responsible for the high mortality rate. In a limited series, they found a mortality rate of 7.5% and a limb salvage rate of 67%. Overall, their recommendations fit nicely into the management scheme for patients with acute arterial thrombosis who have viable limbs; most surgeons continue to favor prompt embolectomy for patients with an acute arterial embolus.

15. What is the role of thrombolytic therapy?
Because thrombolytic therapy often requires from 24–72 hours to achieve clot lysis, it is not appropriate for the patient with significantly acute ischemia who requires immediate embolectomy and/or revascularization to preserve limb viability. In addition, the older and more-organized clot typically present in an embolus may be more resistant to thrombolysis than a recent thrombus. Therefore, an embolus is much more easily and effectively treated by expeditious operation.

BIBLIOGRAPHY

1. Asinger RW, Mikell FL, Elsperger J, et al: Incidence of left ventricular thrombosis after acute transmural myocardial infarction: Serial evaluation by two-dimensional echocardiography. N Engl J Med 305:297–302, 1981.
2. Blaisdell FW, Steele M, Allen RE: Management of acute lower extremity arterial ischemia due to embolism and thrombosis. Surgery 84:822–834, 1978.
3. Comerota AJ, Rubin RN, Tyson RR, et al: Intra-arterial thrombolytic therapy in peripheral vascular disease. Surg Gynecol Obstet 165:1–8, 1987.
4. Connett MC, Murray DH, Wenneker WW: Peripheral arterial emboli. Am J Surg 148:14–19, 1984.
5. Elliott JP, Hageman JH, Szilagyi DE, et al: Arterial embolization: Problems of source, multiplicity, recurrence, and delayed treatment. Surgery 88:833–848, 1980.

6. Kaufman JL, Stark K, Brolin RE: Disseminated atheroembolism from extensive degenerative atherosclerosis of the aorta. Surgery 102:63–70, 1987.
7. Klausner JM, Paterson IS, Mannick JA, et al: Reperfusion pulmonary edema. JAMA 261:1030–1035, 1989.
8. Langdon TJ, Bandyk DK, Olinger GN, et al: Multiple paradoxical emboli. J Vasc Surg 4:284–287, 1986.
9. Meltzer RS, Visser CA, Fuster V: Intracardiac thrombi and systemic embolization. Ann Intern Med 104:689–698, 1986.
10. Sicard GA, Schier JJ, Totty WG, et al: Thrombolytic therapy for acute arterial occlusion. J Vasc Surg 2:65–78, 1985.
11. Tawes RL, Harris EJ, Brown WH, et al: Arterial thromboembolism: A 20-year perspective. Arch Surg 120:595–599, 1985.
12. Walker PM: Pathophysiology of acute arterial occlusion. Can J Surg 29:340–342, 1986.

85. DEEP VENOUS THROMBOSIS OF THE UPPER EXTREMITY

Thomas A. Whitehill, M.D.

1. What is the differential diagnosis of upper-extremity pain and swelling?

Muscle sprain, contusion, lymphedema, cellulitis, fracture, and venous thrombosis.

2. In patients in whom venous obstruction or thrombosis is suspected, what are the usual etiologies?

Upper-extremity venous thrombosis represents only 1–3% of all diagnosed deep venous thrombosis (DVT). Etiologies in order of decreasing frequency include: (1) acute venous thrombosis of the axillary and/or subclavian veins related to venous intimal injury *without* external venous compression (60–70%), i.e., central venous catheter injury; (2) venous thrombosis secondary to external trauma or compression (20–30%), i.e., effort thrombosis/thoracic outlet compression; (3) thrombosis related to rheologic factors, infection, malignancy, or hypercoagulability (5–10%); and (4) intermittent external compression of the axillary-subclavian venous segment without associated thrombosis (<1%).

3. What are common physical findings associated with DVT of the upper extremity?

The majority of patients are asymptomatic, which makes the actual incidence of upper-extremity DVT difficult to determine. Unilateral, nonpitting edema of the arm is often the only sign. Many patients report a deep aching sensation about the shoulder and clavicular region, most likely due to the local inflammation that surrounds the phlebitic vein. Continued physical exertion may worsen the venous congestion and give rise to a "bursting," heavy, or full sensation in the arm accompanied by a cyanotic discoloration (dependent rubor). Prominent superficial venous collaterals may also appear in the affected arm and about the shoulder.

4. What is the association between central venous catheterization and upper-extremity DVT?

Long-term intravenous access of the central venous circulation for hemodynamic monitoring or parenteral nutrition has become a widespread practice. Catheter-induced thrombosis probably represents the largest etiologic process of upper-extremity DVT. Prospective angiographic examination of patients undergoing total parenteral nutrition via the subclavian venous route has revealed an 80–90% incidence of venous thrombosis, but the clinical syndrome of acute DVT occurred in only 25–30% of these patients. This low morbidity rate relates to the limited extent of the thrombus or to its gradual evolution, which permits time for adequate collateral flow to develop. Catheters that develop a sleeve thrombus or cause occlusion without hemodynamic effects do not prompt investigation.

5. What is the Paget-Schroetter syndrome?

Spontaneous, effort-induced thrombosis of the subclavian vein, or Paget-Schroetter syndrome, has been recognized for more than 100 years. The classic case occurs in an otherwise healthy young adult male. It is brought about by repetitive, intermittent venous compression in the costoclavicular space between the first rib and the clavicle and is related to prolonged use of the arm in motions that result in hyperabduction or extensional rotation of the arm at the shoulder or a position with the shoulder back and depressed as in the military salute. In two-thirds to three-fourths of these patients, the form of strenuous activity responsible for initiation of thrombosis is identifiable—tennis, baseball, swimming, painting, waiting tables, or farming (pitching hay).

6. Which anatomic abnormalities can be major factors in the development of subclavian vein thrombosis?

Anatomic abnormalities such as cervical ribs, clavicular or first rib hyperostosis, an axillopectoral muscle, a prevenous phrenic nerve, or compression by pectoralis major or minor tendons may play a role.

7. Which diagnostic test is used most commonly to define the extent and significance of upper-extremity DVT?

Diagnosis of upper-extremity DVT can be deceiving and difficult. The axillary-subclavian venous segment can contain a significant thrombus and yet have normal physical and Doppler examinations due to the potential collateral venous network. Standard venography is the best invasive diagnostic test. The digital subtraction technique can be used to decrease the amount of contrast medium required to visualize the great veins. Duplex venous scanning has made noninvasive diagnosis reliable with actual visualization of the thrombus; its exact diagnostic role is presently being defined.

8. Once the diagnosis of acute DVT of the upper extremity has been established, what is the standard treatment plan?

Standard therapy includes rest, elevation of the affected extremity, and intravenous anticoagulation with heparin. The arm should be maintained in a relaxed position, elevated on pillows, with the shoulder flat in bed. This posture maximizes the hydrostatic gradient for drainage without causing compression of the remaining collaterals at the shoulder. Heparinization is adjusted to maintain partial thromboplastin time two to three times the control value. The heparin infusion is continued for 10–14 days. Catheter-induced venous thrombosis mandates immediate removal of the central line.

9. Is there a role for long-term anticoagulation?

The frequency of pulmonary emboli arising from upper-extremity DVT is probably higher than that reported, but the overall prevalence appears to be somewhat lower than for major leg vein thrombosis. Anticoagulation therapy decreases the incidence of both pulmonary emboli and long-term disability from upper-extremity postphlebitic syndrome if the anticoagulant is administered within the first week after onset of symptoms. Warfarin is started early during the course of heparin therapy at appropriate maintenance doses and adjusted to maintain a prothrombin time of 1.3–1.5 times the control value. This oral anticoagulation therapy continues for 3–6 months to facilitate recanalization of the thrombosed vein(s) before the drug is stopped. If the thrombosis is thought to be secondary to a central line, shorter-term anticoagulation (1–2 months) is adequate, provided the central line has been removed.

CONTROVERSIES

10. Is there a place for thrombolytic therapy in the management of patients with DVT of the upper extremity?

Effort-induced axillary-subclavian venous thrombosis in young patients can produce long-term disability because of failure of the thrombosed vein(s) to recanalize. In a few trials, thrombolytic therapy with streptokinase or urokinase plus anticoagulant therapy was superior to anticoagulant therapy alone in the dissolution of symptoms if considered and used early in the management of these patients. This approach to therapy of thrombi related to external venous compression or for the rare case of impending venous gangrene is appealing; follow-up phlebography may reveal a constrictive lesion that is readily amenable to surgical correction. Recurrent thrombosis is common following clot dissolution; thus, heparin/coumadin therapy is begun as soon as the infusion of thrombolytic agent is stopped. Individuals with *any* contraindication to thrombolytic therapy are excluded. There has been no reported increase in the incidence of therapy-related pulmonary emboli.

11. When would operative therapy be appropriate?

The role of thrombectomy, first rib resection, and subclavian venous bypass procedures is controversial. Following thrombectomy alone, successful maintenance of long-term venous patency is uncommon. Early decompression of the thoracic outlet (first rib resection/ scalenectomy) with venous thrombectomy has been advocated in patients with effort thrombosis; again, postoperative thrombosis is common. In patients with persistent symptoms of disabling venous claudication or even greater severity, several authors have described successful internal jugular to proximal axillary vein bypass operations.

BIBLIOGRAPHY

1. AbuRahma AF, Sadler D, Stuart P, et al: Conventional versus thrombolytic therapy in spontaneous (effort) axillary-subclavian vein thrombosis. Am J Surg 161:459–446, 1991.
2. Donayre CE, White GE, Mehringer SM, et al: Pathogenesis determines late morbidity of axillosubclavian vein thrombosis. Am J Surg 152:179–184, 1986.
3. Gloviczki P, Kazmier FJ, Hollier LH: Axillary-subclavian venous occlusion: The morbidity of a non-lethal disease. J Vasc Surg 4:333–337, 1986.
4. Harley DP, White RA, Nelson RJ, et al: Pulmonary embolism secondary to venous thrombosis of the arm. Am J Surg 142:221–224, 1984.
5. Hill SL, Berry RE: Subclavian vein thrombosis: A continuing challenge. Surgery 108:1–9, 1990.
6. Horattas MD, Wright DJ, Fenton AH, et al: Changing concepts of deep venous thrombosis of the upper extremity: Report of a series and review of the literature. Surgery 104:561–567, 1988.
7. Raju S: New approaches to the diagnosis and treatment of venous obstruction. J Vasc Surg 5:876–878, 1987.
8. Roos DB: The place for scalenectomy and first-rib resection in thoracic outlet syndrome. Surgery 92:1077–1085, 1982.
9. Rutherford RB: Surgical management of chronic venous insufficiency of the upper extremities. Semin Vasc Surg 1:124–130, 1988.
10. Taylor LM, McAllister WR, Dennis DL, et al: Thrombolytic therapy followed by first rib resection for spontaneous ("effort") subclavian vein thrombosis. Am J Surg 149:644–647, 1984.
11. Valerio D, Hussey JK, Smith FW: Central vein thrombosis associated with intravenous feeding: A prospective study. JPEN 5:240–242, 1981.

86. PNEUMOTHORAX

Michael E. Hanley, M.D.

1. What are the major etiologic classifications of pneumothoraces?
Pneumothoraces are classified as spontaneous or traumatic. Spontaneous pneumothoraces occur without antecedent trauma or other obvious cause. A spontaneous pneumothorax that occurs in a previously healthy individual is termed a primary spontaneous pneumo-thorax. A secondary spontaneous pneumothorax occurs as a complication of underlying lung disease. Traumatic pneumothoraces result from direct or indirect trauma to the chest and are further classified as iatrogenic or noniatrogenic.

2. What are the major etiologic causes of spontaneous pneumotharaces?
Primary spontaneous pneumothoraces result from rupture of subpleural emphysematous blebs. These blebs may be congenital or due to a genetic predisposition to bleb formation, possibly related to abnormalities in collateral ventilation. Cigarette smoking may contribute to bleb formation by inducing small airways disease.

Secondary spontaneous pneumothoraces occur as a complication of underlying lung disease. The most common lung disease associated with this type of pneumothorax is chronic obstructive pulmonary disease (COPD) related to smoking tobacco, accounting for up to 67% of cases. Other lung diseases associated with secondary spontaneous pneumo-thoraces include asthma, cystic fibrosis, Marfan's syndrome, pulmonary alveolar proteinosis, pulmonary infarction, *Pneumocystis carinii* pneumonia, granulomatous diseases such as tuberculosis, sarcoidosis and berylliosis, and interstitial lung diseases including idiopathic pulmonary fibrosis, scleroderma, rheumatoid lung disease, eosinophilic granuloma, lymphangiomyomatosis and tuberous sclerosis.

3. What are the major causes of iatrogenic pneumothoraces?
The most common causes include transthoracic needle aspiration, subclavicular needlestick, thoracentesis, transbronchial biopsy, pleural biopsy, positive pressure ventilation, supra-clavicular needlestick, and cardiopulmonary resuscitation.

4. What are the clinical manifestations of pneumothoraces?
Dyspnea and chest pain (usually localized to the side of the pneumothorax) are the most common symptoms in primary spontaneous pneumothorax. The most common physical signs are tachycardia and an abnormal chest exam. The latter includes ipsilateral expansion of the chest and decreased or absent tactile fremitus. Chest percussion reveals ipsilateral hyperresonance and decreased or absent breath sounds. The trachea may be deviated toward the contralateral side.

The symptoms in secondary spontaneous pneumothoraces are more severe than for primary pneumothoraces because the pulmonary reserve is already compromised by under-lying lung pathology. Dyspnea occurs more frequently and commonly appears to be out of proportion to the size of the pneumothorax. Cyanosis and hypotension are more common. Because the chest examination is already abnormal and many of the physical signs asso-ciated with the underlying lung disease are similar to those associated with pneumothoraces, side to side differences in the examination of the chest may not be as apparent.

5. What are the major pathophysiologic features associated with pneumothoraces?
They include a decrease in vital capacity and abnormal gas exchange due to anatomic shunts and ventilation-perfusion imbalance in partially atelectatic lung. Arterial blood gases usually reveal a decrease in PaO_2 and/or an increase in the alveolar-arterial oxygen

gradient in patients without underlying lung disease. However, in patients with significant underlying lung disease, the decrease in vital capacity may result in ventilatory insufficiency with alveolar hypoventilation and respiratory acidosis..

6. How is the diagnosis of pneumothorax established in the critically ill patient?

A pneumothorax should be suspected in any critically ill patient who develops unexplained hypoxemia, dyspnea, or chest pain or who has physical findings consistent with the condition. In addition, the diagnosis should be considered in mechanically ventilated patients who develop unexplained agitation ("fighting the ventilator") or a sudden increase in peak and plateau airway pressures. The diagnosis is established by demonstrating typical chest roentgenographic findings, including a thin pleural line and the absence of lung parenchymal markings between the pleural line and chest wall. However, when the chest roentgenogram is obtained with the patient in the supine position, free pleural air will collect anteriorly and may not be readily apparent. The presence of a pneumothorax in these cases is suggested by evidence of an increase in the size of the ipsilateral hemithorax, including contralateral shift of the mediastinum and heart, as well as depression of the ipsilateral hemidiaphragm. In such cases, chest roentgenograms obtained at expiration or in the lateral decubitus position may be useful in confirming the presence of free pleural air.

7. What is the treatment of a pneumothorax?

Most pneumothoraces in the critically ill patient are either secondary spontaneous or traumatic. Tube thoracostomy should be performed in almost all secondary spontaneous or noniatrogenic, traumatic pneumothoraces, especially if mechanical ventilation is required. Proper positioning of the thoracostomy tube is important in obtaining complete evacuation of the free pleural air. The tube should be directed to an anterior/apical position in a patient at bed rest. Tube thoracostomy should also be performed for all iatrogenic pneumothoraces due to positive pressure ventilation. Other forms of iatrogenic penumothorax require tube thoracostomy only if the pneumothorax is (1) large (greater than 40%), (2) associated with significant symptoms or arterial blood gas abnormalities, (3) progressively enlarges, or (4) does not respond to simple aspiration.

8. What is the management of a persistent bronchopleural fistula?

Management focuses on minimizing air flow through the fistula while maintaining complete evacuation of the pleural space. This is primarily accomplished in patients breathing spontaneously (negative pressure ventilation) by altering the level of suction applied to the pleural space. The optimal amount of suction must be determined on an individual basis, as the level of suction at which gas flow through the fistula is minimized varies.

Gas flow across a bronchopleural fistula in a mechanically ventilated patient is also determined by peak inspiratory and mean airway pressures. In these patients management is also directed at minimizing airway pressures while maintaining adequate ventilation. This is accomplished by minimizing or eliminating positive end-expiratory pressure, tidal volume, number of mechanically delivered breaths per minute, and inspiratory time. Mechanical ventilation should be discontinued as soon as possible.

If a bronchopleural fistula does not close after 5–7 days of chest tube drainage or if adequate ventilation cannot be maintained because of the size of the air leak, open thoracotomy with suturing or resection of the fistula and scarification of the pleura should be performed. The decision to perform this procedure should include a consideration of the operative risk to the patient. Prolonged chest tube drainage, intrabronchial bronchoscopic instillation of materials (Gelfoam or tissue adhesives such as cyanoacrylate-based or fibrin glues) designed to occlude the fistula, differential lung ventilation, or synchronized chest tube occlusion should be considered in patients whose operative risk is increased by significant underlying lung disease or other medical problems.

9. What is reexpansion pulmonary edema? What is the risk of its occurrence following expansion of a pneumothorax? How can the risk be minimized?

Reexpansion pulmonary edema involves the development of unilateral pulmonary edema following reexpansion of a collapsed lung. The risk and severity of reexpansion pulmonary edema appear to be related to the duration of the pneumothorax as well as the magnitude of negative pressure applied to the pleural space to reexpand the lung.

The exact incidence of reexpansion pulmonary edema following treatment of pneumothoraces in humans is unknown but it is quite rare. However, the associated mortality is between 10% and 20%.

The risk can be minimized by withholding pleural suction during the immediate treatment of pneumothoraces of either unknown duration or duration greater than 3 days. If a pneumothorax does not reexpand after 24–48 hours of water seal or if significant respiratory compromise requires more rapid reexpansion, low levels of negative pressure (less than 20 mm Hg) may be applied to the pleural space. Nonetheless, reexpansion pulmonary edema has been reported even under these conditions.

10. What is a tension pneumothorax? What are its clinical manifestations?

A tension pneumothorax occurs when the pleural pressure within a pneumothorax is greater than atmospheric pressure throughout expiration and often during inspiration. Tension pneumothoraces generally result from a one-way valve phenomenon and most frequently occur in patients receiving positive pressure ventilation.

Clinical manifestations include sudden deterioration with rapid, labored breathing, cyanosis, and respiratory distress. The patient is commonly diaphoretic with cardiovascular instability characterized by tachycardia and hypotension. Physical examination demonstrates the findings typically associated with a pneumothorax, but with evidence of a marked increase in the size of the ipsilateral hemithorax, including contralateral shift of the trachea. Arterial blood gases commonly demonstrate severe hypoxemia and occasionally hypercapnia with respiratory acidosis.

11. What is the treatment for a tension pneumothorax?

Untreated tension pneumothoraces are associated with a high mortality and therefore represent medical emergencies. When the diagnosis is suspected and the patient exhibits significant hemodynamic instability, time should not be wasted pursuing roentgenographic confirmation. High levels (FiO_2 = 100%) of supplemental oxygen should be administered and the free pleural air evacuated. This is best accomplished by the insertion into the pleural space of a large-bore needle attached to a three-way stopcock and 50-ml syringe partially filled with sterile saline. The needle is inserted under sterile conditions through the second anterior intercostal space in the midclavicular line while the patient is supine. After the needle has been inserted, the plunger is withdrawn from the syringe. The presence of a tension pneumothorax is confirmed if air bubbles up through the saline. When a tension pneumothorax is present, the needle should be left in place until air ceases to bubble through the saline and a tube thoracostomy is performed. If air does not bubble up into the syringe, a tension pneumothorax is not present and the needle may be removed.

CONTROVERSIES

12. What size chest tube is required when performing a tube thoracostomy for pneumothoraces?

Small:

1. Small catheters may be safely inserted using the trocar method, require little nursing care after insertion, and readily allow ambulation when suction is not required if combined with a Heimlich valve.

2. Small chest tubes successfully evacuated 90% of pneumothoraces in two studies of selected patients. Failures were attributed to kinking, inadvertent removal by patient, occlusion of tube by pleural fluid (two), malposition, and presence of a large bronchopleural fistula.

3. Although rare, insertion of large tubes is associated with lacerations of the diaphragm, lung, and liver.

Large:

1. Almost 50% of pneumothoraces were not successfully managed by small chest tubes in one series. Occlusion or external kinking of the catheter was implicated as the reason for failure in most of the cases.

13. Is high-frequency jet ventilation (HFJV) effective in managing large bronchopleural fistulas?

Yes:

1. In experimental animal models, HFJV decreased gas flow through bronchopleural fistulas and improved gas exchange.

2. Carlon and colleagues[4] described 15 of 20 patients with large, proximal bronchopleural fistulas but otherwise normal lungs who had failed conventional ventilation, but who were successfully ventilated with HFJV.

3. Turnbull and associates[16] described 8 of 12 patients with large bronchopleural fistulas but normal lung parenchyma who had failed conventional mechanical ventilation, but who were successfully ventilated with HFJV. However, four patients with significant parenchymal lung disease and bronchopleural fistulas could not be ventilated with HFJV.

No:

1. Albeda and coworkers[1] reported that although gas flow through bronchopleural fistulas decreased in two of seven patients ventilated with HFJV, it increased in several patients and significant falls in arterial oxygen saturation occurred in five patients.

2. Bishop and associates[3] found no change in gas flow through bronchopleural fistulas in seven patients with acute respiratory failure who were ventilated with HFJV. In addition, gas exchange worsened in six of the patients when HFJV was initiated.

3. HFJV is a rarely performed mode of ventilation that is labor intensive; proper application requires a high level of familiarity by physicians and respiratory therapists.

BIBLIOGRAPHY

1. Albeda SM, Hansen-Flaschen JH, Taylor E, et al: Evaluation of high-frequency jet ventilation in patients with bronchopleural fistulas by quantification of the air leak. Anesthesiology 63:551–554, 1985.
2. Baumann MH, Sahn SA: Medical management and therapy of bronchopleural fistulas in the mechanically ventilated patient. Chest 97:721–728, 1990.
3. Bishop MJ, Benson MS, Sato P, Pierson DJ: Comparison of high-frequency jet ventilation with conventional mechanical ventilation for bronchopleural fistula. Anesth Analg 66:833–838, 1987.
4. Carlon GC, Ray C, Pierri MK, et al: High-frequency jet ventilation: Theoretical considerations and clinical observations. Chest 81:350–354, 1982.
5. Casola GC, vanSonnenberg E, Keightley A, et al: Pneumothorax: Radiologic treatment with small catheters. Radiology 166:89–91, 1988.
6. Conces DJ Jr, Tarver RD, Gray WC, Pearcy EA: Treatment of pneumothoraces utilizing small caliber chest tubes. Chest 94:55–57, 1988.
7. Light RW: Pleural Diseases, 2nd ed. Philadelphia, Lea and Febiger, 1990, pp 237–262.
8. Light RW, O'Hara VS, Moritz TE, et al: Intrapleural tetracycline for the prevention of recurrent spontaneous pneumothorax: Results of a Veteran's Affairs cooperative study. JAMA 264:2224–2230, 1990.
9. Mahfood S, Hix WR, Aaron BL, et al: Re-expansion pulmonary edema. Ann Thorac Surg 45:340–345, 1988.

10. Miller KS, Sahn SA: Chest tubes: Indications, technique, management and complications. Chest 91:258–263, 1987.
11. Orlando R III, Gluck EH, Cohen M, Mesologites CG: Ultra-high-frequency jet ventilation in a bronchopleural fistula model. Arch Surg 123:591–593, 1988.
12. Pavlin DJ, Raghu G, Rogers TR, Cheney FW: Re-expansion hypotension: A complication of rapid evacuation of prolonged pneumothorax. Chest 89:70–74, 1986.
13. Petersen GW, Baier H: Incidence of pulmonary barotrauma in a medical ICU. Crit Care Med 11:67–69, 1983.
14. Powner DJ, Cline CD, Rodman GH: Effect of chest tube suction on gas flow through a bronchopleural fistula. Crit Care Med 13:99–101, 1985.
15. So S, Yu D: Catheter drainage of spontaneous pneumothorax: Suction or no suction, early or late removal? Thorax 37:46–48, 1982.
16. Turnbull AD, Carlon GC, Howland WS, Beattie EJ: High-frequency jet ventilation in major airway or pulmonary disruption. Ann Thorac Surg 32:468–474, 1981.

87. FLAIL CHEST AND PULMONARY CONTUSION

Frederick A. Moore, M.D., and James B. Haenel, R.R.T.

1. What is a flail chest? How is it diagnosed?

A flail chest may occur when three or more consecutive ribs or costal cartilages are fractured bifocally. These circumscribed segments, having lost continuity with the rigid thorax, move inward with inspiration and push outward with exhalation, thus moving paradoxically. Presenting symptoms of pain, tachypnea, dyspnea, and thoracic splinting, along with chest wall contusions, tenderness, crepitance, and palpable rib fractures, are suggestive, but **paradoxical chest wall motion** is the diagnostic *sine qua non*. Detection often requires careful inspection of the two hemithoraces throughout the respiratory cycle to appreciate subtle paradoxical movement. Mechanical ventilation eliminates this abnormal motion because of positive pressure throughout the respiratory cycle, and subcutaneous emphysema, obesity, or large breasts may obscure the involved segment. Flail chest is frequently not conspicuous upon emergency department presentation because of secondary muscle splinting. With time, the flail becomes apparent as pain relief is achieved and the underlying pulmonary contusion worsens. The latter causes decreased pulmonary compliance. For effective ventilation, greater transthoracic pressure is required, which accentuates paradoxical motion. Consequently, patients sustaining severe blunt chest trauma must be carefully observed for at least 24 hours to detect a flail segment, which may herald respiratory failure. The chest film is helpful in identifying multiple displaced rib fractures, but will not reveal cartilaginous disruptions. The major value of routine chest x-ray lies in detecting associated chest injuries such as pneumothorax, hemothorax, or early pulmonary contusion.

2. What are the three most common anatomic distributions of flail chest injuries? How do they relate to mechanism of injury?

Flail segments can be located anteriorly, laterally, or posteriorly. **Anterior flails** are due to blows to the sternum—typically from a steering wheel following frontal impact. They may occur following vigorous cardiopulmonary resuscitation. The result is multiple bilateral anterior rib fractures or costrochondral disruptions with or without sternal involvement. **Lateral flails** occur following broadside (T-bone) impacts or anteroposterior crush mechanisms. Multiple rib fractures or costrochondral disruptions anteriorly are associated with a posterior row of rib fractures. **Posterior flails** result from a direct blow to the back and are characterized by simultaneous fractures along the midaxillary line and the rib neck. Splinting by the posterior thoracic muscles and the scapula plus a supine position effectively limit paradoxical motion.

3. What is a pulmonary contusion? How is it diagnosed?
The spectrum of lung parenchymal injury following a blunt chest impact ranges from simple contusion to frank laceration. Pulmonary contusion, by far the most frequent variant, is merely a bruise of the lung, direct injury causing pulmonary vascular damage with secondary alveolar hemorrhage. In the early phase, these flooded alveoli are poorly perfused; consequently, little shunt exists. However, tissue inflammation develops rapidly and the resultant surrounding pulmonary edema produces regional alterations in compliance and airway resistance, leading to localized ventilation-perfusion mismatch.

The diagnosis is radiologic. The classic finding is a nonsegmental pulmonary infiltrate that occurs within 12–24 hours of injury. The infiltrate may consist of irregular nodular densities that are discrete or confluent, a homogeneous consolidation, or a diffuse patchy pattern. If seen on early chest x-ray, a more severe contusion is likely. In most cases the infiltrates do not become apparent until after fluid resuscitation. Pulmonary contusions tend to worsen over 24–48 hours and then slowly resolve unless complicated by infection, ARDS, or cavitation (see question #16).

4. What causes a pulmonary contusion?
The basic argument is whether shear stress (tearing tissues) or bursting forces (popping the balloons) cause the tissue injury; it is likely that both elements are operational. It has been demonstrated in an animal model that impact velocity and chest wall displacement determine the severity and distribution of parenchymal injury. A high-velocity, low-displacement impact (T-bone motor vehicle accident) causes peripheral alveolar lung injury, whereas a low-velocity, high-displacement impact (crush) produces central parenchymal and major bronchial disruptions.

5. In their severe forms, flail chest and pulmonary contusion often coexist. What is the incidence of other concomitant injuries?
More than 90% of patients have associated intrathoracic injuries, and three out of four require tube thoracostomy for hemopneumothorax. Extrathoracic injuries are common: head injuries occur in 40%, major fractures in 40%, and intraabdominal injuries in 30%.

6. What is the mortality rate and cause of death in combined flail chest/pulmonary contusion injuries?
Despite tremendous advances in trauma and critical care, current mortality is 25%. Improved prehospital care no doubt contributes to this persistently high mortality by delivering more severely injured patients to the reporting trauma centers. Early deaths are due to hemorrhage and head injury; late mortality relates to sepsis and multiple organ failure. Factors that portend a poor outcome include presence of shock (blood pressure < 90 mm Hg), high Injury Severity Score (ISS > 25), associated head injury (Glasgow coma scale < 7), falls from great heights (>20 feet), preexisting disease (atherosclerotic heart disease, COPD, Laennec's cirrhosis), and advanced age (>65 yr).

7. What are the initial priorities in the management of patients with severe blunt chest trauma?
Patient management is prioritized according to the physiologic need for survival. The initial ABCs (airway, breathing, circulation) of advance trauma life support (ATLS) are directed

at establishing peripheral oxygen delivery before a specific diagnosis is made. Prophylactic tube thoracostomy for suspected hemopneumothorax, empirical tracheal intubation, and mechanical ventilation are clearly warranted in the unstable, multisystem-injured patient with chest injuries. If time permits, cervical spine fractures should be excluded so that a large-bore orotracheal tube can be placed safely. Volume resuscitation is initiated promptly since hypovolemia is the most likely cause of reversible postinjury shock. The early use of crystalloid versus colloid is an unresolved controversy, and both will leak through damaged capillary endothelium. Most authorities agree that albumin or artificial plasma expanders are no more effective in restoring tissue perfusion than when adequate sodium is provided. Moreover, colloids are costly and may aggravate pulmonary complications in the setting of disrupted capillary membranes. We prefer isotonic saline for emergent resuscitation and reserve colloid solutions for ICU resuscitation. When crystalloid infusions exceed 50 cc/kg in the ER, blood is administered to increase oxygen-carrying capacity. The next step is to assess life-threatening sources of hemorrhage as well as the presence of cardiogenic shock. Patients who cannot be resuscitated quickly in the ER must be treated definitively in the OR. Once life-threatening injuries have been treated, all efforts are directed at completing resuscitation. Core hypothermia is reversed, metabolic acidosis corrected, and mechanical ventilation is optimized.

8. Do all patients with flail chest require mechanical ventilation? Why or why not?

No. Only selected patients with flail chest require mechanical ventilation. Recent studies have shown that patients who are not intubated but are treated with aggressive pulmonary care have significantly shorter ICU stays, less pneumonia, and reduced mortality.

Roughly 20% need short-term ventilation for nonthoracic indications, primarily head injuries or major operative intervention, and another 40% are mechanically ventilated because of respiratory failure. Standard intubation criteria can be used. Inadequate oxygenation is defined as PaO_2/FiO_2 ratio < 250 or alveolar-arterial oxygen gradient > 400 mm Hg. Measures of impaired ventilation include respiratory rate > 35 breaths per minute, $PaCO_2$ > 50 mm Hg, or respiratory acidosis with a pH < 7.25. Other factors to consider are mental status, physiologic reserve (age, chronic disease), and metabolic stress (shock, associated injuries, ISS).

9. What is the long-term morbidity in flail chest injuries?

Long-term disability has not been well studied. In a recent review of 32 patients with flail chest with a mean follow-up of 5 years, only 12 (38%) had returned to full-time employment. Most complaints were subjective, such as chest tightness, pain, and decreased activity level. Another study reported on 22 patients with isolated flail chest injuries. Follow-up was 2 months to 2 years. Two-thirds experienced long-term morbidity. Persistent chest wall pain, dyspnea on exertion, and chest wall deformity were the most frequent complaints. Five (22%) remained disabled. Additional studies are clearly needed.

10. What is the optimal mode of ventilation for patients with flail chest or pulmonary contusion?

Optimal mode of ventilation continues to be discussed. Intermittent mandatory ventilation (IMV) versus assist control (AC) are the debated conventional modes. IMV may decrease respiratory alkalosis, cardiac depression, asynchronous ventilation, and respiratory muscle dysfunction, and when used properly, shorten weaning time, but cannot respond to changes in clinical status. Multisystem resuscitation is a dynamic phenomenon. CO_2 production may increase abruptly (resuscitation, hypermetabolism, sepsis) or CO_2 elimination may deteriorate suddenly (mucous plug, bronchospasm, ARDS), both sharply increasing minute ventilation demands. In the IMV mode, the patient is required to supply added work of breathing (increased VO_2), and consequently must be monitored closely for hypoventilation (respiratory acidosis). The chest-injured patient is particularly vulnerable to fail the IMV mode because the work of breathing is high (decreased compliance, increased airway resistance) plus the ability to contribute added ventilation is limited by chest wall pain and mechanics.

Initially, we prefer to provide full ventilatory support with the AC mode. Once cardiopulmonary stability is achieved, partial ventilator support is delivered by continuous flow IMV with continuous positive airway pressure (CPAP) or by a combination of intermittent mandatory ventilation/pressure support ventilation (IMV/PSV). Pure pressure support (PS) ventilation, which is becoming a popular weaning mode, should not be used in the acute setting because as compliance worsens, tidal volumes will decrease, and there will be progressive loss of lung volume.

11. What is the role of positive end-expiratory pressure (PEEP) in the management of blunt chest trauma?

For the past two decades PEEP has been an invaluable adjunct to ventilator management of hypoxic postinjury respiratory failure. Improvement in arterial oxygenation results from an increase in alveolar size and recruitment. Presumptive application in multisystem trauma may limit atelectasis, decrease exposure to high inspired oxygen concentration, and even attenuate the natural history of acute lung injury, but indiscriminate use may have profound adverse effects. In the hypovolemic patient, PEEP can embarrass cardiac work. It also produces barotrauma, raises intracranial pressure, promotes accumulation of lung fluid, and increases pulmonary vascular resistance. In flail chest/pulmonary contusion where regional differences in compliance and airway resistance exist, PEEP can accentuate V/Q mismatch. When volume status is judged adequate in the young patient without head injury, we routinely apply 5 cm H_2O PEEP. If FiO_2 cannot be lowered to at least 0.60 within 12 hours, additional PEEP is used. If PEEP exceeds 12 cm H_2O, a formal PEEP trial is performed to identify the optimal level of PEEP, defined as that which provides the best peripheral oxygen delivery. As acute respiratory failure resolves, PEEP levels are weaned.

12. Are there alternative means to avoid intubation/mechanical ventilation in patients with severe blunt chest trauma?

Mask CPAP is particularly attractive for the patient who initially does not require emergent intubation. CPAP restores functional residual capacity, improves compliance, and stabilizes the flail segment until the underlying pulmonary contusion resolves, thus eliminating the need for intubation/mechanical ventilation. Ideally, mask CPAP should be applied prior to severe hypoxemia and there should be no evidence of CO_2 retention. The patient should be alert with a functioning nasogastric tube to prevent serious aspiration. Patients with maxillofacial injuries may not tolerate the tightly applied mask and are at risk for pneumocephalus if a basilar skull fracture exists.

13. What are the pitfalls in pain mangement of nonintubated patients with blunt chest trauma?

Sufficient pain control is the vital adjunct that permits patient mobilization, deep breathing, and secretion clearance. Pain from multiple rib, long bone, and pelvic fractures is surprisingly variable and difficult to evaluate clinically. The traditional approach of intramuscular high-dose narcotics given at 3–4 hour intervals is not rational. The large dose initially oversedates and it depresses respiratory efforts and cough reflex, while the long intervals allow the patients to experience cycles of significant pain and anxiety. Participation in respiratory care is thus limited to both ends of this dosing regimen. Small parenteral dosing at short intervals is preferred. We have found the patient controlled analgesia (PCA) device to be invaluable in achieving this goal. But irrespective of how sophisticated we become in delivering sytemic analgesia, the primary limitation is depression in respiratory drive, and therefore regional anesthetic techniques have been aggressively pursued for the spontaneously breathing, chest-injured patient. Intercostal nerve blocks are highly effective for simple rib fractures, but are not suitable for flail chest injuries because of the multiple ribs involved and the repetition that is therapeutically necessary. Although intercostal and intrapleural catheter infusions of anesthetics have been described, the most convincingly successful application of regional anesthesia in chest trauma is continuous epidural infusion of local anesthetics or narcotics.

14. Which respiratory therapy procedure(s) should be ordered for patients with significant blunt chest trauma?

Vigorous ambulation remains the best method of restoring normal respiratory physiology; early removal of monitoring lines, chest tubes, and Foley catheters should be considered to achieve this goal.

Loss of lung volume is the major mechanism contributing to postsurgical pulmonary complication, and maximal lung expansion can best be achieved with the **incentive spirometer** (IS), which permits maximal inspiration without resistance while it provides visual quantification of the patient's efforts. This "incentive" encourages the patient to repeat the effort frequently. A major advantage is that IS can be performed with little supervision at frequent enough intervals (10 times per hour) to maintain lung volume. It also provides an effective means of monitoring a patient's progress. An abrupt setback may signal inadequate pain relief, progression of the pulmonary contusion, or onset of a new problem such as lobar collapse or pneumothorax.

Intermittent positive-pressure breathing (IPPB) is labor intensive and is reserved for patients who cannot generate adequate inspiratory lung volume with IS. It is generally performed at 4-hour intervals to promote coughing and improve ventilation as well as deliver bronchodilators.

Chest physiotherapy (CPT) is another frequently employed modality and consists of postural drainage, enhanced coughing maneuvers, chest vibration, and chest percussion. Despite its widespread use, prospective studies have shown no advantage of routine CPT in postsurgical prophylaxis, and it may actually worsen oxygenation. We limit its use to patients with tenacious secretions as well as adjunct to the treatment of lobar collapse.

Obviously chest percussion will not be tolerated in the face of multiple rib fractures, but **positional drainage and coughing** can be quite effective.

15. Are prophylactic antibiotics indicated in severe chest trauma?
No clear data address this issue in the severely injured patient. Most pneumonias and virtually all empyemas occur late; thus, a short early course of antibiotics is unlikely to be beneficial, whereas longer coverage selects out a more virulent host flora. In some large retrospective reviews of chest trauma, the incidence of pneumonia is doubled in patients receiving antibiotics, whereas others have observed the opposite—a one-third reduction in pulmonary sepsis.

We do not administer prophylactic systemic antibiotics except to patients undergoing thoractomy. Patients with combined flail chest/pulmonary contusion typically have both evolving pulmonary infiltrates and hypermetabolism, which are difficult to distinguish from sepsis. Daily chest x-rays and surveillance sputum sampling are essential. When clinical judgment suggests an infection, patients are treated with a short course of antibiotics. Early infections (<72 hours) are caused by staphylococcal species or normal oropharyngeal flora amenable to a single agent, whereas late pneumonias generally are due to resistant, hospital-acquired, gram-negative organisms requiring double coverage.

16. What is a posttraumatic pulmonary pseudocyst (PPP)? How is it managed?

PPP describes an air- or fluid-filled intraparenchymal that occurs in the setting of blunt chest trauma. PPP, although unusual, should be considered in all adults sustaining a serious pulmonary contusion. The pseudocyst typically evolves over the first week as a nonspecific air- or fluid-filled loculation seen on plain films. CT scanning of the chest is critical to define air-fluid levels seen on plain films, but its use should be limited to patients with signs of sepsis. In our experience with adult patients, infected pseudocysts are not responsive to antibiotics. Prompt diagnostic aspiration is valuable. Simple infected pseudocysts should be drained percutaneously; complex pseudocysts should be considered for early thoracotomy with the anticipation that formal lobectomy may be necessary.

BIBLIOGRAPHY

1. Bolliger CT, Van Eden SF: Treatment of multiple rib-fractures randomized controlled trial comparing ventilatory with nonventilatory management. Chest 97:943–948, 1990.
2. Covino BG: Intrapleural regional analgesia. Anesth Analg 67:427–429, 1988.
3. Clark GC, Shecter WP, Trunkey DD: Variables affecting outcome in blunt chest trauma: Flail chest vs. pulmonary contusion. J Trauma 28:298–304, 1988.
4. Crossely AWA: Intercostal chatheterization an alternative approach to the paravertebral space? Anesthesia 48:163–164, 1988.
5. Hurst JM, Dehaven CB, Branson RD: Comparison of conventional mechanical ventilation and synchronous independent lung ventilation (SILV) in the treatment of unilateral lung injury. J Trauma 25:766–787, 1985.
6. Mackersie RC, Shackford SR, Hoyt DB, et al: Continuous epidural fentanyl analgesia: Ventilatory function improvement with routine use in treatment of blunt chest injury. J Trauma 27:1207–1212, 1987.
7. Moore FA, Haenel JB, Moore EE, et al: Auto-PEEP in the multisystem injured patient: An elusive complication. J Trauma 30:1316–1321, 1990.
8. Moore FA, Moore EE: Initial assessment and resuscitation of the injured patient. In Wilmore DW, Brenan MF, Harken AH, et al (eds): American College of Surgeons Care of the Surgical Patients. New York, Scientific American, 1988.
9. Moore FA, Moore EE, Haenel JB, et al: Post-traumatic pulmonary pseudocyst in the adult: Pathophysiology, recognition, and selective management. J Trauma :1380–1385, 1989.
10. Shackford SR: Blunt chest trauma in the intensivist's perspective. J Intens Care Med 1:125–136, 1986.
11. Shapiro BA, Cane RD, Harrison RA: Positive end-expiratory pressure therapy in adults with special reference to acute lung injury: A review of the literature and suggested clinical correlations. Crit Car Med 12:127–141, 1984.

88. FAT EMBOLISM SYNDROME

Mark W. Geraci, M.D.

1. What is the fat embolism syndrome (FES)?

Fat embolism syndrome (FES) is a clinical condition that can occur after fractures of long bones or other instances of bone marrow disruption. It is characterized by the appearance of free fat and fatty acids in the blood, lungs, brain, kidneys, and other organs. The classic triad of acute respiratory failure with diffuse pulmonary infiltrates, global neurologic dysfunction, and petechial rash occurs in only 0.5–2% of solitary long bone fractures; however, the incidence approaches 5–10% in multiple fractures with pelvic involvement.

2. When was FES first recognized?

The first description of the FES was offered by Zenker in 1862. He described the findings of microscopic fat emboli in the lungs of a patient who had been killed after being crushed between two railroad cars, and proposed that the ensuing respiratory compromise was the cause of death.

3. What is the pathogenesis of FES?

The pathogenesis is controversial. The most cogent and widely accepted theory holds that embolic marrow fat derived from the fracture site is the central inciting agent. The fat is concentrated in the pulmonary bed and serves to activate the clotting cascade, increase platelet function and fibrinolytic activity, and induce catecholamine-mediated mobilization of free fatty acids. These free fatty acids directly increase capillary permeability. Along with the release of inflammatory mediators, the final common pathway results in critical impairment of gas exchange, and a form of adult respiratory distress syndrome.

4. Who is at risk for FES?

Fat embolism to the lungs and peripheral microcirculation occurs in over 90% of long bone fractures; however, only some 2–5% of patients develop the clinical syndrome. The incidence in children is 100 times less frequent than in adults with comparable injuries. Certain clinical conditions cause increased liquid marrow fat content and medullary cavity enlargement, which can predispose to the FES. These disorders include myelodysplastic syndromes, collagen vascular diseases, osteoporosis, and immobilization for long periods of time. FES is most commonly associated with fractures, but has also been reported after prosthetic joint replacement, lipectomy, bone marrow transplantation, acute hemorrhagic pancreatitis, carbon tetrachloride poisoning, and external cardiac massage.

5. What is the clinical presentation?

The clinical presentation is usually marked by a latency period of 12–72 hours. Respiratory impairment leads to hypoxemia in up to 30% of patients. The chest x-ray often shows diffuse pulmonary infiltrates. Cerebral symptoms may occur in 60% of patients and tend to follow the pulmonary symptoms. Central nervous system impairment may range from restlessness, confusion, and focal deficits to seizures and coma. A petechial rash appears in 50% of patients and is usually found on the neck, axilla, trunk or conjunctivae. The rash is short-lived, usually lasting for only 6 hours.

6. How is the diagnosis made?

The diagnosis is made on clinical grounds and diagnostic criteria are varied. The two most widely accepted criteria are presented. Gurd's (1970) criteria are grouped into major and minor features. Major features include respiratory insufficiency, cerebral involvement, and petechial rash. The minor features are pyrexia, tachycardia, retinal changes, jaundice, renal involvement, and fat macroglobulinemia. Schonfeld (1983) advocates a fat embolism index score (greater than 5 is diagnostic) as follows: petechia = 5, alveolar infiltrates = 4, hypoxemia = 3, and confusion, fever, tachycardia, and tachypnea each = 1.

7. Are there specific tests to aid in the diagnosis of FES?

There is no single test to diagnose FES, but a pattern of biochemical abnormalities may be seen. Hematologic studies may reveal decreased hematocrit and platelets, whereas fibrin degradation products, prothrombin time, erythrocyte sedimentation rate, and C5a levels are often all elevated. Biochemical abnormalities include lowered calcium and the presence of fat microaggregates in samples of clotted blood. In a large series studied prospectively, the commonly held tenet of fat globules presenting in the urine was not found in any patient with FES. Recently, bronchoalveolar lavage (looking for fat droplets) has been found to be sensitive and specific for detecting FES.

8. How is FES treated?

A number of treatment modalities have been studied. The use of ethanol, heparin, low-molecular-weight dextran, and hypertonic glucose has shown inconsistent results and none is currently advocated. The first successful treatment of FES with corticosteroids was reported by Ashbaugh and Petty in 1966. In a well-designed, prospective, randomized, double-blind study of patients at high risk for FES, Schonfeld et al. demonstrated that prophylactic use of methylprednisolone, 7.5 mg/kg intravenously every 6 hours for 12 doses, significantly reduced the incidence of the FES. Lindeque et al. found similar results even with less stringent diagnostic criteria. In both studies, the use of steroids had no adverse effects on fracture healing. The mechanism of steroid effectiveness likely involves membrane stabilization, limitation in the rise of plasma free fatty acids, and inhibition of the complement-mediated leukocyte aggregation. The effectiveness of steroids other than for prophylaxis remains to be tested. In short, the treatment includes aggressive supportive care, early ventilatory support, and early steroid use.

9. Does early operative intervention change outcome?

Retrospective studies seem to confirm that early operative stabilization of fractures within the first 24 hours reduces the incidence of adult respiratory distress syndrome (ARDS) from 75% for delayed surgery to 17% for early surgery. Obviating the development of ARDS provides a survival advantage and decreases morbidity as well as hospital stay.

10. What is the prognosis for patients with FES?

Mortality often depends on the underlying extent of injury. For uncomplicated FES, though, the mortality is often much less than for other types of ARDS, and is most often quoted as 10%. FES is self-limited, and, provided oxygenation is maintained, pulmonary function can be expected to return to normal. Most of the long-term morbidity is associated with cerebral complications, particularly focal neurologic deficits.

BIBLIOGRAPHY

1. Ashbaugh DG, Petty TL: The use of corticosteroids in the treatment of respiratory failure associated with massive fat embolism. Surg Gynecol Obstet 123:493–500, 1966.
2. Chastre J, Fagon JY, Soler P, et al: Bronchoalveolar lavage for rapid diagnosis of the fat embolism syndrome in trauma patients. Ann Intern Med 113:583–588, 1990.
3. Gosling HR, Pellegrini VD: Fat embolism syndrome: A review of the pathophysiology and physiological basis of treatment. Clin Orthop 165:68–82, 1982.
4. Gurd AR: Fat embolism: An aid to diagnosis. J Bone Joint Surg 52:732–737, 1970.
5. Johnson KD, Cadambi A, Seibert GB: Incidence of adult respiratory distress syndrome in patients with multiple musculoskeletal injuries: Effects of early operative stablilization of fractures. J Trauma 25:375–384, 1985.
6. Lindeque BGP, Schoeman HS, Dommisse GF, et al: Fat embolism and the fat embolism syndrome: A double blind therapeutic study. J Bone Joint Surg 69B:128–131, 1987.
7. Peltier LE: Fat embolism: A perspective. Clin Orthop 232:263–270, 1988.
8. Schonfeld SA, Ploysongsang Y, DiLisio R, et al: Fat embolism prophylaxis with corticosteroids: A prospective study in high-risk patients. Ann Intern Med 99:438–443, 1983.
9. Van Besouw JP, Hinds CJ: Fat embolism syndrome. Br J Hosp Med 42:304–311, 1989.
10. Zenker FA: Beitrage zur normalen and pathologischen Anatomie der Lunge. Dresden, J Braunsdorf, 1862.

89. MYOCARDIAL CONTUSION

Eugene E. Wolfel, M.D.

1. What causes cardiac injury in blunt chest trauma?

Nonpenetrating cardiac trauma can result from vehicular impact during an automobile accident, particularly if the steering wheel is involved. Chest injuries account for 25% of the 50,000–60,000 deaths per year in auto accidents and contribute significantly to another 25% of deaths. Other causes include a direct blow to the chest from a blunt object or missile, a clenched fist, sporting equipment such as a hard baseball, or a kick of a large animal. Falls from moderate height and cardiopulmonary resuscitation may cause cardiac injuries. Almost any cardiac structure has been reported to be damaged by blunt chest trauma. Damage to the pericardium, myocardium, coronary arteries, cardiac valves, and aorta can occur, but damage to the myocardium itself (myocardial contusion) is probably the most common and often overlooked injury.

2. What is myocardial contusion?

Myocardial contusion is the result of direct damage to the myocardium without involvement of the coronary arteries. Pathologically there is evidence of tissue injury with cell necrosis, edema, and often hemorrhage. Often there is only subendocardial or subepicardial damage without transmural changes. Clinically, myocardial contusion refers to transient or permanent myocardial dysfunction that includes evidence of myocardial necrosis. The term "myocardial concussion" has been used to describe transient myocardial dysfunction, such as the presence of a wall motion abnormality on an echocardiogram without evidence of tissue necrosis. This finding could be another example of "stunned myocardium" as seen in coronary artery disease with transient severe ischemia. Because of the proximity to the anterior chest wall, the right ventricle is more susceptible to these injuries.

3. Are there other myocardial injuries associated with blunt chest trauma besides myocardial contusion?

Most other injuries of the myocardium associated with blunt chest trauma usually have accompanying myocardial contusion. These complications are quite rare and include laceration and/or rupture of the ventricular wall (atrial rupture is much more common), perforation of the intraventricular septum, and ventricular aneurysm or pseudoaneurysm formation. Direct injury to the coronary arteries resulting in thrombosis or dissection can result in myocardial damage similar to the setting of atherosclerotic myocardial infarction.

4. Are there associated chest injuries that make myocardial contusion more likely after blunt chest trauma?

Severe cardiac injury can occur with minimal or absent external signs of chest injury. However, in general, 75% of patients with myocardial contusion have some signs of external chest injury. In one large series of chest injuries, incidences of myocardial contusion were: upper rib and clavicle fractures (50%), pulmonary contusion (44%), pneumothorax (33%), hemothorax (30%), flail chest (18.5%), sternal fracture (7%), and great vessel injury (7%). With any blunt trauma to the chest, the level of suspicion should be high for possible cardiac injury.

5. What clinical features associated with blunt chest trauma suggest myocardial contusion?

Myocardial contusion is usually clinically silent. Chest pain is not uncommon but is usually related to other thoracic injuries. The pain of classic angina or myocardial infarction is unusual. Unexplained sinus tachycardia or hemodynamic instability could be signs of myocardial dysfunction, but should alert the clinician to the possibility of pericardial tamponade from pericardial injury and hemorrhage. The presence of ventricular ectopic activity in the absence of hypoxemia or electrolyte imbalance may indicate myocardial contusion, especially early in the clinical course. Shock is rare and if related to a cardiac cause usually represents pericardial tamponade or cardiac rupture.

6. What is the role of electrocardiography (EKG) in the diagnosis of myocardial contusion?
Routine EKG is generally not useful because it has poor sensitivity. The most common finding is nonspecific ST-T wave changes. Reported EKG findings with myocardial contusion include sinus tachycardia (poor specificity), peaking of T waves, prolonged QT interval, concave ST elevation indicating pericarditis, and right bundle branch block (RBBB). RBBB, if acute, is felt to be related to right ventricular injury and can be a useful indication of possible contusion. Ventricular arrhythmias, if present, can be a reasonable indicator of myocardial contusion if they occur in the absence of other known arrhythmogenic factors.

7. What is the role of cardiac enzyme determinations in the diagnosis of myocardial contusion?
The use of the MB fraction of creatine kinase is felt to be the most sensitive routine test in the diagnosis of myocardial necrosis. Its efficacy is well established in the diagnosis of routine myocardial infarction. Because myocardial contusion pathologically requires myocyte necrosis, an elevation in the MB fraction should be a useful test to diagnose this condition. Unfortunately, its sensitivity is quite low and often its specificity is suboptimal. In patients with obvious wall motion abnormalities of the right or left ventricle on echocardiography, the cardiac enzymes are often normal. This may represent myocardial concussion rather than contusion. In most series the sensitivity of an elevated MB fraction ranges from 29–47%. Damage to the right ventricle may release only minute quantities of the MB component of creatine kinase. Also total creatine kinase levels are often significantly elevated owing to other skeletal muscle injuries; therefore a higher percentage of the MB fraction ($>5\%$ of the total) should be used. In addition, certain skeletal muscles such as the tongue and diaphragm have higher percentages of MB, increasing the likelihood of a false-positive test for myocardial injury. Although serial determinations may be useful, this test alone cannot make the diagnosis of myocardial contusion.

8. How is echocardiography used in the diagnosis and management of myocardial contusion?
The use of two-dimensional echocardiography along with Doppler ultrasound is probably the best noninvasive tool for the evaluation of blunt chest trauma. The presence of a ventricular wall motion abnormality suggests myocardial contusion or concussion. Other cardiac structures such as the pericardial space and cardiac valves also can be evaluated. Potential complications of myocardial contusion, such as right ventricular mural thrombus, aneurysm and pseudoaneurysm, can also be recognized. This procedure is portable, with bedside capabilities; however, 15–25% of patients with blunt chest trauma have technically inadequate studies, limiting the usefulness of this technique.

9. Does imaging of the heart with radioisotopes help in the diagnosis of myocardial contusion?
Three major types of radioisotopes have been used in the diagnosis of myocardial contusion:
   1. **Technetium pyrophosphate (infarct scanning).** This radioisotope is taken up by newly necrotic myocardium and results in a "hot spot" in the area of myocardial injury. Unfortunately, this technique is too insensitive to detect nontransmural damage. The optimal time for imaging is between 24 and 72 hours after the injury, thereby prolonging

the hospital stay in patients with minimal injuries. Thus, this technique has no usefulness in establishing the diagnosis of myocardial contusion.

   2. **Thallium scintigraphy.** Thallium is taken up by normal myocardium in relation to the degree of coronary blood flow; thus, abnormal areas of myocardial necrosis would appear as "cold spots" on the image of the heart. Use of this isotope in the diagnosis of myocardial contusion has been limited because the isotope is not readily available (produced by a cyclotron with a short isotope half-life), is expensive, and usually requires sophisticated quantitative analysis for optimal diagnostic accuracy. This technique also cannot evaluate the right ventricle, a common site of myocardial contusion.

   3. **Radionuclide ventriculography.** This is the most frequent radioisotopic means of studying patients with blunt chest trauma. The technique involves labeling the blood pool with technetium pyrophosphate, and both global ventricular function as measured by ejection fraction as well as wall motion analysis can be performed. Both the right and left ventricles can be studied. It is a relatively rapid, sensitive, and noninvasive method, and technical limitations are fewer than in echocardiography. The sensitivity is somewhat better than echocardiography for wall motion abnormalities. The disadvantages of the technique are that it also is expensive and requires nuclear medicine support with sophisticated equipment. Unlike echocardiography, radionuclide ventriculography cannot evaluate other cardiac structures, such as the pericardium and cardiac valves, which also may have sustained injuries. False-negative studies can result if the patient receives positive inotropic agents.

10. What are the indications for invasive cardiac diagnostic studies in myocardial contusion?
Invasive studies generally are not used to make this diagnosis. If there is a strong suspicion of coronary involvement, with pathologic Q waves appearing on the EKG in an evolutionary pattern or the presence of a continuous cardiac murmur from a possible coronary arteriovenous fistula, then coronary arteriography is indicated. Right heart catheterization with a balloon flotation pulmonary artery catheter may be useful in a patient with hemodynamic instability. The equilibration of intracardiac pressures, particularly with elevated right atrial and pulmonary capillary wedge pressures, strongly supports the diagnosis of percardial tamponade. Significant right ventricular injury, left ventricular dysfunction, and pulmonary hypertension can be diagnosed with this technique. Sampling of blood for oxygen saturations from the various right heart chambers can also provide the diagnosis of a traumatic intracardiac left-to-right shunt. All these conditions are relatively uncommon and often can be diagnosed by clinical parameters or a cardiac echo-Doppler study.

11. Based on the above information, what is the optimal approach to the diagnosis of myocardial contusion?
A high level of suspicion is most important. All patients with blunt chest trauma should have a 12-lead EKG. Although the findings are often nonspecific, if there are frequent unexplained ventricular ectopic beats or the presence of RBBB, then myocardial contusion should be strongly considered. All patients should have at least two sets of cardiac enzymes drawn at least 4 hours apart. If the MB fraction of the total creatine kinase activity is greater than 5%, myocardial contusion should also be considered. In a select group of patients who have elevations of the MB fraction, an echocardiogram should be performed. Indications include the presence of frequent ventricular arrhythmias, hemodynamic instability, a new cardiac conduction defect, an abnormal cardiac physical exam, associated severe chest trauma requiring surgical correction, and unusual cardiopulmonary symptoms. Patients with normal cardiac enzymes should not receive echocardiograms. Although some patients may have wall motion abnormalities (? "myocardial concussions"), the clinical significance of these findings in the absence of other signs and symptoms of cardiac dysfunction makes this test unnecessary. Also the outcome appears to be excellent in these patients.

12. What is the standard treatment of myocardial contusion?

In the vast majority of patients with myocardial contusion, there is no significant hemodynamic or electrical abnormality. These patients are usually placed on telemetry monitors for 24–36 hours to exclude significant arrhythmias. After that, the hospital course and recovery are dictated by the extent of noncardiac injuries. Patients can return to normal activity in a short period of time without increased cardiac risk. The risk of general anesthesia is low despite the presence of a recent myocardial contusion, a situation quite different from the risk after a recent classic myocardial infarction. If hemodynamic instability is found, then standard therapy for ventricular dysfunction is indicated. Anticoagulation is contraindicated even in the presence of known mural thrombus due to the precipitation or aggravation of intramyocardial or intrapericardial hemorrhage as well as aggravating hemorrhage in noncardiac injuries. Usually no specific cardiac follow-up is indicated in the usual uncomplicated cardiac clinical course. In patients with a wall motion abnormality discovered at the time of the injury, a repeat echocardiogram can be performed at 4–6 weeks to exclude the rare late complications of aneurysm or pseudoaneurysm. Usually the wall motion abnormalities resolve in about 86% of patients with initial abnormal findings.

CONTROVERSIES

13. Routine hospitalization with EKG monitoring is required in all cases of blunt chest trauma with a suspicion of myocardial contusion.

For:

1. Some patients will have unrecognized significant myocardial injury that may result in serious ventricular arrhythmias or other cardiac complications.

2. Because myocardial dysfunction has been evident on echocardiograms even in the presence of a normal 12-lead EKG and no elevation of cardiac enzymes, all patients should be observed for possible adverse cardiac events.

Against:

1. The prognosis in these patients is excellent and their clinical course is dicatated by noncardiac injuries; therefore, in patients with no other injuries, a short period of monitoring in the emergency room is sufficient.

2. Several clinical factors can be used to designate a higher risk group for further observation: the elderly, presence of arrhythmias or conduction defects, hemodynamic abnormalities, and significant abnormalities on chest x-ray or EKG. These are the patients who should be admitted and have further diagnostic studies.

14. Echocardiograms and/or radionuclide studies should be used in the standard evaluation of patients with blunt chest trauma for possible myocardial contusion.

For:

1. These studies are the most sensitive means of determining injury to the myocardium and are useful in detecting possible serious cardiac complications from this injury.

2. These studies will affect the subsequent length of hospitalization and further treatment of patients with blunt chest trauma.

Against:

1. These studies are relatively insensitive and have no value in determining the clinical outcome of these patients.

2. The prognosis in uncomplicated patients with blunt chest trauma is excellent, and these studies only add to the expense of the evaluation. Even if a wall motion abnormality is found, it resolves in 85% of cases on follow-up.

3. The clinical outcome of these patients is determined by the extent of the noncardiac injuries. Only cardiac rupture has a profound effect on survival and most of these patients expire before they arrive at the emergency room.

BIBLIOGRAPHY

1. Baxter BT, Moore EE, Synhorst DP, et al: Graded experimental myocardial contusion: Impact on cardiac rhythm, coronary artery flow, ventricular function, and myocardial oxygen consumption. J Trauma 28:1411–1417, 1988.
2. Dubrow TJ, Mihalka J, Eisenhauer DM, et al: Myocardial contusion in the stable patient: What level of care is appropriate? Surgery 106:267–274, 1989.
3. Fabian TC, Mangiante EC, Patterson CR, et al: Myocardial contusion in blunt trauma: Clinical characteristics, means of diagnosis, and implications for patient management. J Trauma 28:50–56, 1988.
4. Healey MA, Brown R, Fleiszer D: Blunt cardiac injury: Is this diagnosis necessary? J Trauma 30:137–146, 1990.
5. Hossack KF, Moreno CA, Vanway CW, Burdick DC: Frequency of cardiac contusion in nonpenetrating chest injury. Am J Cardiol 61:391–394, 1988.
6. Liedtke AJ, DeMuth W. Nonpenetrating cardiac injuries: A collective review. Am Heart J 86:687–697, 1973.
7. Lindenbaum G, Carroll S, Block E, Kapusnick R: Value of creatine phosphokinase isoenzyme determinations in the diagnosis of myocardial contusion. Ann Emerg Med 17:885–889, 1988.
8. Miller FA, Seward JB, Gersh BJ, et al: Two-dimensional echocardiographic findings in cardiac trauma. Am J Cardiol 50:1022–1027, 1982.
9. Miller FB, Shumate CR, Richardson JD, Myocardial contusion: When can the diagnosis be eliminated? Arch Surg 124:805–808, 1989.
10. Mooney R, Niemann JTT, Bessen HA, et al: Conventional and right precordial ECGs, creatine kinase, and radionuclide angiography in post-traumatic ventricular dysfunction. Ann Emerg Med 17:890–894, 1988.
11. Potkin RT, Werner JA, Trobaugh GB, et al: Evaluation of noninvasive tests of cardiac damage in suspected cardiac contusion. Circulation 66:627–631, 1982.
12. Reid CL, Kawanishi DT, Rahimtoola SH, Chandraratna AN: Chest trauma: Evaluation by two-dimensional echocardiography. Am Heart J 113:971–976, 1987.
13. Ross P, Degutis L, Baker CC: Cardiac contusion: The effect on operative management of the patient with trauma injuries. Arch Surg 124:506–507, 1989.
14. Sinkinson CA, Hossack KF, Waxman K: The perplexities of diagnosing cardiac contusion. Emerg Med Rep 9:121–127, 1988.
15. Sturaitis M, McCallum D, Sutherland G, et al: Lack of significant long-term sequelae following traumatic myocardial contusion. Arch Intern Med 146:1765–1769, 1986.
16. Tenzer ML: The spectrum of myocardial contusion: A review. J Trauma 25:620–627, 1985.

90. HEART TRANSPLANTS

Robert M. Claytor, III, R.N., B.S.N.

1. How are potential recipients evaluated for transplantation?

Evaluation includes an echocardiogram, cardiac catheterization, pulmonary function tests; renal, hepatic hematologic and general metabolic studies as well as a financial and psychosocial assessment. All information is scrutinized by a medical review board, and, if accepted, the person's name is entered into the national donor computer along with weight, ABO type, distance the procurement team can travel, and status (from 1 to 6, 1 being working or attending school to 6 being in an ICU on circulatory and/or ventilatory support to include ventricular assist devices). Because this treatment is no longer considered experimental, insurance companies and some government programs will provide reimbursement. The age of potential recipients may range from newborn to 70. The candidate's chronologic age is not as important as physiologic age.

2. What conditions warrant consideration for heart transplantation?
Cardiomyopathy, coronary artery disease, valvular disease, congenital heart disease, myocarditis, and graft rejection.

3. What are contraindications to heart transplantation?
The National Heart, Lung, and Blood Institute's Special Advisory Group specifies the following contraindications to heart transplantation:
    1. **Advancing age** (beyond which the patient has decreased ability to adapt to the stresses of surgery)
    2. **Pulmonary hypertension:** pulmonary vascular resistance > 6 Wood units or pulmonary artery systolic pressure over 65–70 mm Hg and exceeding pulmonary capillary wedge pressure by 40 mm Hg
    3. **Irreversible severe hepatic or renal dysfunction**
    4. **Active systemic infection**
    5. **Any systemic disease** that may impair survival and rehabilitation potential
    6. **Psychiatric illness** likely to interfere with compliance to a rigorous therapeutic regimen
    7. **Pulmonary infarction** either recent or unresolved
    8. **Insulin-dependent diabetes**
    9. **Severe peripheral or cerebrovascular disease**
    10. **Acute peptic ulcer disease**
    11. **Absence of an adequate psychosocial support system**

4. What are donor criteria for heart transplantation?
Most commonly, heart transplant donors are victims of blunt or penetrating trauma from motor vehicle accidents, gunshot wounds, or cerebrovascular disease. The California Donor Network specified that the following criteria must be met for heart donation:
    "• Age: newborn to 60 years
    • Evaluate preexisting heart disease and family history.
    • No evidence of severe cardiothoracic trauma or cardiac puncture; chest tubes *do not* preclude donation.
    • Additional testing: chest x-ray, EKG, echocardiogram, ABGs, CPK with isoenzymes, and blood, urine and sputum cultures.
    • Cardiology consult.
    • Arteriogram may also be necessary depending on donor age or medical condition.
    • If the heart cannot be used for transplant, it still may be recovered for valves.
    • Bradycardia, tachycardia and hypertension/hypotension resulting from brain death *do not* contraindicate heart donation.
    • Ideally, dopamine level should be kept below 10 mg/kg/min. *Do not* disqualify a donor based on dopamine level alone."

5. How are potential donors managed?
Intensive care is required to monitor hemodynamics, as brain death leads to extreme lability of autoregulatory function. With loss of brainstem function, the body loses its ability to maintain vascular tone, leading to increased intravascular capacitance, hypotension, and decreased venous return, producing hypovolemic shock. Invasive monitoring includes an arterial line, central venous pressure (CVP) line, and a Foley catheter as well as two large-bore peripheral IVs for rapid fluid resuscitation and maintenance of adequate preload. Maintenance of a CVP between 10 and 12 mm Hg is recommended. Preservation of the heart often is at cross purposes with end-stage CNS-preserving therapies such as osmotic diuretics. Dopamine at 5–10 μg/kg/min may be used to maintain a systolic blood pressure of 100 mm Hg if volume replacement and electrolyte/acid-base regulation fail to maintain an adequate blood pressure.

6. What is the surgical technique for heart transplantation?

There are two types of heart transplants: orthotopic, or removing the recipient's old failing heart and replacing it with the donor heart; and heterotopic, or simply adding the donor heart in "piggyback" fashion to serve as an adjunct to the diseased heart's function. During **orthotopic transplantation**, a median sternotomy is performed on the recipient and cardio-pulmonary bypass is initiated. Following determination of donor heart suitability (the absence of congenital or traumatic lesions), the main pulmonary artery and ascending aorta are transected. An incision is then made along the recipient's atria, leaving the posterior walls in place and the inferior and superior vena cava intact. The donor heart is removed in toto and its atria are "carved" to fit the remnant atria within the recipient. Anastomoses are made between the donor atria and the recipient's atrial cuff, followed by aortic and pulmonary artery end-to-end anastomoses. During **heterotopic transplantation**, the donor heart is placed parallel to the recipient heart in the mediastinal cavity. Anastomoses are made between both aortas, the atria, and pulmonary arteries.

7. What are the indications for heterotopic versus orthotopic transplants?

Where possible, orthotopic transplanation is performed, as it is associated with lower mortality. Heterotopic transplants may be indicated when the donor heart is significantly smaller than the recipient's or in the setting of elevated pulmonary vascular resistance. Heterotopic transplant recipients must be anticoagulated secondary to the higher incidence of thromboembolism from the native heart. They also may experience ongoing postoperative angina. Surgically the operation is technically more difficult because of the multiple anastomoses and the use of prosthetic graft material. Future cardiac catheterizations are also technically more difficult.

8. How is rejection diagnosed?

Hyperacute rejection occurs immediately upon implantation of the donor heart and necessitates retransplantation of mechanical assistance until a suitable heart can be located. It is usually as a result of ABO incompatibility or a lymphocyte reaction (the donor heart acts as an antigen to preformed antibodies in the recipient). **Acute rejection** occurs within 3 months of transplant and is cell mediated by activation of T lymphocytes. It results in interstitial and perivascular mononuclear cell infiltrates that may lead to cellular necrosis if untreated. It is diagnosed by transmyocardial biopsy, initially performed weekly for 6 weeks, then biweekly, monthly, bimonthly, and eventually 3 or 4 times per year. **Chronic rejection** occurs after the first 3 months. It is characterized by a diffuse pattern of atherosclerosis throughout the length of the coronary arteries. Because of its diffuse nature, this condition is refractory to percutaneous transluminal angioplasty or surgical revascularization. The incidence of this phenomenon makes yearly cardiac catheterizations mandatory to monitor for atherosclerotic changes.

9. How is rejection treated?

Variations exist among institutions in methods employed and in what order or combination. The treatments for mild, moderate, or severe rejection include **high-dose steroids** (to blunt the immune response proximally by suppression of interleukin-1 production), **OKT3** (a monoclonal antibody that removes lymphocytes from circulation), an increase in cyclosporine blood levels, and **rabbit antithymocyte globulin** or antithymocyte serum (an antibody to lymphocytes involved in the rejection process).

10. How does heart transplantation affect conduction?

In the normal heart, sympathetic and parasympathetic nerve fibers extend to both sino-atrial (SA) and atrioventricular (AV) nodes. Sympathetic stimulation causes increased speed of conduction through the AV node (increased dromotropic effect) as well as increased heart rate (increased chronotropic effect). Likewise, parasympathetic stimulation leads to slowed SA node firing and prolonged AV conduction. Because the sympathetic and parasympathetic nerves are transected during harvest, heart transplantation results in total denervation of the transplanted heart in situ within the recipient. Afferent or sensory fibers from the pericardium, adventitia, and myocardial wall are also severed, preventing the recipient from experiencing chest pain from myocardial ischemia. (There is, however, some evidence of reinervation of these sensory pathways, as evidenced by reports of angina in the post-transplant population). Therefore, Valsalva maneuvers, carotid massage, or body position changes no longer affect heart rate. On the whole, heart transplant recipients have faster heart rates than the general population secondary to loss of vagal innervation. They do not, however, respond with the usual reflex tachycardia associated with increased oxygen demands.

11. Which pharmacologic agents are effective or ineffective in persons with heart transplants?

Atropine is ineffective in treating bradycardia secondary to transection of the vagus nerve.

Digoxin will continue to act as a positive inotrope due to its direct effect on the myocardium and it will slow conduction through the AV node. However, its negative chronotropic effects through vagal stimulation are not preserved. It is therefore not indicated in the treatment of acute supraventricular tachycardias.

Edrophonium (Tensilon), an anticholinesterase, will not produce heart-rate-lowering effects because it relies on intact vagal innervation to the SA node.

Ephedrine will have very little effect on heart rate because of a lack of sympathetic innervation to the SA node; however, because it causes release of norepinephrine stores with direct adrenergic stimulation, it will achieve increased strength of myocardial contractions and vasoconstriction.

Quinidine loses its anticholinergic (blocking vagal impulses to the AV node) effect but retains its class 1 antiarrhythmic effects of depressing myocardial irritability and contractility.

Isoproterenol is a synthetic substance that acts directly on β-adrenergic sites to increase heart rate as well as contractility. Because it acts directly on β_1 and β_2 receptors in the cardiac muscle, it does not depend on innervation to achieve a clinical response. Thus stroke volume, heart rate (chronotrope), speed of conduction (dromotrope), coronary blood flow, venous return, and work are all increased as a result. Also, because it acts only on higher ventricular foci, it allows a more normal pacemaker to take over. It may frequently be used in conjunction with temporary pacing.

12. How is the cardiac output of the transplanted heart maintained in the immediate post-operative period?

Because of ischemia to the donor organ during harvest and transport, the implanted myocardium is stiff and noncompliant. Increasing cardiac output by enhancing stroke volume or contractility meets with limited success, as the donor heart has limited contractile reserve. Drug therapy is used to maximize what contractility is available. Positive inotropes such as dopamine, dobutamine, epinephrine, amrinone, and enoximone serve this purpose either individually or in combination. Increasing heart rate is the more effective way to increase cardiac output in the fresh heart transplant patient, because cardiac output equals stroke volume times heart rate: stroke volume will be maximized through the use of beta agonists such as dobutamine, amrinone, and enoximone; and heart rate will be maintained at a sinus tachycardia with the use of AV sequential pacing and/or isoproterenol.

13. Why do heart transplant recipients experience right ventricular failure?

Neurogenic pulmonary edema/fluid overload. In cerebral ischemia it is common for the donor's pulmonary system to experience neurogenic pulmonary edema. This, coupled with a propensity of donor managers to run their patients "wet" to preserve other organs and avoid the use of inotropic support, leads to early and often unnoticed stresses on the right ventricle of the donor heart.

Ischemic time. With current practices in use for preservation of the donor heart during transit, the myocardial tissue can be expected to perform reasonably well with up to 4 hours of ischemic time between removal from the donor and implantation into the recipient. Even under the best of circumstances, however, the donor heart will perform as ischemic myocardium because of handling and cooling and the preservative solution used.

Recipient's pulmonary system. Patients with normal or slightly elevated pulmonary artery pressures (many times evaluated months prior to transplantation) may, for reasons unclear, have elevated pulmonary artery pressure at the time of transplantation or may have an extremely "reactive" pulmonary system, leading to pulmonary hypertension and concomitant right ventricular stress and failure.

Right ventricular anatomy. The right ventricle differs from the left ventricle in that it has a much thinner freewall, less muscle tissue, and less contractile reserve, leading to early fatigue as cardiac muscle fibers become overdistended. The right ventricle also has biphasic perfusion in that it receives oxygenated blood during systole as well as diastole. With greater demands for contraction during systole, the right ventricle can lose as much as 50% of its perfusion.

14. What are the long-term complications of heart transplants?

Infection is the primary complication of any treatment involving immunosuppression, especially in the lung. Chronic rejection from an ongoing "immune-mediated" process results in a generalized diffuse pattern of atherosclerotic changes that are refractory to any kind of medical or surgical treatment. The only alternative is retransplantation.

15. What are typical sites of infection?

The lungs are the most common site of postoperative infection, although no body system is immune to opportunistic pathogens.

16. What are the mortality statistics for heart transplants?

For adult orthotopic heart transplant recipients worldwide, operative mortality (occurring in the first 30 days after transplant) is 10–12%. One-year survival is 81%. At 5 years, 72% of recipients will survive.

17. What is the quality of life for a heart transplant recipient?

When compared with the general population, 75% of heart transplant recipients rate themselves just as highly on indices of well-being. They report greater feelings of achievement, decision-making abilities, and independence. They are generally optimistic about the future, although some qualify this optimism with the statement, "If things stay just as they are, I'll be happy." One quarter of recipients report no improvement in quality of life after transplant. They relate low self-esteem, fatigue, difficulty with concentrating, and mood swings.

BIBLIOGRAPHY

1. Addonzio LJ, Gersony WM, Robbins RC: Elevated pulmonary vascular resistance and cardiac transplantation. Circulation 76(Suppl V):V52–V55, 1987.
2. Carleton RA, Heller SJ, Najafi H, et al: Hemodynamic performance of a transplanted human heart. Circulation 40:447–452, 1969.
3. Futterman LG: Cardiac transplantation: A comprehensive nursing perspective. Parts I and II. Heart & Lung 17:499–510; 631–638, 1988.
4. Kriett JM, Kaye MP: The Registry of the International Society for Heart Transplantation: Seventh official report. Heart Transplant 9:323–330, 1990.

5. Ley SJ: Right ventricular failure following cardiac transplantation: Nursing assessment and intervention. Proceedings of the 7th Annual National Teaching Institute of the AACN, San Francisco, CA, May 21–24, 1990.
6. Lough ME: Quality of life for heart transplant recipients. J Cardiovasc Nurs 2:11–22, 1988.
7. Macdonald SN, Naucke NA: Heart transplantation. In Smith SL (ed): Tissue and Organ Transplantation: Implications for Nursing Practice. St. Louis, Mosby-Year Book, 1990.
8. Mohanty PK, Capehart JR, Lower RR: Afferent reinnervation of canine cardiac autotransplant. Am J Coll Cardiol 3:509, 1984.
9. Morrison DM, Goldman S, Wright AL, et al: The effect of pulmonary hypertension on systolic function of the right ventricle. Chest 84:250–257, 1983.
10. Young JB, Leon CA, Short HD, et al: Evolution of hemodynamics after orthotopic heart and heart-lung transplantation: Early restrictive patterns persisting in occult fashion. J Heart Transplant 6:34–43, 1987.

91. POSTOPERATIVE CARE OF THE CARDIOTHORACIC SURGERY PATIENT

Jeffrey S. Cross, M.D., and Michael R. Johnston, M.D.

1. Why are epicardial leads placed during cardiac surgery?

Temporary epicardial leads are placed because of the well-recognized disturbances of cardiac rhythm and conduction that occur in the postoperative period. Using leads placed on the atrium, an atrial electrogram can be obtained, which often assists in the diagnosis of tachyarrhythmias. Atrial pacing through these same leads can many times suppress premature atrial or ventricular contractions or override atrial tachycardias. Bradycardia of any origin can be treated effectively with either atrial or ventricular pacing. The ventricular epicardial leads are less versatile but more reliable. They are primarily used for brady-arrhythmias and tend to stay functional throughout the postoperative period. Use of both atrial and ventricular leads in conjunction with an atrioventricular (AV) sequential pacemaker is useful in patients with AV block who need coordinated atrial contractions for optimal ventricular performance. These leads are easily removable at the bedside prior to the patient leaving the hospital, and complications from their placement are extremely rare.

2. How should a patient be evaluated upon arrival to the ICU following a cardiothoracic procedure?

In addition to hemodynamic monitoring, the patient should be evaluated for correct endotracheal tube position, equal breath sounds, proper connection and functioning of chest tubes, and visual assessment of the presence and quantity of an air leak through the chest tube system. Arterial blood gases should be analyzed to manage proper changes in ventilator settings. A chest x-ray should be performed immediately to evaluate the position of the endotracheal tube, nasogastric tube, and any invasive monitoring lines. The x-ray should be closely inspected for the status of lung inflation, including the presence of a pneumothorax or a hemothorax and for abnormal shifting of the mediastinum. These x-rays are typically difficult to evaluate unless the physician has firsthand knowledge of the procedure performed.

3. What is the most common postoperative complication in cardiac surgical patients?

Cardiac dysrhythmias are the most common and occur in approximately 50% of patients. When a dysrhythmia occurs, the initial concern is the hemodynamic stability of the patient.

In the unstable patient, a quick reading of the monitor and an appropriate response is crucial. If the patient is tolerating the dysrhythmia in terms of the resultant hemodynamics, a more leisurely analysis of the rhythm and therapy directed to the underlying cause is then appropriate.

4. What other complications may occur following cardiopulmonary bypass?

Atelectasis (60–84% of patients), pneumothorax, bronchospasm (evaluate for protamine reaction, noncardiogenic pulmonary edema), pulmonary edema, pulmonary embolus, pleural effusion (may occur in 72% of patients but frequently resolves spontaneously), pneumonia and phrenic nerve paralysis (1.5% of patients). Phrenic nerve palsy may be related to the topical iced-slush poured into the pericardial sac during surgery. The diagnosis of phrenic nerve palsy can be confirmed by observing diaphragmatic movement under fluoroscopy. Coagulation defects may be dilutional or may result from prolonged cardiopulmonary bypass. Neurologic deficits have been reported to occur in 16% of patients on the first postoperative day but resolved in all but 6.4% by the tenth postoperative day. Cerebral vascular accidents may result from microemboli of air, fat, or atheromatous plaque. Brachial plexus injury is unusual and is probably related to the sternal retractor. Although severe acute renal failure after cardiac surgery occurs in 7% of patients, it has an associated mortality of 65%. Risks for acute renal failure include advanced age, left ventricular dysfunction, prolonged hypotension, bypass time, and excessive hemolysis.

5. What is the incidence of postoperative atrial fibrillation or atrial flutter following lung resection?

The incidence of atrial arrhythmias after lung resection ranges from 3.4–30%. The most common arrhythmias are atrial fibrillation and atrial flutter, likely related to hypoxia, to alterations in vagal control of the heart, and to shifting of the mediastinum. Risks include advanced age, preexisting cardiovascular disease, and pneumonectomy. Prophylactic administration of digitalis decreases both the incidence and the severity of the arrhythmia.

6. What are the surgical indications for positive pressure ventilation (PPV) in the postoperative thoracic surgical patient?

None. Continued postoperative PPV should be used only for standard indications of postoperative respiratory failure, including inadequate CO_2 elimination and insufficient oxygenation. In patients who have undergone large chest-wall resections, fatigue and CO_2 retention may develop insidiously many hours after a routine extubation. This is due to the mechanical instability of the resected area. Posterior defects are generally much better tolerated than anterior or lateral defects.

7. What parameters should be met prior to extubation?

Vital capacity should be at least 10 ml/kg body weight and the negative inspiratory force greater than or equal to 25 cm H_2O. A trial of spontaneous breathing with continuous positive airway pressure (CPAP) is sometimes helpful.

8. What is the differential diagnosis of hypoxemia in the immediate postoperative period following lung resection?

Pneumothorax, hemothorax, upper airway obstruction, malpositioned endotracheal tube, atelectasis secondary to mucous plugging or inspissated secretions, cardiac herniation (if the pericardium has been opened), and lung torsion should all be considered. Auscultation and a chest x-ray will diagnose most conditions, but emergent bronchoscopy or possibly thoracotomy are occasionally necessary.

9. What are the likely causes of hypoxemia in the immediate postoperative period following cardiopulmonary bypass?

Pneumothorax, hemothorax, cardiac tamponade, low cardiac output, pulmonary edema, malpositioned endotracheal tube, ventilation/perfusion mismatch secondary to cardiopulmonary bypass, and bronchospasm secondary to drug or blood product reactions are all possibilities. Stabilization of hemodynamics and rapid diagnosis of the inciting cause are crucial.

10. A patient is admitted to the ICU in septic shock 6 weeks following a pneumonectomy. What is the differential diagnosis?

The two most common causes of sepsis in this situation are pneumonia and a postpneumonectomy empyema, although a late wound infection and an intraabdominal source need also be considered. Pneumonia or empyema may be secondary to a bronchopleural fistula, in which case both may occur simultaneously. If the patient has a history of a productive cough and if the chest x-ray shows a decrease in the fluid level in the pneumonectomy space, a diagnosis of a bronchopleural fistula is confirmed. The remaining fluid in the pleural space should be drained with a large-bore chest tube, cultures of blood, pleural fluid, and sputum obtained, and the patient started on appropriate antibiotics. The general condition of the patient, the size of the hole in the bronchial stump as determined by bronchoscopy, and the underlying pathologic process are all factors in deciding the long-term management of the bronchopleural fistula.

11. What acute abdominal complications may occur following cardiopulmonary bypass?

Pinson and Alberty noted 142 general surgical complications in a total of 82 patients after 5,682 cardiac operations. The most common complication was acute cholecystitis, whereas the most lethal complications involved hemorrhage and perforation of the gastroduodenal area. The mortality rate of these abdominal complications is 23% if it occurs within 6 weeks of cardiac surgery and 2% after 6 weeks. Pancreatitis is an uncommon complication associated with a very high mortality. Prolonged cardiopulmonary bypass, the low cardiac output syndrome, and inadequately treated or unrecognized pancreatitis in the early postoperative period portend a poor outcome.

12. What are indications for the use of the flow-directed pulmonary artery catheter in the postoperative period following lung resection?

It may be used to optimize fluid management or inotropic support in the management of either cardiogenic or noncardiogenic pulmonary edema as well as to evaluate therapy with mechanical ventilation, vasoactive drugs, hemodialysis, or assisted circulation. Complications are most commonly related to the insertion of the catheter and include carotid artery puncture (1.9%), pneumothorax (0.5%), and dysrhythmias (72%). Premature ventricular contractions are the most common dysrhythmia and often resolve with adjustment of the catheter-tip position. Knotting of the catheter, hydrothorax, and line sepsis are less common. Pulmonary artery perforation is rare but is associated with a high mortality. Risk factors include pulmonary hypertension, anticoagulation, and hypothermia.

13. What are the indications for tracheostomy in the postthoracotomy patient?

Prolonged respiratory failure requiring ventilatory support, and inability to handle pulmonary secretions are the two main indications for tracheotomy. A tracheostomy tube provides quick access for frequent pulmonary toilet and decreases patient effort related to clearing secretions. It is particularly useful in debilitated or severely compromised patients.

14. What is a tracheoinnominate artery fistula? How should it be managed?

This fistula most often occurs following erosion of a tracheostomy tube or the cuff of that tube into the innominate artery. It should be suspected in any patient who develops bleeding through the tracheostomy tube. Usually a premonitory "herald" bleed occurs first, followed at a variable period of time by massive hemoptysis. When the condition is first suspected, fiberoptic bronchoscopy should be performed, making sure to remove the tracheostomy tube so that the area of the trachea in contact with the tube can be carefully examined. Massive hemorrhage is controlled with digital pressure in the pretracheal space or by hyperinflation of the tracheostomy tube cuff. The fistula must then be emergently controlled surgically. The mortality for untreated tracheoinnominate erosion is 100%, but with appropriate surgical therapy drops to approximately 25%. Prevention includes use of a high-volume, low-pressure cuff and placement of the tracheostomy at the level of the second or third tracheal ring.

CONTROVERSY

15. What are the minimum pulmonary function criteria for performing a pneumonectomy? Although no test or physical sign can predict who will best tolerate a pneumonectomy, a maximum voluntary ventilation (MVV) of greater than 55% of predicted value and a forced expiratory volume in 1 sec (FEV_1) exceeding 2 liters are the requirements most commonly considered adequate for a pneumonectomy. CO_2 retention greater than 45 mm Hg and moderate to severe pulmonary hypertension are relative contraindications to pneumonectomy. Because numerous studies show no direct correlation between these tests and operative morbidity and mortality following pneumonectomy, a number of other tests have been proposed. These include ventilation/perfusion scan of the lung to determine the percentage of functional lung to be resected compared to functional lung remaining after resection, the maximal oxygen consumption (VO_2max), and pulmonary vascular resistance at both rest and exercise. Although correlation of these studies with postoperative morbidity and mortality appear to be more precise, adequate experience in a large group of patients is not yet available.

BIBLIOGRAPHY

1. Angelini P, Feldman MI, Lufschanowski R, et al: Cardiac arrhythmias during and after heart surgery: Diagnosis and management. Prog Cardiovasc Dis 16:469, 1974.
2. Gale GD, Teasdale SJ, Sanders DE, et al: Pulmonary atelectasis and other respiratory complications after cardiopulmonary bypass and investigation of aetiological factors. Can Anaesth Soc J 26:15, 1979.
3. Hilberman M, Myers BD, Carrie BF, et al: Acute renal failure following cardiac surgery. J Thorac Cardiovasc Surg 77:880, 1979.
4. Kirsh MM, Rotman H, Behrendt DM, et al: Complications of pulmonary resection. Ann Thorac Surg 20:216–236, 1975.
5. Marco JD, Hahn JW, Barner HB: Topical cardiac hypothermia and phrenic nerve injury. Ann Thorac Surg 23:235, 1977.
6. Markland ON, Moorthy SS, Mahomed Y, et al: Postoperative phrenic nerve palsy in patients with open-heart surgery. Ann Thorac Surg 39:68, 1985.
7. Miller JI, Grossman GD, Hatcher CR: Pulmonary function test criteria for operability and pulmonary resection. Surg Gynecol Obstet 153:893–895, 1981.
8. Morin JE, Long R, Elleder MG, et al: Upper extremity neuropathies following median sternotomy. Ann Thorac Surg 34:181, 1982.
9. Nelems JM: Tracheo-innominate artery fistula. Am J Surg 141:526–527, 1981.
10. Pinson CW, Alberty RE: General surgical complications after cardiopulmonary bypass surgery. Am J Surg 146:133–137, 1983.
11. Rose DM, Ranson JH, Cunningham JN: Patterns of severe pancreatic injury following cardiopulmonary bypass. Ann Surg 199:169–172, 1984.
12. Shah KB, Rao TLK, Laughlin S, El-Etr AA: A review of pulmonary artery catheterization in 6245 patients. Anesthesiology 61:271–275, 1984.
13. Waldo AL, MacLean WAH, Cooper TB, et al: Use of temporarily placed epicardial atrial wire electrodes for the diagnosis and treatment of cardiac arrhythmias following open heart surgery. J Thorac Surg 76:500–505, 1978.

92. LIVER TRANSPLANTATION

Teresa DeLong, R.N., M.S.N.

1. Which conditions may necessitate liver transplantation in adults and in children?

Adults	Children
Chronic active hepatitis	Biliary hypoplasia
Primary biliary cirrhosis	Alpha-1-antitrypsin deficiency
Sclerosing cholangitis	Tyrosinemia
Budd-Chiari syndrome	Galactosemia
Wilson's disease	Protoporphyria
Hemochromatosis	Glycogen storage disease
Cryptogenic cirrhosis	Chronic active hepatitis
Primary hepatomas	Fulminant hepatitis
Hemangiomas	Cryptogenic cirrhosis
Familial hypercholesterolemia	Drug-induced hepatic failure
Polycystic liver disease	Benign tumors
Alpha-1-antitrypsin deficiency	Crigler-Najjar syndrome
Fulminant hepatitis	Neonatal hepatitis
Cholangiocarcinoma	Wilson's disease
	Hepatoma/hepatoblastoma

2. What are the criteria for selecting candidates for liver transplantation?

Criteria vary for each transplant center, but two common factors for candidacy are (1) irreversible chronic liver disease for which all forms of therapy have been exhausted, and (2) a life expectancy of less than a year.

3. When should patients be considered potential candidates for liver transplantation?

Indications include any one of the following clinical manifestations: serum bilirubin concentrations greater than 10 mg/dl, serum albumin concentrations less than 2.5 gm/dl, ascites refractory to medical therapy, encephalopathy refractory to medical management that significantly impairs the patient's lifestyle, variceal hemorrhage refractory to sclerotherapy, hepatorenal syndrome, and coagulopathy unresponsive to vitamin K therapy.

4. How are potential candidates for liver transplantation evaluated?

An extensive physical and psychological health profile is evaluated by the liver transplant physicians, a cardiologist, anesthesiologist, psychiatrist, dentist, nutritionist, social worker, transplant coordinator, and financial counselor. The goal of this evaluation is to (1) confirm the etiology and evaluate the severity of the liver disease; (2) assess the existence of contraindications; (3) evaluate the patient's financial status; and (4) assess the patient's psychosocial support and willingness to comply to a lifelong medical regimen.

5. What are the contraindications to liver transplantation?

The two categories of contraindications, absolute and relative, depend on each center's guidelines. **Absolute contraindications** (eliminate a transplant candidate) may include a positive human immunodeficiency virus (HIV) test, advanced cardiopulmonary or cerebrovascular disease, active infection/sepsis, active alcohol or drug abuse, malignant disease outside the hepatobiliary system, or inability of the patient or his or her support system to cope with the demands of the immunosuppression regimen. **Relative contraindications** (may or may not exclude a patient from transplantation) may include renal failure, age over 60 years, cholangiocarcinoma, positive test for hepatitis B surface antigen, or portal venous thrombosis.

6. How is the donor liver selected?
The largest limiting factor is availability, particularly in the pediatric population. Although ABO compatibility is not essential, ABO mismatching is associated with decreased patient survival. The size of the donor liver must match that of the recipient. Too large an organ can lead to respiratory compromise and pressure necrosis of the graft, whereas too small an organ may present problems with vessel size mismatch and result in relative stenosis.

7. What are the major postoperative complications following liver transplantation?
Hemodynamic instability due to bleeding and fluid volume shifts, infection, rejection, vascular thrombosis, biliary leakage, renal dysfunction, and psychological impairment.

8. What is included in the immediate postoperative assessment, care, and management of these patients?
Continual assessments include cardiac monitoring, vital signs, hemodynamic monitoring, cardiac output, arterial blood gas, bile volume and consistency, abdominal fluid volume from drains, abdominal girth, weight, blood glucose and electrolytes, coagulation, and blood count. The nurse to patient ratio is usually 2:1 in the first 12–24 hours postoperatively because of the need for hourly multisystem assessments.

9. What are the predominant problems immediately postoperatively? How are these assessed and managed?
The predominant problem is hemodynamic instability due to bleeding and fluid volume shifts. Until the transplanted liver effectively produces coagulation factors, blood products are replaced on the basis of a combination of factors, including the amount and consistency of fluid draining from the abdominal drains, hemodynamic parameters such as blood pressure, heart rate and central venous pressure, blood count, and blood coagulation findings. Bleeding can also occur from rupture of the anastomosis, thrombocytopenia, or stress ulcers. Fluid volume shifts occur rapidly postoperatively. Hypertension is treated with intravenous administration of an antihypertensive drug that can be rapidly titrated. Hypotension is treated with fluid challenge and blood products if indicated. When replacing fluid, central venous pressure should remain below 12 mm Hg to avoid venous congestion in the transplanted liver.

10. Are any pulmonary complications specific to this population of patients?
Atelectasis, ventilation-perfusion imbalance, and right-sided pleural effusions are likely to occur immediately postoperatively because of the massive insult from the surgical procedure inflicted on the diaphragm as well as the prolonged general anesthetic course and immobility. Compounding the situation is the prior development of arteriovenous collateral vessels in the pulmonary circulation as a result of advanced liver disease and portal hypertension, which shunts unoxygenated blood into the systemic circulation. Mechanical ventilation is necessary initially in the postoperative period for the maintenance of adequate lung volume and normal gas exchange. High levels of positive end-expiratory pressure (PEEP), greater than 10 cm H_2O, should be avoided because such pressure might reduce venous return to the heart and cause fluid congestion in the liver.

11. How long are most liver transplant patients intubated postoperatively?
Most patients are extubated within 12–48 hours after surgery. Narcotics and sedation are either held or used sparingly during that period to promote early extubation to assess neurologic status. Most liver transplant patients report minimal or no incision pain in the immediate postoperative period.

12. Why are liver transplant patients in the ICU usually maintained on low-dose dopamine or diuretics?

Acute renal failure can occur in conjunction with the hypovolemia and hypotension of surgery or in the immediate postoperative period. Antibiotic therapy and cyclosporine (CSA) immunosuppression can also precipitate renal failure. Intravenous furosemide is given to overcome sodium retention and is used in conjunction with low-dose dopamine to increase renal perfusion. If urinary output remains low, CSA is discontinued for a brief period and then restarted at lower doses.

13. Why do serum electrolytes and blood glucose need to be measured so frequently?

Hypokalemia results from flushing of the donor allograft with Collins solution and diuretic therapy. Hypocalcemia results from the massive transfusion of blood preserved with calcium-binding calcium citrate. Both potassium and calcium need to be replaced frequently based on the laboratory data. Blood glucose is elevated from steroid therapy and patients may require an insulin drip.

14. What is the incidence of infection following liver transplantation?

Almost all patients will experience at least one bacterial infection following transplantation. There is a 40–50% chance of developing a fungal or viral infection. These infections are primarily related to immunosuppressive drug therapy.

15. What are the sources of infection?

The main sources of bacterial infection are the biliary tree, intraabdominal abscess, pneumonia, and central venous catheters. The most common viral infections are from the herpes family. For herpes prophylaxis, all patients are treated with acyclovir.

16. What are the signs and symptoms of rejection? How often does this occur?

There are four types of rejection: hyperacute, accelerated, acute, and chronic. Hyperacute occurs immediately and accelerated occurs within the first 24–36 hours following surgery; both require immediate retransplantation. Both types are rare. As many as 80% of liver transplant recipients experience some type of rejection during their lifetimes. Chronic rejection occurs several months to years following transplantation and may be ongoing for years before retransplantation is required. By far the most common type of rejection seen in critical care units is acute rejection. Acute rejection occurs 7–10 days following surgery and may be associated with fever ($\geq 38°$C), graft tenderness, malaise, hypertension, fluid retention, and an increase in liver function tests. Diagnosis is based on a combination of biopsy results, laboratory findings (coagulation and liver function tests), and clinical findings. Drugs such as OKT3 and antilymphocyte globulin (ALG) reduce the need for retransplantation following an episode of acute rejection to less than 5% at most centers.

BIBLIOGRAPHY

1. Asher NL: Selection criteria for liver transplantation donors. Transplant Proc 21:3482–3483, 1989.
2. Bass PS, Bindon-Perler PA, Lewis R: Liver transplantation: The recovery phase. Critic Care Nurs Q 13:51–61, 1991.
3. Coleman J, Mendoza M, Bindon-Perler P: Liver diseases that lead to transplantation. Crit Care Nurs Q 13:41–50, 1991.
4. Davis F: Organ procurement and transplantation. Nurs Clin North Am 24:823–836, 1989.
5. Miller H: Liver transplantation postoperative ICU care. Crit Care Nurs 8:19–31, 1988.
6. Overman J, Cox D, Buchl L, et al: Role of the nurse in the multidisciplinary team approach to care of liver transplant patients. Mayo Clin Proc 64:690–698, 1989.
7. Shaw BW: Exclusion criteria in liver transplant recipients. Transplant Proc 21:3484–3486, 1989.
8. Sheets L: Liver transplantation. Nurs Clin North Am 24:881–889, 1989.
9. Whiteman K, Nachtmann L, Biondo M, Formella L: Liver transplantation. Am J Nurs, 1990, pp 68–72.

XIII: Anesthesia

93. USE OF PARALYTIC AGENTS IN THE ICU

Jean-François Pittet, M.D.

1. What are the two major types of muscle relaxants?

Depolarizing (e.g., succinylcholine). These act by binding to acetylcholine receptor sites and depolarizing the postjunctional membrane, preventing further muscle action potentials. This results in the relaxation of skeletal muscle. These drugs act very quickly but the effect is brief.

Nondepolarizing (e.g., pancuronium, atracurium, vecuronium). These act by competing with acetylcholine for binding to the nerve endplate, but they prevent depolarization of the nerve. These agents tend to be intermediate- to long-acting relative to the depolarizing agents.

2. When should succinylcholine be used?

Critically ill patients frequently require emergent intubation. Because some patients will have full stomachs (e.g., newly admitted patients) or delayed gastric emptying (abdominal trauma, ileus, sepsis, etc.), it is imperative that intubation be done quickly in a well-controlled setting. Succinylcholine causes muscle relaxation within 30 seconds, which generally lasts 10–15 minutes, making it useful in these situations.

3. What are the contraindications to the use of succinylcholine?

Succinylcholine causes serum potassium to increase, so it should not be used in patients with hyperkalemia. Other patients at risk for an exaggerated increase in serum potassium levels include those with renal failure, burns, or crush injury.

4. What are the indications for nondepolarizing muscle relaxants in the ICU?

Improved forms of mechanical ventilation and optimal administration of sedatives and analgesics have decreased the need for muscle relaxants. The major indications include:

- Control of shivering after cardiopulmonary bypass surgery
- Temporary control of agitated, sedated, ventilated patients
- Facilitation of mechanical ventilation in patients with severely impaired lung mechanics
- Patients in status asthmaticus who fail to respond to conventional therapy
- Control of intracranial pressure in ventilated neurosurgical or neurologic patients
- Control of painful cramps in patients with tetanus

5. What are the risks related to use of nondepolarizing muscle relaxants in the ICU?

Prolonged use is associated with (1) inability to clear pulmonary secretions secondary to the suppression of cough, (2) atrophy of skeletal muscles, (3) venous thrombosis and pulmonary embolism, (4) osteoporosis with impairment of calcium-phosphorus balance, (5) psychic trauma if the patient is not adequately sedated while paralyzed, (6) skin breakdown, and (7) injuries to nerves and limbs secondary to poor positioning.

The patient's safety rests entirely with the medical staff and the available hemodynamic monitors, so all alarms should be activated and quickly heeded. Close attention should be paid to any changes in vital signs, as they may provide subtle clues to significant changes in clinical status.

6. Is it true that patients paralyzed with muscle relaxants are "unconscious"?
No. These patients are awake and can feel pain, so it is imperative that they receive adequate sedation and analgesia.

7. What are the most useful nondepolarizing muscle relaxants for ICU patients?
Pancuronium (Pavulon), atracurium (Tracrium), and vecuronium (Norcuron).

8. How do you decide which agent to use?
Atracurium. This drug is spontaneously degraded in plasma rather than eliminated by the kidneys or liver, so it may be the drug of choice for patients with renal or hepatic failure. One potential serious side effect is substantial histamine release; thus it may be relatively contraindicated in patients with significant cardiovascular disease, asthma, or anaphylactoid reactions.
Vecuronium. This drug does not produce histamine release or cardiovascular instability, so it is potentially useful in patients with bronchospasm or cardiovascular disease. The drug is primarily metabolized by the liver and excreted in bile, and thus is useful for patients with renal failure. Prolonged neuromuscular blockade may occur in patients with hepatic failure.
Pancuronium. This drug does not produce histamine release and prevents vagally mediated bradycardia, so it may be useful in patients with cardiovascular disease; however, tachycardia develops occasionally, which must be considered. Because 90% of the drug is renally excreted and 10% is metabolized by the liver, renal and hepatic function need to be monitored closely.

9. What are the recommended dosages for nondepolarizing agents?

	Pancuronium	**Atracurium**	**Vecuronium**
IV bolus:	0.06 mg/kg	0.3–0.6 mg/kg	0.07 mg/kg

10. How do you decide when a patient is adequately paralyzed?
Muscle twitch response to peripheral nerve stimulation can be monitored. Normally the goal is to decrease the twitch response by 90%

11. Are there any clinically significant interactions between muscle relaxants and other drugs used in the ICU?
Yes. The following drugs have been shown to potentiate neuromuscular blockade: furosemide, type 1 antidysrhythmics, calcium channel blockers, magnesium, aminoglycosides, clindamycin, lithium, and nitroglycerin. Other drugs such as theophylline, azathioprine, and possibly steroids have been shown to decrease the level and duration of neuromuscular blockade.

12. What is the best way to terminate the actions of muscle relaxants?
The best way is to ventilate the patients and wait until these drugs are metabolized or excreted. Assessment of the level of neuromuscular blockade by a nerve stimulator may be useful in some circumstances.

13. Which drugs can be used to terminate the action of muscle relaxants?
Nondepolarizing muscle relaxants may be antagonized by anticholinesterase drugs, which block the hydrolysis of acetylcholine. As a result, acetylcholine accumulates at the neuromuscular junction and antagonizes the blockade.

14. What is the usual dosage of anticholinesterase drugs?

The following drugs may be administered in an IV bolus: Neostigmine: 0.03–0.06 mg/kg; pyridostigmine: 0.1–0.2 mg/kg; edrophonium: 0.5–1.0 mg/kg.

15. What are the most common side effects of anticholinesterase drugs?

The most common side effect is excessive stimulation of cholinergic receptors in the peripheral nervous system, which elicits bradycardia, vasodilation, contraction of ureter and bronchioles, increased gastrointestinal motility and secretion of hydrogen chloride from gastric parietal cells, increased secretory gland activity, and miosis. To counteract these effects, it is customary to administer anticholinesterase drugs in combination with atropine (0.01–0.02 mg/kg IV) or glycopyrrolate (0.01 mg/kg IV). The duration of action of glycopyrrolate is twice that of atropine, and, in contrast to atropine, it has no effect on the central nervous system.

BIBLIOGRAPHY

1. Clyburn PA, Marshall RD: Control of ventilation by continuous infusion of pancuronium bromide. Anesthesia 36:860, 1981.
2. Gilston A: Paralysis or sedation for controlled ventilation. Lancet 1:480, 1980.
3. Green D: Paralysis or sedation for controlled ventilation. Lancet 1:715, 1980.
4. Lumb PD: Sedatives and muscle relaxants in the intensive care unit. In Fuhrman BP, Shoemaker WC (eds): Critical Care: State of the Art, Vol. 10. Fullerton, CA, Society of Critical Care Medicine, 1989, p 145.
5. Miller-Jones CMH: Paralysis or sedation for controlled ventilation. Lancet 1:312, 1980.
6. Partridge BL: Clinical use of muscle relaxants: Avoiding the complications. Prog Anesthesiol 4:314–323, 1990.
7. Schapera A: The use of neuromuscular blocking agents in the intensive care unit. Pulmonary and Critical Care Update 5:1–7, 1990.

94. PAIN MANAGEMENT IN THE ICU

Jean-François Pittet, M.D.

1. Is the pain relief generally adequate in ICU patients?

Probably not. Many studies have reported that inadequate pain relief is common after surgery. The potential for inadequate analgesia is probably greater in ICU patients, who are often confused, paralyzed, or unable to communicate.

2. Why do ICU patients often receive inadequate analgesia?

Physicians frequently underestimate the amount of pain patients are experiencing and are overly concerned about side effects of treatment.

3. Why is it important to provide adequate pain relief?

Aside from humanitarian reasons, there are a number of benefits of providing adequate analgesia:

- Prevention of deep venous thrombosis and lung embolism by earlier patient mobilization.
- Attenuation of the stress response and more rapid normalization of the overactivity of the nervous system (tachycardia, hypertension, increased systemic vascular resistance and oxygen consumption), which is poorly tolerated by critically ill or geriatric patients.

4. Are pain-stimulating factors present in the ICU environment?
Yes. Admission to an ICU provokes anxiety, which leads to sleep deprivation and discomfort and increases the perception of pain. Noise, a common problem in the ICU, interferes with sleep and has been found to increase analgesic requirements.

5. What methods can be used for relieving pain in the ICU?
Narcotic or nonnarcotic analgesics and regional nerve blocks are the classic methods. Other methods such as electroanalgesia, psychotherapy, or hypnosis should also be considered.

6. What are the indications for narcotic analgesics in the ICU?
Narcotics are administered most often for pain relief. Narcotics are used for their beneficial side effects, including sedation, depression of respiratory drive, and attenuation of psychologic discomfort.

7. How can narcotic analgesics be administered to ICU patients?
Narcotic analgesics are administered to ICU patients as repeated boluses or continuous infusions intravenously or in the epidural space.

8. Does the achievement of pain relief correlate to the blood level of narcotic analgesics?
Yes. It is generally accepted that analgesia occurs when a definite blood level of narcotics has been achieved (analgesia threshold). This blood level is not the same for all patients. Therefore, the concept of a minimum effective analgesic concentration (MEAC) has been proposed and corresponds to the minimal blood level of narcotic that provides effective analgesia for an individual patient. Each patient has a different MEAC, which changes as the intensity of pain changes.

9. What are the advantages and disadvantages of intermittent IV bolus and continuous IV infusion of narcotics analgesics?
Intermittent IV boluses of narcotics can relieve pain effectively if the patient is observed closely to determine when the blood level of narcotic is below the MEAC. This method prevents drug accumulation and allows rapid drug elimination when the drug is stopped. In practice, close evaluation of a patient's pain is seldom possible because ICU nurses are busy.

Continuous IV infusion of narcotics easily maintains a blood drug level above the MEAC. This technique needs minimal nursing care and often provides good analgesia. However, excessive drug accumulation may occur, particularly in patients with hepatic or renal failure. The use of newer narcotics, such as alfentanil or sulfentanil, with more rapid onset and shorter half-lives may be advantageous. The most difficult problem when using continuous IV infusion of narcotics is determining the appropriate dose. An objective clinical assessment of analgesia is difficult and the patient should therefore be consulted about his or her level of pain relief.

10. What is patient-controlled analgesia (PCA)?
PCA is a system that allows the patient to monitor his or her own blood level of narcotic analgesia by its effect on pain, and to self-administer the drug to achieve pain relief. This system was developed about 20 years ago, but became more popular recently with the wide availability of commercial devices.

11. What is the goal of PCA?
The goal of PCA is to produce a relatively stable and effective level of narcotics by allowing the patient to receive multiple small boluses of opiate following an initial loading dose. This allows the patient to maintain his or her narcotic blood level above the MEAC. PCA may also be used with continuous IV infusion of narcotics.

12. What are the characteristics of PCA devices?

PCA devices are microprocessor-based pumps that can deliver narcotics on demand. The following parameters can be set on the pump: the dose administered when the patient pushes the button, the lock-out interval or length of time between doses, the maximal dose to be given, the initial loading dose, and a bolus dose that can be used for extreme pain.

13. Do patients receive more narcotics when using PCA than they do with other traditional techniques?

No. Studies have shown that PCA patients used more narcotics on the first day, but then less on subsequent days. The risk of addiction is minimal. Patients prefer this pain-relief technique because they control their analgesia administration.

14. What are the undesirable side effects of intravenous narcotics?

They include respiratory depression, euphoria and development of addiction, a withdrawal syndrome when narcotics are administered over a long period (0.1 mg IV clonidine, twice daily, may be helpful in this situation), increased gastric, pancreatic, and biliary secretions, increased tone in anal, biliary, and ileocolic sphincters, release of histamine (morphine, meperidine), and development of seizures (fentanyl, sulfentanil), particularly in patients with chronic renal failure.

15. What is the rationale for using epidural opioid analgesia in the ICU?

Administration of narcotics into the epidural space produces safe and effective analgesia equal or superior to that produced by conventional analgesic techniques. However, epidural opioid analgesia has been associated with less sedation, greater improvement in postoperative pulmonary function, earlier ambulation, decreased morbidity, and shorter hospital stay compared with other analgesic techniques.

16. How can narcotics be administered in the epidural space?

Techniques of epidural opioid administration include intermittent boluses, continuous infusion, or epidural PCA. Although adequate analgesia may be obtained with all of these techniques, continuous epidural infusion of narcotics allows a more selective titration of analgesia, and the use of more lipophilic opioids with short duration of action and less intrinsic risk of respiratory depression. The concomitant use of local anesthetics is performed more safely (stable sympathetic blockade) with this technique than with repeated boluses.

17. What are the undesirable side effects of epidural narcotics? How are they managed?

Respiratory depression, particularly in elderly patients, is the most serious side effect. Respiratory depression following epidural morphine has been reported to be biphasic: an early phase resulting from absorption in epidural veins and circulatory redistribution to the brain, and a late phase resulting from the cephalic movement of the morphine in the cerebrospinal fluid. Avoidance of large doses of epidural narcotics, careful titration of analgesia, and use of lipophilic narcotics may significantly increase the margin of safety with this technique.

Side effects of epidural narcotics include itching, nausea and vomiting, urine retention, decreased gastrointestinal motility. Itching, nausea and vomiting may be treated by very small IV doses of naloxone (0.04–0.08 mg), which do not completely antagonize the epidural analgesia and do not produce the undesirable side effects (hypertension, cardiac arrhythmias, lung edema, and sudden death) observed after greater doses (0.4 mg). Cisapride, a gastric and intestinal prokinetic drug, has been reported to be more effective than metoclopramide in treating the morphine-induced delay in gastric emptying, and may be useful in treating the gastrointestinal effects of epidural opioids.

18. What is the rationale for using nonnarcotic analgesics in the ICU?

Nonnarcotic analgesics (prostaglandin inhibitors) are particularly effective in reducing muscular and skeletal pain and may decrease the need for narcotics. They are often more effective than narcotics in reducing pain from pleural or pericardial rubs, a pain that responds poorly to narcotics. They are also useful in providing analgesia for neurosurgical patients who are not ventilated, because narcotics may reduce respiratory drive and lead to CO_2 retention and increased intracranial pressure in patients with poor cerebral compliance.

Most of these compounds decrease platelet function and therefore may interfere with hemostasis. Prostaglandins are involved in the regulation of the renal function. Their inhibition by nonnarcotic analgesics may lead to sodium and water retention, hyperkalemia, increased blood pressure, and impaired response to diuretics.

19. What are the advantages of regional blocks for ICU patients?

The greatest advantage of regional anesthesia is the production of pain relief superior both in quality and duration to that obtained by IV narcotics. In particular, regional blocks provide sufficient analgesia for movement and physiotherapy, whereas narcotics only eliminate pain at rest. Other advantages include greater improvement in respiratory function by inhibition of muscle spasms, a sedation that facilitates neurologic assessment, less constipation, and a possible reduction in the incidence of thromboembolic phenomena.

20. What are the limitations to regional anesthesia in the ICU?

Regional blocks are time-consuming, difficult to perform, and contraindicated in patients with a coagulopathy or receiving anticoagulants. Epidural or other catheters used to administer local anesthetics continuously may become infected. Local anesthetics have a low therapeutic/toxic ratio and may accumulate easily, particularly in patients with renal or hepatic failure. Finally, tachyphylaxis is likely to occur, especially with short-acting local anesthetics.

21. Are hypnosis and relaxation-associated strategies useful for treating acute pain in the ICU?

Yes. Hypnotic strategies have been used successfully for treating acute pain in the ICU, particularly for patients suffering extensive burns. Hypnosis has been hypothesized to reduce pain through mechanisms such as attentional control or dissociation. During hypnosis, suggestions are combined with imagery to enhance the feeling of comfort.

22. Does hypnosis decrease acute pain in every ICU patient?

No. The reduction of pain depends on the suggestibility of the patient. Moreover, it appears that effective pain reduction is consistently achieved when patients have had sufficient practice with such techniques.

BIBLIOGRAPHY

1. Bion JF, Logan BK, Newman PM, et al: Sedation in intensive care: Morphine and renal function. Intens Care Med 12:359, 1986.
2. Cohen AT, Kelly DR: Assessment of alfentanil by intravenous infusion as long-term sedation in intensive care. Anaesthesia 42:545, 1987.
3. Donovan M, Dillon P, McGuire L: Incidence and characteristics of pain in a sample of medical-surgical inpatients. Pain 30:69, 1987.
4. Ferrante FM, Orav EJ, Rocco AG, et al: A statistical model for pain in patient-controlled analgesia and conventional intramuscular opioid regimens. Anesth Analg 67:457, 1988.

5. Forrest WH, Smethurst PWR, Kienitz ME: Self-administration of intravenous analgesics. Anesthesiology 33:363, 1970.
6. Hansell NH: The behavioral effect of noise on man: The patient with "intensive care unit psychosis." Heart Lung 13:59, 1984.
7. Jones J, Hoggart B, Withey J, et al: What the patient says: A study of reactions to an intensive care unit. Intens Care Med 5:89, 1979.
8. Peck CL: Psychological factors in acute pain management. In Cousins MJ, Phillips GD (eds): Acute Pain Management. New York, Churchill Livingstone, 1985, pp 251.
9. Pflug AE, Murphy TM, Butler SH, et al: The effects of postoperative peridural analgesia on pulmonary therapy and pulmonary complications. Anesthesiology 41:8, 1974.
10. Rowbotham DJ: Cisapride and anesthesia. Br J Anaesth 62:121, 1989.
11. Yeager MP, Glass DD, Neff RK, et al: Epidural anesthesia in high-risk surgical patients. Anesthesiology 66:729, 1987.

95. UPPER AIRWAY OBSTRUCTION

Jean-François Pittet, M.D.

1. Define upper airway obstruction.

Upper airway obstruction is the blockage of air between the nose and the mouth and the tracheal bifurcation. It may be complete or incomplete and is often life-threatening when it occurs below the hypopharynx, where the cross-sectional diameter of the airway is the smallest.

2. What is the clinical presentation of upper airway obstruction?

Three phases of physiologic change occur in acute airway obstruction before death:

1. The first phase (1–3 min duration) is characterized by a marked sympathetic response with an increase in blood pressure, pulse, and respiratory rate, and an increase in the work of breathing. Then, PaO_2 decreases and $PaCO_2$ increases, causing a fall in pH. The patient is still conscious and choking, making paradoxic respirations that do not result air movement. The patient rapidly becomes cyanotic.

2. During the second phase (2–5 min duration), blood pressure and heart rate fall rapidly, respiratory movements diminish, and the patient loses consciousness.

3. The third and terminal phase (5–8 min after beginning the airway obstruction) is characterized by asystole; the cardiac rhythm degenerates from sinus to nodal bradycardia, then to idioventricular rhythms, and terminates in asystole or ventricular fibrillation.

The same physiologic changes occur in partial upper airway obstruction but more slowly and to lesser degrees. However, when symptoms are present, the obstruction should be considered as substantial because mild obstruction is generally asymptomatic.

3. Do the signs of upper airway obstruction depend on its location?

Yes. Airway obstruction produces different anatomic and physiologic changes depending on whether it is fixed or variable, extrathoracic or intrathoracic. An extrathoracic obstruction with a mobile airway wall produces more symptoms during inspiration because the airway lumen is normally more narrow during inspiration in its extrathoracic portion. A mobile intrathoracic obstruction causes more symptoms during expiration. However, if the airway obstruction is fixed, both inspiratory and expiratory flow will be limited equally, because changes in transmural pressure cannot modify the diameter of the airway.

4. What should be included in the physical examination of a patient presenting with an upper airway obstruction?

The oral cavity is inspected, avoiding instrumentation in patients with suspected epiglottitis and severe airway obstruction. Auscultation over the larynx, trachea, and both lungs is done to exclude tension pneumothorax. Flail chest, which may mimic airway obstruction, also should be excluded. The physician should listen for stridor, which may be inspiratory (supraglottic obstruction), expiratory (infraglottic obstruction), or both. Its presence signifies an airway diameter of 5 mm or less in adults.

5. Can upper airway obstruction be precisely localized?

Yes. Neck and chest x-rays (anteroposterior and lateral views), airway tomography, CT scan, pulmonary function testing, and, if necessary, bronchoscopy can localize the airway obstruction.

6. What causes upper airway obstruction?

The site of an upper airway obstruction may be extrathoracic or intrathoracic, and localized within the lumen, in the wall, or extrinsic to the wall of an anatomic or artificial airway. The following clinical conditions may be associated with upper airway obstruction:

- Infection: acute epiglottitis, tonsillitis, peritonsillar and retropharyngeal abscess, diphtheria, Ludwig's angina, and laryngitis
- Mass lesions: benign and malignant tumors, traumatic hematomas and hematomas secondary to anticoagulants
- Head and neck trauma
- Foreign body aspiration (cafe coronary)
- Inflammation: angioneurotic edema, anaphylaxis, inhalation of corrosives and toxins, thermal burns
- Vocal cord pathology: laryngospasm, bilateral vocal cord paralysis
- Cricoarytenoid arthritis
- Sleep apnea syndrome

7. What is the clinical presentation of upper airway infections?

Acute infectious epiglottitis is unusual but not rare in adults. Adults have a longer prodromal state than children, as more inflammatory edema is needed to produce symptoms at the larger glottic opening. As in children, *Hemophilus influenzae* is the most common organism, but pneumococcus, Staphylococcus, and Streptococcus have been incriminated. The initial symptoms are a muffled voice, signs and symptoms out of proportion to the degree of oropharyngeal obstruction, and some early signs of upper airway obstruction. Although indirect laryngoscopy has been considered to be dangerous in patients with severe airway obstruction, this procedure should be performed in patients with milder symptoms in order to establish the diagnosis. **Acute and chronic tonsillitis** can cause an upper airway obstruction and lead to the development of a sleep apnea syndrome associated with snoring, restless sleep, chronic mouth-breathing, daytime hypersomnolence, and morning headache. **Peritonsillar abscess** may threaten the upper airway as an obstructive mass lesion and may also threaten the airway by rupturing and causing pulmonary aspiration. **Ludwig's angina** is an infection of the floor-of-the-mouth, usually due to the spread of infection from the lower molar teeth. It is characterized by rock-hard swelling of this area, with elevation of the base of the tongue and with both paralaryngeal and glottic edema.

8. What is a cafe coronary? Which patients are at risk?

Cafe coronary, or aspiration of partially chewed food, usually occurs in elderly persons with altered consciousness, decreased gag reflexes, or dentures. Individuals who are taking drugs with anticholinergic effects are at risk for swallowing a large bolus of food and having it obstruct the glottis. Although food appears to be the most common obstructing foreign body, dentures, loose teeth, or other objects should be considered.

9. Which patients are at greatest risk for nonpenetrating trauma to the upper airway?

Young adult men with sport injuries and patients who suffer blunt trauma from motor vehicle accidents are at greatest risk. The presence of a cervical spine injury should be considered when the initial mechanism of upper airway injury is associated with dissipation of high energy to the tissues of the neck. These lesions are often characterized by the presence of a large hematoma, subcutaneous emphysema, and the development of stridor.

10. What is the clinical presentation of laryngeal edema?

Laryngeal edema occurs within minutes during an allergic response or as a part of anaphylaxis. There is usually angioneurotic edema of the tongue, the lips, or the supraglottic tissues as well as the subglottic tissues. This edema can result in complete airway obstruction. Some patients may also have a cardiovascular collapse, severe bronchoconstriction, urticaria, and diarrhea. The most frequent etiologies are hymenoptera bites, shellfish allergies, and drug reactions. Laryngeal edema may also occur in patients with extrinsic asthma as part of an acute attack or in patients with C1 esterase inhibitor deficiency (hereditary angioneurotic edema).

11. What is the treatment of foreign body aspiration?

For obstruction of the supraglottic area, the Heimlich maneuver (abdominal thrust) is indicated. If it is not successful, laryngoscopy and extraction of the foreign body by suction and/or by forceps is mandatory. A cricothyroidotomy may be life-saving if the foreign body is impacted in a subglottic site. In the presence of viscous particulate matter, endotracheal intubation (with a long endotracheal tube) may be helpful.

Extraction of foreign bodies from the trachea requires judgment because aggressive treatment may be more detrimental than helpful. If air movement is present, supplemental oxygen should be provided. Then, rigid bronchoscopy should be considered quickly. A mixture of helium and oxygen (80:20) may be administered in certain patients for a short interval to reduce the work of breathing. This gas mixture is given by endotracheal tube or by a tightly fitting, nonrebreathing mask. Such treatment has been reported to decrease airway resistance in normal volunteers by 23% during quiet breathing and to decrease airway resistance by 49% during panting. This decrease in airway resistance may be explained by a reduction in gas density (the density of helium is roughly one-third that of oxygen or air), by elimination of turbulence downstream from the obstruction, and by a reduction in the tendency for the airways to collapse downstream from the obstruction.

12. What is the treatment of trauma to the upper airway?

In complete airway obstruction, transtracheal jet ventilation is probably the best procedure. Various devices have been developed to facilitate this procedure. Basically, a catheter attached to a syringe is inserted into the trachea across the crycothyroid membrane. The transtracheal ventilation system is then attached to the intratracheal catheter. Surgical cricothyroidotomy (opening the cricothyroid membrane with a scalpel and inserting a small endotracheal tube) is an alternative treatment. A classic tracheotomy requires more skill and training and is not the standard technique for managing acute upper airway obstruction. Indeed, the presence of a severe contusion of the neck soft tissues may make tracheotomy particularly difficult. With less severe injuries, endotracheal intubation may exacerbate injuries.

Even in patients with minimal symptoms of airway obstruction, prophylactic intubation may need to be considered, particularly in patients who have suffered thermal burns.

In such cases, endotracheal intubation has to be atraumatic, so the use of a fibroscope may be helpful.

13. What is the treatment of epiglottitis in adult patients?
Endotracheal intubation should be performed early, once the diagnosis becomes clear. Inhalation anesthesia with 100% oxygen is preferable to the use of intravenous hypnotics and muscle relaxants in order for the patient to maintain spontaneous breathing during the whole procedure. Monitoring of oxyhemoglobin saturation with pulse oximetry is highly desirable. After intubation, secure fixation of the endotracheal tube is mandatory. There is no need for mechanical ventilation if the lungs are not involved. Patients should receive antibiotics effective against *Hemophilus influenzae* and may usually be extubated within 2 or 3 days when an air leak exists around the endotracheal tube with a deflated cuff.

14. What is the treatment for laryngeal edema secondary to anaphylaxis?
The management of acute anaphylactic reactions is described in chapter 97 (p. 385) and will not be repeated here. Briefly, the management of severe cases includes endotracheal intubation, or cricothyroidotomy if necessary, and intravenous epinephrine (0.2–0.5 mg). In milder cases, 0.3 mg of epinephrine subcutaneously may be sufficient. The use of corticosteroids and antihistamines is of secondary importance in the acute care of these patients.

BIBLIOGRAPHY

1. Curtis JL, Mahlmeister M, Fink JB, et al: Helium-oxygen gas therapy: Use and availability for the emergency treatment of inoperable airway obstruction. Chest 90:455–457, 1986.
2. DeWeese EL, Sullivan TY, Yu PL: Ventilatory and occlusion pressure responses to helium breathing. J Appl Physiol 54:1525–1531, 1983.
3. Jacobson S: Upper airway obstruction. Emerg Med Clin North Am 7:205–217, 1989.
4. Jorden RC: Airway management. Emerg Med Clin North Am 6:671–686, 1988.
5. Jorden RC: Percutaneous transtracheal ventilation. Emerg Med Clin North Am 6:745–752, 1988.
6. Walls RM: Cricothyroidotomy. Emerg Med Clin North Am 6:725–736, 1988.

96. MONITORING IN THE OPERATING ROOM

Jean-François Pittet, M.D.

1. What monitoring is necessary for patients scheduled for major surgery?
Monitoring patients scheduled for major surgery (>3 hours, blood loss more than 10%, or surgery involving the lungs, central nervous system, or cardiovascular system) should include ECG, pulse oximetry, direct arterial and central venous pressure measurements (in certain patients pulmonary pressure and cardiac output measurements), capnography, urine output and body temperature recording, blood loss measurement, blood gas analysis, serum electrolytes determinations, and clotting tests. In addition, monitoring of neuromuscular function may be suitable, particularly in patients with liver and renal diseases.

2. What is the significance of pulse oximetry and capnography in the OR?
The most preventable disaster in the OR is patient hypoxia, mostly due to the failure to provide adequate ventilation. Therefore, monitoring of patient oxygenation by pulse oximetry and alveolar ventilation by capnography is essential.

3. Can routine use of pulse oximetry facilitate the diagnosis of hypoxia and decrease the incidence of complications during and after anesthesia?
Yes. Two recent studies suggest that the routine use of pulse oximetry in the OR may allow the diagnosis of hypoxia before clinical signs are present and therefore decrease the incidence of major hypoxemic events.

4. What information can a capnograph provide to the anesthesiologist?
Capnography is useful to detect malpositioning of the endotracheal tube, a disconnected breathing circuit, or lack of perfusion of the lungs.

5. What is the normal alveolar-arterial CO_2 gradient?
The alveolar-arterial CO_2 gradient for normal lungs is 2 mm Hg.

6. What does an increase in end-tidal CO_2 concentration measured by capnography mean?
A **gradual increase** in end-tidal CO_2 ($ETCO_2$), without a change in the morphology of the capnograph curve, may be associated with a partial airway obstruction, a rise in body temperature (consider the possibility of malignant hyperthermia!), or a leak in the breathing circuit with hypoventilation. If the increase in $ETCO_2$ is associated with an increase in the baseline value, the possibility of rebreathing the previously exhaled CO_2 should be considered. A **sudden increase** in $ETCO_2$ usually corresponds to an increased CO_2 load transported to lungs for excretion (i.e., sodium bicarbonate administration, release of a tourniquet).

7. What does a decrease in end-tidal CO_2 concentration measured by capnography mean?
A **gradual decrease** in $ETCO_2$ may correspond to a fall in body temperature, slowly decreasing systemic or pulmonary perfusion, or hyperventilation. A **sudden decrease** in $ETCO_2$ may be caused by a cardiac arrest, severe pulmonary hypoperfusion, or embolism.

8. What are the sources of inaccuracy in capnograph monitoring?
    1. Increasing the breathing frequency to more than 15/min may decrease the accuracy of $ETCO_2$ to predict $PaCO_2$, due to the slow response time of many current devices.
    2. Although the alveolar-arterial CO_2 gradient is very low (2 mm Hg), the following factors may affect this gradient: inspired oxygen concentration, tidal volume, inspiratory/ expiratory time ratio, hypotension, and lung disease. In anesthetized patients with lung disease, this gradient may increase up to 13 mm Hg.

9. What information can the EKG provide to the anesthesiologist?
In the operating room, the electrocardiogram may be used as a heart-meter to detect and characterize arrhythmias and to provide some indication of myocardial ischemia.

10. Is the EKG a good indicator of the adequacy of the circulation?
No. The EKG does not provide any indication of the adequacy of the circulation, and may give a false sense of security if it is used as the only continuous monitor of the circulation.

11. What EKG leads should be used in OR?
To detect **myocardial ischemia**, a V lead can be of particular value. If the EKG is designed for monitoring bipolar limb leads only, a modified V_5 lead may be used. A classical

modified V_5 is CM_5: the right arm electrode of lead I is placed over the manubrium sterni, the left arm electrode is placed over the V_5 position (left anterior axillary line of the fifth intercostal space), and the ground electrode is placed on the left shoulder. Moreover, the sensitivity of EKG for detecting ischemia is related to the number of leads used: more ischemic changes are detected with a 12-lead system than with a regional 3-lead system.

Accuracy in detecting **arrhythmias** is improved by using a variety of leads. Of primary importance is the presence and configuration of the P wave. The EKG must also allow the determination of the QRS form. To distinguish between right and left bundle branch block patterns, a V_1 lead may be useful.

12. What are the two methods of monitoring blood pressure in the OR? What are the advantages and disadvantages of each?

Arterial pressure can be monitored by direct arterial cannulation or by Doppler measurements. Direct measurement of arterial pressure requires arterial invasion but also allows blood gas sampling for accuracy. The pressure transducer is accurately calibrated, the transducer is at the same level as the patient, and the pressure transducer has been zeroed. The Doppler measurements of arterial pressure are accurate and noninvasive. The pressure exerted by the inflated cuff may cause peripheral nerve injury of the arm.

13. Do changes in respiratory pressures influence the measurement of the right atrial pressure?

Yes, particularly in patients with low right atrial pressure and low lung compliance. As a result, right atrial pressure may be overestimated or underestimated (with controlled and spontaneous respiration, respectively) by as much as 4 mm Hg. The most accurate measurement may be obtained by determining the pressure at the peak of the a-wave, at the end of expiration, with a lung volume equal to the functional residual capacity.

14. What are the temperature differences between different regions of the body?

Oral and axillary temperatures are usually about 0.4 and 0.7° C, respectively, lower than pulmonary artery temperature. Esophageal temperature is similar to PA temperature, and rectal temperature is about 0.25° C greater than PA temperature.

15. What is the rationale for monitoring neuromuscular transmission during general anesthesia?

Up to 40% of patients entering the recovery room may have inadequate neuromuscular transmission. Inadequate recovery from neuromuscular blockade also has been identified as an important factor in anesthesia-related mortality because patients vary extensively in their sensitivity to nondepolarizing muscle relaxants.

16. How can the neuromuscular transmission be assessed in the OR?

The classic assessment of neuromuscular transmission is based on the electrical stimulation of the ulnar nerve (using a monophasic rectangular pulse lasting 0.2 msec) and the measurement of the electrical or mechanical response of the corresponding muscle (adductor pollicis). Although the use of a nerve stimulator is always advantageous during general anesthesia, it is the most useful in patients with renal or liver disease in the period just before and immediately after the reversal of competitive neuromuscular blockade, and in the assessment of patients with hypoventilation after surgery.

BIBLIOGRAPHY

1. Cooper JB, Cullen DJ, Nemeskal R, et al: Effects of information feedback and pulse oximetry on the incidence of anesthesia complications. Anesthesiology 67:686, 1987.

2. Cote CJ, Goldstein EA, Cote MA, et al: A single blind study of pulse oximetry in children. Anesthesiology 68:184, 1988.
3. Ilsley AH, Rutten AJ, Runciman WB: An evaluation of blood pressure measurement. Anesth Intens Care 9:314, 1981.
4. Lunn JN, Hunter AR, Scott DB: Anaesthesia related surgical mortality. Anesthesia 38:1090, 1982.
5. Runciman WB. Monitoring. In Nimmo WS, Smith G (eds): Anesthesia. London, Blackwell Scientific Publications, 1989, pp 460–491.
6. Runciman WB, Rutten AJ, Ilsley AH: An evaluation of blood pressure measurement. Anesth Intens Care 9:314, 1981.
7. Schnapp LM, Cohen NH. Pulse Oximetry: Uses and abuses. Chest 98:1244, 1990.
8. Sykes MK. Essential monitoring. Br J Anaesth 59:901, 1987.
9. Tiret L, Desmonts LM, Hatton F, et al: Complications associated with anesthesia—a prospective study in France. Can Anesth Soc J 33:336, 1986.
10. Vibe-Mogensen J, Chraemmer-Jorgensen B, Ording H: Residual curarization in the recovery room. Anesthesiology 50:539, 1979.
11. Whitesell R, Asidao C, Gollman D, et al: Relationship between arterial and peak expired carbon dioxide pressure during anesthesia and factors influencing the difference. Anesth Analg 60:508, 1981.

97. COMPLICATIONS OF GENERAL ANESTHESIA

Jean-François Pittet, M.D.

1. What is the incidence of complications due to general anesthesia?

In a review of 112,000 anesthetic procedures, Cohen et al. reported an 8–10% rate of complications during and after general anesthesia; the incidence of life-threatening complications was less than 1%. Many postoperative problems described as complications of anesthesia are a combination of preexisting disease and extent of surgery, regardless of the anesthetic technique.

2. What are the causes of CNS dysfunction after general anesthesia?

CNS dysfunction may be due to decreased oxygen availability, increased oxygen consumption, or a specific drug effect. Decreased oxygen availability is the most common cause and results generally from problems with anesthesia equipment. The increased use of monitors to measure the oxygenation (as pulse oximeters) should reduce the incidence of this tragic complication.

3. What measures should be taken if a patient suffers a cerebral insult during general anesthesia?

First, attempt to keep the patient hemodynamically stable. The following techniques specific to resuscitation of the brain may be used: (1) Improve cerebral perfusion pressure by maintaining an adequate systemic arterial pressure. (2) Lower intracranial pressure by decreasing cerebral blood flow by increasing the respiratory rate (thereby decreasing arterial PCO_2) and decreasing free brain water with diuretics (mannitol, furosemide). (3) Improve venous return by keeping the head elevated to 30° or greater and by avoiding positive end-expiratory pressure if oxygenation is not compromised. (4) Administer drugs to decrease the cerebral metabolic rate (barbiturates, phenytoin).

4. What causes changes in heart rate during general anesthesia?

Abnormalities in heart rate are defined as a sinus rhythm less than 50 beats/min (bradycardia) or more than 100 beats/min (tachycardia). In general, tachycardia is more deleterious, due to the reduction of diastolic filling time of the coronary circulation. The cause of sinus tachycardia is usually increased sympathetic activity secondary to inadequate anesthesia. Preoperative conditions such as anxiety, cardiac disease, fever, burns, or hyperthyroidism may also cause tachycardia. Intraoperatively, drug effect (atropine, pancuronium, isoflurane), hyperthermia, thyroid storm, and pheochromocytoma should be considered in the differential diagnosis.

Bradycardia is important when the decrease in cardiac output leads to impairment of organ perfusion. The most common causes are increased vagal tone from traction or pressure on body tissues with vagal innervation (i.e., mesenteric traction), and drug effects (i.e., suxamethonium, halothane, high-dose opioids). Treatment includes stopping the vagal stimulus, administering IV atropine (0.5–1 mg), and reducing the inspired concentration of the halogenated agent.

5. Which arrhythmias should be treated?

Cardiac dysrhythmias may occur in 60% or more of patients undergoing anesthesia when continuous methods are used for surveillance. All arrhythmias produce some decrease in cardiac output and should be treated if there is a significant decrease in cardiac output. Treatment should be instituted for arrhythmias causing hypotension, or those resulting in myocardial ischemia, or when ventricular fibrillation or asystole is present.

6. What is the treatment of supraventricular tachyarrhythmias observed during general anesthesia?

Treatment depends on the rate and rhythm and the degree of decrease in cardiac output. Adequate oxygenation and ventilation and sufficient anesthetic depth are of paramount importance. If the arrhythmia persists, IV adenosine (6–12 mg) may be the drug of choice. Verapamil (5 mg infused over 1–2 min) and propranolol (0.5–1 mg IV) may also be used to slow the ventricular response.

7. Can general anesthesia make preexisting conduction blocks worse?

Yes. In such cases, the risk of asystole and sudden death must be weighed against the morbidity of placing a temporary or permanent pacemaker. Pacing is not indicated in asymptomatic patients with type I AV block or congenital heart block. Patients with asymptomatic type II AV block as well as those with symptomatic bradycardia require a pacemaker.

8. Are ventricular arrhythmias common during general anesthesia?

Yes. The most frequent cause is sympathetic overactivity of endogenous or exogenous origin. Endogenous causes are anxiety, primary hypertension, pheochromocytoma, and surgical stimulation. Exogenous causes are hypoxia, hypercapnia, and drug interactions (i.e., epinephrine and volatile anesthetics). Lidocaine (IV bolus of 50–100 mg) is the drug of choice for emergency treatment of acute ventricular arrhythmias.

9. Do electrolytes disturbances induce ventricular arrhythmias?

Yes, specifically acute hypokalemia. Hyperventilation lowers serum potassium by 0.5 mmol/L for every 9.7 mm Hg reduction in $PaCO_2$. The safe level of serum potassium is around 3.5 mmol/L, and may be higher in patients taking digitalis or with ischemic myocardial disease. Oral replacement consists of 25 mmol KCl every 6–8 hr. Intravenous administration of KCl should not exceed 0.5 mmol $\cdot$ kg^{-1} $\cdot$ hr^{1} or 240 mmol/24 hr for patients with normal renal function. Transport of potassium in cells is facilitated by concomitant administration of 10% glucose with insulin (0.5 unit/2 gm of glucose). EKG monitoring is essential during this treatment.

10. Does cardiac arrest occur without preceding signs during general anesthesia?
Generally, there are warning signs. Cardiac arrest is normally preceded by a progressive bradycardia. The incidence of cardiac arrest during general anesthesia is estimated to be 6–10 per 10,000 anesthesia. The most important causes include overdose of anesthetics, inadequate ventilation, long periods of hypotension, or anaphylactoid reaction to anesthetic agents or other drugs.

11. What is the risk of myocardial infarction (MI) during anesthesia?
The risk of MI is low (0.1%) in patients without preoperative cardiac disease. In patients with a previous MI, the risk decreases as the time interval to surgery increases. During the first 3 months after an MI, the risk of reinfarction during anesthesia is 5–6%, with an overall mortality of 35% for a patient optimally monitored and treated. This risk decreases to 2% after 6 months. Elderly patients (more than 70 years old) undergoing noncardiac surgery who have chronic stable angina, previous MI, or EKG signs of myocardial ischemia are at increased risk for perioperative MI or cardiac death. In patients with coronary artery disease, early postoperative myocardial ischemia is an important correlate of adverse cardiac outcome. These recent studies suggest that prevention and therapy for preoperative and postoperative myocardial ischemia may be important to reduce perioperative cardiac morbidity.

12. Does anesthetic technique play a significant role in the development of perioperative MI?
No. No study has demonstrated a difference in the risk of perioperative MI between patients undergoing general or regional anesthesia with sufficient intravenous sedation. The general aim with either technique is to maintain a slightly depressed mean arterial pressure and to avoid tachycardia, hypertension, and severe hypotension.

13. What are the most important causes of changes in systemic arterial pressure during anesthesia?
The causes of arterial hypotension during anesthesia include a change in cardiac rate, rhythm or contractility, a decrease in systemic vascular resistance, or a decrease in circulating blood volume. The causes of arterial hypertension during general anesthesia include increased cardiac contractility or increased systemic vascular resistance. The latter is the result of increased sympathetic tone, either endogenous (anxiety, pain) or exogenous (inadequate anesthesia, ketamine).

14. What are the most important respiratory complications observed during general anesthesia?
Laryngospasm, bronchospasm, obstruction of the endotracheal tube, and pneumothorax.

15. What are the causes and treatment of laryngospasm?
Laryngospasm may result from edema of the airway, a reflex response to local irritation (i.e., presence of secretions), or inadequate anesthesia. Laryngospasm may be partial or complete. Partial spasm is audible if the airway has narrowed to 4 mm or less (in adults). Treatment includes ventilation with 100% oxygen and a low level PEEP (5 cm H_2O), correction of the cause, and deepening of anesthesia. A short-acting neuromuscular blocking agent may be used to relieve the spasm.

16. What are the causes and treatment of bronchospasm?
Factors predisposing to bronchospasm include preoperative wheezing, endotracheal intubation of inadequately anesthetized patient, placement of the endotracheal tube near or

at the carina, surgical stimulus, or aspiration of gastric contents. Treatment includes ventilation with 100% oxygen and aerosol of a beta-agonist through the endotracheal tube to relieve the spasm. Increasing the concentration of volatile anesthetics is helpful, although halothane has the potential of causing cardiac arrhythmias in a hypoxic, hypercapnic patient. Isoflurane is probably the volatile agent least likely to trigger such arrhythmias.

17. When is a pneumothorax a problem intraoperatively?
A small pleural leak will rapidly increase under the effect of positive pressure ventilation and the influx of nitrous oxide into the pleural space. Pneumothoraces frequently accompany central line placements, nephrectomies, thoracotomies, median sternotomies, and abdominal procedures adjacent to the diaphragm.

18. Does anesthesia contribute to postoperative abnormalities in gas exchange?
Yes. Postoperative abnormalities in gas exchange present in two temporal patterns:
   1. Transient postoperative hypoxemia is mostly due to the reduction of the postoperative hypoxic and hypercapnic drive induced by narcotics used for induction and maintenance of anesthesia (particularly in elderly patients), a residual effect of muscle relaxants used intraoperatively, the loss of pulmonary hypoxic vasoconstrictive reflexes following the administration of volatile anesthetic agents, and increased oxygen consumption due to hypertonic muscles and shivering.
   2. A second pattern lasts several hours to days, due to the effect of anesthesia and surgery on the chest-wall system, and this pattern appears to be an important factor contributing to the postoperative morbidity of anesthesia and surgery.

19. What is the effect of general anesthesia on the lung–chest-wall system?
Induction of anesthesia, within 5 minutes, causes the development of compression atelectasis in the dependent part of the lung in 90% of supine subjects without preexisting lung diseases. Application of 10 cm H_2O of PEEP eliminates the atelectasis, which then reappears within 1 minute after discontinuation of PEEP. Compression atelectasis is due to a reduction in functional residual capacity, probably secondary to the relaxation of the chest wall muscles (rib cage and diaphragm) caused by the induction of anesthesia.

20. Does a correlation exist between the extent of atelectasis and impairment of gas exchange during anesthesia?
Yes. In subjects with healthy lungs, a strong correlation was found during anesthesia between the amount of atelectasis and the percentage of shunt. In patients who did not develop atelectasis, there was no increase in shunt and no impairment of gas exchange during general anesthesia.

21. What is the most frequent cause of postoperative nausea?
The presence of nitrous oxide in the stomach is one of the major causes of postoperative nausea. At an alveolar nitrous oxide concentration of 75%, bowel volume increases by 0.5 L/hr. Another important cause of postoperative nausea is the administration of narcotics for postoperative analgesia.

22. Does the anesthetic technique influence the liver blood supply?
Yes. Both regional and general anesthesia produce a decrease in hepatic blood flow in a dose-dependent fashion. If volatile anesthetic agents are used, isoflurane is the drug of choice to ensure maintenance of hepatic oxygenation. As hypocapnia also decreases hepatic blood flow, arterial PCO_2 should be carefully controlled.

23. Does anesthesia influence the immune response of the patient?

Yes. Anesthesia may produce underactivity or overactivity of the immune response. All anesthetic agents produce a short-term and reversible decrease in chemotactic migration, phagocytic activity, and bactericidal function of neutrophils. However, antibody production remains unchanged. The drug the most frequently implicated is nitrous oxide, which inactivates the methionine synthetase, leading to oxidation of vitamin B_{12}, an important compound in DNA synthesis.

Overactivity of the immune system during general anesthesia is characterized by anaphylactoid reactions to intravenous anesthetic agents. Specific mechanisms by which the majority of anaphylactoid reactions occur are anaphylaxis (type 1 hypersensitivity), activation of complement system (classic or alternate pathway activation), and direct histamine liberation. Irrespective of the initial mechanism, the final pathway of an anaphylactoid response is the degranulation of mast cells with release of mediator substances. Mediator release is triggered by calcium transport through specific channels into the mast cells. Mediators are preformed or membrane-derived. Preformed granule substances include histamine, eosinophil chemotactic factors of anaphylaxis (ECF-A), and neutrophil chemotactic factor. Membrane-derived factors are leukotrienes and prostaglandins, both formed from arachidonic acid as part of the process that triggers calcium influx.

24. When are such anaphylactoid reactions observed?

More than 90% of reactions occur within 5 minutes after drug administration. Delayed hypersensitivity (type 4) reactions are rare.

25. What are the target organs of anaphylactoid reactions during general anesthesia?

Principal target organs are the skin, and the cardiovascular, respiratory, and gastrointestinal systems. Skin is involved in 75% of major hypersensitivity reactions (erythema with or without urticaria or angiodema). Hypotension occurs in 80% of patients due to H1- and H2-receptor activation and intravascular volume depletion secondary to translocation of fluid by capillary leakage. Cardiac arrhythmias are reported in 10–15% of patients as a result of effect of histamine on cardiac conduction system, endogenous release and exogenous administration of catecholamines, concurrent administration of volatile anesthetic agents, and presence of hypoxia, hypercarbia, and acidosis. Bronchospasm occurs in 30% of patients. It is mediated by the effect of histamine on H1 bronchial smooth muscle receptors, prostaglandins D_2 and F_2-alpha, and leukotrienes C_4 and D_4. Pulmonary edema occurs rarely. Abdominal pain, diarrhea, and vomiting are frequent during the recovery period, possibly due to a histamine-enhanced peristaltic activity.

26. Which drugs are implicated in anesthetic anaphylactoid reactions?

Although all agents given during general anesthesia may induce the release of mediators from mast cells, the following agents are most frequently implicated in major anaphylactoid reactions: neuromuscular blocking agents (suxamethonium, alcuronium, gallamine, and tubocurarine), barbiturates (thiopental and methohexital), colloid solutions (gelatin, dextrans, hetastarch), local anesthetics (procaine), and a polyoxylated castor oil (Cremophor EL) used to solubilize many anesthetic agents.

BIBLIOGRAPHY

1. Atlee JL, Bosnjack ZJ: Mechanisms for cardiac dysrhythmias during anesthesia. Anesthesiology 72:347–374, 1990.
2. Cohen MM, Duncan PG, Pope WDB, Wolkenstein C: A survey of 112,000 anesthetics at one teaching hospital (1975–1983). Can Anaesth Soc J 33:22, 1986.
3. Davies JM: Complications of general anesthesia. In Nimmo WS, Smith G (eds): Anesthesia. London, Blackwell Scientific Publications, 1989, pp 502–521.

4. Frost AM: Management of head injury. Can Anaesth Soc J 32:S32, 1985.
5. Haagensen R, Steen PA: Perioperative myocardial infarction. Br J Anaesth 61:24, 1988.
6. Mangano DT, Browner WS, Hollenberg M, et al: Association of perioperative myocardial ischemia with cardiac morbidity and mortality in men undergoing noncardiac surgery. N Engl J Med 323:1781, 1990.
7. McGovern B: Hypokalemia and cardiac arrhythmias. Anesthesiology 63:127, 1985.
8. Palazzo MGA, Strunin L: Anesthesia and emesis. I. Etiology. Can Anaesth Soc J 31:178, 1984.
9. Rao TLK, Jacobs KH, El-Etr AA: Reinfarction following anesthesia in patients with myocardial infarction. Anesthesiology 59:449, 1983.
10. Shah KB, Kleinman BS, Rao TLK, et al: Angina and other risk factors in patients with cardiac diseases undergoing noncardiac operations. Anesth Analg 70:240, 1990.

98. MALIGNANT HYPERTHERMIA

Jean-François Pittet, M.D.

1. What is malignant hyperthermia?

Malignant hyperthermia (MH) is a myopathy, usually subclinical, that induces acute loss of intracellular control of calcium. Normally, the wave of depolarization transferred to the sarcoplasmic reticulum results in the release of calcium. This increase in cytoplasmic calcium removes the troponin inhibition from the contractile elements, resulting in muscle contraction. Then, intracellular calcium pumps rapidly transfer calcium back into the sarcoplasmic reticulum, resulting in relaxation when the Ca^{++} concentration is less than the mechanical threshold. MH is characterized by this alteration of the sarcoplasmic reticulum, resulting in an abnormal release of calcium. This leads to a massive increase in the energy demand needed to maintain the cellular homeostasis of calcium.

2. What are the characteristics of this clinical syndrome?

The development of MH is characterized by a massive increase in aerobic and anaerobic metabolism, resulting in an intense production of heat, carbon dioxide, and lactate, and associated respiratory and metabolic acidosis. Whole body rigidity is observed in 75% of cases. Body temperature may exceed 43.5°C (109.4°F), $PaCO_2$ may be greater than 100 mm Hg, and arterial pH may be less than 7. Sympathetic hyperactivity is often the first sign of increased metabolism (tachycardia, sweating, hypertension). As MH progresses, cellular permeability may increase, with the development of hyperkalemia, hypercalcemia (ionized calcium), hypernatremia, and generalized edema, including acute cerebral edema. Finally MH may lead to disseminated intravascular coagulopathy, renal, liver and cardiac failure, and death.

3. Does the presence of one suggestive clinical sign indicate development of MH?

No. When clinical signs such as muscle rigidity, tachycardia, or fever are present, there is a close association with MH only if more than one of these signs is present. When there is only one suggestive clinical sign, the diagnosis is usually not MH.

4. Is this opinion also true when masseter spasm (trismus) is observed after the administration of succinylcholine?

Until recently, most people believed that trismus signified the development of MH in most patients. However, recent studies have documented a 1% incidence of trismus in children given succinylcholine after induction of anesthesia with halothane. None of these children developed MH. Therefore, some people believe that trismus may be a benign response in many cases and that anesthesia can be continued safely; however, nontriggering anesthetic agents should then be used. Some believe that anesthesia should be stopped and the patient carefully observed for other signs of MH. It is extremely important that patients who develop trismus undergo testing for MH susceptibility.

5. What causes an episode of MH?

The development of an acute episode of MH depends on three variables: a genetic predisposition (autosomal dominant with variable penetrance), the absence of inhibiting factors, and the presence of a sufficiently potent anesthetic or nonanesthetic trigger.

6. Which anesthetic drugs can trigger an acute episode of MH?

Halothane, enflurane, isoflurane, sevoflurane, methoxyflurane, cyclopropane, and ether, as well as succinylcholine and decamethonium.

7. What is the predictability and time course of an acute episode of MH?

MH-susceptible persons respond less predictably than swine to anesthetic triggers. Some patients may previously have tolerated potent anesthetic triggers without problem. The onset of MH can be acute and rapid, particularly during the induction of anesthesia when inhaled anesthetics or succinylcholine are used. However, the onset of MH may be delayed for hours and may be observed only when the patient is awake in the recovery room. This may be related to the use of induction agents or nondepolarizing muscle relaxants that delay or partially mask early manifestations of MH.

8. Is it possible to observe an episode of MH in awake patients?

Several findings suggest that human MH may be unrelated to anesthesia. In particular, MH-susceptible persons may have an increased incidence of unexplained sudden deaths. There is also a series of case reports relating heat stroke, sudden and unexpected death, unusual stress and fatigue, and myalgia to possible awake MH episodes. However, the incidence of such cases is rare and precautions are now recommended for anesthetic administration.

9. Is MH associated with other disorders?

Yes, particularly with other myopathies such as Duchenne's muscle dystrophy, central spinal cord disease, and a rare syndrome, the King-Denborough syndrome, which is characterized by short stature, musculoskeletal abnormalities, and mental retardation. There is also an inconstant association between MH and other disorders such as sudden infant death syndrome, neuroleptic malignant syndrome, or heat stroke.

10. What is the differential diagnosis of MH?

Other disorders with similar clinical signs such as hyperthyroidism, pheochromocytoma, neuroleptic malignant syndrome, and a rare familial fever syndrome must be excluded in patients in whom an acute episode of MH is suspected.

11. Does a specific treatment for MH exist?

Yes. Dantrolene sodium blocks the release, but not the reuptake, of calcium from the sarcoplasmic reticulum. To be effective, the patient must have adequate muscle perfusion. Dantrolene has no serious side effects when given for a short period of time.

12. What is the therapy for an acute episode of MH?

(1) Discontinue all anesthetic agents and hyperventilate the patient with 100% oxygen.
(2) Give dantrolene, 2 mg/kg every 5 minutes to a total dose of 10 mg/kg. Dantrolene should probably be repeated every 10–15 hours for several doses until no signs of recurrence

are present. (3) Administer sodium bicarbonate, 2–4 mEq/kg, to control the continuous production of lactate by skeletal muscles. (4) Control fever by all disposable means (ice fluids, surface cooling, cooling of body cavities, eventually heat exchanger). (5) Monitor urine output to prevent acute tubular necrosis. (6) Some recommend steroids in large doses. (7) Perform blood studies: electrolytes, liver profile, BUN, lactate, glucose, coagulation profile, and serum and urine hemoglobin and myoglobin.

13. If present, how should acute hyperkalemia be treated?
In MH, hyperkalemia should be treated slowly. The most effective way to decrease serum potassium level is reversal of MH by effective doses of dantrolene. The administration of calcium is indicated only for related arrhythmias or poor cardiac function.

14. Which drugs are ineffective for treating MH?
Calcium and beta-sympathetic antagonists. Calcium antagonists act primarily on surface membranes of cardiac or smooth muscles. They do not increase the survival of MH-susceptible swine and may interact with dantrolene to produce hyperkalemia. Beta-sympathetic antagonists do not increase the survival of MH-susceptible swine and may prevent the increase in myocrdial oxygen consumption. This is not desirable because increased cardiac function is necessary for survival during an acute episode of MH.

15. Is it necessary to administer dantrolene before giving anesthesia for MH-susceptible patients?
The present consensus is not to administer dantrolene preoperatively in most instances because the use of nontriggering anesthetic agents is associated with uneventful anesthesia. If dantrolene is administered, it should be given intravenously (2 mg/kg) just before the induction of anesthesia. Orally administered dantrolene requires higher dosage with the risk of prolonged weakness or enhancement of the effects of nondepolarizing muscle relaxants.

16. Are some anesthetics safe for MH-susceptible patients?
Yes. In MH-susceptible patients, anesthesia should consist of nitrous oxide, barbiturates, opiates, tranquilizers, and nondepolarizing muscle relaxants. Etomidate and propofol are probably safe but their use in MH-susceptible patients has not been reported.

17. Is regional anesthesia safe for MH-susceptible patients?
Yes. Regional anesthesia may be preferred for some surgical procedures in MH-susceptible patients.

18. Is it true that amide anesthetics should be considered dangerous in MH-susceptible patients?
No. Several reports demonstrated lack of danger of amide anesthetics for MH-susceptible patients. It is true that amide anesthetics may increase the efflux of calcium from the sarcoplasmic reticulum. However, these effects require millimolar concentrations of these drugs, much greater than the plasma values achieved in clinical usage.

19. Is it necessary to provide an uncontaminated anesthesia machine for MH-susceptible patients (by flushing with oxygen for many hours)?
No. Removal of the vaporizers, replacement of the fresh gas outlet hose, and use of a disposable circle with a flush of 6 L/min for 5 minutes are sufficeint.

20. Which tests should be used to evaluate MH susceptibility?
Measurements of blood creatine phosphokinase (CK) level in the resting and fasting patient without recent trauma provide a basic screening tool. When blood CK concentration is

increased in a close relative, such a patient should be considered to be susceptible to MH. A normal blood CK level has no predictive value. In such cases, a muscle biopsy may be necessary for in vitro studies. Muscle biopsy studies are 95% reliable in predicting MH susceptibility, and no false-negative results have been reported.

BIBLIOGRAPHY

1. Brownell AKW: Malignant hyperthermia: Relationship to other diseases. Br J Anaesth 60:303, 1988.
2. Flewellen EH, Nelson TE, Jones WP, et al: Dantrolene dose response in awake man: Implications for management of malignant hyperthermia. Anesthesiology 59:275, 1983.
3. Gronert GA, Thompson RL, Onofrio BM: Human malignant hyperthermia: Awake episodes and correction by dantrolene. Anesth Analg 59:377, 1980.
4. Gronert GA, Theye RA: Halothane-induced porcine malignant hyperthermia: Metabolic and hemodynamic changes. Anesthesiology 44:36, 1976.
5. Gronert GA, Mott J, Lee J: Aetiology of malignant hyperthermia. Br J Anaesth 60:253, 1988.
6. Gronert GA, Rosenberg H: Management of patients in whom trismus occurs following succinyl-choline. Anesthesiology 68:653, 1988.
7. Gronert GA, Schulman SR, Mott J: Malignant hyperthermia. In Miller R (ed): Anesthesia. New York, Churchill Livingstone, 1990.
8. Harriman DGF: Malignant hyperthermia myopathy—a critical review. Br J Anaesth 60:309, 1988.
9. Harrison GG: Dantrolene—dynamics and kinetics. Br J Anaesth 60:279, 1988.
10. Larach MG, Rosenberg H, Larach DR, et al: Prediction of malignant hyperthermia susceptibility by clinical signs. Anesthesiology 66:547, 1987.
11. Ording H: Diagnosis of susceptibility to malignant hyperthermia in man. Br J Anaesth 60:287, 1986.
12. Rubin AS, Zablocki AD: Hyperkalemia, verapamil , and dantrolene. Anesthesiology 66:247, 1987.

XIV: Radiology

99. PORTABLE RADIOGRAPHY

Marsha J. Heinig, M.D., Ph.D.

1. When is a portable chest x-ray indicated for an ICU patient?
(1) Daily for patients on ventilators, as the physical examination is often difficult and unreliable. (2) Following invasive line placement (e.g., central venous catheter, endotracheal tube, nasogastric tube, or feeding tube). (3) For an abrupt change in clinical status.

2. Is there a justifiable diagnostic yield for the daily portable chest x-ray?
Yes. Unexpected findings in cardiopulmonary status or tube position have been reported in 35–65% of portable radiographs. Routine daily films significantly affect patient management in at least 24%.

3. What is the average radiation exposure for a single view of the chest?
Portable chest x-ray: 0.01–0.02 rads (average dose per view of the chest in the radiology department is 0.05 rads).

4. What is the most important source of radiation exposure from portable x-rays to personnel and other patients? What is the best way to minimize this exposure?
The largest source of radiation exposure is scatter from the patient. The best way to minimize exposure is to increase distance from the patient, remembering that radiation intensity decreases as $1/r^2$. A distance of 2 meters from the patient will decrease scattered radiation intensity to $1/10^6$ of the incident radiation. Thus, a distance of about 6 feet from the patient is considered safe.

5. What are the limitations of portable x-rays compared with posteroanterior and lateral films taken in the radiology department?
- Portable radiographs have less mediastinal penetration because they are taken at a lower kilovoltage. Thus, evaluation of the mediastinum is limited.
- Portable radiographs have less detail, less sharpness, and less signal to noise because they are obtained without a grid and with a faster film-screen combination to minimize motion. Thus, even nodules 1–2 cm in size or interstitial lung disease that may be obvious on radiographs obtained in the department may be completely invisible on portable x-ray.
- Exposures are difficult and often suboptimal. Phototiming is not available as it is in the radiology department.
- Motion is often present, which significantly degrades any image, owing to a combination of longer exposure time and limited degree of cooperation of a critically ill patient.
- Radiographs are often obtained with the patient in supine or semi-upright position, which has a significant effect on anatomy and diaphragm position. Thus, layering pneumothoraces or pleural effusions are easily missed.
- Degree of inspiration is often limited.

Thus, portable chest x-rays permit limited, gross evaluation of the lungs and pleura.

6. Are portable abdominal x-rays useful?
Portable abdominal films are extremely limited in value. Proper exposures are difficult and detail is lacking. Uncontrollable patient motion (breathing) is often present, destroying diagnostic quality. Portable abdominal films may be useful for checking tube placements, but are very poor for detail of bowel, intraabdominal organs or masses, or free air. If an abdominal problem is a significant clinical concern, the patient should be brought to the radiology department or a CT scan considered (see chapter 100).

7. What common errors in tube and line placements are seen radiographically? What should be checked on the portable film?
   1. **Chest tubes:** side holes (seen as a gap in the radiopaque marker) should be in the patient. The tube may be in the lung or a fissure (sometimes confirmable only by CT scan). A lateral film may be needed to demonstrate anterior or posterior position.
   2. **Endotracheal tubes:** most common malpositions are in the right main bronchus or esophagus. Esophageal position may be confirmed or ruled out by a film obtained in slight (about 25°) right posterior oblique position, which separates the trachea and esophagus.
   3. **Feeding tubes** may enter the right or left main bronchus, perforate the lung, and end up in the pleural space. Feeding tubes perforating the left main bronchus and ending up in the left pleural space have been mistaken for positioning in the stomach with fatal results following feeding.
   4. **Central venous catheters** may track into the internal jugular vein, left superior intercostal vein, or opposite brachiocephalic vein. Swan-Ganz catheters may coil in the superior vena cava, right atrium, etc. It is important to follow meticulously the course of all invasive lines.

8. What is the radiographic appearance of air space disease?
Fluffy or ill-defined infiltrates, extensive regions of consolidation (solid white appearance), and air bronchograms. Air bronchograms can be distinguished from spared aerated lung by the fact that bronchi become smaller as they branch peripherally.

9. What are the common causes of air-space filling disease (consolidation) in ICU patients? Can these be distinguished radiographically?
Edema (particularly from congestive heart failure or ARDS), atelectasis, pneumonia, and occasionally hemorrhage are common causes and cannot be distinguished radiographically. The time course of onset or clearing may be helpful to distinguish them.

10. How can pleural effusion be distinguished from parenchymal disease on a portable radiograph? What are some pitfalls in diagnosing pleural disease from a supine film?
Pleural effusion may cause a diffuse haze over a hemithorax, blunting of a costophrenic sulcus, or meniscus appearance of its border. A pleural effusion demonstrates no air bronchograms. Very importantly, a pleural effusion should change with position of the patient; therefore, upright or decubitus views are often helpful. Chronic pleural thickening, left lower lobe atelectasis (without air bronchograms), and a hazy hemidiaphragm from nonparallel beam orientation may simulate a pleural effusion.

11. What is the most common location for atelectasis in the ICU patient? What are its signs on a supine chest film?
Left lower lobe. Its signs are triangular density behind the heart, obscuration of the left hemidiaphragm, depression of the left hilum, air bronchograms, and occasionally obscuration of the left costophrenic sulcus. Subsegmental atelectasis appears as streaky regions of increased density sometimes referred to as "plate-like" atelectasis.

12. (a) Where does free pleural air commonly collect in a supine patient? (b) What are the signs of pneumothorax on a supine chest film? (c) Which views may help in the diagnosis of a pneumothorax?

(a) Free pleural air collects in the lower anterior chest, which is the highest point in the chest in a supine patient. Air, which is lighter than water or lung, will tend to collect at the highest point.

(b) Although a thin pleural line may be visualized over the apex or laterally, one must check the diaphragmatic surface. There may be a loculated lucency (black area) between the lung base and diaphragm. The **anterior sulcus sign** is lack of visualization of the normal hemidiaphragm and a very lucent lower hemithorax and upper abdomen. This may indicate a significant amount of tension.

(c) Upright, particularly expiratory, views and decubitus views with the side of interest up may help to demonstrate the thin visceral pleural line (white) displaced away from the chest wall.

13. (a) What are the characteristic features of pneumomediastinum? (b) Can it always be distinguished from pneumopericardium? (c) Which views may be helpful to distinguish pneumomediastinum from air in other spaces? (d) What causes a pneumomediastinum in the critically ill patient?

(a) A pneumomediastinum usually appears as a thin lucency (black area), usually along the left heart border and extending superiorly along the left mediastinal contour. Just lateral to this thin lucency is a thin white line that represents the displaced parietal pleura. Streaky lucencies may be seen extending into the neck.

(b) A pneumomediastinum can be difficult to distinguish from pneumopericardium, but pneumomediastinum is much more common. If the lucent air extends above the origins of the great vessels (where the pericardium ends), it is mediastinal. If the air is continuous under the heart, it is probably pericardial.

(c) A cross-table lateral view may be very helpful in demonstrating air outlining the anterior mediastinum and extending above the origin of the ascending aorta. A decubitus view (usually left side up) may help distinguish a pneumomediastinum from a medial pneumothorax, as the air should shift laterally if it is pleural.

(d) The most common cause of pneumomediastinum in the ICU patient is barotrauma. The mechanism is rupture of an alveolus with escape of air into the peribronchovascular interstitium, which then tracks centrally to the hilum and thence to the mediastinum. In the trauma patient, early or delayed development of a pneumomediastinum is worrisome for a bronchial rupture.

14. What is the radiographic appearance of acute respiratory distress syndrome (ARDS)?
Initially, ARDS looks like fluid overload, with interstitial edema manifested by fuzzy bronchovascular markings and septal lines. With progression, there is patchy air-space filling disease, with fluffy infiltrates. Finally, there is dense consolidation with a characteristic (but not pathognomonic) appearance. A combination of interstitial and air-space processes produces a ground-glass appearance that is quite homogeneous. The fact that all parts of the lungs look the same helps to distinguish ARDS from pneumonia, which tends to be patchy, or edema, which tends to be central.

15. What are the common signs of pneumoperitoneum on a supine abdominal radiograph?
- **Football sign**—free air collecting in the mid abdomen (highest point; seen only with massive pneumoperitoneum).
- Very well-defined bowel wall appearing as a stark white line (about 2–3 mm thick) representing air on both sides of the bowel wall.

- Air surrounding structures that are not usually seen. The falciform ligament may be visualized as an oblique white line just to the right of the spine in the right upper quadrant. The liver edge, or Morrison's pouch, may be unusually well defined.

16. What is the most sensitive view for demonstrating a pneumoperitoneum?

An upright chest x-ray in the radiology department is the most sensitive. It may demonstrate as little as 1–2 ml of free air. An "upright" portable film is significantly less sensitive. In the ICU setting, a left-side-down decubitus view is helpful. It will demonstrate small amounts of free air collecting lateral to the liver, whose soft tissue density provides good contrast. However, the patient must be on his left side for *at least* 10 minutes to allow air to flow to the least dependent position.

17. What are the characteristic plain film findings of mechanical small bowel obstruction? How is it distinguished from adynamic ileus?

The characteristic finding of either mechanical obstruction or adynamic ileus is dilatation of bowel (diameter greater than 3 cm). Mechanical small bowel obstruction often demonstrates differential air-fluid levels with a stair-step appearance on upright or decubitus views: there may or may not be gas in the colon, which is not dilated. In adynamic ileus, the colon is often dilated as well and there tends to be less fluid. However, the distinction may not always be made. Dilated, fluid-filled loops of small bowel are difficult or impossible to identify on plain films. A left-side-down, vertical-beam radiograph may be helpful to demonstrate air in the rectum and exclude low colonic obstruction.

18. What is the gastrointestinal contrast agent of choice for demonstration of a small bowel obstruction?

Barium (approximately 60% w/v). High-osmolarity water-soluble contrast (meglumine diatrizoate, Gastrografin) is osmotically active and becomes very dilute in the small bowel, resulting in difficulty in demonstrating the point of obstruction. Gastrografin is contraindicated in small bowel obstruction because of induction of significant fluid and electrolyte abnormalities due to outpouring of fluid into the small bowel with the high osmotic load. There is also a risk of aspiration into the lungs in the critically ill patient, which can result in significant chemical pneumonitis, pulmonary edema, and occasionally death.

CONTROVERSY

19. What is the best method for localizing a pleural effusion?

a. (Decubitus) chest x-ray
   Advantages: Inexpensive; easily performed at bedside.
   Disadvantages: Difficult to mark fluid for drainage.
b. Ultrasound
   Advantages: Can be performed portably; site of pleural effusion can be marked on the skin for thoracentesis; more sensitive for small pleural effusions.
   Disadvantages: Difficult to find loculated effusion: somewhat operator dependent for small effusions; hypoechoic abdominal structures or peritoneal fluid may be mistaken for pleural fluid.
c. CT
   Advantages: Extremely sensitive; localization is accurate; may be used to guide placement of percutaneous drainage catheters.
   Disadvantages: Expensive; patients must be transported to CT suite.

BIBLIOGRAPHY

1. Bekemeyer WB, Crapo RO, Calhoon S, et al: Efficacy of chest radiography in a respiratory intensive care unit. Chest 88:691, 1985.
2. Goodman LR, Putman CE: Intensive Care Radiology. St. Louis, C.V. Mosby, 1978.
3. Iannuzzi M, Petty TL: The diagnosis, pathogenesis, and treatment of adult respiratory distress syndrome. J Thorac Imag 1:1, 1986.
4. Kohan JM, Poe RH, Israel RH, et al: Value of chest ultrasonography versus decubitus roentgenography for thoracentesis. Am Rev Respir Dis 133:1124, 1986.
5. Ovenfors CO, Hedgcock MW: Intensive care unit radiology: Problems of interpretation. Radiol Clin North Am 16:407, 1978.
6. Rhea JT, VanSonnenberg E, McLoud TC: Basilar pneumothorax in the supine adult. Radiology 133:593, 1979.
7. Smith GM, Reed JC, Choplin RH: Radiographic detection of esophageal malpositioning of endotracheal tubes. AJR 154:23, 1990.
8. Swensen SJ, Peters SG, Leroy AJ, et al: Radiology in the intensive care unit. Mayo Clin Proc 66:396, 1991.
9. Wechsler RJ, Steiner RM, Kinori I: Monitoring the monitors: The radiology of thoracic catheters, wires, and tubes. Semin Roentgenol 23:61, 1988.
10. Zylak CJ, Littleton JT, Durizch ML: Illusory consolidation of the left lower lobe: A pitfall of portable radiography. Radiology 167:653, 1988.

100. CT SCANNING IN THE ICU SETTING

Marsha J. Heinig, M.D., Ph.D.

1. Is CT scanning of the chest useful in the ICU patient, especially considering problems of patient transport, monitoring, etc?

Yes. In select groups of patients, CT scanning has contributed additional information and altered management in up to 70% of those scanned.

2. What are indications for CT scanning of the chest in the ICU patient?

- When clinical course is not explained by plain chest x-ray findings.
- To distinguish pleural from parenchymal disease; diagnosis of lung abscess vs. empyema.
- To determine presence or position of a pneumothorax, particularly a loculated one, and document position of chest tubes.
- To further define equivocal findings on plain x-ray: for example, possible cavity or pneumatocele vs. spared lung, pulmonary nodules, possible mediastinal abnormalities.

3. How does CT scanning of the chest add information not readily detectable by portable radiography?

The combination of contrast resolution over a wide range of densities and thin (usually 1 cm or less) axial sectioning provides excellent anatomic detail of the mediastinum, lungs, and pleura. The problem of confusing, overlapping shadows is eliminated.

4. What are some findings on chest CT scans that may be unsuspected on portable chest radiographs and that may significantly affect patient management?

Pneumothorax, pleural effusion, pericardial effusion, lung abscess, cavity, lung laceration, empyema, mediastinal abnormalities (hematoma, adenopathy, abscess), atelectasis (especially left upper lobe, which may be difficult to evaluate on a plain AP portable film), and abnormal chest tube position. Occasionally, diffuse edema or focal pneumonia may be more readily detected by CT.

5. When is CT scanning of the abdomen indicated in the critically ill patient?
Indications include suspected abscess, abdominal symptoms not explained by physical examination, and persistent and unexplained acidosis following surgery or trauma.

6. What are some findings on abdominal CT scan that may not be apparent on plain films?
Abscess, organomegaly, pancreatic pseudocyst or phlegmon, small bowel obstruction (especially with fluid filled bowel), bowel wall edema or pneumatosis, free intraperitoneal air, air in portal veins or biliary tree, ascites, abdominal aortic aneurysm, and retroperitoneal processes. Chest processes such as pneumothorax, pleural effusion, or lower lobe pneumonia may also be identified on the upper slices.

7. When is iodinated intravenous contrast indicated in CT of the chest or abdomen?
   Chest: mediastinal abnormalities, vascular vs. nonvascular, evaluation of hilar adenopathy vs. enlarged pulmonary arteries, thoracic aortic dissection, or aneurysm. Contrast is *not* needed for evaluation of pleural vs. parenchymal disease, lung nodules, abscesses, etc.
   Abdomen: in general, contrast is helpful in evaluating liver, spleen, pancreas, kidneys, and bladder for focal abnormalities. It is generally used in multiple trauma. Abdominal aortic aneurysm and possible leak are well evaluated with contrast-enhanced CT. However, abdominal CT without intravenous contrast may still be quite valuable if contrast is contraindicated.

8. What are the risks of intravenously administered iodinated contrast? What are the contraindications?
   Risks: (1) Allergic reaction is usually mild. Severe reactions occur in about 1/3,000–1/14,000 cases, and death as a result of contrast material has been reported in about 1/14,000–1/117,000 cases. (2) Renal failure may occur, but this risk in the normal patient is small. Risk is increased in patients with dehydration, previously existing renal disease, and diabetes with abnormal creatinine. (3) Extravasation of contrast into soft tissues may produce tissue necrosis.
   Contraindications: Previous severe reaction or preexisting nephropathy, particularly in a diabetic.

9. How may the risks of intravenous contrast be minimized?
   Renal failure. Adequate hydration is extremely important. In patients with mild preexisting nephropathy, mannitol may be administered immediately prior to and following the procedure. Creatinine should be measured in patients at risk; with significant elevation of creatinine, alternative diagnostic methods should be sought. CT with oral contrast only may still be an extremely useful diagnostic procedure.
   Allergic reaction. Pretreatment with corticosteroids (e.g., 32 mg of methylprednisolone orally 12 and 2 hours prior to administration) has been reported to decrease the incidence of allergic reactions but remains controversial. Low-osmolality nonionic contrast materials appear to be associated with a significantly decreased incidence of allergic reaction; however, their cost is approximately 10 times greater than that of conventional ionic contrast media.

10. What is the value of oral contrast in CT scanning of the abdomen? Which oral contrast agent is used?
Oral contrast is essential to distinguish fluid-filled loops of bowel from abnormal collections, such as abscess or tumor, which both are soft-tissue density by CT. Very dilute

(1–2% w/v) barium or water-soluble contrast (diatrizoate or ioxaglate at about 2% iodine) is used. Meticulous attention to administration (orally or nasogastrically) is necessary for good GI contrast. Ideally, 1000 cc should be administered in 3–4 doses every 20–30 minutes to opacify the entire bowel. If pelvic or paracolic gutter pathology is of particular interest, dilute barium or water-soluble enema may be given just prior to the CT scan.

11. What previous studies interfere with CT scanning of the body?
Barium in the GI tract from a prior study will cause marked degradation of the CT image. Barium is so dense to the scanner that extensive streak artifact is created, in the same manner that a piece of metal creates streak artifact. This artifact may also degrade images of the lung bases on a chest CT scan. CT scanning should be delayed until barium is cleared from the GI tract. Certain procedures performed prior to CT scanning may create iatrogenic abnormalities. For example, diagnostic peritoneal lavage prior to abdominal CT scanning may introduce pneumoperitoneum and free intraperitoneal fluid, which are indistinguishable from findings secondary to bowel perforation.

12. How may subsequent studies be affected by prior CT with intravenous or oral contrast?
Intravenous contrast administers a large (about 30 gm) load of iodine to the body. A significant amount is taken up by the thyroid, and the thyroid becomes saturated with iodine. Iodine-uptake studies or thyroid scanning with radioactive iodine may be affected for up to 2 years.

Closely administered doses of intravenous contrast (e.g., for CT and angiography) will increase the incidence of renal failure, especially in patients with underlying nephropathy. It is best to try to schedule contrast studies at least several days apart, ensuring adequate hydration between examinations.

The oral contrast for CT, although it is very faint on plain films, will affect visibility of mucosal detail on subsequent GI examinations. GI examinations should be scheduled after oral contrast has cleared the GI tract.

CONTROVERSIES

13. What is the best imaging technique for diagnosis of an abdominal abscess?
a. CT scanning

Advantages: Overall probably the most accurate; most specific; sensitive for fluid collections; can be used to guide percutaneous drainage.

Disadvantages: Patient must be transported; not as sensitive as nuclear medicine scanning; diffuse process may be more difficult to detect; uninfected fluid may not always be distinguishable from abscess.

b. Ultrasound

Advantages: May be done portably; no ionizing radiation; fairly sensitive for fluid collections.

Disadvantages: Least sensitive (particularly in left upper quadrant and mid abdomen); very dependent on operator skill; retroperitoneum not well visualized; infected and uninfected fluid may not be distinguishable.

c. Gallium scanning

Advantages: Very sensitive; can detect diffuse inflammation; whole body imaging.

Disadvantages: Imaging after 24–72 hours; extensive overlapping physiologic uptake; less anatomic resolution; less specific (e.g., uptake in neoplasms, uninfected inflammatory processes); best in chronic infection.

d. Indium-labelled leukocyte imaging

Advantages: Very sensitive; more specific for infection than gallium; best in acute infectious processes.

Disadvantages: Images at 24 hours; less anatomic resolution; less specific than CT; overlapping physiologic uptake limits diagnosis.

The conclusion is that, depending on clinical suspicion and condition of the patient, more than one technique may provide complementary information in diagnosis of abscess.

14. What is the procedure of choice for diagnosing thoracic aortic dissection?

a. Dynamic, contrast-enhanced CT

Advantages: Noninvasive (arterial puncture not required); may be more sensitive than angiography; demonstrates accompanying pathology (e.g., periaortic hematoma from rupture or pericardial effusion).

Disadvantages: Intimal flap may be obscured by motion because of exposure time (about 2 seconds); involvement of coronary and brachiocephalic arteries cannot be accurately assessed; does not demonstrate aortic insufficiency.

b. Aortography

Advantages: Rapid film sequence demonstrates the timing of filling of true and false lumens; intimal flap may be better demonstrated; anatomy of coronary arteries and great vessels better delineated; demonstrates aortic insufficiency.

Disadvantages: Invasive; higher risk; less sensitive for intramural hematoma.

c. Magnetic resonance imaging

Advantages: Contrast not required; imaging in any plane; no ionizing radiation.

Disadvantages: Less experience with this technique; limitations on emergency availability; limits on life-support equipment; long imaging times requiring the patient to lie very still; cannot image intimal calcifications; difficult to distinguish slow flow from thrombus; may be the least sensitive with current imaging techniques.

In summary CT is useful in excluding dissection when the index of suspicion is low, the chest x-ray is abnormal, or in a debilitated patient. Aortography may be the initial study in surgical candidates when there is a high suspicion of dissection. When there is a strong suspicion of dissection but the initial study is normal or nondiagnostic, both CT and angiography may be necessary to make the diagnosis.

BIBLIOGRAPHY

1. Cohan RH, Dunnick NR: Intravascular contrast media: Adverse reactions. AJR 149:665, 1987.
2. Gagliardi PD, Hoffer PB, Rosenfield AT: Correlative imaging in abdominal infection: An algorithmic approach using nuclear medicine, ultrasound, and computed tomography. Semin Nuc Med 18:320, 1988.
3. Godwin JD: Conventional CT of the aorta. J Thorac Imaging 5:18, 1990.
4. Jasinski RW, Glazer GM, Francis IR, Harkness RL: CT and ultrasound in abscess detection at specific anatomic sites: A study of 198 patients. Comput Radiol 11:41, 1987.
5. Katayama H, Yamaguchi K, Kozuka T, et al: Adverse reactions to ionic and nonionic contrast media. Radiology 175:621, 1990.
6. Lasser EC: Pretreatment with corticosteroids to prevent reactions to IV contrast material: Overview and implications. AJR 150:257, 1988.
7. Mirvis SE, Tobin KD, Kostrubiak I, Belzberg H: Thoracic CT in detecting occult disease in critically ill patients. AJR 148: 685, 1987.
8. Posniak HV, Olson MC, Demos TC, et al: CT of thoracic aortic aneurysms. Radiographics 10:839, 1990.
9. Snow N, Bergin KT, Horrigan TP: Thoracic CT scanning in critically ill patients: Information obtained frequently alters management. Chest 97:1467, 1990.
10. Stark DD, Federle MP, Goodman PC, et al: Differentiating lung abscess and empyema: Radiography and computed tomography. AGR 141:163, 1983.

101. ULTRASONOGRAPHY

Julia A. Drose, B.A., R.D.M.S., and Suzanne Z. Barkin, M.D.

GENERAL CONCEPTS

1. Which abdominal structures are best evaluated by ultrasound?

Ultrasound can evaluate any solid, soft-tissue organ. In the abdomen, this includes liver, spleen, and kidneys. It is also useful to evaluate fluid-filled structures such as the gallbladder, bile ducts, and abdominal vasculature (e.g., aorta, inferior vena cava). Ultrasound is not useful in evaluating air-filled structures such as bowel, or lung, or bone.

2. Which structures in the pelvis are best evaluated by ultrasound?

Ultrasound is useful in evaluating the uterus and ovaries for the presence of solid masses or fluid-filled structures such as ovarian cysts. Because of the large amount of bowel located in the pelvis, the patient must have a full urinary bladder in order to permit evaluation of the uterus and ovaries when scanning transabdominally. A transvaginal ultrasound may be performed, obviating the need for a full urinary bladder. This entails using an endovaginal transducer, which is placed inside the vagina next to the cervix. A closer evaluation of the uterus, ovaries, and fallopian tubes can be achieved with this method in some cases. Some structures such as early gestational sacs or hydrosalpinx, which may not be evident by transabdominal sonography, may be seen by using an endovaginal probe.

3. When is ultrasound useful in evaluation of the chest?

Although ultrasound is not able to evaluate lungs, it can identify pleural fluid and guide a needle for thoracentesis. Some chest masses such as mediastinal lymph nodes may be evaluated, although CT is the modality of choice. Ultrasound is an excellent tool for evaluating structure and function of the heart.

4. Which vascular structures can be evaluated by ultrasound?

Almost any vascular structure that is not surrounded by air or bowel can be evaluated using diagnostic ultrasound. In the abdomen this includes evaluating the aorta for aneurysm, the inferior vena cava and renal veins for clot, and the renal arteries for stenosis. Peripheral vasculature that can be evaluated by ultrasound includes the carotid arteries and jugular veins in the neck, subclavian and axillary veins of the upper torso, and the iliac and femoral arteries and deep venous system of the lower extremities.

5. When is Doppler ultrasound useful?

Doppler ultrasound can be used to evaluate any vascular structure for presence, direction, and velocity of flow, and to differentiate type of flow, i.e., arterial vs. venous.

6. When is ultrasound valuable intraoperatively?

Intraoperative ultrasound is useful in the brain to help identify the location of a tumor and to assist in ventricular shunt placement. It may also be useful in locating tumors of the spinal cord or abdomen, in evaluating the carotid artery following arthrectomy, or in evaluating function after cardiac valve replacement to assure that appropriate blood flow has been established.

7. How good is portable ultrasound compared with studies done in the radiology department?

All real-time ultrasound units are portable, but there are still drawbacks to doing a portable examination. First, the ultrasound machines with the best resolution are usually large and often do not fit into small spaces such as ICUs or nurseries. Other problems include monitors that the patient has on, which can interfere with the sound transmission of the ultrasound transducer. Also, many intensive care patients have tubes, lines, or bandages that limit access of the ultrasound transducer.

VASCULAR APPLICATIONS

8. What noninvasive modalities can be used to evaluate a patient with deep venous thrombosis (DVT)?
The most frequently used techniques are impedance plethysmography, Doppler ultrasonography, and iodine-125 fibrinogen leg scanning. The veins and thrombi can be directly visualized with real-time ultrasound. Duplex color Doppler imaging is now available, and in many institutions high-quality ultrasound examinations have replaced contrast venography.

9. Can the veins distal to the popliteal vein in patients with suspected DVT be visualized using ultrasound?
The calf veins are not well visualized with ultrasound; however, the proximal segment of the anterior tibial and posterior tibial-peroneal trunks can frequently be studied.

10. Can ultrasound be used as a primary modality to evaluate the carotid arteries for stenosis and plaque identification and characterization?
Yes. Traditionally, the diagnostic evaluation of atherosclerotic disease in the extracranial carotid arteries has been with carotid angiography; however, with sonographic imaging using duplex or color Doppler instruments, plaque morphology and flow characteristics can be assessed.

ABDOMINAL APPLICATIONS

11. When is ultrasound better than CT scanning in the abdomen?
Ultrasound is inherently better than CT scanning when looking for gallstones or deciding when the consistency of a mass is cystic vs. solid. It is also the method of choice for evaluating hydronephrosis and vascular flow patterns. Both ultrasound and CT are equally good when evaluating abdominal aortic aneurysms; however, ultrasound is less expensive and does not use ionizing radiation. When evaluating the pancreas or looking for an abscess or bowel lesions, CT is the method of choice because of the inability of ultrasound to penetrate bowel.

12. What is the role of ultrasound in the diagnosis of appendicitis?
Historically, appendicitis has been a clinical diagnosis. However, in equivocal cases, ultrasound with graded compression is of definite value. An inflamed appendix on ultrasound is differentiated from normal bowel by size, shape, location, and absence of peristalsis. It is also difficult to compress and is relatively rigid. Wall-thickening and fluid around the appendix are other signs. The McBurney sign, producing moderate tenderness with the ultrasound transducer, is frequently seen.

13. Which modality is best for evaluating hepatic pathology?
Ultrasonography is probably the best method of screening patients for suspected hepatic pathology. It is noninvasive, can be performed rapidly, provides excellent results, and is the least expensive of available imaging tests. It is also usually better in characterizing lesions that have been detected, in distinguishing simple cysts from noncystic lesions, and in

diagnosing anatomic variants. CT may be needed as a secondary imaging modality once an abnormality has been identified.

14. What is the differential diagnosis of a solid hepatic lesion?

A single, solid lesion in the liver statistically represents a cavernous hemangioma. These are usually small and found in patients who are asymptomatic. A large solid lesion may be more indicative of neoplasm, with hepatocellular carcinoma being the most common primary malignant tumor of the liver. Multiple solid lesions may also represent cavernous hemangiomas or, more likely, metastatic disease. Other possibilities include hepatic adenomas or focal nodular hyperplasia.

15. When is ultrasound useful in evaluating the biliary system?

Ultrasound is the procedure of choice for evaluating the biliary system because of its high sensitivity and accuracy in detecting gallstones and for detecting biliary dilatation.

16. What other gallbladder abnormalities can be detected by ultrasound?

Sonography can be used to detect diffuse wall thickening, which is diagnosed when the wall is more than 3 mm thick. Polyps or masses of the gallbladder may also be identified as foci that do not move or shadow. Other conditions seen by ultrasound include echogenic bile or sludge, or pericholecystic fluid, most often due to acute cholecystitis.

17. When should ultrasound be used to evaluate the pancreas?

Ultrasound is valuable in examining the size and echotexture of the pancreas and accompanying lesions and the presence of a dilated pancreatic duct. However, adequate visualization of the pancreas is often obscured by the ribs, stomach, and colon. Therefore, a CT scan may be the modality of choice.

GENITOURINARY APPLICATIONS

18. When is ultrasound useful in evaluating urinary tract abnormalities?

Ultrasound is usually the modality of choice when evaluating the kidneys. Renal anatomy can be well delineated with the superior resolution provided by currently available ultrasound units. The internal architecture of the kidney is now routinely displayed with a clarity approaching that of the cut surface of a gross anatomic specimen. Not only can the kidney be evaluated for anatomic abnormalities, but with the use of Doppler and color flow imaging, renal blood flow alterations can be identified and studied. Furthermore, with ultrasound guidance, biopsy of renal masses or renal parenchyma can be performed and fluids aspirated. Ultrasound is very useful in identifying and following dilatation of the renal pelvis and dilated ureters. The urinary bladder may also be evaluated for the presence of masses. Nephrolithiasis, however, is still best evaluated by excretory urography.

19. When a patient presents with an acutely painful scrotum, which imaging studies are most helpful in making the diagnosis?

It is important to differentiate torsion of the testis from epididymitis when there is no history of trauma, because torsion requires immediate surgical intervention. A nuclear medicine scan in the acute setting should be performed first with technetium 99m sodium pertechnetate. This study is 95% accurate in the first 6 hours in distinguishing torsion from epididymitis. Ultrasound can be done following the nuclear medicine study.

Clinically, torsion and epididymitis may be difficult to differentiate; however, ultrasonographically they are very different. Torsion on ultrasound may appear as an enlarged testis with normal echogenicity, whereas epididymitis appears as an enlarged epididymis with a normal testis.

When an intratesticular lesion is considered with a palpable scrotal mass, ultrasonography is excellent and is the first imaging study that should be ordered. However, there is no way to delineate malignant from benign lesions, except with surgery. Any intratesticular lesion should be considered malignant until proved otherwise.

GYNECOLOGIC APPLICATIONS

20. What are the advantages of transabdominal versus transvaginal sonography?
Transabdominal and transvaginal ultrasound are best used in an additive fashion. Transvaginal ultrasound may be able to detect an intrauterine pregnancy earlier than transabdominal. It also enables visualization of structures sometimes missed by transabdominal ultrasound such as an ectopic pregnancy, tubal ovarian abscess, and small fibroids. However, large ovarian masses or fibroids, especially those located high in the pelvis, may be missed by transvaginal ultrasound because they are too far from the transvaginal probe to be visualized. Bowel may also obscure normal ovaries and ovarian masses when using a transvaginal probe, whereas a full bladder and a transabdominal probe may facilitate their visualization.

21. What are the ultrasound findings in pelvic inflammatory disease?
They are usually nonspecific and therefore cannot definitively make the diagnosis, but a constellation of sonographic findings may be present. Because the infection affects the endometrium, early findings may include a prominent and hyperechoic endometrium surrounded by a hypoechoic ring, or a definitive fluid collection may be seen within the endometrium. A subtle hypoechogenicity of the uterus may signal early uterine infection. Indistinct borders of pelvic structures and posterior cul-de-sac fluid may also be present. As the infection ascends, acute salpingitis results. When this occurs, dilated cystic or complex structures may be seen, representing a hydrosalpinx or pyosalpinx. Pyosalpinx is usually a unilateral process but may be seen bilaterally. Severe pelvic inflammatory disease may appear as an indistinct complex mass.

22. When should you see a gestational sac, fetal pole, and fetal heartbeat by transabdominal ultrasound versus transvaginal ultrasound?
By transabdominal ultrasound, a gestational sac may often be seen as early as 5 weeks' gestational age. The secondary yolk sac becomes visible at approximately 5–5.5 weeks, and shortly thereafter (by 6.5 weeks) a small fetal pole containing a flickering fetal heart can be seen adjacent or near the yolk sac. The use of transvaginal transducers permits these structures to be seen approximately 1 week earlier.

23. What are the ultrasound criteria for an ectopic pregnancy?
The only conclusive criteria for excluding an ectopic pregnancy by ultrasound is to demonstrate a viable intrauterine pregnancy occupying a high fundal position in the endometrium. The coexistence of intrauterine and extrauterine gestations occurs 1 in 6000 cases and is considered a rare phenomenon. The appearance of a sac-like structure within the endometrium itself is not diagnostic of an intrauterine pregnancy because a similar structure termed "pseudogestational sac" can accompany an ectopic pregnancy. Ultrasound may provide a definitive diagnosis of an ectopic pregnancy only if an ectopic gestational sac is visualized outside of the uterus and fetal heart movements are demonstrable within it.

24. What is the sonographic appearance of hydatidiform mole?
A variable appearance is possible by ultrasound. Some first-trimester moles may simulate anembryonic gestation, missed abortion, degenerating fibroid, or hydropic placenta. Others may appear as an echogenic mass filling the entire uterine cavity. The more advanced

hydatidiform mole, which contains numerous hydropic villi, can be well visualized by sonography. It appears as a large, soft-tissue mass containing cystic spaces of various sizes. Large multiseptated ovarian cysts (theca lutein cysts) may be present. Whenever these criteria are seen, careful clinical correlation is important in differentiating the possible causes.

BIBLIOGRAPHY

1. Berland LL, Lawson TL, Folley WD: Porta hepatis: Sonographic discrimination of bile ducts from arteries with pulsed Doppler with new anatomic criteria. AJR 138:833, 1982.
2. Bernardino NE, Thomas JL, Maklad N: Hepatic sonography: Technical considerations, present applications, and possible future. Radiology 142:249, 1982.
3. Carroll BA, Gross DM: High frequency scrotal sonography. AJR 140:511–515, 1983.
4. Cronan JJ, Dorfman GS, Scola FH, et al: Deep venous thrombosis: US assessment using vein compression. Radiology 162:191–194, 1987.
5. Goldstein SR, Snyder JR, Watson C, et al: Very early pregnancy detection with endovaginal ultrasound. Obstet Gynecol 72:200–204, 1988.
6. Graif M, Mannor A, Itzchak Y: Sonographic differentiation of extra- and intrahepatic masses. AJR 141:553, 1983.
7. Grant EG: Duplex ultrasonography: Its expanding role in noninvasive vascular diagnosis. Radiol Clin North Am 23:563–582, 1985.
8. Grant EG, Raqavendra N, McNamara RO: Color Doppler depicts flow patterns in legs. Diagn Imaging 11:140–146, 1990.
9. Groseman H, Rosenberg ER, Bowey JD, et al: Sonographic diagnosis of renal cystic diseases. AJR 140:81, 1983.
10. Hessler PC, Hill DS, Detorie FM, Rocco AF: High accuracy sonographic recognition of gallstones. AJR 136:157, 1981.
11. Hill MC: Pancreatic sonography: An update. In Saunders RC (ed): Ultrasound Annual. New York, Raven Press, 1982.
12. Kane RA: Sonographic anatomy of the liver. In Raymond HW, Zwiebel WJ (eds): Seminars in Ultrasound, vol. 2. New York, Grune and Stratton, 1981.
13. Mendelson EB, Bohm-Velez M, Neiman HL, et al: Transvaginal sonography in imaging. Semin Ultrasound CT MR 9:102–121, 1988.
14. Mittlestaedt CA: Abdominal Ultrasound. New York, Churchill Livingstone, 1987.
15. Renz J, Merritt CRM, Bluth EI: Sonographic evaluation of carotid plaque. Appl Radiol 8:29–32, 1990.
16. Rifkin MD, Kurtz AB, Goldberg BB: Epididymis examined by ultrasound. Radiology 151:187–190, 1984.
17. Rosenfield AT: Ultrasound evaluation of renal parenchymal disease and hydronephrosis. Urol Radiol 4:125, 1982.
18. Rumack CM, Wilson SR, Charboneau JM: Diagnostic Ultrasound. St. Louis, Mosby-Year Book, 1991.
19. Sarti D: Diagnostic Ultrasound: Text and Cases, 2nd ed. Chicago, Year Book Medical Publishers, 1987.
20. Sexton CC, Zeman RK: Correlation of computed tomography, sonography and gross anatomy of liver. AJR 141:711, 1983.

XV: Emergency Medicine

102. TETANUS

Peter T. Pons, M.D.

1. What is tetanus?

Tetanus is acute infection with *Clostridium tetani* (gram-positive anaerobic rod), which produces a neurotoxin (exotoxin) whose primary action is to cause profound skeletal muscle hypertonicity. In the most severe form, the muscle spasms can cause respiratory failure and death. *C. tetani* can be introduced into any wound or open tissue; it proliferates in necrotic or compromised tissue, then elaborates the exotoxin.

2. How does the exotoxin/neurotoxin cause the disease?

C. tetani manufactures three exotoxins: tetanospasmin, tetanolysin, and nonconvulsive neurotoxin. Most clinical manifestations appear to be produced by tetanospasmin. This exotoxin becomes concentrated in the anterior horn of the spinal cord and blocks neurotransmitter release at presynaptic sites of inhibitory neurons, thus causing increased muscle tone, hypertonicity, and muscle spasms. Tetanolysin is a hemolytic toxin that may cause hemolysis and myocardial injury and dysfunction. The role of the third toxin, nonconvulsive neurotoxin, has not been well defined. The toxins spread via lymphatics, blood vessels, and neural pathways to the target organ, alpha motor neurons.

3. What is the epidemiology of tetanus?

Incidence and geographic distribution. In the United States, there are approximately 80 cases of tetanus each year; worldwide, there are between 250,000 and 500,000 cases. In the U.S., the disease occurs most commonly in the Southeast; however, the organism is ubiquitous in dirt and dust and is found worldwide. It is less common in cold climates.

Incubation period: varies between 2 and 14 days with a median of 7 days.

Prognosis. The mortality rate is 30% in the U.S. and 40–60% worldwide. The mortality is 100% if the disease becomes manifest within 2 days of injury and infection. Worldwide, 90% of deaths occur in infants.

4. Who is prone to developing tetanus?

General. Most at risk are individuals who have never been or are inadequately immunized against tetanus. It is estimated that 50–90% of patients in the U.S. are inadequately protected (in most cases, immigrants or adults over the age of 50–60 years who never completed the immunization series).

Neonates. Newborns can acquire tetanus following nonsterile transection of the umbilical cord. In many countries, local remedies such as cow dung, garlic, coffee, and ashes are applied to the umbilical stump to facilitate healing, only to produce tetanus.

Drug abusers. Parenteral drug abusers who administer their drugs by "skin popping" are prone to acquiring tetanus by developing subcutaneous abscesses that support the growth of *C. tetani.*

Septic abortion. Women who have undergone septic abortion are prone to the development of tetanus.

Acne. Cephalic tetanus has been reported as a complication of acne.

5. What sort of wound is prone to infection with *C. tetani?*

Most cases result from accidental soft-tissue injury, such as lacerations or puncture wounds, which may occur indoors or outdoors. The Centers for Disease Control reported that almost 50% of wounds resulting in tetanus occurred indoors. Many wounds appear quite minor and sometimes cannot be found at the time of presentation of clinical tetanus. *C. tetani* is a strict anaerobe and proliferates only in tissue with low oxygen tension. Necrotic tissue, foreign bodies, and associated infection are predisposing factors. Tetanus has been reported after elective surgery, burn injury, and chronic skin ulceration. The organism itself is not invasive; thus the infection is localized. Once the exotoxin is produced, however, the toxin is transported systemically.

6. What are the clinical manifestations of tetanus?

The most dramatic and obvious findings in tetanus are in the musculoskeletal system. Initial findings are characterized by increased muscle tone, which is usually first noticed in the face and jaw. Trismus, difficulty swallowing, and facial distortion from the muscle spasms (risus sardonicus) develop. Over the next 24–48 hours, generalized muscle hypertonicity develops and muscle spasms may occur. These spasms may be initiated by external stimuli such as loud noises or touch. Spasms of neck and back muscles result in opisthotonic posturing. Other findings are low-grade elevation in temperature and pulse, increased or decreased blood pressure, pain associated with the muscle spasms, rigid abdominal wall (also due to muscle spasms but mimicking an acute abdomen), and clear mentation during these episodes. The disease remains "stable" for the next 5–7 days, followed by recovery over the next 7–10 days. Muscle stiffness may remain for up to 2 months. In neonates, the disease is characterized by irritability, difficulty nursing and swallowing, and hypertonicity of the muscles. If the patient survives, recovery occurs without permanent sequelae. The disease does not confer immunity; therefore survivors must be immunized to prevent recurrence.

7. What are the four types of tetanus?

1. **Generalized.** This is the most common form and is manifested by the full constellation of symptoms and signs. Overall mortality is approximately 50%.

2. **Neonatal.** Newborns may acquire tetanus from contamination of the umbilical stump. Immunization of the mother can prevent the disease in neonates. The mortality in infants is 50–60%.

3. **Local.** This form is characterized by increased muscle tone near the inoculation site that usually resolves over time. Progression to the generalized form is uncommon but possible.

4. **Cephalic.** This rare form presents with trismus and cranial nerve paralysis (VII most commonly, also III, IV, VI, and XII). Generalized tetanus follows in approximately two-thirds of cases.

8. Are any laboratory studies diagnostic of tetanus?

Virtually all laboratory studies yield nonspecific, nondiagnostic results. Approximately one-third of patients have mild to moderate granulocytosis. Decreased hematocrit may be noted, probably secondary to the hemolysin exotoxin. Electrolyte and calcium levels should be normal. As the disease progresses, however, 7% of patients develop the electrolyte picture of inappropriate antidiuretic hormone secretion (SIADH), including decreased sodium and serum osmolality. Arterial blood gases should be monitored to assess pulmonary function. Of note, cultures for *C. tetani* were positive in only one-third of patients diagnosed with tetanus clinically.

9. Which diseases are included in the differential diagnosis?

Hypocalcemia. Decreased serum calcium can produce tetany. Laboratory evaluation is usually diagnostic.

Oral infection or abscess. Infection or abscess in and about the oral cavity (e.g., peritonsillar or dental abscess) can result in trismus or difficulty opening the mouth. Physical examination usually reveals localized swelling and tenderness.

Phenothiazine reaction. Dystonic reactions secondary to phenothiazines may cause muscle rigidity or torticollis. The history usually reveals recent drug use; relief of symptoms occurs with intravenous diphenhydramine.

Black widow spider bite. Pain and muscle spasm are usually acute in onset. Careful physical examination may reveal the telltale spider bite. Administration of calcium intravenously usually relieves the symptoms.

Rabies. Rabies involves the respiratory muscles and muscles of glutition without causing trismus. As the disease progresses, there is progressive alteration in the level of consciousness and increasing fever.

Strychnine poisoning. Muscle spasms (usually involving the upper extremities) and opisthotonus occur; however, facial muscle involvement develops later in the course. Suicidal ideation or possible homicide attempt may be evident by history.

Hyperventilation. Physical examination reveals carpopedal spasm. Arterial blood gas evaluation shows respiratory alkalosis.

10. What are the complications of tetanus?

Spasm of laryngeal muscles, the diaphragm, and other muscles of respiration may produce hypoxia or respiratory arrest. The compromise in respiratory function may lead to atelectasis and pneumonia. Other complications include vertebral subluxation or compression fracture as a result of the profound muscle contractions (usually in children), dehydration, pulmonary edema, and SIADH.

11. How is tetanus treated once it becomes manifest?

The four primary goals of treatment are (1) relief of muscle spasms, (2) support of respiratory status and prevention of complications, (3) treatment of the infection (remove toxin production), and (4) neutralization of any unbound toxin.

1. **Relief of muscle spasms.** The patient should be placed in a darkened room with minimal external stimulation. Diazepam, administered intravenously, is useful for relieving muscle spasms. Oral muscle relaxants such as meprobamate can be used in mild cases or during convalescence. In severe cases not responding to diazepam, chemical paralysis (with intubation and mechanical ventilation) using pancuronium is indicated. The addition of a sedative is helpful in reducing the effect of external stimulation, but careful monitoring of respiratory status is necessary.

2. **Support of respiratory status and prevention of complications.** Close monitoring of the patient's respiratory function is imperative because spasm of laryngeal muscles, the diaphragm, and muscles of respiration can lead to respiratory failure and suffocation. If necessary, endotracheal intubation and mechanical ventilation should be performed. Formal tracheostomy may be needed if intubation cannot be accomplished. Secretions should be suctioned frequently and the patient positioned to minimize aspiration (and decubiti).

3. **Treatment of the infection (remove toxin production).** When a wound or site of infection is identifiable, any necrotic tissue or foreign material should be removed and any abscess drained. Antibiotics are administered in the hope of preventing further proliferation of the organism and therefore decreasing toxin production, but there is little evidence that the course of the diisease is affected. Penicillin is the drug of choice, and tetracycline may be used in penicillin-allergic patients.

4. **Neutralization of unbound toxin.** Human tetanus immune globulin is the medication of choice for neutralization of free exotoxin. The antiserum will not have any effect on toxin already bound in neurons. Equine antiserum can be used if human antiserum is not

available; however, hypersensitivity, anaphylaxis, and serum sickness are serious complications. Following recovery, active immunization is necessary because immunity is not acquired by having the disease.

12. Can tetanus be prevented?

Tetanus is easily prevented by immunization and could be virtually eradicated worldwide by an aggressive immunization campaign. Neonatal tetanus is also preventable if the mother is protected because the antibody can pass through the placental barrier. Part of every routine history should include a review of tetanus immunization. Unimmunized patients or those with unclear histories should undergo active immunization with absorbed tetanus toxoid. The first dose should be given at the time of contact, the second dose 1–2 months later, and the third dose 6–12 months after the second dose.

Tetanus Prophylaxis After Injury

IMMUNIZATION HISTORY	TOXOID[1]	ANTITOXIN	
		NON-TETANUS PRONE	TETANUS PRONE
None	Yes	No	Yes
Uncertain or < 3 doses	Yes	No	Yes
3 or more doses	No[2]	No	No

[1] If patient age is less than 7 years, administer toxoid as diphtheria-tetanus-pertussis (DPT).
  If patient age is greater than 7 years, administer toxoid as tetanus-diphtheria (Td).
[2] Yes if last prior immunization was greater than 5 years and tetanus-prone wound or 10 years and non–tetanus-prone wound.
When both toxoid and antitoxin are indicated, they may be given at the same time without concern that one will interfere with the action of the other, but separate injection sites should be used.

BIBLIOGRAPHY

1. American College of Emergency Physicians: Tetanus immunization recommendations for persons seven years of age and older. Ann Emerg Med 15:1111–1112, 1986.
2. American College of Emergency Physicians: Tetanus immunization recommendations for persons less than seven years old. Ann Emerg Med 16:1181–1183, 1987.
3. Bowen V, Johnson J, Boyle J, et al: Tetanus: A continuing problem in minor injuries. Can J Surg 31:7–9, 1988.
4. Brand D, Acampora D, Gottlieb LD, et al: Adequacy of antitetanus prophylaxis in six hospital emergency rooms. N Engl J Med 309:636–639, 1985.
5. Centers for Disease Control: Tetanus—United States, 1985–1986. MMWR 36:477–481, 1987.
6. Dixon AM, Bibby JA: Tetanus immunization state in a general practice population. Br Med J 297:598, 1988.
7. Hinman A, Foster S, Wassilak S: Neonatal tetanus: Potential for elimination in the world. Pediatr Infect Dis J 6:813–816, 1987.
8. Jagoda A, Riggio SY, Burguieres T: Cephalic tetanus: A case report and review of the literature. Am J Emerg Med 6:128–130, 1988.
9. Potgieter PD: Inappropriate ADH secretion in tetanus. Crit Care Med 11:417–418, 1983.
10. Searl S: Minor trauma, disastrous results. Surv Ophthalmol 31:337–342, 1987.
11. Stair TO, Lippe MA, Russell H, et al: Tetanus immunity in emergency department patients. Am J Emerg Med 7:563–566, 1989.
12. Trujillo MH, Castillo A, Espana JV, et al: Impact of intensive care management on the prognosis of tetanus. Chest 92:63–65, 1987.
13. Weber LE, Greenhouse AH: Update on tetanus. Semin Neurol 3:88–94, 1983.
14. Williams WW, Hickson MA, Kane MA, et al: Immunization policies and vaccine coverage among adults: The risk for missed opportunities. Ann Intern Med 108:616–625, 1988.

103. ANAPHYLAXIS

Vincent Markovchick, M.D.

1. What is anaphylaxis?

Anaphylaxis is a systemic immediate hypersensitivity reaction of multiple organ systems to an antigen-induced IgE-mediated immunologic mediator release in previously sensitized individuals.

2. What are the most common causes?

Ingestion, inhalation or parenteral injection of antigens that sensitize predisposed individuals. Common antigens include drugs (e.g., penicillin), foods (shellfish, nuts, egg whites), insect stings (hymenoptera) and bites (snakes), diagnostic agents (ionic contrast media), and physical and environmental agents (exercise and cold).

3. What are the most common "target" organs?

The most common organ systems involved are the skin (urticaria, angioedema), mucous membranes (edema), upper respiratory tract (edema and hypersecretions), lower respiratory tract (bronchoconstriction), and cardiovascular system (vasodilatation).

4. What are the most common signs and symptoms?

The clinical presentation ranges from mild to life threatening. Mild manifestations that occur in most people include urticaria and angioedema. Life-threatening manifestations involve the respiratory or cardiovascular systems. Respiratory signs and symptoms include acute upper airway obstruction presenting with stridor or lower airway manifestations of bronchospasm with diffuse wheezing. Cardiovascular collapse presents in the form of syncope, hypotension, tachycardia, and arrhythmias.

5. What is the role of diagnostic studies?

There is no role for diagnostic studies in anaphylaxis because diagnosis and treatment are based solely on clinical signs and symptoms. There is a role for skin testing either prior to administration of an antigen or in follow-up referral to determine exact allergens involved.

6. What is the differential diagnosis?

Anaphylaxis may be confused with septic and cardiogenic shock, asthma, croup and epiglottitis, vasovagal syncope, and myocardial or any acute cardiovascular or respiratory collapse of unclear etiology.

7. What is the most common form of anaphylaxis? How is it treated?

Urticaria, either simple or confluent, is the most benign and, fortunately, the most common clinical manifestation. This is thought to be due to a capillary leak mediated by histamine release. It may be treated by the administration of antihistamines (PO, IM or IV) or epinephrine (subcutaneous).

8. What is the initial treatment for life-threatening forms of anaphylaxis?

    1. Upper airway obstruction with stridor and edema should be treated with high-flow nebulized oxygen, racemic epinephrine, and IV epinephrine. If airway obstruction is severe or increases, endotracheal intubation or cricothyroidotomy should be performed.

    2. Acute bronchospasm should be treated with epinephrine. Mild to moderate wheezing in patients with a normal blood pressure may be treated with .01 mg/kg of 1:1000 epinephrine administered subcutaneously or IM. If the patient is in severe respiratory

distress or has a "quiet" chest, IV epinephrine should be administered via a drip infusion: 1 mg epinephrine in 250 cc D5W at an initial rate of 1 $\mu g/min$.

3. Cardiovascular collapse presenting with hypotension should be treated with a constant infusion of epinephrine, titrating the rate to attain a systolic BP of 100 mm Hg or mean arterial pressure of 80 mm Hg.

4. For patients in full cardiac arrest, administer 0.1–0.2 mg/kg of 1:10,000 epinephrine slow IV push or via endotracheal tube. In addition, immediate endotracheal intubation or cricothyroidostomy should be performed.

9. What are the adjuncts to initial epinephrine and airway management?

If intubation is unsuccessful and cricothyroidostomy is contraindicated, percutaneous transtracheal jet ventilation via needle cricothyroidostomy should be considered, especially in small children. Intravenous diphenhydramine (2 mg/kg) should be administered to all patients. Simultaneous administration of H2 blocker such as cimetidine, 300 mg IV, may be helpful. Aerosolized bronchodilators such as metaproterenol are useful if bronchospasm is present. Corticosteroids are usually given but do not have an immediate positive effect. For refractory hypotension, pressors such as norepinephrine or dopamine may be administered. Glucagon, 1 mg IV q 5 min, may be helpful in "epinephrine-resistant" patients who are on long-term beta-adrenergic blocking agents such as propranolol.

10. What are the complications of bolus IV epinephrine administration?

When epinephrine 1:10,000 is administered via IV push in patients who have an obtainable blood pressure or pulse, there is significant potential for overtreatment and the potentiation of hypertension, tachycardia, chest pain, and ventricular arrhythmias. Extreme care must be exercised in elderly patients and in those with underlying coronary artery disease. It is much safer to administer IV epinephrine by a controlled titratable drip infusion with continuous monitoring of cardiac rhythm and blood pressure.

11. Is there a role for prophylactic treatment in anaphylaxis? How is this performed?

When the potential benefits of treatment or diagnosis outweigh the risks (e.g., administration of antivenom for life- or limb-threatening snake bites), informed consent should be obtained if the patient is competent. Pretreatment with IV Benadryl and corticosteroids should be carried out. An IV epinephrine infusion should be prepared. The patient should be in an ICU setting with continuous monitoring of blood pressure, cardiac rhythm, and oxygen saturation. Full intubation and cricothyroidomy equipment should be at the bedside. Administration of the antigen (e.g., rattlesnake antivenom) should be started very slowly with a physician at the bedside who is capable of immediately administering IV epinephrine and managing the airway. Nonionic contrast medium for diagnostic imaging studies should be administered to patients with a history of anaphylaxis to ionic contrast material.

12. What is the prehospital treatment of anaphylaxis?

Patients who are known to be at high risk (e.g., previous anaphylactic reaction to hymenoptera) should be prescribed and educated in the self-administration of epinephrine at the first sign of anaphylactic symptoms. In addition, self-administration of oral diphenhydramine is indicated for the treatment of mild reactions such as urticaria or concomitant with the administration of epinephrine.

BIBLIOGRAPHY

1. Jacobs RL, et al: Potentiated anaphylaxis in patients with drug-induced beta-adrenergic blockage. J Allergy Clin Immunol 68:125, 1981.
2. Lee ML: Glucagon in anaphylaxis (letter). J Allergy Clin Immunol 69:331, 1981.

3. Lindzon RD, Silvers WS: Anaphylaxis. In Rosen P (ed): Emergency Medicine: Concepts and Clinical Practice, 2nd ed. St. Louis, C.V. Mosby, 1988, pp 203–231.
4. Lucke WC: Anaphylaxis. Emergindex, Vol. 67, Denver, Micromedex Inc., 1991.
5. Lucke WC, Thomas H: Anaphylaxis: Pathophysiology, clinical presentations and treatment. J Emerg Med 1:83–95, 1983.
6. Phanuphak P, Schocket A, Kohler PF: Treatment of chronic idiopathic urticaria with combined H_1 and H_2 blockers. Clin Allergy 8:429, 1978.
7. Roberts JR, Greenberg MI: Endotracheal epinephrine in cardiorespiratory collapse. JACEP 8:515–519, 1979.
8. Silverman JH, Van Hook C, Haponik EF: Hemodynamic changes in human anaphylaxis. Am J Med 77:341–344, 1984.
9. Weiszer I: Allergic emergencies. In Patterson R (ed): Allergic Diseases: Diagnosis and Management. Philadelphia, J.B. Lippincott, 1980, pp 374–394.

104. HYPOTHERMIA

John A. Marx, M.D.

1. How is hypothermia defined?
Specifically, hypothermia is a core temperature of $< 35°C$ or $95°F$. Physiologically, it is a clinical state of subnormal temperature in which the body is unable to generate sufficient heat to function efficiently. When hypothermia is suspected, it is imperative that thermometers be capable of measuring core temperatures accurately. Many thermometers have a lower limit of 34–35°C.

2. What is the function of shivering? When does it occur?
Shivering is an early response to cold stress and is able to increase the basal metabolic rate two- to fivefold. It is operative between 30 and 37°C. Shivering is modulated by the posterior hypothalamus and spinal cord and is limited by fatigue and glycogen depletion.

3. What is the J-wave?
This electrocardiographic feature, also known as the Osborn wave or hypothermic hump, is seen at the junction of the QRS and ST segments and appears at any temperature below 32°. It is most often seen in leads II and V6, but in more severe hypothermia may be seen in V3 or V4. Its size increases with temperature depression. It is not specific for hypothermia and can be seen in cardiac ischemia, sepsis, and certain CNS lesions, particularly of the hypothalmus.

4. What are the indications to initiate cardiopulmonary resuscitation (CPR) in the field in a patient with suspected hypothermia?
Peripheral pulses are difficult to palpate in patients with profound bradycardia and vasoconstriction. At least 1 minute should be spent in determining whether spontaneous pulse is present because extreme bradydysrhythmias may be sufficient to meet the very depressed metabolic needs of the hypothermic patient. Moreover, unnecessary handling is a purported cause of arrhythmias. If no evidence of perfusion can be discerned, an arrest rhythm should be presumed and CPR initiated. Respiratory minute volume is also significantly depressed and careful scrutiny is required to distinguish apnea. A patent airway should always be established. If the patient is in respiratory arrest, ventilation should also be instituted.

CPR in hypothermia is contraindicated under the following circumstances: any signs of life are present, lethal (non-hypothermia-related) injuries are obvious, chest wall compression is impossible due to loss of elasticity, or "do not resuscitate" status is verified.

5. What are the current recommendations for rate and technique in CPR?

With regard to duration, it is clear that prolonged closed chest compressions have resuscitated many severely hypothermic patients to normal neurologic status. It is recommended that resuscitative measures continue until a core temperature of 35° has been reached before a patient is declared dead.

Optimal guidelines for rate and techniques are evolving. In an animal model of hypothermic cardiac arrest, cardiac output and cerebral and myocardial blood flows of 50%, 55%, and 31%, respectively, of those produced during normothermic closed chest compression were achieved. These compare well with the reduced metabolic demands of the hypothermic patient. Because chest wall elasticity and pulmonary compliance are decreased, more force is needed for chest wall compressions in order for adequate intrathoracic pressure gradients to be generated.

6. What is the preferred mode of therapy for ventricular fibrillation in the setting of hypothermia?

Most dysrhythmias of any type will convert spontaneously during rewarming. Ventricular fibrillation occurs at temperatures below 32°C and is most likely to occur at 28°C. The recommended approach to ventricular fibrillation begins with one attempt at cardioversion with 2 watt-sec/kg up to 200 watt-sec. It is unlikely that this will be successful until the core temperature reaches 28–30°C. Bretylium tosylate is the pharmacologic defibrillator of choice for ventricular fibrillation. Magnesium sulfate has also been used successfully in this setting. Lidocaine and propranolol, although not harmful, have little to no efficacy. Procainamide has been reported to increase the incidence of ventricular fibrillation in hypothermia and should not be used. In hypothermia, the fraction of drug bound to protein increases and liver metabolism is decreased. Thus, toxic levels of antiarrhythmics may develop with rewarming. Optimal dosages in this setting are not well established.

7. What are the basic types of rewarming?

Passive external rewarming (PER). PER minimizes the normal process of heat loss while it allows the body to rewarm spontaneously via shivering thermogenesis. It is indicated for patients with all levels of hypothermia and is sufficient by itself for mild illness. The technique is to cover the patient with an insulating material in an ambient temperature that exceeds 21°C. In order to be effective, the patient should have a core temperature of 30–32° (i.e., shivering thermogenesis intact), sufficient glycogen stores, and operative metabolic homeostasis. Advantages of the technique include its noninvasiveness, simplicity, and maintenance of peripheral vasoconstriction.

Active rewarming. Active rewarming includes techniques that directly transfer heat and is divided into **external (AER)** or **internal core (ACR)** methods. Active rewarming is indicated for patients with moderate or severe hypothermia (< 32°C), cardiovascular instability, endocrine failure, impaired thermoregulation, mild hypothermia with failure to rewarm with PER, and peripheral vasodilatation (traumatic, toxicologic).

AER. In AER, exogenous heat is transferred to the skin via heating pads, heating blankets, radiant light sources, warm water immersion, hot water bottles, and the like. It is not recommended as the sole method of rewarming for patients with moderate to severe hypothermia, but may be successful when combined with ACR methods. The heat source should be applied only to the thorax because heat application to the extremities often produces thermal injury to vasoconstricted and hypoperfused skin and increases the metabolic requirements of the periphery, thus increasing cardiovascular demands.

ACR. These techniques minimize pathophysiologic consequences of rewarming. ACR methods include airway rewarming, heated irrigation (gastric, colonic, chest, mediastinal), diathermy, and extracorporeal rewarming (cardiopulmonary bypass, hemodialysis).

8. What are the preferred methods of ACR?

A widely employed algorithm for ACR in hypothermia is as follows:

Airway rewarming and heated intravenous fluids can be administered safely and effectively in virtually all patients. Those *in extremis* should, in addition, be submitted to cardiopulmonary bypass (CPB) or hemodialysis. Other ACR modalities have less efficacy (heated irrigation), significant complication rates (peritoneal dialysis), or limited experience in humans (diathermy).

A rewarming rate of 1–2.5° C/hour can be achieved with heated (42–44°), humidified oxygen delivery. Heat exchange is augmented depending on technique (endotracheal superior to mask) and volume of minute ventilation. Advantages include technical ease, avoidance of temperature afterdrop, assured oxygen delivery, decreased viscosity of pulmonary secretions, decreased cold-induced bronchorrhea, and modification of the amplitude of shivering, which in severe cases decreases the metabolic demands of the periphery.

Cardiopulmonary bypass, when available, should be instituted in patients with minimal or absent mechanical cardiac activity. CPB can increase core temperature 1–2° C every 5 minutes with a bypass flow rate of 2–3 L/min. Hemodialysis, although less rapid and effective, will become more practical with the development of two way flow catheters.

9. What stabilizing measures should prehospital care providers undertake?

The patient should be handled as gently and carefully as possible because ventricular fibrillation has been ascribed to excessive mechanical stimulation. In cases of immersion, wet clothing should be removed. Further heat loss should be limited by provision of a dry and insulated environment. Blankets, sleeping bags, or aluminum-coated foils can be used for this purpose. Ethanol should not be given because it suppresses shivering thermogenesis, promotes peripheral vasodilatation and can prompt hypoglycemia in these typically glycogen-depleted patients. Massage of the extremities provides unnecessary physical stimulation and, like ethanol, can mitigate both shivering and appropriate peripheral vasoconstriction. If venous access can be acquired, 50 cc of 50% dextrose, 2 mg of naloxone, and 100 mg of thiamine are appropriate. A fluid challenge of D5 0.9% normal saline, 250–500 cc (preferably heated), is indicated, as the majority of patients with moderate to severe hypothermia have sustained cold-induced diuresis. Lactated Ringer's solution is a less preferred crystalloid because the hypothermic liver is less able to metabolize lactate.

AER measures are safe in the minimally hypothermic patient but unnecessary. In the patient with moderate to profound hypothermia, these may increase morbidity and should not be used. The only method of ACR appropriate in the field is heated, humidified oxygen. Several portable devices are available for this purpose.

10. What procedures are hazardous in the management of the hypothermic patient?

In patients with moderate and severe hypothermia, cardiac monitoring is indicated and harmless. Central venous pressure catheters can provide useful information and will not precipitate cardiac arrhythmias unless they are inserted into the heart. The placement of pulmonary artery catheters can be quite hazardous in this regard. Nasogastric tubes and Foley catheters are frequently required and are safe to place.

Endotracheal intubation was thought to create a higher risk of arrhythmias. However, these reported sequelae were likely coincidental to, rather than caused by, this procedure. Numerous reports have failed to elicit a single case of arrhythmia provoked by endotracheal intubation. Factors that may be responsible for arrhythmias in the immediate post-intubation period include physical stimulation of the patient, acid-base or electrolyte disturbances, and failure to preoxygenate the patient adequately.

11. Are prophylactic antibiotics indicated for hypothermic patients?

Infection, including septicemia, may be the cause of (e.g., gram-negative sepsis in adults), coincident with, or sequel of hypothermia. Even in the recovery phase of hypothermia, fever as well as other signs of infection are typically absent. Shaking chills caused by sepsis may unwittingly be ascribed to the shivering of hypothermia. Leukocytosis is often absent due to compromised bone marrow release and circulation of neutrophils.

The incidence of infection in hypothermic neonates is quite high and ranges from 41–53% in two series. Pulmonary infections are most commonly found and bacteriology is likely to reveal Enterobacteriaceae, Hemophilus, Staphylococcus or Streptococcus species. In adults, soft-tissue and pulmonary infections are most likely. Occult CNS bacteremia appears to be rare. Gram-negative bacteria, gram-positive cocci, Enterobacteriaceae, and oral anaerobes are likely to be found. The elderly patient with thermoregulatory failure should be considered to have sepsis until proved otherwise.

The key to management is repeated physical examination during and following rewarming. Culture specimens should be secured early in the emergency department course. Lumbar puncture is indicated in adults with persistent altered mental status following rewarming and should be employed more liberally in neonates and the elderly. Antibiotic prophylaxis is recommended for neonates and the elderly. Routine prophylaxis does not appear warranted in hypothermic adults who have no obvious manifestations of infection.

12. What is the relationship of alcohol to hypothermia?

Ethanol has social and pathophysiologic consequences. It is the most frequent associated cause of heat loss in urban hypothermia. Alcoholics are more vulnerable to the hazards of climate because of altered perception due to acute intoxication, inadequate clothing, and insufficient shelter. Heat loss is promoted by peripheral vasodilatation, impaired shivering thermogenesis, and decreased subcutaneous fat caused by malnutrition. There is a strong association between alcohol-induced hypoglycemia and ethanol. An unusual clinical presentation of Wernicke-Korsakoff syndrome is profound hypothermia. This is due to thiamine-depletion-induced hemorrhage in the hypothalamus. The clinical presentation is heralded by hypothermia, bradycardia, hypotension, miosis, and depressed deep tendon reflexes. Therefore, thiamine, 100 mg intravenously, is indicated in hypothermic patients. Magnesium, a necessary co-factor for thiamine, is often depleted in the alcoholic and repletion is required in order for thiamine administration to be effective.

CONTROVERSY

13. Active external rewarming is an effective and safe means of therapy in hypothermia.

For: Certain series report excellent success with the use of AER. The preponderance of data, however, indicate that AER, as an isolated measure of rewarming, is associated with high morbidity and mortality in patients with severe hypothermia. Candidates for AER are previously healthy patients who develop acute hypothermia (e.g., immersion), in whom minimal pathophysiologic changes have occurred. AER in the patient with minimal hypothermia is probably not harmful. The combination of truncal AER with core rewarming has been successful in patients who have more serious hypothermic conditions.

Against: Pathophysiologic consequences of AER in moderate and severe hypothermia include sudden peripheral vasodilatation accompanied by shock, afterdrop in core temperature, suppressed shivering thermogenesis with decreased overall rate of core rewarming, increased peripheral metabolic demands, and decreased threshold for ventricular fibrillation due to myocardial thermal gradients. AER should not be used alone in the patient with moderate to severe hypothermia. If AER is used, it should be restricted to the torso to prevent core temperature afterdrop and thermal injury to the extremity.

BIBLIOGRAPHY

1. Brunette DD, et al: Comparison of gastric and closed thoracic cavity lavage in the treatment of severe hypothermia in dogs. Ann Emerg Med 16:1222, 1987.
2. Danzl DF, et al: Multicenter hypothermia survey. Ann Emerg Med 16:1042, 1987.
3. Kramer MR, Vandijk J, Rosin AJ: Mortality in elderly patients with thermoregulatory failure. Arch Intern Med 149:1521, 1989.
4. Maningas PA, et al: Regional blood flow during hypothermic arrest. Ann Emerg Med 15:390, 1986.
5. Maresca L, Vaska JS: Treatment of hypothermia by extracorporeal circulation and internal rewarming. J Trauma 7:89, 1987.
6. Murphy K, Nowak RM, Tomlanovich MC: Use of bretylium tosylate as prophylaxis and treatment in hypothermic ventricular fibrillation in the canine model. Ann Emerg Med 15:1160, 1986.
7. Otto RJ, Metzler MH: Rewarming from experimental hypothermia: Comparison of heated aerosol inhalation. Crit Care Med 16:869, 1988.
8. Potts DW, Sinopoli A: Infection, hypothermia, and hemodynamic monitoring. Ann Intern Med 102:869, 1985.
9. Reuler JB, Girard DE, Cooney TG: Wernicke's encephalopathy. N Engl J Med 312:1035, 1985.
10. Solomon A, Barish RA, Browne B, et al: The electrocardiographic features of hypothermia. J Emerg Med 7:169, 1989.

105. HEAT STROKE

Stephen V. Cantrill, M.D.

1. What is heat stroke?
Heat stroke is a rectal temperature of approximately $40.6°C$ ($105°F$) or greater in a person with a history of exposure to exercise or increased temperature and humidity with accompanying neurologic disturbance, usually in the form of altered mental status. Anhidrosis (lack of sweating) is not a criterion, as sweating may or may not be present.

2. Why is a rectal temperature of $40.6°C$ selected as the threshold?
A body temperature of this magnitude or greater implies that the body's mechanisms for dealing with an increased heat load have been overwhelmed and the pathologic effects of increased temperature may occur.

3. What are the two types of heat stroke? How do they present?
Classic heat stroke is not associated with exercise, but rather with exposure to high heat and humidity over time. This form of heat stroke has a slow onset, often developing over days. It is common in the elderly and the chronically ill, who may present with anorexia, nausea, vomiting, headache, dizziness, confusion, and hypotension. Anhidrosis is common. **Exertional heat stroke** usually affects young people in good health who are exercising in a hot, humid environment. It is rapid in onset. Nausea, dizziness, and confusion are common. Fatigue, ataxia, coma, and nuchal rigidity or posturing may also occur. Patients often are sweating at the time of presentation.

4. Which populations are at greater risk for heat stroke?
- Extremes of age—due to relatively poor temperature regulation in the young and old
- Chronically ill—especially those on drugs that predispose to heat illness
- Military recruits—especially unacclimated northerners training in the South
- Athletes—most commonly football players and runners
- Laborers—especially if water losses have not been replaced
- Obese individuals—heat dissipation is compromised
- Persons dressed inappropriately for environment or activity level

5. Which drugs predispose a person to heat stroke?
Drugs increasing heat production through increased activity: cocaine, amphetamines, phencyclidine, lysergic acid diethylamide
Drugs decreasing thirst: haloperidol
Drugs decreasing sweating: antihistamines, anticholinergics, phenothiazines, beta-blockers

6. What is the most effective measure of the effect of heat in the environment on a human subject?
The commonly measured ambient air temperature is a poor gauge because it does not measure the effect of humidity, wind velocity, and radiational heating. Research has shown that an entity known as the wet bulb globe temperature (WBGT) is a much more accurate measure. The WBGT combines the wet bulb temperature (measuring the effect of humidity and wind velocity), the black globe temperature (measuring radiational heating), and the dry bulb temperature (measuring ambient air temperature). Although rarely used in the civilian world, the WBGT is commonly used by the military as a guide to determine the allowable level of activity.

7. What is the mortality rate of heat stroke?
Mortality rates vary from zero to 76% in different reports. This high variability is due to the differences in the populations studied. Young, healthy individuals with exertional heat stroke usually do quite well, whereas the elderly, chronically ill suffering classic heat stroke fare quite poorly.

8. What differential diagnosis should be considered in patients presenting with a rectal temperature greater than 40.6° C?

Meningitis	Hypothalamic lesion
Typhus	Neuroleptic malignant syndrome
Falciparum malaria	Malignant hyperthermia
Rocky Mountain spotted fever	

9. Name some end-organ effects in heat stroke.

Skeletal muscle:	rhabdomyolysis
Cardiac:	hemorrhage, necrosis
Respiratory:	adult respiratory distress syndrome
Renal:	acute tubular necrosis
Hepatic:	centrolobular hepatocellular degeneration
Coagulation:	thrombocytopenia, disseminated intravascular coagulation
Central nervous system:	edema, petechial hemorrhages

10. What is the most important aspect in the treatment of heat stroke?
Rapid cooling. Heat stroke is a true medical emergency where minutes count. Poor patient outcome is related more to the length of time the temperature remains elevated than to the absolute degree of hyperpyrexia.

11. What treatment modalities are effective for rapid cooling?
Immersion in ice water is effective, although many feel this must be accompanied by vigorous skin massage to counteract the cutaneous vasoconstriction that may actually impede heat loss. This modality may not be appropriate in the comatose or combative patient. Aggressive evaporative cooling, consisting of treatment with water spray and a forced air stream from a fan, has proved successful. Ice packs and massage may be used. Techniques such as iced gastric lavage and peritoneal lavage have also been reported. Cooling efforts should be ceased when the patient's temperature falls to 38.5°C (101.3°F) to avoid temperature undershoot and shivering.

12. What additional steps should be taken in dealing with heat stroke?
Continuous monitoring of rectal temperature
Supplemental oxygen
Active airway management as indicated
Cardiac monitor and electrocardiogram
Central line placement with CVP monitoring
Cautious fluid replacement: normal saline in the hypotensive patient; otherwise
    D5–0.5% normal saline
Foley catheter and nasogastric tube placement
Restraints as needed

13. Which laboratory studies are appropriate in the severely ill heat stroke patient?

Arterial blood gases	LFTs, CK
Serum electrolytes, BUN, creatinine, glucose	Urinalysis
Complete blood count with platelet count	Serum calcium, magnesium,
PT/PTT, fibrin split products	phosphate

14. What complications may occur in patients with heat stroke?
Emesis—especially in the comatose patient
Electrolyte disorders—hypokalemia, hyperkalemia, hyponatremia
Shivering—treat with diazepam, 5 mg IV
Seizures
Acidosis—treat with sodium bicarbonate if severe
Cardiogenic shock—treat with isoproterenol; avoid alpha agents
Decreased urinary output—treat with mannitol if necessary
Pulmonary edema—from injudicious fluid replacement
Clotting disorders—may require fresh frozen plasma, heparin, or platelets
Combative, psychotic behavior—IV sedation may be necessary

15. Are there prognostic signs that help to indicate outcome?
Yes. The longer the duration of the elevated temperature, the poorer the prognosis. Coma, hypotension, hyperkalemia and an SGOT of greater than 1,000 units are all associated with a poor prognosis.

16. What steps can be taken to prevent heat stroke?
Adequate fluid intake during periods of high temperature, high humidity, or increased
    activity levels
Decreased levels of activity as mandated by the WBGT
Control of ambient temperature and humidity if possible
Appropriate dress for the weather
Prudence during acclimation to a hotter environment
Adjustment of dosages of predisposing drugs, if possible, during hot weather
Awareness of symptoms of impending heat stroke

CONTROVERSIES

17. Is dantrolene sodium effective in treating heat stroke?
Dantrolene sodium uncouples the heat-generating mechanism in muscle and is the drug of choice in treating malignant hyperthermia and neuroleptic malignant syndrome, which cause excessive muscular heat production. The potential benefit of this drug in treating heat stroke has been debated. Many investigators are of the opinion that no benefit would accrue, because once treatment has begun, the problem is not heat production but rather heat dissipation. Dog studies have confirmed that administration of dantrolene sodium has no effect on passive cooling rates, pathologic changes, or clinical outcome. However, a recent human trial has demonstrated a significant improvement in cooling rates in patients treated with dantrolene. This trial, however, failed to demonstrate any difference in clinical outcome. These data, however, raise some interesting questions concerning the pathophysiology and treatment of heat stroke and deserve further study. Routine use of dantrolene sodium in heat stroke patients does not appear to be warranted at this time.

18. What is the most effective means of inducing rapid cooling?
Much discussion has centered on use of immersion, iced gastric lavage, or evaporative cooling of the heat stroke patient, either singly or in combination. Iced peritoneal lavage has also been anecdotally reported. Controlled comparison studies have most commonly used a dog model, which may not adequately represent the human response. At this time, there does not appear to be a "best" method, although many favor evaporative (water spray and forced air) cooling as the best compromise for ease of use, speed of cooling, and patient safety.

BIBLIOGRAPHY

1. Barthel HJ: Exertion-induced heat stroke in a military setting. Milit Med 155:116, 1990.
2. Callaham M: Heat illness. In Rosen P, et al (eds): Emergency Medicine: Concepts and Clinical Practice. St. Louis, C.V. Mosby, 1988, pp 693–717.
3. Channa AB, et al: Is dantrolene effective in heat stroke patient? Crit Care Med 18:290, 1990.
4. Costrini A: Emergency treatment of exertional heatstroke and comparison of whole body cooling techniques. Med Sci Sports Exerc 22:15, 1990.
5. Horowitz BZ: The golden hour in heat stroke: Use of iced peritoneal lavage. Am J Emerg Med 7:616, 1989.
6. Hubbard RW, et al: Novel approaches to the pathophysiology of heatstroke: The energy depletion model. An Emerg Med 16:1066–1075, 1987.
7. Hubbard RW: Heatstroke pathophysiology: The energy depletion model. Med Sci Sports Exerc 22:19, 1990.
8. Knochel JP: Environmental heat illness: An eclectic review. Arch Intern Med 133:841–864, 1974.
9. McElroy C, Auerbach PS: Heat illness: Current perspectives. In Auerbach PS, Geehr EC (eds): Management of Wilderness and Environmental Emergencies. New York, Macmillan, 1983, pp 64–81.
10. Shibolet S, et al: Heat stroke: A review. Aviat Space Environ Med 47:280–301, 1976.
11. Sprung CL, et al: The metabolic and respiratory alterations of heat stroke. Arch Intern Med 140:665–669, 1980.
12. Vicario SJ, Okabajue R, Haltom T: Rapid cooling in classic heatstroke. Am J Emerg Med 4:394–398, 1986.
13. White JD, et al: Evaporative versus iced gastric lavage treatment of heatstroke: Comparative efficacy in a canine model. Crit Care Med 15:748–750, 1987.

XVI: Obstetrics

106. ACUTE OBSTETRIC COMPLICATIONS

Polly E. Parsons, M.D., and Sue Anne Murahata, M.D.

1. What are the obstetric causes of disseminated intravascular anticoagulation (DIC)?
Abruptio placentae, intrauterine demise, amniotic fluid embolism, eclampsia, and acute fatty liver of pregnancy are the more common causes. Saline-induced abortion, molar pregnancy, and ruptured uterus may also cause DIC.

2. What is the differential diagnosis of acute pulmonary edema in the peripartum period?

Postpartum cardiomyopathy	Amniotic fluid embolism
Valvular heart disease	Venous air embolism
Preeclampsia	Pulmonary embolism
Tocolytic-induced pulmonary edema	Aspiration pneumonia/ARDS

3. What is peripartum cardiomyopathy?
It is a dilated cardiomyopathy that occurs during the last trimester of pregnancy or within the first 3–6 postpartum months. Risk factors include maternal age, multiparity, twins, and eclampsia. The etiology is unclear.

4. What is amniotic fluid embolism?
Amniotic fluid presumably enters the maternal circulation either during labor or immediately postpartum, causing acute pulmonary injury. Patients present with acute dyspnea, hypoxia, and hypotension. The diagnosis is frequently made at autopsy, as the mortality is approximately 80%, but may be made in some patients by obtaining blood from a central line or pulmonary artery catheter and examining it for the presence of fetal squamous cells or debris. The only therapy is supportive care.

5. What is tocolytic-induced pulmonary edema?
Up to 4% of patients receiving beta-agonist therapy to suppress premature labor may develop noncardiogenic pulmonary edema either while receiving the drug or within 12 hours of its cessation. There is not an absolute association between the total dose of drug received and the development of the syndrome. Most patients respond to stopping the tocolytic agent and instituting oxygen and diuretic therapy.

6. What are the major causes of abnormal liver function tests during the late stages of pregnancy?
Fatty liver of pregnancy, intrahepatic cholestasis, hepatitis, eclampsia, HELLP (*H*emolysis, *E*levated *L*iver function, *L*ow *P*latelets) syndrome, gallstones, cirrhosis, and normal pregnancy.

7. There are multiple diagnoses to consider when evaluating a pregnant patient with an acute abdomen:
a. Which diagnoses occur with the same frequency in pregnant and nonpregnant persons?
Hepatitis, appendicitis, gastroenteritis, and intrinsic bowel disease.

b. Which diagnoses are more frequent in pregnant persons?
Cholecystitis, pancreatitis, urinary tract infection, ovarian torsion, corpus luteum cyst rupture, intestinal obstruction, and leiomyoma infarction.

c. Which diagnoses are less common in pregnant persons?
Diverticulitis, salpingitis, peptic ulcer disease, and kidney stones.

8. What is the most common nonobstetrical operation performed during pregnancy?
Appendectomy. Although the incidence of appendicitis is not greater during pregnancy, the incidence of appendiceal perforation in pregnancy can be as high as 30–70%, so it is important to be vigilant in the care of a pregnant patient with abdominal pain.

9. What is the most common lower pelvic process presenting as an acute abdomen early in pregnancy?
Ectopic pregnancy, which occurs in approximately 1% of pregnancies. Approximately 0.1% of ectopic pregnancies are associated with maternal death. The major cause of death from an untreated ruptured ectopic pregnancy is hemorrhage, so that immediate surgery is required in patients with an ectopic pregnancy with hemorrhage. The clinical findings of ruptured ectopic pregnancy may mimic those of a hemorrhagic corpus luteum; however, with significant hemorrhage, the treatment is the same for both entities.

10. List the common infections in the postpartum period.
Endometritis, urinary tract infection, pneumonia, wound infection, and mastitis.

11. What percentage of women develop acute pyelonephritis?
1–2%. A small number of these patients develop serous complications, including septic shock, adult respiratory distress syndrome, renal insufficiency, and anemia.

12. What is the approach to the pregnant patient with severe asthma?
The goal is to prevent the development of maternal hypoxemia. Although none of the pharmacologic agents used to treat asthma has been classified A by the Food and Drug Administration (posing no risk during pregnancy), standard asthma medications (epinephrine, terbutaline, theophylline, and steroids) are generally considered safe and are used in pregnant women with severe asthma.

BIBLIOGRAPHY

1. Cunningham FG, MacDonald PC, Grant NF (eds): Williams' Obstetrics. Norwalk, CT, Appleton & Lange, 1989.
2. Durfee RB, Pernoll ML: Early pregnancy risks. In Pernoll ML (ed): Obstetrics and Gynecologic Diagnosis and Treatment. Norwalk, CT, Appleton & Lange, 1991.
3. Greenberger PA: Asthma during pregnancy. J Asthma 27:341–347, 1990.
4. Homan DC: Peripartum cardiomyopathy. N Engl J Med 312:1432–1435, 1985.
5. Kapernick PS: Postpartum hemorrhage and the abnormal puerperium. In Pernoll M (ed): Obstetrics and Gynecologic Diagnosis and Treatment. Norwalk, CT, Appleton & Lange, 1991.
6. Newton ER: The acute abdomen in pregnancy. In Sciarra JJ (ed): Gynecology and Obstetrics. Philadelphia, J.B. Lippincott, 1991.
7. Parsons PE: Pulmonary disease in pregnancy. In Frederickson HL, Wilkins-Haug L (eds): Ob/Gyn Secrets. Philadelphia, Hanley & Belfus, 1991.
8. Pisani RJ, Rosenow EC: Pulmonary edema associated with tocolytic therapy. Ann Intern Med 110:714–718, 1989.

107. ECLAMPSIA

Sue Anne Murahata, M.D.

1. What is eclampsia?
Eclampsia is the occurrence of convulsions and/or coma in a patient suffering from preeclampsia. One way of looking at eclampsia is to consider it the extreme end point of the disease spectrum of preeclampsia (preeclampsia being the triad of hypertension, pathologic edema and proteinuria in a pregnant woman).

2. Who is at risk for eclampsia?
Eclampsia is primarily, but not exclusively, a disease of young primigravidas. There is also an increased incidence in women over 35 years of age and in pregnancies of multiple gestations. Circumstances in which it may develop in the multiparous patient include diabetes, fetal hydrops, underlying chronic hypertension, chronic renal disease, and molar pregnancy. There is also an increased incidence when there is a strong family history present.

3. How common is eclampsia? Preeclampsia?
It occurs in roughly 0.05–0.2% of all deliveries and 3.6% of twin deliveries. Preeclampsia occurs in 6–7% of all pregnancies in the United States.

4. How is the diagnosis made?
The criterion for making the diagnosis of eclampsia is the development of convulsions in a patient suffering from preeclampsia after the 20th week of gestation or within 48 hours postpartum. Although the course of eclampsia may be gradual, the actual onset of generalized convulsions may be quite abrupt and is a life-threatening medical emergency. Symptoms to watch for are complaints of headaches, blurred vision, photophobia, epigastric pain, right upper quadrant pain, and the finding of hyperreflexia.

5. What else could cause the convulsions?
The differential should include cerebrovascular accidents, hypertensive encephalopathy, pheochromocytoma, brain tumor/abscess, infectious disease, metabolic imbalances, or epilepsy.

6. What are the laboratory findings?
The diagnosis of eclampsia does not depend on any specific set of laboratory results. Some common laboratory abnormalities include an elevated serum uric acid level (greater than 6.2 mg/dl), elevated 24-hour urine total protein, and decreased creatinine clearance. A complete blood count often shows an abnormally high hematocrit (a sign of hemoconcentration) and low platelets. Liver enzymes (SGOT, SGPT, LDH) are elevated. An electroencephalogram is acutely abnormal in the immediate postictal period but the pattern is not pathognomonic of eclampsia. HELLP syndrome (see p. 417) occurs in roughly 10% of eclamptic patients.

7. What causes preeclampsia/eclampsia?
Of the many theories proposed (including immunologic phenomena, placental endocrine dysfunction, maternal hormonal abnormalities, coagulation abnormalities, and dietary factors), the most widely accepted at present is a relative increase in thromboxane over prostacyclin derived from placental sources. The excess thromboxane leads to increased vasoconstriction and platelet aggregation. Eclamptic patients exhibit hypersensitivity to angiotensin II and catecholamines.

8. What actually causes the convulsions?

This is also not specifically known. Suggested mechanisms include cerebral vasospasm, cerebral hemorrhage, cerebral ischemia, cerebral edema, hypertensive encephalopathy, and metabolic encephalopathy.

9. When in pregnancy does it occur?

Approximately 50% of cases are antepartum, 25% during labor, and 25% postpartum. In most studies, the majority of cases occur during the third trimester (from 28 weeks to delivery).

10. How is the eclamptic patient managed?

The goals are to control the convulsions and prevent further convulsions, support maternal vital functions, control hypertension, correct hypoxemia or acidemia, and arrange for delivery. During the convulsions, precautions should be taken to avoid physical injury (insert padded tongue blade into the mouth). Oxygen should be administered as soon as feasible.

1. The most routinely used anticonvulsant agent is magnesium sulfate. A loading dose 4 gm is administered intravenously over 10 minutes followed by a continuous infusion (via pump) of 2–3 gm/hr. (As with any medical regimen there are variations.) A therapeutic serum magnesium level is 4–6 mEq/L. The patient must be watched closely for signs of magnesium toxicity. Patellar reflexes disappear at 8–10 mEq/L and severe respiratory depression can develop at 12 mEq/L. Calcium gluconate should be kept at the bedside as an antidote. High levels of magnesium may also be a temporary nephrotoxin. Urine output should be maintained at 25–30 cc/hr. If oliguria occurs, the infusion of magnesium should be decreased or temporarily discontinued. The magnesium infusion is generally continued for at least 24 hours postpartum (perhaps longer, depending on the clinical situation).

2. Hypertension can be controlled with IV boluses of hydralazine, 5 to 10 mg every 20 minutes as needed, until the systolic pressure is between 140 and 150 mm Hg or diastolic pressure is between 90 and 100 mm Hg. To maintain control of blood pressure, a continuous infusion of hydralazine may also be required. Although these patients are hypertensive, they are often intravascularly volume depleted. Whether fluid therapy is of benefit is controversial; central venous monitoring is often helpful in making this decision.

3. Arterial blood gas measurements should be made to assess maternal PO_2 and pH. A chest x-ray should be obtained to rule out aspiration.

4. The patient should now be delivered. If the cervix is favorable, steps should be taken to induce labor. It is critical to have continuous monitoring of fetal heart tones as well as periodic fetal scalp pH monitoring to assure that the fetus continues to do well. If there are signs of fetal distress, a cesarean delivery should be performed. Other reasons for cesarean delivery include abnormal fetal presentation, placental abruption leading to fetal distress (this is reported in 5–25% of eclamptic pregnancies), or extreme prematurity.

11. Are there other considerations with regard to delivery?

One must keep in mind that many of these women have blood clotting abnormalities and/or thrombocytopenia. This is particularly important when considering what type of analgesia to use. Many feel that IV narcotics for labor or general anesthesia for cesarean is safer than regional anesthesia because of the risk of bleeding at the epidural/spinal site and the dramatic fluid shifts (and subsequent blood pressure fluctuations) that can occur.

12. What about perinatal outcome?

Reported mortality rates range from 10–28%. Many variables other than maternal illness determine outcome, among which are degree of intrauterine growth retardation, degree of fetal hypoxia, and extreme prematurity.

13. And maternal outcome?

Maternal prognosis is generally quite good. Although maternal mortality rates in the past have been from 0–14%, in recent years it has been closer to 5%. Potential maternal complications related to eclampsia are disseminated intravascular coagulopathy, intracerebral hemorrhage, pulmonary edema, aspiration pneumonia, acute renal tubular necrosis, retinal detachment, and ruptured liver.

14. Are there long-term sequelae?

Hypertension may persist until 2 weeks postpartum but is generally normal at the 6-week postpartum visit. In long-term follow-up studies, there is a considerable increase in chronic hypertension in patients who have previously suffered eclampsia.

15. Does eclampsia occur with each pregnancy?

As stated previously, it tends to occur in first pregnancies. If a previously eclamptic woman has a problem in a subsequent pregnancy, it tends to be in the form of mild preeclampsia.

16. Can eclampsia be prevented?

Because eclampsia is the extreme form of preeclampsia, with careful close follow-up and aggressive management of patients suffering from preeclampsia, the incidence of eclampsia can be decreased. It must be remembered, however, that some women develop eclampsia abruptly without warning signs or symptoms. Some studies have shown a benefit in increasing dietary calcium to as much as 1.5 gm/day. Others are looking at low-dose aspirin (one baby aspirin per day) as a preventive measure. Some have studied the amount of dietary protein and salt, but none of these studies is definitive.

BIBLIOGRAPHY

1. Crowther C: Magnesium sulphate versus diazepam in the management of eclampsia: A randomized controlled trial. Br J Obstet Gynecol 97:110–117, 1990
2. D'Addesio JP: Postpartum eclampsia. Ann Emerg Med 18:1105–1106, 1989.
3. Garner PR, D'Alton ME, Dudley DK, et al: Preeclampsia in diabetic pregnancies. Am J Obstet Gynecol 163:505–508, 1990.
4. Hernandez C, Cunningham FG: Eclampsia. Clin Obstet Gynecol 33:460–466, 1990.
5. Miles JF, Martin JN, Blake PG, et al: Postpartum eclampsia: A recurring perinatal dilemma. Obstet Gynecol 76:328–331, 1990.
6. O'Brien WF: Predicting preeclampsia. Obstet Gynecol 75:445–452, 1990.
7. Sibai BM: Magnesium sulfate is the ideal anticonvulsant in preeclampsia-eclampsia. Am J Obstet Gynecol 162:1141–1145, 1990.
8. Sibai BM: The HELLP syndrome (hemolysis, elevated liver enzymes, and low platelets): Much ado about nothing? Am J Obstet Gynecol 162:311–316, 1990.
9. Van Dam PA, Renier M, Baekelandt M, et al: Disseminated intravascular coagulation and the syndrome of hemolysis, elevated liver enzymes, and low platelets in severe preeclampsia. Obstet Gynecol 73:97–102, 1989.
10. Villar MA, Sibai BM: Eclampsia. Obstet Gynecol North Am 15:355–377, 1988.
11. Watson CJE, Thomson HJ, Calne R: HELLP—it's not cholecystitis. Br J Surg 77:539–540, 1990.

XVII: Psychiatry

108. MANAGEMENT OF THE DANGEROUS PATIENT IN THE ICU

Edmund Casper, M.D., and Jonathan Ritvo, M.D.

1. What kind of patient is at highest risk for violent behavior toward self or others while in the ICU?

The delirious patient, especially the agitated, overactive, delirious patient.

2. What behavioral signs indicate or suggest impending violence?

Threatening words

Increasingly loud, intense, and threatening speech

Increased motor activity

Easily startled

Inability to be calmed by or respond reasonably to verbal intervention

3. What are the behavioral manifestations of delirium?

Delirious patients may be underactive or overactive. Delirious patients may appear depressed, anxious, paranoid, manic, or irritable. Delirious patients, particularly overactive, agitated patients, are at risk for violence to self and others.

4. Should the delirious patient who is considered dangerous to himself or others be placed on "mental health hold" (involuntary civil commitment status) or restrained?

Restraints should be used early if the delirious patient is considered dangerous. A mental health hold is not necessary. Delirium should be considered a medical, not a mental, illness. The physician should document the signs and symptoms of delirium and the need for restraints to prevent dangerous behavior or allow treatment (e.g., prevent pulling out IV lines).

5. What interventions are available in the delirious patient who is agitated, combative, and paranoid?

Agitated, delirious patients seldom respond to verbal interventions alone. Constant presence of a known and trusted relative, friend or nurse can help. Pharmacologic and physical intervention (restraint) needs to be considered. The drug of choice in such patients is haloperidol (Haldol). Haloperidol is an excellent drug for use in critically ill patients. It has little anticholinergic activity and does not cause hypotension or respiratory depression. Initial doses are 0.5–10 mg, with lower doses used for the elderly and higher doses for more severely agitated patients. Oral potency is half of IM or IV potency. (IV use is not FDA approved.) Doses can be doubled and repeated in 30 minutes. If the patient is not settling down after 2–4 doses, 0.5–1 mg of lorazepam can be added IV or IM. In alcohol, sedative, or hypnotic withdrawal, benzodiazepines should be used first and haloperidol added if psychotic symptoms (delusions or hallucinations) are present.

6. What are the common immediate side effects of haloperidol? How are they treated?

Akathisia (restlessness) may paradoxically increase agitation. This is one rationale for adding lorazepam. Benzodiazepines alleviate akathisia. Lorazepam is better absorbed IM than other benzodiazepines. Propranolol and anticholinergics such as Cogentin (see below) have cardiac effects. Anticholinergics may exacerbate delirium.

Dystonias (tonic muscular contractions) include torticollis, opisthotonos, oculogyric crisis, and tongue dystonias. They occur during the first several days of neuroleptic administration. They can be alleviated with Benadryl, 50 mg IV or IM, after which the patient should be treated prophylactically with Cogentin, 1–2 mg PO or IM bid for 3–5 days.

7. What factors increase the risk of suicide? What are the indications for psychiatric hospitalization after a suicide attempt?

Age, male gender, lack of social support, concomitant psychiatric diagnoses (such as major depression, bipolar disorder, schizophrenia, alcoholism, drug abuse/dependence), hopelessness, lethality of means chosen or used, likelihood of attempt being discovered, lack of relatedness (i.e., suicide attempt does not appear to be directed at obtaining a response from others), family history of suicide, history of impulsiveness, past near-lethal suicide attempt, chronic illness, recent loss, and evidence of a suicide plan with intent to carry it out.

8. What medical conditions are associated with increased risk of suicide?

Severe respiratory disease, chronic hemodialysis, and delirium tremens have been shown to be associated with increased suicide risk. In general, suicide risk should be kept in mind in cases of chronic illness and agitated delirium.

9. Following an overdose of a number of medications, a patients awakens in the ICU. The patient denies attempting suicide and relates, "I got confused and took too many medications by accident." The patient wants to sign out and leave the hospital. How do you handle?

Any patient who needs the ICU for treatment for an overdose of medications should be considered dangerous until proved otherwise.

This patient should have an immediate psychiatric consultation. If the patient refuses to wait for the psychiatric consultant, the patient should be placed on a mental health hold immediately. In most states, this allows adequate psychiatric evaluation of dangerousness. It is always prudent to request a psychiatric consultation whenever a patient wants to sign out of the hospital against medical advice.

10. How can a person who is a potential suicide risk be approached in a therapeutic manner?

Be direct, honest, and to the point in the discussion of suicide with any patient. The majority of patients with suicidal thoughts or behavior welcome the opportunity to discuss the feelings that led to their suicidal behavior. This discussion of feelings will often diminish the suicidal impulse. Keep in mind that suicidality is not static. Suicidal intent varies from moment to moment. All suicide attempts are marked by ambivalence; that is, there is a wish to die and a wish to live. Encourage collaboration of family, friends, significant others both for their input in the evaluation and then in support of the patient. Try to answer these two questions: (1) Has this behavior changed anything in the patient's life? (2) Are there alternative solutions that have been offered and can be accepted by the patient?

11. What are the diagnostic signs and symptoms of major depression?

The diagnosis requires a predominantly sad or depressed mood or loss of interest over a period of 2 weeks. The diagnostic criteria for depression are summarized by the mnemonic **SIGECAPS**:

S = Sleep disturbance (insomnia or hypersomnia)
I = loss of **I**nterest in usual activities
G = preoccupation with **G**uilt or other cognitive features (worthlessness, hopelessness, helplessness)
E = lack of **E**nergy
C = impaired memory or **C**oncentration
A = **A**ppetite disturbance
P = **P**sychomotor agitation or retardation
S = **S**uicidal ideation (thoughts about death)

Five of these criteria are required for the diagnosis. Depressed mood or loss of interest must be one of the five criteria.

12. Is major depression a normal reaction to medical illness?

No. Obviously some signs of depression may accompany major physical illness, especially sleep disturbance, loss of appetite, and loss of energy. The following associated features of depression have been shown to be useful in recognizing depression in the medically ill: sense of failure, loss of social interest, feeling punished, suicidal ideation, dissatisfaction, indecision, and crying. However, consideration should be given to pharmacologic treatment when this diagnosis is entertained. As many as 33% of severely ill patients may have depression.

13. Under what conditions can a patient be placed on a mental health hold?

Any patient who exhibits behavior that is dangerous to himself or to others due to mental illness can be placed on a mental health hold. Some states include grave disability due to mental illness as a criterion for a mental health hold.

14. Under what conditions can a patient suffering from a psychiatric illness or mental illness be placed in restraints?

Restraints can be applied to a patient suffering from a psychiatric illness when the patient's behavior presents a threat or danger to himself or to others around him. A mental health hold should be initiated or already in place before placing restraints. In an emergency, restraints should be applied immediately and a mental health hold initiated.

A clear note in the chart should document the patient's behavior and the actions taken, including writing a mental health hold and placing restraints. In all cases the minimum number of restraints should be two, usually the opposing arm or leg. One restraint should never be applied to a patient. It leads to a false sense of security. Patients have been known to injure themselves or others, including successful suicides and homicides, while in one-point restraint.

15. What information should be conveyed to a patient when obtaining informed consent for a procedure?

(1) The nature of the procedure. (2) The dangers or potential complications of such a procedure. (3) The potential consequences of not undergoing the procedure. (4) Side effects that may accompany the procedure. (5) Any alternative methods of treatment and their potential risks. Basically, the risks, benefits, and alternatives of the procedure should be understood by the patient.

16. Under what conditions is informed consent not required?

In an emergency situation with immediate need for medical treatment to preserve life or limb, treatment should be administered despite a lack of consent.

17. Should medical information be kept from a patient because of concern that the patient will be overwhelmed by the information?

Therapeutic privilege may be invoked to limit full disclosure. In this situation responsible relatives should document the reason for limiting disclosure and the informing of relatives.

18. What is competency to consent to treatment?

According to common law, all persons of adult age are presumed to be competent to make medical treatment decisions until they are shown to be otherwise through a court hearing or some other means. Several issues are generally involved in determination of competency:

- The patient evidences a choice about treatment; that is, the patient is able to express a choice, either for the treatment or against it.
- The patient's choice is deemed to be reasonable and based on a sound reasoning capacity.
- The patient is able to understand the risks and benefits and alternatives involved in the treatment, and the patient manifests an understanding and appreciation of the information presented to him.

A consideration of the relative risk/benefit ratio for the treatment is a good guide to how rigorously competency needs to be proved. If risk is low and benefit high, a reasonable choice (acceptance of the treatment) is usually accepted as competent. An unreasonable choice (refusal of low risk/high benefit treatment) may lead to further investigation, including examination of reasoning capacity, understanding, and appreciation. For higher risk/benefit ratios, more rigorous demonstration of competency may be required.

19. When should guardianship be obtained through the court?

When the patient is deemed incompetent, the treatment decision is not urgent, and either the patient is refusing a reasonable, needed (low risk/high benefit) treatment or a high risk/low benefit treatment is being considered. Examples include refusal of nursing home placement by a demented patient (low risk/high benefit) and discontinuation of life support for a brain-dead patient (high risk/low benefit). Acute medical treatment is usually too urgent to suffer delay for guardianship, in which case hospital policy for obtaining substitute consent from next of kin or (if kin unavailable) from a hospital administrator should be followed.

20. How should the patient who refuses all treatment be managed?

The patient should be determined to be competent or incompetent. The incompetent patient is discussed above. The competent patient who refuses to follow a specific treatment plan may be acting out of panic, denial of the illness, or anger about loss of control. Patients who are in an ICU are virtually helpless and powerless. When a patient asks questions, staff may become defensive. The approach to such a patient should be firmly informative and should attempt to enlist the patient's participation in the treatment. If the underlying issues or feelings can be recognized, they should be addressed and plans modified to assist the patient. Psychiatric consultation should be obtained if the refusal is not resolved quickly.

21. How should the overreacting, inappropriately reacting, or overly demanding family be managed?

Family members should be oriented in a calm, firm manner away from the patient in order to prepare the family members for multiple procedures, personnel, and modern-day technology used in the treatment of patients. What is an accepted environment for the medical team in an ICU is a completely foreign atmosphere for most families and patients.

BIBLIOGRAPHY

1. Baker JE: Monitoring of suicidal behavior among patients in the VA health care system. Psychiatr Ann 14:272–275, 1984.
2. Cassem EH: Depression secondary to medical illness. In Frances AJ, Hales RE (eds): Review of Psychiatry, Vol. 7. Washington, D.C., American Psychiatric Press, Inc., 1988.

3. Cavanaugh S, Clark DC, Gibbons RD: Diagnosing depression in the hospitalized medically ill. Psychosomatics 24:809–815, 1983.
4. Clark DC, Cavanaugh SV, Gibbons RD: The core symptoms of depression in medical and psychiatric patients. J Nerv Ment Dis 171:705–713, 1983.
5. Cohen-Cole SA, Stoudemire A: Major depression and physical illness. Psychiatr Clin North Am 10:1–17, 1987.
6. Glickman LS: Psychiatric Consultation in the General Hospital. New York, Marcel Dekker, 1980.
7. Keller CH, Best CL, Roberts JM, et al: Self-destructive behavior in hospitalized medical and surgical patients. Psychiatr Clin North Am 8:279–289, 1985.
8. Roth LH, Meisel A, Lidz CW: Tests of competency to consent to treatment. Am J Psychiatry 134:279–284, 1977.
9. Schwartz HI, Roth LH: Informed consent and competency in psychiatric practice. In Tasman A, Hales RE, Frances AJ (eds): Review of Psychiatry, Vol. 8. Washington, D.C., American Psychiatric Press, Inc., 1989.
10. Shapiro S, Waltzer H: Successful suicides and serious attempts in a general hospital over a 15 year period. Gen Hosp Psychiatry 2:118–126, 1980.
11. Soloff PH: Emergency management of violent patients. In Frances AJ, Hales RE (eds): Psychiatry Update: The American Psychiatric Association Annual Review, Vol. 6. Washington, D.C., American Psychiatric Press, Inc., 1987.

109. DELIRIUM

Marshall Thomas, M.D.

1. What are the organic mental disorders?

The organic mental disorders are psychological and behavioral syndromes that are caused by transient or permanent brain dysfunction. The organic mental disorders are subdivided into nine categories, the boundaries of which are not well demarcated and tend to overlap. **Delirium**, the most common organic mental disorder, is characterized by widespread cerebral dysfunction, a fluctuating level of consciousness, and most often an acute or subacute onset. The other organic mental disorders tend to represent more selective and/or more stable forms of dysfunction. They include dementia, organic mood syndrome, organic affective syndrome, organic amnestic syndrome, organic delusional syndrome, organic hallucinosis, organic personality syndrome, and atypical/mixed syndromes.

2. What is "ICU psychosis"?

It is a nonspecific and somewhat misleading term. The stress of being in an ICU, with the unfamiliarity of the surroundings, the disruption in sleep/wake cycle, and the admixture of sensory overload and deprivation, can worsen an underlying organic mental disorder. Most patients with ICU psychosis are delirious and require further medical evaluations to determine the cause of delirium. A few of the many other terms used and misused to connote delirium include acute organic brain syndrome, metabolic encephalopathy, toxic psychosis, cerebral insufficiency, acute confusional state, and toxic encephalopathy. None of these terms should be thought of as suggesting an etiologic diagnosis.

3. Describe the clinical features of delirium.

The clinical features of delirium are protean and fluctuate over time. In the prodromal phase, the delirious patient may be restless, anxious, irritable, and beginning to show disturbances in sleep/wake pattern. As delirium progresses, there are increasing **deficits in**

attention and concentration with a **fluctuating level of arousal** that is sometimes interspersed with **lucid intervals**. The worsening of attention and concentration contributes to the evolving memory impairment (especially recent), disorientation, and disorganization of thought and speech.

Behaviorally, the patient may be **hypoactive** and thus appear apathetic or somnolent, or **hyperactive** as evidenced by agitation, but most often demonstrates a **mixed picture** with swings between these two states. The delirious patient is **emotionally labile**, showing a range of affect that fluctuates and changes rapidly. Perceptual disturbances such as **illusions, delusions, and hallucinations** are common and are frequently paranoid in content. Motorically, **dysgraphia**, action tremor, myoclonus, asterixis, and muscle tone changes may occur.

4. How is delirium diagnosed?

The diagnosis of delirium is based on the clinician's familiarity with the presenting features of the syndrome and on a thorough assessment of the patient's mental and physical state. An accurate **history** is helpful in assessing whether there is a change from baseline mental status. Because the delirious patient is often a poor historian, the history is augmented by a **thorough chart review** and histories obtained from past physicians, family, and friends. Such detective work may uncover the cause of delirium—for example, a medication error, a previously unsuspected medical disorder, or a covert alcohol or drug problem. The patient's physical status is further assessed by obtaining **serial physical and neurologic exams**, laboratory studies, and vital signs. A **mental status exam** that assesses level of arousal, attention, concentration, orientation, thought processes, affect, and performance ability (praxis, writing, naming) is performed and serially repeated.

5. Describe the patient groups at increased risk for delirium.

Approximately one-third of hospitalized medical patients are delirious at some point in their hospitalization. Elderly patients, children, postcardiotomy patients, burn patients, patients with drug and alcohol addictions, and patients with preexisting brain disease are at increased risk for developing delirium. Common examples in the latter category include elderly patients with dementia and younger patients with HIV infection. In general, the elderly represent the highest risk category, with the risk of delirium increasing progressively with age. Increasing severity of physiologic stressors, such as more extensive burns or longer operations, further increase the risk of delirium.

6. What laboratory studies are indicated in the work-up of delirium?

The basic studies are complete blood count, SMA-6, SMA-12, urinalysis, arterial blood gases, chest x-ray, and EKG. Clinical judgment is used in deciding the appropriateness of studies such as drug levels, toxicology screens, lumbar puncture (LP), electroencephalogram (EEG), MRI, or CT scans. In persistent, unexplained delirium, the laboratory work-up may extend to include thyroid function tests (including TSH), VDRL, sedimentation rate, HIV, ANA, thiamine and folate levels, urinary porphobilinogen, and a screen for heavy metals.

7. What are the indications for CT scan, MRI, EEG, and LP in the work-up of delirium?

Because delirium is usually caused by toxic-metabolic disorders, the majority of patients will not require these studies. A **CT scan or MRI** of the head is performed early in the work-up of delirium if there are signs of increased intracranial pressure (papilledema or meningeal irritation), focal neurologic findings, significant recent headache or head trauma, or in the presence of coma. An **EEG** may be helpful in detecting seizure activity or a focal lesion, or in confirming the diagnosis of delirium. Most but not all patients with delirium show generalized diffuse background slowing on EEG that correlates with the severity of the delirium. A **lumbar puncture** may be difficult to perform in the delirious patient, but is indicated if acute bacterial or fungal meningitis is suspected, and in the evaluation of mental status changes associated with fever of unknown origin, possible subarachnoid hemorrhage, encephalitis, neurosyphilis, or unexplained seizures.

Although CT scan, MRI, EEG, and LP are not always needed in the work-up of acute delirium, they are usually indicated in the work-up of prolonged delirium of indeterminate etiology.

8. Discuss the differential diagnosis of delirium.

It is extensive. Complicating the issue is the fact that frequently there are multiple causes of cerebral dysfunction. Each potential cause is assessed and pursued individually, with priority being given to the more life-threatening and emergent causes. The mnemonic **I Watch Death** covers an extended differential diagnosis.

Causes of Delirium (I Watch Death)

I	= Infection	Encephalitis, meningitis, syphilis
W	= Withdrawal	Alcohol, barbiturates, sedatives-hypnotics
A	= Acute metabolic	Acidosis, alkalosis, electrolyte disturbance, hepatic failure, renal failure
T	= Trauma	Heat stroke, postoperative state, severe burns
C	= CNS pathology	Abscesses, hemorrhage, normal pressure hydrocephalus, seizures, stroke, tumors, vasculitis
H	= Hypoxia	Anemia, carbon monoxide poisoning, hypotension, pulmonary/cardiac faliure
D	= Deficiencies	B12, hypovitaminosis, niacin, thiamine
E	= Endocrinopathies	Hyper(hypo)adrenalcorticism, hyper(hypo)glycemia
A	= Acute vascular	Hypertensive encephalopathy, shock
T	= Toxins/drugs	Medications, pesticides, solvents
H	= Heavy metals	Lead, manganese, mercury

From Wise MG: Delirium. In Hales RE, Yudofsky SC (eds): Textbook of Neuropsychiatry. Washington D.C., American Psychiatric Press, 1987.

9. Give an expanded list of the drugs that are most likely to be associated with delirium.

Delirium can be associated with any number of drugs. Polypharmacy contributes to delirium in several ways: (1) drugs compete for metabolism, thereby prolonging half-lives; (2) protein displacement changes bioavailability; (3) additive effects occur such as in the simultaneous use of more than one anticholinergic agent. Drug levels should be monitored, but patients with already compromised brain function may experience CNS toxicity at "therapeutic levels" (as with aminophylline, digitalis, and lithium). Other acutely ill patients may experience the accumulation of certain drugs (as in the excess accumulation of meperidine and its active metabolite normeperidine in patients with renal failure). The following is a partial list of drugs that may cause delirium in the ICU:

Anesthetics—all (especially fentanyl)
Antibiotics
   Penicillin (high-dose)
   Cephalosporins (especially in patients with renal failure)
Anticholinergics—all
   Atropine/scopolamine/belladonna
   Tricyclic antidepressents (especially amitriptyline)
   Phenothiazines (especially thioridazine and chlorpromazine)
   Antiparkinsonian agents (benztropine, biperiden, trihexyphenidyl)
   Over-the-counter agents (Compoz, Excedrin P.M., Sleep-eze, Sominex)

Analgesics
  Opiates
  Synthetic narcotics (especially
    meperidine)
Anticonvulsaants
  Barbiturates
  Carbamazepine
  Phenytoin
  Sodium valproate
Antihistaminics
  Nonselectives: diphenhydramine
              chlorpheniramine
              promethazine
  H2 blockers: cimetidine
              ranitidine
              famotidine
Anti-inflammatory drugs
  ACTH
  Corticosteroids
  Nonsteroidal anti-inflammatory drugs
  Ibuprofen
  Indomethacin
  Naproxen
  Phenylbutazone
  Sulindac
  Tolmetin
  Salicylates

Cardiac agents
  Antiarrhythmics: lidocaine
                  mexiletine
                  procainamide
                  quinidine
                  tocainide
  Antihypertensives: methyldopa
                  beta-blockers
                  (propranolol)
                  diuretics
                  reserpine
  Inotropics: L-dopa
                  cardiac glycosides
                  digitalis
Pulmonary drugs
  Aminophylline
  Theophylline
Sedatives hypnotics—all
  Barbiturates
  Benzodiazepines
Miscellaneous
  Hypoglycemic agents
  Disulfiram
  Lithium
  Metrizamide
  Metronidazole
  Podophyllin (by absorption)

10. What is the course of delirium?

The outcome of delirium may be full recovery, development of a more chronic organic brain syndrome, or death. Although the most common outcome is recovery, morbidity and mortality are high. Delirious patients are at risk for seizures, coma, and medical complications related to agitation (e.g., fractures, subdural hematomas, and pulling out of intravenous and intra-arterial lines). Conservatively estimated, 25% of hospitalized delirious patients will die within 3–4 months.

11. How is delirium treated?

The first goal of treatment is to determine the cause(s) of the disorder; then, specific treatments can be instituted. The patient with hypertensive encephalopathy can be treated with antihypertensive agents, the patient with alcohol withdrawal can be treated with a benzodiazepine, and the patient with hypoxia and pneumonia can be treated with oxygenation and antibiotics.

In the absence of a specific diagnosis and until the delirium resolves, the patient requires close and frequent supervision. As the diagnostic search continues, nonessential medications are discontinued while vital signs, input and output, laboratory studies, and adequacy of oxygenation are followed. Attempts are made to orient and reassure the patient, provide appropriate levels of environmental stimulation, reestablish a more normal day/night sleep cycle (i.e., dimming the lights at night), and keep the patient in contact with familiar objects, family and friends. The agitated delirious patient may or may not respond to verbal interventions and thus may require physical restraint and/or pharmacologic intervention to ensure safety.

12. Describe the pharmacologic management of delirium.

Although controlled studies are lacking, consensus opinion holds haloperidol as the treatment of choice in managing delirium while or until more specific treatment is initiated.

Haloperidol is a high-potency neuroleptic agent whose acute side effects include extra-pyramidal symptoms, dystonia, and akathisia. In contrast to other psychotropic agents, haloperidol causes little sedation, orthostatic hypotension, or cardiac or anticholinergic effects.

Usually well-tolerated in the medically ill, haloperidol is prescribed in doses of 2, 5, or 10 mg for younger patients, and 0.5, 1, or 2 mg for elderly patients with mild, moderate, or severe agitation, respectively. Doses can be repeated every 30 minutes until the patient is sedated or calm. Once adequate control is achieved, relatively more of the dose can be given at night to help reestablish a normal sleep/wake pattern. As the patient improves, usually the dose is tapered over several days rather than abruptly discontinued.

The acute dystonia and parkinsonian rigidity associated with neuroleptic agents can be treated with diphenhydramine (25–50 mg PO or IM), or benztropine (1–2 mg PO or IM). Akathisia, a potentially troublesome side effect that may actually worsen agitation, is more likely to respond to low-dose propranolol (40 mg per day in divided doses) or lorazepam (1–4 mg per day in divided doses).

13. What are the psychiatric and neurologic sequelae of cardiac arrest?

Overt neurologic sequelae are unusual, but patients may experience subtle signs and symptoms of persistent cognitive, mood, or behavioral dysfunction. Common symptoms include fatigue, distractibility, inability to learn new skills, impaired recall, apathy, irritability, petulance, emotional disinhibition, and disturbances in impulse control, insight, empathy, judgment, and social perceptiveness.

14. Describe the psychological and behavioral consequences of mild to moderate head injury or the "postconcussive syndrome."

Epidemiologically, traumatic brain injury is one of the most common causes of organic mental disorders. Patients with "minor" closed head injuries frequently have somatic, cognitive, perceptual, and emotional symptoms that sometimes result in prolonged disability. In "milder" forms of closed head injury, symptoms include anxiety, depression, irritability, headache, dizziness, fatigue, insomnia, memory difficulties, impaired concentration, tinnitus, and sensitivity to noise and light. In more severe cases, traumatic brain injuries can precipitate full-blown delirium, psychosis, depression, mania, and aggressive syndromes.

15. What is Wernicke-Korsakoff syndrome? How is it treated?

Wernicke-Korsakoff syndrome represents a spectrum of neurologic dysfunction associated with thiamine deficiency. Although most often associated with alcoholism, the thiamine deficiency associated with Wernicke-Korsakoff can also be caused by malabsorption syndromes, severe anorexia, upper GI obstruction, prolonged IV feeding, and hemodialysis. **Wernicke's encephalopathy** is an acute life-threatening condition characterized by oculomotor disturbances (nystagmus to complete gaze palsy), cerebellar ataxia (truncal), and mental confusion. The general confusional state can progress to stupor and coma. Morbidity, if left untreated, includes a significant mortality rate (17%) and progression to Korsakoff's psychosis. **Korsakoff's psychosis** is a debilitating chronic condition that includes retrograde amnesia, anterograde amnesia, and usually but not always confabulation. Punctate lesions in the periventricular and periaqueductal regions of the brain stem and diencephalon are seen at autopsy and can sometimes be picked up on CT or MRI scan.

Wernicke's encephalopathy is treated acutely with doses of parenteral thiamine, 100 mg IM, until ophthalmoplegia resolves. Patients are also given magnesium sulfate, 1 to 2 mg IM in a 50% solution. Symptoms of Korsakoff's psychosis, once established, are irreversible and overlap somewhat with chronic alcohol dementia.

CONTROVERSY

16. What is the role of benzodiazepines as adjunctive treatment in the agitated, delirious patient?

Excluding alcohol and sedative hypnotic withdrawal, high-potency neuroleptics are considered the treatment of choice in managing the agitation associated with delirium. Some controversy exists about the adjunctive use of benzodiazepines in this situation.

For: High-potency neuroleptics are specific antipsychotic agents that are not particularly sedating. The agitated delirious patient may require high doses of a high-potency neuroleptic to achieve sedation or to become calm. High doses of neuroleptics increase the risk for potentially serious side effects such as neuroleptic malignant syndrome and tardive dyskinesia. Short- or intermediate-acting benzodiazepines can be used in this situation for their sedating effects, thereby allowing for the use of a relatively lower dose of the antipsychotic agent.

Against: Some argue that the short-term use of antipsychotic agents in the medically ill population is usually safe and that the use of a benzodiazepine can contribute to respiratory depression and worsening of delirium.

BIBLIOGRAPHY

1. Andreason JC: Neurospychiatric complications in burn patients. Int J Psychiatr Med 5:161–171, 1974.
2. Folstein MF, Folstein SE, McHugh PR: (Mini-Mental State): A practical method for grading the cognitive state of patients for the clinician. J Psychiatr Res 12:189–198, 1975.
3. Goldstein MJ: Intensive care syndromes. In Stoudemire A, Fogel BS (eds): Principles of Medical Psychiatry. New York, Grune and Stratton, 1987, pp 403–421.
4. Layne OL, Yudofsky SC: Postoperative psychosis in cardiotomy patients: The role of organic and psychiatric factors. N Engl J Med 289:518–520, 1971.
5. Perry SW, Markowicz J: Organic mental disorders. In Talbot JA, Hales RE, Yudofsky SC (eds): Textbook of Psychiatry. Wasington D.C., American Psychiatric Press, 1988, pp 279–311.
6. Salzman C, Green AI, Rodriguez-Vela F, et al: Benzodiazepines combined with neuroleptics for acute and severe disruptive behavior. Psychosomatics 27 (Suppl):17–21, 1986.
7. Slaby AE, Cullen LO: Dementia and delirium. In Stoudemire A, Fogel BS (eds): Principles of Medical Psychiatry. New York, Grune and Stratton, 1987, pp 135–175.
8. Trepacz PT, Teague GB, Lipowski ZJ: Delirium and other organic mental disorders in a general hospital. Hosp Psychiatry 7:101–106, 1985.
9. Wettington WW: The mortality of delirium: An underappreciated problem? Psychosomatics 23:1232–1235, 1982.
10. Wise MG: Delirium. In Hales RE, Yudofsky SC (eds): Textbook of Neuropsychiatry. Washington D.C., American Psychiatric Press, 1987, pp 89–106.
11. Wise MG, Cassem NH: Psychiatric consultation to critical care units. In Tasman A, Goldfinger SM, Kaufmann CA (eds): Review of Psychiatry, vol. 9. Washington D.C., American Psychiatric Press, 1990, pp 413–432.
12. Yudofsky SC, Silver JM: Psychiatric aspects of brain injury: Trauma, stroke, and tumor. In Hales RE, Frances AJ (eds): American Psychiatric Association Annual Review. Washington D.C., American Psychiatric Press, 1985, pp 142–158.

110. ANXIETY AND AGITATION IN THE ICU

Marshall R. Thomas, M.D.

1. How are anxiety and agitation diagnosed?
Anxiety and agitation are nonspecific symptoms that indicate an underlying problem(s) that requires further exploration and differential diagnosis. Anxiety can have both psychological (excessive apprehension and fear) and physiologic components (including signs of motor tension, autonomic hyperactivity, and hypervigilance) Agitation is a behavioral symptom of excessive motor activity that indicates internal discomfort. Both anxiety and agitation can be caused by a broad array of medical and psychiatric conditions, or may reflect a more purely "psychological reaction" to the circumstances that surround ICU admission. In the ICU, agitation, for example, is most commonly caused by delirium, but may also result from anxiety, fear, pain, psychosis, or akathisia.

2. Which medical conditions are associated with anxiety and agitation?
Listed below in the table are medical conditions that tend to present with prominent symptoms of anxiety with or without concomitant delirium.

Medical Conditions Associated with Anxiety

Coronary insufficiency	Hypocalcemia (hypoparathyroidism)
Cardiac arrhythmias (PAT)	Hyper and hypothyroidism
Hypoxia	Post-concussive syndromes
Drug toxicities (stimulants, xanthines, sympathomimetics)	Hyperventilation (e.g., that associated with pulmonary emboli)
Drug (sedative-hypnotic, opiate, TCA) and alcohol withdrawal	Mitral valve prolapse
Hypercortisolism	Pheochromocytoma
Hyperparathyroidism/hypercalcemia	Partial complex seizures
Hypoglycemia	Tumors in the area of the third ventricle
	Inadequately treated pain

3. Give an expanded list of drugs that are associated with anxiety in the medical setting.

Sympathomimetics	Bronchodilators	Calcium channel blockers
Phenylephedrine	Isoetharine	Verapamil
Epinephrine	Isoproterenol	Nifedipine
Phenylpropanolamine	Metaproterenol	Diltiazem
Stimulants	Albuterol	Excess thyroid supplement
Amphetamines	Antiarrhythmics	Steroids
Cocaine	Lidocaine	L-dopa
Methylphenidate	Tocainide	Baclofen
Xanthines	Flecainide	Cycloserine
Theophylline	Mexiletine	Indomethacin
Caffeine	Quinidine	Quinacrine
		Neuroleptics
		Metoclopramide ⎫ drugs that can
		Fluoxetine ⎬ cause akathisia
		Amoxapine ⎭

4. Describe the symptoms and syndromes associated with alcohol withdrawal.
Alcohol withdrawal should be considered in any patient who develops extreme anxiety within the first several days of admission to a hospital service; 30–50% of hospitalized medical patients are thought to have a problem that in some way relates to alcohol abuse,

dependence, or withdrawal. In the ICU, the presence of other medical conditions or the use of concomitant medications (analgesics, beta blockers, and narcotics) may alter the clinical presentation and obscure the diagnosis of acute alcohol withdrawal. The common and **early signs of alcohol withdrawal** typically occur within 24 hours of cessation or reduction in drinking and include anxiety, irritability, tremulousness, nausea, and vomiting. Other symptoms are malaise, tachycardia, elevations in blood pressure, sweating, and orthostatic hypotension. In milder forms of withdrawal, symptoms peak within 24–48 hours and subside within 5–7 days.

Between 1 and 10% of hospitalized alcoholics develop delirium associated with alcohol withdrawal. **Alcohol withdrawal delirium** (delirium tremens, DTs) is associated with confusion, disorientation, fluctuating and clouded consciousness, delusions, paranoia, vivid hallucinations, marked autonomic arousal, mild fever, agitation, and insomnia. The usual onset is 3–4 days after cessation of drinking, with a peak intensity of symptoms occurring on the fourth and fifth days. The syndrome is usually self-limited (3–5 days), but in rare cases may extend longer (4–5 weeks). With more modern medical interventions, the previously reported high rate of fatality (20%) is now less than 1%.

Alcohol withdrawal seizures tend to occur within 48 hours after last alcohol use. In patients with seizures, more than half have multiple seizures (two to six grand mal), but the development of status epilepticus is rare (less than 3%). In addition to acute cessation of long-term alcohol use, alcohol withdrawal seizures may be more common in patients with hypomagnesemia, respiratory alkalosis, and hypoglycemia.

Alcohol hallucinosis is a syndrome in which vivid hallucinations (usually auditory) occur shortly after cessation of alcohol, but in the presence of an otherwise clear sensorium and with a relative paucity of autonomic symptoms. In the majority of cases, symptoms recede within a few hours to a few days, but in a small proportion of cases the symptoms become chronic.

5. What is the medical treatment of acute alcohol withdrawal?

Benzodiazepines, a class of drugs cross-tolerant with alcohol, are the treatment of choice for moderate to severe alcohol withdrawal. The standard treatment for withdrawal using the longer-acting benzodiazepines, chlordiazepoxide (Librium) and clorazepate (Tranxene), may be inappropriate in the acute-care setting where the longer half-lives of these agents may combine with medical complications (liver failure and drug interactions) to cause prolonged obtundation, respiratory depression, and worsening or obscuration of a co-morbid delirium. In this setting, intermediate-acting agents, lorazepam (Ativan) or oxazepam (Serax), may be easier to titrate because of their shorter half-lives. Lorazepam may be given in doses of 1–4 mg q 6–8 hr, and oxazepam, 15–60 mg q 8 hr. Oxazepam has the added advantage of primary renal excretion without reliance on intermediate liver metabolism.

Benzodiazepines not only treat autonomic hyperactivity, but also decrease the likelihood of alcohol withdrawal delirium (DTs) and alcohol withdrawal seizures. As a result, anticonvulsants are not indicated except in patients with preexisting or underlying seizure disorders. Antipsychotics (e.g., haloperidol) are sometimes used to treat alcohol hallucinosis but are used cautiously in patients undergoing alcohol withdrawal because of their ability to lower seizure threshold. Vitamin deficiencies and electrolyte disturbances are addressed, and in patients with severe nutritional deficit the acute administration of thiamine, 100 to 200 mg IM, prior to glucose infusion may prevent the development of the potentially irreversible Wernicke-Korsakoff syndrome.

6. Describe the syndrome of sedative-hypnotic withdrawal.

Sedatives-hypnotics include benzodiazepines, barbiturates, and miscellaneous other CNS depressants (including chloral hydrate, ethchlorvynol, glutethimide, meprobamate, and paraldehyde). Sedative-hypnotic withdrawal is virtually identical to alcohol withdrawal. It is not uncommon, in fact, for a patient to be simultaneously dependent on alcohol and another sedative-hypnotic. The time of onset and duration of the syndrome differ in accordance with the half-life of the agent abused. With alprazolam (Xanax), for example, the onset of withdrawal is 8–12 hours, whereas for the longer-acting diazepam (Valium), the onset of withdrawal may take 5–7 days. The frequently problematic **alprazolam withdrawal syndrome** can be treated by a slow tapering of alprazolam or by switching the patient to clonazepam (Klonopin), a high-potency benzodiazepine with a longer half-life, and then tapering. Alprazolam can be converted to clonazepam at a rate of 0.5 mg of clonazepam for every 1 mg of alprazolam.

7. What is the opiate withdrawal syndrome? What are the symptoms?
Opiate withdrawal occurs in the hospital when addicted patients no longer have access to their supply or iatrogenically when pain medications are tapered too rapidly. Patients switched to narcotics with mixed agonist-antagonist properties, such as pentazocine, may also experience withdrawal. Symptoms include intense anxiety, rhinorrhea, lacrimation, goose flesh, mydriasis, abdominal pain, nausea, vomiting, diarrhea, fever, and leukocytosis. Although intensely uncomfortable, opiate withdrawal is less medically serious than sedative-hypnotic and alcohol withdrawal. Opiate withdrawal can be treated through a more gradual tapering of the opiate or mitigated by adjunctive use of clonidine, a centrally-acting alpha$_2$-adrenergic agonist.

8. What are the symptoms of antidepressant withdrawal?
Both tricyclic antidepressants (TCAs) and monoamine oxidase inhibitors (MAOIs) are associated with a withdrawal syndrome following abrupt cessation. Symptoms include anxiety, agitation, anorexia, nausea, vomiting, abdominal pain, diarrhea, myalgias, night-mares, insomnia, hyperreflexia, akathisia, and delirium. Abrupt withdrawal from anticho-linergic TCAs can lead to a syndrome of cholinergic overdrive characterized by sialorrhea, abdominal cramping, and diarrhea. Symptoms usually begin within a couple of days of cessation of medication and can last for up to 2 weeks. Reinstitution of the antidepressant with more gradual tapering is effective in treating the withdrawal syndrome.

9. What is the differential diagnosis of anxiety and agitation that results from a primary psychiatric disorder versus that from delirium or another organic mental disorder?
Once organic mental disorders have been ruled out, a wide variety of primary psychiatric disorders may present with the prominent symptom of anxiety. The patient's past psychiatric history may reveal a mood, anxiety, psychotic, or character disorder. Individually and as a group, anxiety disorders, mood disorders, and substance abuse disorders are the most prevalent psychiatric disorders in the general population.

Anxiety is a frequent concomitant of **depression**. Anxiety and agitation are particularly common in severe depression and **mania**. Patients with other forms of **psychosis**, including schizophrenic, schizophreniform, and paranoid disorders, may appear fearful, anxious, and agitated, especially if left unmedicated. Under severe stress, patients with **character disorders** show symptoms of excessive anxiety, agitation, hostility, dependence, or psychosis. Patients with borderline, narcissistic, histrionic, schizotypal, and antisocial personalities may be more prone to severe regressions.

A diagnosable anxiety disorder is present in 10–15% of the general population. In the acute-care setting, patients with **panic disorder, acute and chronic PTSD**, and **hyperventilation syndrome** may be more likely to present management problems. Patients with generalized anxiety disorder, obsessive-compulsive disorder, and phobic disorders, though common, are more likely to have chronic symptoms that will be detected only after a careful interview. All anxiety disorders demonstrate high rates of co-morbidity with affective and substance abuse disorders. Additionally these patients are at risk for having their preexisting anxiolytic or antidepressant medications unwittingly discontinued, thereby creating an iatrogenic withdrawal syndrome.

10. What is panic disorder? How is it treated?
Approximately 10% of the population experiences panic attacks, whereas 1% of the population has a diagnosable panic disorder. Patients wtih panic disorder experience the sudden onset of extreme anxiety characterized by physical symptoms of intense autonomic arousal and extreme apprehension and fear. Initially, attacks may be linked to psychological and physiologic stressors, such as loss, separation, trauma, severe illness, hyperventilation, and ingestion of illicit drugs. In true panic disorder, panic attacks can develop spontaneously and appear to "come out of the blue." Panic attacks are usually short-lived (5–20 minutes) yet intensely uncomfortable. During an attack, patients are afraid that they are going to die, lose control, or go crazy. Once panic attacks develop, many patients develop **anticipatory anxiety** as they worry about future attacks and **phobic avoidance** as they attempt to avoid situations that they fear might provoke another attack. In between episodes, panic disorder patients appear "high-strung" and hypochondriacal. Because of the prominence of physiologic symptoms (shortness of breath, dyspnea, palpitations, nausea, and vertigo), many patients seek medical help from emergency rooms, cardiologists, neurologists, and pulmonary specialists.

Panic disorder is treated with a combination of supportive psychotherapy, cognitive behavioral interventions, and pharmacotherapy. Patients are reassured that they are not going to die, educated about the disorder, taught relaxation techniques, and progressively desensitized to phobic stimuli. Pharmacologically, panic disorder is treated with either high-potency benzodiazepines (typically alprazolam or clonazepam), TCAs (imipramine, nortriptyline, or desipramine), MAOIs (phenelzine or tranylcypromine), or some combination of the above medications. Untreated panic disorder is associated with high rates of morbidity and mortality.

11. What are the signs, symptoms, and treatment of acute and chronic posttraumatic stress disorder (PTSD)?
PTSD occurs in reaction to overwhelmingly traumatic events and can result in psychic numbing, autonomic hyperarousal, and intrusive re-experiencing of the event as with recurrent recollections, daydreams, and nightmares. Associated symptoms vary, but they include anxiety, irritability, anger, hostility, depression, guilt, emotional withdrawal, dissociation, hypervigilance, exaggerated startle response, difficulty falling asleep, lack of trust, and a feeling of meaninglessness.

The patient admitted to the ICU who has just suffered a rape, beating, or automobile accident may be suffering acutely from PTSD in addition to the medical and surgical problems that result. Acute symptoms, such as anxiety, irritability, fearfulness, guilt, hypervigilance, nightmares and exaggerated startle, may be most prominent. Patients with chronic forms of PTSD, such as those that result from childhood physical or sexual abuse or neglect, or from some other previous traumatic experience, are at risk for being retraumatized by the current situation and have difficulty tolerating the helplessness and loss of control associated with being a critically ill patient. Potentially problematic in the management of such patients are the understandable difficulties they may have in trusting care-givers and in modulating anger and fear.

In the acute management of patients with PTSD, an atmosphere of concern, safety, and understanding is crucial. Frequently, if the physician is able to deal calmly with an initial onslaught of anxiety or hostility without reacting in kind, an unintentional yet significant test has been passed. An understanding of the symptoms associated with PTSD and a willingness to share this information with the patient can be helpful. In acute PTSD, early psychiatric intervention may prevent the development of a more severe or chronic disorder.

12. What is the hyperventilation syndrome?

Anxiety can lead to hyperventilation, and hyperventilation can worsen anxiety. Associated symptoms include light-headedness, weakness, paresthesias, and carpopedal spasm. Hyperventilation leads to respiratory alkalosis, cerebral artery constriction and substantial reductions ($\geq$40%) in cerebral blood flow. Many patients are unaware that they are hyperventilating, but once established, respiratory alkalosis is easily maintained. Some patients with panic disorder are chronic hyperventilators and can have full-blown "panic attacks" provoked by hyperventilation. The diagnosis of hyperventilation syndrome is suspected by clinical presentation and can be confirmed by ruling out organic causes (for example, recurrent pulmonary emboli) and by reproduction of symptoms while voluntarily overbreathing. Hyperventilation syndrome can be treated with patient education and reassurance, a conscious decrease in respiratory rate, and rebreathing (i.e., into a paper bag) when necessary.

13. Describe common psychological reactions to admission to the ICU. How can they be managed?

Anxiety is probably ubiquitous in noncomatose patients (and their loved ones) admitted to the ICU. Fears of death, abandonment, isolation, loss of control, physical disability, and loss of role function are common. The seriousness of the patient's medical condition, the omnipresent monitors and alarms, the lack of accurate medical information, and inherent difficulties in communication all contribute to worsen anxiety.

In the face of overwhelming anxiety, patients may regress and fall back on earlier more primitive and more rigid defenses. Denial and projection or vacillations between extreme passivity and defiant assertions of control may emerge. Defenses are simultaneously adaptive and maladaptive. In the acute post-MI patient, for example, some degree of denial is associated with a decrease in anxiety and perhaps with a better prognosis in the immediate postinfarction period. Acutely, a physician's attempts to interfere with denial usually serve to increase anxiety and are counterproductive.

Although anxiety is common in the ICU setting, each individual assigns personal and private meanings to the experience. Interest in the patient as an individual and attention to his concerns can be helpful. A willingness to support the patient's attempts to cope, to share information, to help distinguish fantasy from reality, and to restore the patient's sense of control are useful. Questions like, "What is it like for you to . . ." may give the patient a chance to express his feelings while leaving his defensive structure intact. The physician's alliance with the patient's family and sensitivity to the impact of the current crisis on the family system can help in decreasing anxiety. A sense of the physician's concern and availability greatly decrease anxiety for both the patient and the family. Allowing the patient access to family members can decrease fears of abandonment and isolation.

14. What is the pharmacologic treatment of anxiety in the ICU?

In using psychotropics in the ICU, one must take care not to further impair cognition or obscure the diagnosis of developing delirium. In general, nonpharmacologic interventions are used to manage the psychological reactions to ICU admission. Exceptions might include the acute coronary care patient in whom adequate treatment of anxiety may improve survival, or the severely agitated patient in whom agitation is interfering with necessary treatment. Patients with preexisting psychiatric disorders may have been receiving neuroleptics, antidepressants, or benzodiazepines on an outpatient basis. These drugs can be associated with both psychiatric and physiologic withdrawal syndromes, and although dosages may need to be adjusted, they should be continued when possible.

Anxiety and agitation arising from delirium are best treated by identifying and treating the underlying disorder and, when necessary, with the symptomatic use of a high-potency antipsychotic such as haloperidol. Neuroleptics may also be used in the pharmacologic management of the anxious patients where respiratory depression is a concern.

The benzodiazepines increase levels of drugs such as phenytoin and digoxin and may potentiate respiratory depression associated with narcotics. Benzodiazepines are used in alcohol and/or sedative-hypnotic withdrawal and may be used adjunctively in the treatment of severe agitation. Intermediate and short-acting benzodiazepines are preferred.

Other anti-anxiety agents of use in selected patients include beta blockers, antihistamines, and narcotics.

BIBLIOGRAPHY

1. Dubovsky SL: Pharmacologic treatment in neuropsychiatry. In Hales RE, Yudofsky SC (eds): Textbook of Neuropsychiatry. Washington D.C., American Psychiatric Press, 1987, pp 411–438.
2. Dubovsky SL, Weissberg MP: Anxiety. In Clinical Psychiatry in Primary Care, 2nd ed. Baltimore, Williams & Wilkins, 1982, pp 57–79.
3. Frances RJ, Franklin JE: Alcohol-induced organic mental disorders. In Hales RE, Yudofsky SC (eds): Textbook of Neuropsychiatry. Washington D.C., American Psychiatric Press, 1987, pp 141–156.
4. Gold PW, Goodwin FK, Chrousos GP: Clinical and biochemical manifestations of depression: Relation of neurobiology to stress. Parts I and II. N Engl J Med 319:348–353, 1988; 319:413–420, 1988.
5. Goldstein MG: Intensive care syndromes. In Stoudemire A, Fogel BS (eds): Principles of Medical Psychiatry. New York, Grune and Stratton, 1987, pp 403–421.
6. Goldberg RJ: Anxiety in the medically ill. In Stoudemire A, Fogel BS (eds): Principles of Medical Psychiatry. New York, Grune and Stratton, 1987, pp 177–203.
7. Hollander E, Liebowitz MR, Gorman JM: Anxiety disorders. In Talbott JA, Hales RE, Yudofsky SC (eds): Textbook of Psychiatry. Washington D.C., American Psychiatric Press, 1988, pp 443–492.
8. Silver JM, Yudofsky SC: Psychopharmacology and ECT. In Talbott JA, Hales RE, Yudofsky SC (eds): Textbook of Psychiatry. Washington D.C., American Psychiatric Press, 1988, p 767–854.
9. Tesar GE, Stern TA: Evaluation and treatment of agitation in the intensive care unit. J Intens Care Med 1:137–148, 1986.
10. Van der Kolk BA: The psychological consequences of overwhelming life experiences. In Van der Kolk BA (ed): Psychological Trauma. Washington D.C., American Psychiatric Press, 1987, pp 1–30.
11. Wise MG: Delirium. In Hales RE, Yudofsky SC (eds): Textbook of Neuropsychiatry. Washington D.C., American Psychiatric Press, 1987, pp 89–106.
12. Wise MG, Cassem NH: Psychiatric consultation to critical care units. In Tasman A, Goldfinger SM, Kaufmann CA (eds): Review of Psychiatry, vol. 9. Washington D.C., American Psychiatric Press, 1990, pp 413–432.

111. NEUROLEPTIC MALIGNANT SYNDROME

James L. Jacobson, M.D.

1. What is neuroleptic malignant syndrome?

Neuroleptic malignant syndrome (NMS) is an acute, potentially fatal, idiosyncratic reaction to neuroleptic medications (which primarily are antipsychotic medications). The principal manifestations are due to disorders of thermoregulation and skeletal muscle metabolism mediated via central mechanisms. The usual presentation consists of four primary features: (1) hyperthermia, (2) extreme generalized regidity, (3) autonomic instability, and (4) altered mental status. The overall appearance is of a profoundly ill individual with an alert frightened stare.

2. What are the specific criteria for diagnosis of NMS?

The diagnosis of NMS requires the presence of specific historical information, physical signs, symptoms, and exclusionary criteria. There must be a **recent history of exposure** to neuroleptic medication. Usually this exposure is acute and occurs within 7–10 days of onset of the syndrome. However, NMS can occur in chronic usage. **Temperature elevation** can be mild or severe. **Autonomic instability** is indicated by labile hypertension (less often hypotension) and tachycardia. **Mental status** is always **altered**, typically in the form of delirium, which may progress to stupor, obtundation, and coma. Extreme **muscular rigidity** has been characterized as "lead-pipe rigidity" and is present in all skeletal muscle. **Diaphoresis** is always present. **Sialorrhea** is often present, as is **dysphagia**. Alternative etiologies for these symptoms must be excluded by history, examination, and laboratory studies.

3. Are there specific laboratory findings for NMS?

No laboratory findings are pathognomonic for NMS, but certain studies are important both to support the diagnosis of NMS and to exclude other systemic illnesses. Common laboratory findings are elevated creatinine phosphokinase (muscle fraction), leukocytosis, and a low serum iron. Electrolyte disturbances that may occur secondarily, as well as hypocalcemia, hypomagnesemia, and hypophosphatemia, may require therapy. Urinalysis often reveals proteinuria and myoglobinuria from rhabdomyolysis. Cerebrospinal fluid (CSF) studies should be normal. An EEG may show diffuse slowing without focal abnormalities. To evaluate a patient with suspected NMS, the following studies should be done to exclude a systemic illness: CBC with a differential WBC; serum electrolytes; creatinine and BUN; muscle and hepatic enzymes; thyroid function tests; urinalysis; EKG; appropriate cultures for infection; and brain imaging, EEG, CSF studies (when indicated).

4. What is the differential diagnosis of NMS?

The differential diagnosis includes several processes that can cause increased temperature due to abnormal thermoregulation, and these are divided into primary CNS disorders and systemic disorders.

Differential Diagnosis of NMS

PRIMARY CNS DISORDERS	SYSTEMIC DISORDERS
Infections (viral encephalitis, postinfectious encephalitis, HIV)	Infections
	Metabolic conditions
	Endocrinopathies (thyrotoxicosis, pheochromocytoma)
Tumors	Autoimmune disease (SLE)
Cerebrovascular disease	Heat stroke
Head trauma	Toxins (CO, phenols, strychnine, tetanus)
Seizures	Drugs (salicylates, dopamine inhibitors and antagonists,
Major psychoses (lethal catatonia)	stimulants, psychedelics, MAOIs, anesthetics, anticholinergics, alcohol or sedative withdrawal)

From Caroff SN, et al: Neuroleptic malignant syndrome: Diagnostic issues. Psychiatr Ann 21:130–147, 1991, with permission.

5. What causes NMS?

The specific antidopaminergic activity of antipsychotic medications appears to be the predominant cause of NMS. Central dopaminergic systems are involved in thermoregulation as well as regulation of muscle tone and movement. The relatively infrequent occurrence of NMS, however, suggests the concurrence of other factors. Speculations have included imbalances with other neurotransmitter systems, abnormalities in second messenger systems, and the presentation of particular risk factors. Currently, all of the antipsychotic medications have been reported to cause NMS, including a recent report implicating the atypical antipsychotic medication, clozapine. NMS also has been reported with some antiemetic medications such as prochlorperazine maleate and metoclopramide, which are also neuroleptics.

6. Which risk factors predispose to the development of NMS?

Suggested risk factors include dehydration, a primary diagnosis of affective disorder (especially bipolar disorder and psychotic depression), concurrent presence of an organic brain syndrome, use of other neuroactive medications, higher relative doses and parenteral administration of neuroleptics, prior history of NMS, electrolyte disturbances, any medical or neurologic illness, and a recent history of substance abuse or dependence.

7. How common is NMS?

Rates as low as 0.02% and as high as 2.5% have been reported, but overall the rate appears to be about 1%.

8. What is the mortality associated with NMS?

Mortality from NMS has been declining since its original description in 1968. The earliest reports suggested mortality rates as high as 75%. In the early 1980s mortality rates declined to 20–30%. Current studies suggest that the mortality rate declined further, probably to less than 15%. Early recognition and familiarity with the syndrome are the most likely reasons for this hopeful trend.

9. What are the treatments for NMS?

Early recognition is crucial. Increased temperature, elevated blood pressure, tachycardia, muscle stiffness not responsive to antiparkinsonian agents, clustering of risk factors, dysphagia, and severe diaphoresis early in the course of treatment with neuroleptic medication should alert the physician to the possible emergence of NMS. Neuroleptic and other neurotoxic medications must be stopped. Supportive measures to lower temperature and ensure good fluid intake are essential. Electrolyte disturbances must be corrected. The patient should be closely monitored for signs of impending respiratory failure secondary to severe muscle rigidity and inability to handle oral secretions. Renal function should be monitored closely. Although there is no evidence that osmotic diuresis hastens recovery from NMS, it may help to maintain renal function.

Pharmacologic intervention has tended to be reserved for severe cases. Dopamine agonists (bromocriptine and amantadine) and/or direct muscle relaxants (dantrolene) have been used; decreased mortality rates have been reported with both types. Dosages vary widely, but doses of bromocriptine have been documented between 2.5 and 35 mg/day. Dopamine agonists, particularly in higher doses, can cause psychosis and/or vomiting, which clearly can complicate the picture and compromise the patient. The only data available on direct-acting muscle relaxants are for dantrolene. Doses of up to 10 mg/kg have been used. The goal is to decrease muscular rigidity in order to decrease the hypermetabolic state in skeletal muscle, which is partially responsible for the hyperthermia in NMS. Dantrolene can cause hepatoxicity, which can lead to overt hepatitis and death. Combinations of dantrolene and dopamine agonists have been used, although there is no evidence that they further decrease mortality. Anticholinergic medications commonly used to treat pseudoparkinsonism have little benefit. Although there is no clear evidence to support the use of benzodiazepines in the treatment of NMS, they can be useful in managing an agitated hyperactive patient once NMS has begun to resolve. No currently available drug therapy has been shown to shorten the course of NMS. One study suggested that therapy may prolong the total period of disability from NMS. However, because only the most severe cases have been treated with medication, the apparently longer disease course may be a manifestation of the initial severity of the illness.

10. Will NMS recur with subsequent use of neuroleptic medication?

The risk of recurrence decreases with time. Of patients rechallenged with neuroleptics prior to 2 weeks after resolution of NMS, there is a high recurrence rate. Those cautiously rechallenged 2 weeks or longer after resolution of NMS often tolerated neuroleptics without difficulty. A low-potency neuroleptic agent is chosen for the rechallenge. Dosing should be conservative and increased gradually. Recent interest in the concurrent use of the calcium channel blocker nifedipine has also shown promise in prevention of recurrence, although the data are still incomplete. Some individuals are prone to NMS and, of course, close attention to early symptoms is crucial.

Guidelines for Managing Patients After NMS

---

1. History of a previous episode of NMS confirmed?

   Yes: Go to (2)
   No: Speak with patient, family, and treating physician(s). Retrieve pertinent medical records to confirm the diagnosis of NMS.

2. Based on careful review of the psychiatric history and previous response to treatment, is neuroleptic therapy essential?

   Yes: Go to (3)
   No: Treat accordingly, without neuroleptics.

3. Two or more episodes of NMS with more than one neuroleptic?

   Yes: Go to (4)
   No: Wait 1–2 weeks after recovery from NMS. Rechallenge with a low-potency neuroleptic. If a low-potency neuroleptic originally caused NMS, rechallenge with a low-potency neuroleptic from a different chemical class.

4. Have prophylactic agents—bromocriptine, dantrolene, or nifedipine—been used in conjuction with neuroleptics?

   Yes: Go to (5)
   No: Consider such a trial, or go to (5)

5. Alternatives to conventional neuroleptic therapy:

   (a) clozapine, (b) benzodiazepines, (c) electroconvulsive therapy, (d) anticonvulsants, and (e) lithium.

From Lazarus et al: Beyond NMS: Management after the acute episode. Psychiatr Ann 21:165–174, with permission.

11. Is there any way to prevent NMS?

No. Early recognition and, when clinically warranted, lower dosing, avoidance of parenteral neuroleptic medication, avoidance of rapid increases in dosage, and minimization of the other risk factors (e.g., good hydration) may decrease the incidence of NMS.

12. Are there alternatives to neuroleptic treatment for the acutely psychotic patient?

There are a number of treatment options. Benzodiazepines may help in the management of the hyperactive psychotic patient and lower the absolute dose of neuroleptic needed. When the primary diagnosis is affective disorder (as in a significant percentage of patients developing NMS), aggressive treatment of the manic or depressive illness with antidepressants, lithium carbonate, or carbamazepine is indicated. It is usually necessary to administer neuroleptic medications concomitantly when psychotic symptoms are present. Electroconvulsive therapy is a viable alternative for manic psychosis and depressive psychosis, and it may alleviate catatonia.

BIBLIOGRAPHY

1. Caroff SN (ed): Neuroleptic malignant syndrome. Psychiatr Ann 21:128–180, 1991.
2. Castillo E, Rubin R, Holsboer-Truacster E: Clinical differentiation between lethal catatonia and neuroleptic malignant syndrome. Am J Psychiatry 145:324–328, 1989.
3. Levenson JL: Neuroleptic malignant syndrome. Am J Psychiatry 142:1137–1145, 1985.
4. Pope HG Jr, Aizley HG, Keck PE, McElroy SL: Neuroleptic malignant syndrome: Long-term follow-up of 20 cases. J Clin Psychiatry 52:208–212, 1991.
5. Pope HG Jr, Keck PE Jr, McElroy SL: Frequency and presentation of neuroleptic malignant syndrome in a large psychiatric hospital. Am J Psychiatry 143:1227–1232, 1986.
6. Shalev A, Heresh H, Munitz H: Mortality from neuroleptic malignant syndrome. Clin Psychiatry 50:18–22, 1989.
7. Susman VL, Addonizio G: Recurrence of neuroleptic malignant syndrome. J Nerv Ment Dis 176:234–241, 1988.
8. Rosebush P, Stewart T: A prospective analysis of 24 episodes of neuroleptic malignant syndrome. Am J Psychiatry 146:717–725, 1989.
9. Rosebush PI, Stewart TD, Gelenberg AJ: Twenty neuroleptic rechallenges after neuroleptic malignant syndrome in 15 patients. J Clin Psychiatry 50:295–298, 1989.

XVIII: Ethics

112. ETHICS

Georgia H. Couderc, R.N., B.S.N., and Julie A. Dearwater, R.N., B.S.N.

1. What is the legal principle on which judicial decisions regarding withdrawal of life support are based?

The law of informed consent to medical care is the foundation of such decisions. Under this law, physicians are legally bound to provide the patient with information about available treatment options and the risk and benefit of these options (including the option of no treatment), and must be confident that the patient understands the information provided.

2. What is an "advanced directive"? Is it legally binding?

It is a form of communication one dictates while competent to express future wishes regarding medical care in the event one becomes incompetent or otherwise unable to make his or her preferences known. Living wills are a popular form of advanced directive, as is the durable power of attorney. Such directives indicate what type of care an individual wishes to receive and may also appoint a party to be responsible for making decisions. Despite the uncertain legal status, courts tend to uphold patients' wishes unless there is a specific reason to doubt the validity of the advanced directive.

3. How does one determine if a patient is competent to make his or her own health care decisions? What action should be taken if it is suspected that the patient is unable to do so?

A competent patient is able basically to understand proposed treatment options and alternatives, and can communicate this understanding and decisions. Examples of incompetent patients are those in vegetative states or severely retarded persons without the intelligence to make such decisions. Some patients, however, are not so obviously imcompetent, in which case the physician may request a psychiatric consultation to determine competency. When a patient is deemed incompetent, it is necessary to appoint a surrogate to make health care decisions. This is usually done quite informally, with a family member or next-of-kin speaking on behalf of the patient. When there is no family, a conservator may need to be appointed by the court.

4. What is the purpose of the hospital Ethics Committee? How does it function?

Ideally, the Ethics Committee is an interdisciplinary group that provides a forum for discussion of ethical issues and consultation on specific cases in the hospital. Ethics Committees commonly review cases, help clarify competency of the patient or the surrogate's understanding of the options and alternatives, and provide support to the members of the health care team involved in difficult ethical decision making. The Ethics Committee does not function to make such decisions but to consult and provide information to guide the decision-makers.

5. What is the physician or nurse's recourse when he or she morally disagrees with a patient's plan of care?

It is advisable to discuss the plan with other caregivers to determine if one's concerns are shared. Health care providers should trust their instincts when uncomfortable with the treatment being provided; there is usually a valid basis for concern. An ethics consult is an excellent means of examining the issue. When these actions fail to reconcile the caregiver to the course of treatment, a request to be removed from the case should be honored, as long as others are available to care for the patient.

6. What strategies can be used to include families in the decision-making process?
When it appears that a patient will be in the hospital for an extended stay, it is advisable to set up weekly meetings between the family spokesperson and the attending physician or intensive care consultant. This helps the family gain confidence in the medical system and opens the doors of communication. If a social worker is available, weekly social service rounds involving both nurses and physicians are an excellent forum to discuss discharge planning, family issues, and plan for the future.

7. Who is ultimately responsible for determining the "code status" of a patient?
The decision to withhold resuscitation attempts should be a collaborative one, determined by the patient, family, and physician. Emotional involvement of the family or the incompetent status of the patient frequently render them incapable of making such a decision, however. It is unfair to place this burden on a grieving family. The objective medical opinion of the attending physician is the determining factor in decisions not to resuscitate.

8. What constitutes "extraordinary" treatment measures?
Extraordinary measures are any treatments that impose a greater burden to the patient than benefit. Therefore, this term can be applied to different treatments for different persons. Such interventions may cause undue pain, expense, or questionable gains.

9. When is it ethically correct to withhold or terminate medical interventions?
When interventions are futile or unable to improve a patient's condition, they often merely prolong life and delay the inevitable demise of the patient. Health care providers are not morally obligated to perform futile actions.

10. Is a "slow-code" a legal order?
The decision to refrain from cardiopulmonary resuscitation should be clear and definite, and communicated to all involved parties via the medical record. A slow-code order is dissimulation, in that it is a contradiction in terms and conveys a confusing message to all members of the health care team.

11. Is it acceptable to deny treatment to patients based on their inability to pay for it?
It is simplistic to believe that socioeconomic considerations should never be allowed to influence patient care decisions; however, the clinician must have the patient's welfare as the primary objective.

12. How does one provide analgesia to a dying patient while ascertaining that euthanasia is not occurring?
Euthanasia, or "good death," can be defined as active or passive, voluntary or involuntary, by commission or omission. Medication for pain relief is appropriate and one of the most important treatments health care providers can offer. In the dying patient, the prolonging of life is no longer a goal. Rather, relief of pain may be the primary goal. To deny analgesia in such a situation, regardless of the fact that it may depress respirations or blood pressure, would be to deny the patient one of the few interventions that can increase comfort at a time he may need it most.

13. How is a dying patient's need for analgesia assessed?
If the patient is conscious, attempts should be made to communicate with him or her. If the patient is unresponsive, pain medication should be administered based on physiologic

responses such as heart and respiratory rate, blood pressure, and facial expression. The nurse should document the physiologic factors that indicated need for analgesia, as well as the patient's response to the pain medication.

14. Are there various methods of administration of analgesia for the dying patient?
The most common method is bolus injection. Continuous intravenous drips of analgesia may be more effective in establishing a stable comfort level because they can be titrated to maintain a particular blood level of medication.

15. What coping strategies can be used by health care providers to ease the emotional burden of caring for patients in a persistent vegetative state?
The humanity of the patient can be emphasized by promoting family involvement and developing an individualized plan of care. Photographs of the patient in the hospital room are invaluable in assisting medical and nursing staff to understand the person in the hospital bed. Most importantly, adhering to the wishes of the patient about extent of medical interventions, when these wishes are known, allows the caregiver to rest assured that the patient is being treated with the greatest dignity possible.

Bonus Question

16. What is PSDA? (*Hint:* It went into effect December 1, 1991.)
The Patient Self-Determination Act of 1990. It is the first federal statute to address advance directives and the right of adults to refuse life-sustaining treatment.[8]

BIBLIOGRAPHY

1. Bone RC, Rackow EC, Weg JG: Ethical and moral guidelines for the initiation, continuation, and withdrawal of intensive care. Chest 97:949–958, 1990.
2. Edwards BS: Does the DNR patient belong in the ICU? Crit Care Nurs Clin North Am 2:473–479, 1990.
3. Goldberg IV, Sprotzer I: Life, death, and liability: Duties of health care providers regarding withdrawal of treatment. Health Care Supervisor 9:33–42, 1990.
4. Jonsen AR, Siegler M, Winslade WJ: Clinical Ethics, 2nd ed. New York, Macmillan, 1986.
5. Levine ME: Ration or rescue: The elderly patient in critical care. Crit Care Nurs Q 12:82–89, 1989.
6. Shoemaker WC, Ayres S, Granvik A, et al (eds): Textbook of Critical Care, 2nd ed. Philadelphia, W.B. Saundres, 1989.
7. Thelan LA, Davie JK, Urden LD: Textbook of Critical Care Nursing. St. Louis, C.V. Mosby, 1990.
8. Wolf SM, Boyle P, Callahan D, et al: Sources of concern about the patient self-determination act. N Engl J Med 325:1666–1671, 1991.

113. WHEN MAY CRITICAL CARE BE TERMINATED?

J. S. *Kobayashi*, M.D.

1. What are the three primary areas of consideration in the legal and ethical aspects of decisions to terminate medical care in the intensive care setting?
(1) Whether the patient is capable or competent to give informed consent (see chapter 112).
(2) If the patient is incapacitated, whether the patient has established an advance directive

such as a living will or durable power of attorney for health care; or, in the absence of these documents, whether there is a clear substitute decision maker, or the need for a court determination of guardianship limited to health care decisions. A physician may not terminate treatment unilaterally simply because the patient is incapacitated. (3) If there is medical consensus that further medical intervention could only be considered **futile care**, there is no ethical obligation to continue or initiate futile treatment or to present treatment alternatives that are considered futile to the family.

2. What is the difference between a living will, a durable power of attorney for health care, and a limited guardianship for medical decisions?
Although specific legislation has not been passed in all states, advance directives are gaining increasing acceptance as means for maintaining patient autonomy under circumstances of incapacitation. They are called advance directives because the patient establishes them while still competent, in anticipation of the possibility of incapacitation (see chapter 112). Physicians can find reassurance in being able to respect the wishes of the patient through the availability of these instruments.

A **living will** is a document that usually specifies the conditions under which a patient with an irreversible medical condition may wish to terminate or limit treatment. A patient may indicate, for example, that he or she does not wish to be maintained on ventilatory support for more than a specified period of time.

A **durable power of attorney for health care** specifies a person designated by the patient as a substitute decision maker who is able to give informed consent for health care decisions in the event the patient is incapacitated.

A **guardian** may be appointed by a court as the medical decision maker for an incapacitated patient when the patient has not designated anyone in advance. If there is no dispute between primary family members and the medical team about the termination of care, a guardian may not need to be formally appointed. Under these circumstances, the physician may allow the family to act as surrogate decision makers in one of several different ways. The physician may accept the family's report of the patient's previously stated preferences about terminating or continuing treatment, or allow them to make a "substituted judgment"—judgment they feel the patient would have made under the circumstances. Or the physician might accept the family's consensus as "in the best interests" of the patient when the patient's preferences are not known.

3. What is futile care?
There has been increasing medical and societal recognition that more care is not always better care. Given the sometimes limited benefits, particularly when frequently associated with significant discomfort, offered by advanced technology and even basic resuscitative efforts, there have been increasing discussions of the circumstances under which medical treatment should be limited or terminated. The most extreme case is when care might be considered futile.
a. What is the definition of futile care?
Futile care is medical treatment that serves only to prolong dying and offers virtually no chance of recovery or even significant actual benefit to the patient. An irreversible condition is present that will lead to the patient's death with or without treatment. Care may be considered futile in two separate ways: physiologic futility, in the sense of no chance for recovery; or futility in the sense of no chance of recovering a meaningful quality of life. Only the first is in the province of medical decision making (see part c).
b. What are criteria for deciding if care is futile?
Some physicians have proposed that if, in the last 100 cases, a medical treatment has been useless, the treatment should be regarded as futile. Others have suggested methods that vary in considering treatment futile when survival was no better than from a lower limit

of 2% to an upper limit of 7%. While these criteria will continue to be debated, sufficient clinical trials have not systematically studied such outcomes in order to provide a strictly scientific basis of judgment. Most would nevertheless agree on beginning to have specialists raise questions about futility of care based on their extensive experience, rather than to try everything simply because the treatments are available.

c. Who should decide if care is futile?

One distinction that is ethically based is that the decision maker should depend on whether the care is considered physiologically futile or futile in the sense of inability to recover a meaningful quality of life. Some argue that the first can only be a medical decision, and even question whether the family should be involved at all (such as in the decision not to initiate cardiopulmonary resuscitation). Quality-of-life decisions, however, involve value judgments about the patient's life and can be evaluated only by the patient or his or her loved ones.

In many cases, however, there is interaction between these two arenas, such as in patients with significant neurologic compromise. The neurologist must first determine, for example, if the patient is in a persistent vegetative state, and the family may then decide if the patient would have wanted to live in that state. A persistent vegetative state is not medically futile in the sense of prognosis for survival, but is futile with regard to recovery.

In some case psychosocial considerations may predominate. For example, there may be medical consensus about physiologic futility, but a decision is made in conjunction with the family to continue treatment until a particular relative or friend could arrive to see the patient.

4. If care is considered futile:

a. Should withdrawing treatment that has already been initiated be considered any differently from withholding treatment that has not been started?
There is no ethical difference. In fact, it might be argued that feeling free to initiate treatment (without worrying about not being able to withdraw it later) affords the opportunity of a clinical trial that could provide the basis for a more accurate decision about the value of withholding or using treatment. While withdrawing and withholding treatment may "feel" or seem like different actions, ultimately they are not ethically different.

b. Is withdrawal of nutrition and hydration considered the same as withdrawal of other medical treatment?
A number of court cases and a number of states have defined nutrition and hydration as medical treatment, which can be withdrawn when an overall decision has been made to withdraw all medical therapies. A competent patient may decide to terminate nutrition and hydration; nutrition and hydration for incapacitated patients often entail involved medical procedures, such as gastrostomies and parenteral nutrition, which may at times be more complicated than the rest of the treatment program. Although withdrawal of nutrition and hydration may "feel" or seem like a different kind of medical intervention, ultimately it is not ethically different.

5. What are the ethical issues in a unilateral DNR order?

Unilateral refers to the discretion of the physician to write a do-not-resuscitate (DNR) order without the formal consent of the family of an incapacitated patient. Although physicians may make unilateral decisions not to proceed with treatment demanded by the family when it is totally inappropriate (such as performing surgery when there is no specific indication), the debate continues as to whether the final decision about a DNR order is, under certain circumstances, entirely within the domain of the physician to make. Most would agree that optimal care entails participation of the family as well as obtaining their consent for any decision; however, some would argue that giving final responsibility for the DNR decision to the family in the name of patient autonomy is actually an abdication of the physician's responsibility for making a decision based on medical expertise, and, in some sense, a less compassionate response.

Clinical aspects include whether most families have unrealistic expectations for resuscitative efforts, on the one hand, and, on the other, are able to withstand the potential guilt of having set a limit to the care of their loved one; and whether physicians are willing to confront and actively address the fact that resuscitation in a particular patient is likely to bring more suffering than benefit. Some studies have pointed out that longer-term outcome measures, such as surviving to hospital discharge, indicate a much less optimistic outcome for cardiopulmonary resuscitation than immediate survival of the arrest, supporting arguments for more specific decision making about withholding resuscitative efforts. Ethical debate continues to focus on whether or not this is paternalism under the auspices of medical expertise, and where the limits of unilateral physician decision making will be.

BIBLIOGRAPHY

1. Baird RM, Rosenbaum SE: Euthanasia: The Moral Issues. Buffalo, Prometheus Books, 1989.
2. Bedell SE, Delbanco TL: Choices about cardiopulmonary resuscitation in the hospital: When do physicians talk with patients? N Engl J Med 310:1089–1093, 1984.
3. Bedell SE, Delbanco TL, Cook EF, et al: Survival after cardiopulmonary resuscitation in the hospital. N Engl J Med 309:569–576, 1983.
4. Blackhall LJ: Must we always use CPR? N Engl J Med 317:1281–1285, 1987.
5. Callahan D: Setting Limits. New York, Simon & Schuster, 1987.
6. Council on Ethical and Judicial Affairs, American Medical Association: Guidelines for the appropriate use of do-not-resuscitate orders. JAMA 265:1868–1871, 1991.
7. Hastings Center: Guidelines on the Termination of Life-Sustaining Treatment and the Care of the Dying: A Report by the Hastings Center. New York, The Hastings Center, 1987, p 30.
8. Kilner JF: Who Lives? Who Dies? Ethical Criteria in Patient Selection. New Haven, Yale University Press, 1990.
9. Lantos JD, Singer PA, Walker RM, et al: The illusion of futility in clinical practice. Am J Med 87:81–84, 1989.
10. Lo B: Unanswered questions about DNR orders. JAMA 265:1874–1875, 1991.
11. Lo B, Mcleod GA, Saika G: Patient attitudes to discussing life-sustaining treatment. Arch Intern Med 146:1613–1615, 1986.
12. President's Commission for the Study of Ethical Problems in Medicine and Biomedical and Behavioral Research: Deciding to Forego Life-Sustaining Treatment. Publication 0-383-515/8673. Washington, D.C., U.S. Government Printing Office, March 1983.
13. Ruark JE, Raffin TA, et al: Initiating and withdrawing life support: Principles and practice in adult medicine. N Engl J Med 318:25–30, 1988.
14. Schneiderman LJ, Spragg RG: Ethical decisions in discontinuing mechanical ventilation. N Engl J Med 318:984–988, 1988.
15. Tomlinson T, Brody H: Ethics and communication in do not resuscitate orders. N Engl J Med 318:43–46, 1988.
16. Youngner SJ: Futility in context. JAMA 264:1295–1296, 1990.

XIX: Toxicology

114. GENERAL APPROACH TO POISONINGS

Ken Kulig, M.D.

1. What are the 12 most common causes of death from acute poisoning reported to poison centers?

The 1989 annual report of the American Association of Poison Control Centers lists the following:

		Total	Percent
1.	Antidepressants	140	.559
2.	Analgesics	126	.078
3.	Stimulants and street drugs	64	.320
4.	Sedative hypnotics	78	.153
5.	Cardiovascular drugs	70	.345
6.	Alcohols	53	.122
7.	Gases and fumes	46	.225
8.	Asthma therapies	34	.265
9.	Hydrocarbons	31	.053
10.	Chemicals	27	.051
11.	Cleaning substances	25	.016
12.	Pesticides (including rodenticides)	14	.023

2. What is the current role of syrup of ipecac in treating acute poisoning?

Although syrup of ipecac induces vomiting within 20–30 minutes in most persons who are administered a therapeutic dose, very little poison is removed; there are more effective means of decontaminating the gastrointestinal (GI) tract. Ipecac may have a role in treating children at home, who frequently can be administered a dose soon after ingestion. By the time most patients present to a hospital, however, too much time has elapsed for syrup of ipecac to be of benefit. Its use also delays the administration of activated charcoal, which needs to be administered as quickly as possible for maximal benefit.

3. What is the current role of gastric lavage in treating acute poisonings?

Gastric lavage has the advantage over ipecac in that it works faster in emptying stomach contents, and activated charcoal can be administered down the lavage tube before it is pulled. Gastric lavage can be accomplished without prior tracheal intubation in most patients, but it is advised that airway equipment, including suction, be immediately available at the bedside. Placing the patient on his or her left side in mild Trendelenburg position will help to prevent aspiration if vomiting occurs. Nasogastric tubes are too small to remove pills or large pill fragments; whenever gastric lavage is performed, a large-bore (36- or 40-French tube in adults) should be placed through the mouth. A bite block with an oral airway will prevent the patient from biting the tube.

4. Is there a role for cathartics in treating acute poisoning?

The theory behind cathartics is that they will speed up GI transit time, allowing activated charcoal to catch up with pills in the bowel, and also prevent desorption of drug from activated charcoal. A single dose of a cathartic is commonly used, although this practice is of unproven benefit. Multiple-dose cathartics should never be used because life-threatening complications from electrolyte imbalance may result. A single dose of a saline cathartic such as magnesium sulfate or magnesium citrate, or a single dose of sorbitol (approximately 1 gm/kg), is unlikely to be harmful and may be of slight benefit.

5. What is the current role of whole-bowel irrigation in the treatment of acute poisoning?
Whole-bowel irrigation uses a polyethylene glycol electrolyte solution such as Golytely or Colyte, which is not adsorbed and will flush drugs or chemicals rapidly through the GI tract. This procedure appears to be most useful when radiopaque tablets or chemicals have been ingested, as their progress through the GI tract can be monitored by radiography. This procedure is also commonly used when packets of street drugs such as heroin or cocaine have been ingested and need to be passed through the GI tract as quickly as possible. The limitations of the procedure are that unless the patient is awake, cooperative, and able to sit on a commode, there is a risk of vomiting and aspiration in addition to the logistical problem of having an unconscious patient in bed with massive diarrhea.

6. What is the role of multiple-dose charcoal in the treatment of acute poisoning?
Multiple-dose charcoal has been shown to enhance the elimination of many drugs that have already been absorbed from the GI tract or that are given intravenously. This process has been called "gastrointestinal dialysis," and has been shown to be quite effective for theophylline and perhaps phenobarbital poisoning. Numerous other drugs have been shown to have their pharmacokinetics altered by multiple-dose charcoal, but it is not clear if this makes a clinical difference. Some of these drugs are listed below; new studies are being currently performed on others. For the majority of acute poisonings in which use of multiple-dose charcoal is being contemplated, it should be borne in mind that the primary reason for giving multiple-dose charcoal is to prevent absorption of drugs from the GI tract, not to enhance their elimination from the blood. In the common case of tricyclic anti-depressant overdose, for example, multiple-dose charcoal should be used when large amounts of the antidepressant have been ingested to prevent its absorption but not necessarily to enhance its elimination. Many of these drugs have large volumes of distribution, and increasing elimination of the small amount present in the blood is unlikely to be of benefit.

Drugs with Altered Pharmacokinetics in Response to Multiple-dose Charcoal

Amitriptyline	Dextropropoxyphene	Meprobamate	Piroxicam
Atrazine	Diazepam	Methotrexate	Porphyrins
Carbamazepine	Digitoxin	Nadolol	Proscillaridin
Chlorpropamide	Digoxin	Nortriptyline	Quinine
Cyclosporine	Doxepin	Phenobarbital	Salicylates
Dapsone	Glutethimide	Phenylbutazone	Sotalol
Desmethyldiazepam	Imipramine	Phenytoin	Theophylline

7. Is forced diuresis of benefit in the treatment of acute poisoning?
Very few drugs are excreted unchanged in the urine, so that even increasing urine flow significantly above baseline is unlikely to be of benefit. However, by manipulating the pH of the urine by infusions of bicarbonate solution along with enhanced urine flow, in certain cases drug elimination can be increased. This is most commonly used for salicylates and phenobarbital. By placing 3 ampules of sodium bicarbonate in a liter of D5W along with potassium chloride, and infusing this solution at rates sufficient to produce at least a normal urine flow and a urine pH of 7.5 or greater, the elimination of salicylate and phenobarbital can be increased. Intake and output and urine pH should be monitored hourly with a Foley catheter in place. In the presence of pulmonary or cerebral edema, alkaline diuresis is dangerous and should not be undertaken.

There is some suggestion that alkaline diuresis will also work in a similar manner for chlorophenoxy herbicides, but acute poisonings by these agents are rare. The use of high-volume normal saline to treat lithium intoxication is common, and it is certainly important to maintain adequate urine output and serum sodium in this scenario. It is not clear, however, that forced-saline diuresis for lithium intoxication is of extra benefit over simply ensuring normal renal flow.

8. When are extracorporeal techniques such as hemodialysis or hemoperfusion indicated?
Drugs can be successfully removed by extracorporeal maneuvers only if they have relatively small volumes of distribution and hence are found in significant quantities in the circulation, as opposed to having rapid and thorough tissue distribution. This is the case for only a few drugs. In practice, the drugs most commonly dialyzed after overdose include aspirin, lithium, and perhaps theophylline. Dialysis has the advantage over hemoperfusion in that it is frequently easier and faster to get started and can correct fluid and electrolyte abnormalities as it removes drugs. Charcoal hemoperfusion may be more effective at removing drugs that are highly bound to plasma proteins, as the affinity for charcoal may be higher than the affinity for the protein carrier. The disadvantage of hemoperfusion is that unless frequently performed in skilled hands, the procedure can result in frequent canister clotting. In addition, hypocalcemia and a precipitous drop in platelet count are quite common. Drugs for which charcoal hemoperfusion is frequently employed include theophylline, phenobarbital, and a handful of other less common agents such as paraquat and amatoxin.

9. How can the diagnosis of a drug overdose be made when the patient is unconscious and history is unavailable?
The diagnosis of acute overdose is sometimes difficult to make and requires some detective work on the part of the physician. All unconscious patients should receive dextrose and naloxone (Narcan), and a positive response to either of these is diagnostic. Whenever possible, examination of the pill bottles available to the patient is important, and it is useful to call the pharmacies where the prescriptions were filled to determine if other prescriptions were filled there for different drugs. Discovering which chemical agents were available to the patient, including street drugs, is always important. If track marks are seen, consider street drugs commonly given intravenously such as opiates, cocaine, and amphetamine. The physical examination is extremely useful in narrowing the diagnosis to a class of drug or chemicals. This concept is commonly called toxic syndromes, the most common of which ar listed below.

The Most Common Toxic Syndromes

Anticholinergic

Common signs: dementia with mumbling speech, tachycardia, dry flushed skin, dilated pupils, myoclonus, temperature slightly elevated, urinary retention, decreased bowel sounds. Seizures and dysrhythmias may occur in severe cases.

Common causes: antihistamines, antiparkinsonism medication, atropine, scopolamine, amantadine, antipsychotics, antidepressants, antispasmodics, mydriatics, skeletal muscle relaxants, many plants (most notably jimson weed).

Sympathomimetic

Common signs: delusions, paranoia, tachycardia, hypertension, hyperpyrexia, diaphoresis, piloerection, mydriasis, hyperreflexia. Seizures and dysrhythmias may occur in severe cases.

Common causes: cocaine, amphetamine, methaphetamine (and derivatives MDA, MDMA, MDEA, DOB), over-the-counter decongestants (phenylpropanolamine, ephedrine, pseudoephedrine). Caffeine and theophylline overdoses cause similar findings secondary to catecholamine release, except for the organic psychiatric signs.

Table continued on next page.

The Most Common Toxic Syndromes (Cont.)

Opiate/Sedative

Common signs: coma, respiratory depression, miosis, hypotension, bradycardia, hypothermia, pulmonary edema, decreased bowel sounds, hyporeflexia, needle marks.

Common causes: narcotics, barbiturates, benzodiazepines, ethchlorvynol, glutethimide, methyprylon, methaqualone, meprobamate.

Cholinergic

Common signs: confusion/CNS depression, weakness, salivation, lacrimation, urinary and fecal incontinence, GI cramping, emesis, diaphoresis, muscle fasciculations, pulmonary edema, miosis, bradycardia (or tachycardia), seizures.

Common causes: organophosphate and carbamate insecticides, physostigmine, edrophonium, some mushrooms (*Amanita muscaria, Amanita pantherina,* Inocybe sp., Clitocybe sp.)

---

10. How can a toxicology screen and other ancillary lab tests make the diagnosis of acute poisoning?

Nontoxicologic laboratory tests that are frequently useful include the electrocardiogram, which can help diagnose overdose of tricyclic antidepressants or cardiac medications; chest radiograph, which if demonstrative of noncardiogenic pulmonary edema would make one think of salicylates or opiates; a KUB, looking for radiopaque material, which would make one suspicious of ingestion of a heavy metal, including iron, phenothiazines, chloral hydrate, or chlorinated hydrocarbon solvents. Liver function tests may help to diagnose ingestion of hepatotoxins such as acetaminophen or carbon tetrachloride. A urinalysis may demonstrate the presence of calcium oxalate crystals, suggesting the diagnosis of ethylene glycol poisoning. The acid-base status of the patient is extremely important. Persistent unexplained metabolic acidosis should always prompt the search for other diagnostic clues to aspirin, methanol, or ethylene glycol poisoning. Many other drugs can cause a persistent unexplained metabolic acidosis, including the ingestion of acids themselves, cyanide, carbon monoxide, theophylline, and others. In the work-up of persistent acidosis, a serum osmolality done by freezing point depression can be very useful if it is elevated. A difference between the measured osmolality and the calculated osmolality of greater than 10 is always significant, although a normal osmolol gap does not rule out toxic ingestion.

The toxicology screen, both blood and urine, should be done on any patient who has significant toxicity and when the diagnosis is uncertain. Alternatives to a full toxicology screen include testing discrete serum levels of the toxins in question, doing a urine qualitative test for drugs of abuse, or drawing specimens but holding them until it is determined that a toxicology screen is definitely indicated. More drugs and chemicals are *not* found on typical toxicology screens than *are* found on the screens, although the majority of drugs that are commonly ingested are found on comprehensive toxicology screens. It is important to communicate with the laboratory about which drugs are suspected, which drugs the patient takes therapeutically, and the clinical condition of the patient. Whenever there is a discrepancy between clinical suspicion and findings from toxicology screen, it is useful to communicate with the toxicology laboratory and assist them in determining if other tests are likely to be of benefit. Toxicology screens are expensive, frequently inexact, and frequently do not give all the information that is expected by the clinician. Therefore it is important to interpret the toxicology screens carefully and to know which drugs and chemicals were not screened for.

11. What are some other useful antidotes for common poisonings?

Naloxone and **dextrose** are the most common antidotes and should be given routinely to unconscious overdose patients. Intravenous administration of 2 mg of naloxone that results in awakening of the patient is diagnostic of acute opiate overdose. Lesser doses may be ineffective and should not be used unless it is known that the patient is an opiate addict and that the 2 mg dose of naloxone will precipitate withdrawal. Many drugs and chemicals can cause hypoglycemia, including ethanol, and for this reason dextrose should likewise be given.

Other common antidotes include **physostigmine** for the anticholinergic syndrome. Physostigmine should be used only when the diagnosis of the anticholinergic syndrome is certain, and should seldom if ever be used to treat tricyclic antidepressant poisoning. Seizures and bradydysrhythmias have been reported when used in this setting. A dose of 1–2 mg given slowly intravenously to an adult is usually sufficient.

Digoxin Immune Fab (Digibind) is a safe and effective antidote for digitalis glycoside poisoning and can rapidly reverse coma, dysrhythmias, and hyperkalemia, which can be life threatening. Unlike naloxone, however, Digibind does not work immediately and a full response to therapy may not be seen until approximately 20 minutes after administration. For a life-threatening digitalis overdose when the dose and the serum level are currently unknown, 10 vials of Digibind should be given.

Atropine and **pralidoxime (Protopam)** are antidotes used for cholinesterase inhibitor toxicity. This group of pesticides includes the organophosphates and carbamates, which are commonly found in even household insecticides. Atropine is used to dry up secretions, primarily pulmonary, and pralidoxime is used primarily to reverse the skeletal muscle toxicity of these agents, including weakness and fasciculations.

Flumazenil is a benzodiazepine antagonist that has been shown to be useful in cases of acute benzodiazepine overdose resulting in significant toxicity. Its approval by the FDA is currently pending.

BIBLIOGRAPHY

1. Hofer P, Scollo-Lavizzari G: Benzodiazepine antagonist Ro 15-1788 in self-poisoning: Diagnostic and therapeutic use. Arch Intern Med 145:663–664, 1985.
2. Hoffman RS, Smilkstein M, Goldfrank CR: Whole bowel irrigation and the cocaine body packer: A new approach to a common problem. Am J Emerg Med 8:523–527, 1990.
3. Kellerman AL, Fihn SD, Logerfro JP, et al: Impact of drug screening in suspected overdose. Ann Emerg Med 16:1206–1216, 1987.
4. Kulig KW, Bar-Or D, Cantrill SV, et al: Management of acutely poisoned patients without gastric emptying. Ann Emerg Med 14:562–567, 1985.
5. Litovitz TL, Schmitz BF, Bailey KM: 1989 Annual Report of the American Association of Poison Control Centers National Data Collection System. Am J Emerg Med 8:394–442, 1990.
6. Merigian KS, Woodard M, Hedges JR, et al: Prospective evaluation of gastric emptying in the self-poisoned patient. Am J Emerg Med 8:479–483, 1990.
7. Olson KR, Pentel PR, Kelley MT: Physical assessment and differential diagnosis of the poisoned patient. Med Toxicol 2:52–81, 1987.
8. Osterloh JD: Utility and reliability of emergency toxicologic testing. Emerg Med Clin North Am 8:693–723, 1990.
9. Smith TW, Butler VP Jr, Haber E, et al: Treatment of life-threatening digitalis intoxication with digoxin-specific Fab antibody fragments: Experience in 26 cases. N Engl J Med 307:1357–1362, 1982.
10. Tenenbein M, Cohen S, Sitar DS: Whole bowel irrigation as a decontamination procedure after acute drug overdose. Arch Intern Med 147:905–907, 1987.

115. ASPIRIN INTOXICATION

Ken Kulig, M.D.

1. Is salicylate intoxication a serious problem in adults? Isn't this a pediatric disease?
In a two-year review of salicylate deaths in Ontario published in 1987, 51 cases of salicylate deaths, all in adults, were discovered. Salicylate-caused deaths were more than twice as numerous as any other single drug death during that time. Despite the fact that many of these patients were obviously significantly salicylate toxic, unaggressive treatment, including not giving activated charcoal or instituting dialysis, resulted in fatal outcomes.

Aspirin intoxication is a serious adult problem, particularly when chronic toxicity occurs in the elderly, or when the diagnosis is delayed. Physicians get a false sense of security from seeing salicylate levels slowly decline, without recognizing that the reason for the decline may be that the salicylate is moving into tissues and thereby worsening toxicity. Salicylate intoxication resulting in mental status changes, pulmonary edema, or persistent metabolic acidosis should always be taken seriously and treated aggressively in an ICU.

2. What is the cause of death when patients die from salicylate intoxication?
Pulmonary edema and/or cerebral edema are the most common causes of death. Persistent severe metabolic acidosis may also contribute to the onset of ventricular dysrhythmias. In some patients, precipitous cardiovascular collapse occurs in the absence of obvious pulmonary or cerebral edema. This is generally a late finding seen in the hospital when the patient has been managed unaggressively for many hours.

3. What are the symptoms and signs of aspirin intoxication?
The earliest symptoms are usually nausea, vomiting, tachypnea (which may be perceived as dyspnea), and tinnitus. These symptoms are self-limited in mild or moderate intoxications. In severe poisonings, persistent vomiting (which may include hematemesis) may occur, and the patient gradually becomes more dyspneic as the acidosis and pulmonary problems worsen. Concomitant mental status changes including confusion, bizarre behavior, hallucinations, seizures and coma may occur. A mild coagulopathy can be seen with even a single acute ingestion of salicylates. Elevated hepatic enzymes can be seen if the ingestion was chronic.

4. What is the toxic dose of aspirin?
A dose of 150–300 mg/kg (or up to approximately 65 regular-strength tablets in an average-size adult) usually results in mild to moderate toxicity after a single acute ingestion; greater than this amount frequently results in more serious toxicity. Oil of wintergreen is a more dangerous source of salicylate—1 teaspoon contains the equivalent of 21 regular-strength adult aspirin tablets—thus oil of wintergreen intoxications must always be taken seriously. The toxic dose of aspirin during chronic therapy varies from individual to individual. The maximum recommeended dose is 8 regular-strength aspirin tablets per day for a normal size adult. Under certain conditions, doses exceeding this may result in cumulative toxicity of aspirin, and can be life threatening.

5. When should salicylate levels be drawn?
It is common practice to wait 6 hours after an acute overdose to draw an aspirin level, in order to plot the level on the Done nomogram. However, if the patient is symptomatic even several hours after an acute overdose, it is useful to draw an immediate salicylate level so

that therapy can begin prior to 6 hours. If the early level is nondetectable in cases of questionable overdose, then it is relatively certain that salicylate was not ingested. Most hospital laboratories can assess salicylate levels rapidly; in any symptomatic patient, getting a level back as soon as possible after presentation yields useful clinical information.

It is imperative that the correct units be used when interpreting levels. Therapeutic salicylate levels in patients taking aspirin for arthritis are 20–30 mg/dl. Some labs report salicylates in μg/ml. The coversion is mg/dl × 10 = μg/ml.

6. What is the Done nomogram? How should it be used?

The Done nomogram was developed by observing the kinetics of aspirin after overdose in children and in experimental animals. Based on extrapolated half-lives seen, the nomogram was touted to be predictive of degree of toxicity after a single acute aspirin overdose. The Done nomogram is frequently misused and misinterpreted. It should not be used when oil of wintergreen, enteric-coated aspirin tablets, or any of the newer variety of slow-release preparations are ingested. It should never be used in chronic aspirin ingestion. The nomogram should not be used to determine expected toxicity in the patient who is already significantly symptomatic. Finally, in all significant aspirin ingestions, at least two determinations of aspirin level are done to ensure that it is falling prior to hospital discharge. The clinical status of the patient is always more important than the salicylate level in guiding therapy.

7. What are the indications for alkaline diuresis to treat aspirin intoxication?

An alkaline diuresis is generally safe and quite effective at eliminating aspirin from the body. It should be undertaken in patients who are significantly symptomatic or who have significantly elevated salicylate levels (greater than 40 mg/dl). Adding 3 ampules of sodium bicarbonate to 1 liter of D5W and the appropriate amount of potassium (most aspirin-intoxicated patients are significantly potassium depleted) and running the fluid at a rate fast enough to induce a urine output at least 2 cc/kg/hr will greatly enhance the excretion of salicylate. Contraindications to alkaline diuresis include pulmonary edema, cerebral edema, or oliguric renal failure.

8. What are the indications for hemodialysis or hemoperfusion for aspirin poisoning?

Hemodialysis is recommended over hemoperfusion because, in addition to rapidly removing aspirin, it can correct electrolyte and acid-base disturbances. Indications for hemodialysis include cerebral edema, pulmonary edema, oliguric renal failure, or severe acid-base abnormalities that are not corrected with the usual measures.

9. Is there a role for multiple-dose charcoal after aspirin ingestion?

Aspirin tablets can form concretions in the GI tract. Because of their chemical nature, they tend to clump together and slowly release salicylate, which can result in steadily rising levels over long periods of time. For this reason, multiple-dose charcoal may be useful in significant ingestions. Charcoal also enhances the elimination of salicylate that has already been absorbed and hence can be used as an adjunct to alkaline diuresis or hemodialysis.

10. When can patients by safely discharged from the ICU after aspirin poisoning?

In addition to having a return to baseline mental status and pulmonary function, patients should have serial determinations of aspirin level to document that it is going down and that it has at least reached low therapeutic levels (15–20 mg/dl). Vital signs should be normal with no residual tachypnea and acid-base status should be normal. Even after having charcoal stools, some patients will continue to absorb aspirin from the GI tract, with late intoxication being seen. If the levels are not falling, the patient should be kept in the ICU.

BIBLIOGRAPHY

1. Anderson RJ, Potts DE, Gabow PA, et al: Unrecognized adult salicylate intoxication. Ann Intern Med 85:745–748, 1976.
2. Chapman BJ, Proudfoot AT: Adult salicylate poisoning: Deaths and outcome in patients with high plasma salicylate concentrations Q J Med 72:699–707, 1989.
3. Done AK: Salicylate intoxication: Significance of measurements of salicylates in blood in cases of acute ingestion. Pediatrics 26:800–807, 1960.
4. Dugandzic RM, Tierney MG, Dickinson GE, et al: Evaluation of the validity of the Done nomogram in the management of acute salicylate intoxication. Ann Emerg Med 18:1186–1190, 1989.
5. Gabow PA, Anderson RJ, Potts DE, et al: Acid-base disturbances in the salicylate-intoxicated adult. Arch Intern Med 138:1481–1484, 1978.
6. Hillman RJ, Prescott LF: Treatment of salicylate poisoning with repeated oral charcoal. Br Med J 291:1492, 1985.
7. Jacobsen D, Wiik-Larsen E, Bredesen JE. Haemodialysis or haemoperfusion in severe salicylate poisoning. Hum Toxicol 7:161–163, 1988.
8. McGuigan MA: A two-year review of salicylate deaths in Ontario. Arch Intern Med 147:510–512, 1987.
9. Prescott LF, Balali-Mood M, Critchley JA, et al: Diuresis or urinary alkalinazation for salicylate poisoning? Br Med J 285:1383–1386, 1982.
10. Riggs BS, Kulig K, Rumack B: Current status of aspirin and acetaminophen intoxication. Pediatr Ann 16:886–898, 1987.
11. Vertrees JE, McWilliams BC, Kelly HW: Repeated oral administration of activated charcoal for treating aspirin overdose in young children. Pediatrics 85:594–598, 1990.
12. Walters JS, Woodring JH, Stelling CB, et al: Salicylate-induced pulmonary edema. Radiology 146:289–293, 1983.
13. Wortzman DJ, Grunfeld A: Delayed absorption following enteric-coated aspirin overdose. Ann Emerg Med 16:434–436, 1987.

116. ACETAMINOPHEN OVERDOSE

Ken Kulig, M.D.

1. What are the symptoms and signs after acetaminophen overdose?

Patients are frequently asymptomatic for the first 8–12 hours after even a massive acetaminophen overdose. However, patients who have taken a very large overdose usually develop severe nausea and vomiting at 8–12 hours after ingestion, which can be protracted for the next several days. The skin color can be very pale or pale green, and the patient is frequently diaphoretic during this period of time. As the hepatic enzymes rise, generally beginning between 18 and 24 hours after ingestion, the liver may become enlarged and tender. In severe cases resulting in fulminant hepatic failure, encephalopathy and coma may be seen. Hypoglycemia should always be ruled out in patients with altered mental status after acetaminophen poisoning.

2. When should an acetaminophen level be obtained after an overdose?

The acetaminophen treatment nomogram can be used only after a single acute overdose when a plasma level is obtained between 4 and 24 hours after ingestion. Levels before 4 hours are difficult to interpret, although if the level is zero, the patient probably has not ingested acetaminophen at all. Levels that are high prior to 4 hours after ingestion may actually fall to below the nomogram line by the time the 4-hour level is obtained. If the time of ingestion is unknown, the acetaminophen level cannot be plotted on the nomogram line. In this case, clinical judgment only must decide whether the antidote is indicated.

3. Should activated charcoal be given after an acetaminophen overdose?

Activated charcoal effectively binds acetaminophen in the GI tract and, when given early enough, can ensure that the patient does not develop a toxic acetaminophen level and therefore require the antidote. Activated charcoal does not prevent the absorption of N-acetylcysteine (NAC, Mucomyst) to a significant degree unless very large doses of charcoal are given concurrently with the antidote. Even if a dose of activated charcoal has been given, antidotal therapy will probably still be effective. The activated charcoal administered does not have to be removed by lavage tube as previously thought. The dose of Mucomyst does not have to be increased after activated charcoal is given. Instead, the standard doses of 140 mg/kg loading dose followed by 70 mg/kg maintenance doses every 4 hours for 72 hours is sufficient therapy if administered early enough, regardless of the presence of activated charcoal.

4. How does the antidote work?

N-acetylcysteine (NAC, Mucomyst) is thought to work by a variety of mechanisms:

1. By acting as a glutathione surrogate, which detoxifies the toxic metabolite that is formed within liver cells.
2. By being converted to glutathione itself.
3. By blunting the inflammatory response that can contribute to hepatic necrosis.
4. By increasing sulfation of acetaminophen, which also prevents the formation of the toxic metabolite.

If the antidote is given within 8 hours of overdose, it is effective even if the overdose has been massive. If given between 16 and 24 hours after ingestion, it is less effective; and between 16 and 24 hours, it is less effective still. However, it is felt that Mucomyst may be of some benefit if started at least up to 24 hours, and in some cases may be useful if begun after 24 hours.

5. How should liver function tests be interpreted after an acetaminophen overdose?

It is not uncommon to see hepatic enzymes rise into the tens-of-thousands after an acute acetaminophen overdose without the development of life-threatening liver failure. When massive hepatic necrosis and hepatic encephalopathy develop, the hepatic enzymes are usually falling 3–5 days after the overdose, whereas the bilirubin and protime continue to rise. This finding is always of concern, particularly when the bilirubin rises above 5 and the protime rises above 20 seconds. At that time, standard therapy for hepatic failure should be instituted.

6. When can the antidote be stopped?

Sufficient data have been gathered in the United States only for the 72-hour oral NAC protocol and the 48-hour IV NAC protocol. No published studies demonstrate that the antidote can be stopped once acetaminophen levels have fallen below the nomogram line. There is some suggestion that this practice is unsafe and can result in late development of hepatic toxicity. The 20-hour IV NAC protocol used in Canada and Europe is probably effective for many patients, but is thought not to be as effective as the two longer protocols used in the United States. NAC should be stopped only when either the 72-hour oral protocol or the 48-hour IV protocol has been completed.

7. Should liver transplant be considered after massive acetaminophen overdose?

The majority of patients who develop even major biochemical evidence of liver damage after acetaminophen overdose do well with supportive and antidotal therapy. However, in a subset of patients who have taken a massive overdose and present to the hospital very late, fulminant hepatic necrosis and death from liver failrue can occur. Patients who have elevated and rising bilirubin levels and protimes and are becoming encephalopathic should be considered candidates for liver transplantation. Allowing the liver transplanation center to participate in the decision early ensures that the possible liver transplant is done expeditiously if required.

8. Is there a role for hemodialysis or hemoperfusion after acetaminophen overdose?
N-acetylcysteine works extremely well in preventing hepatic toxicity if given early enough after an overdose. Even when acetaminophen levels are very high, patients treated early enough with the antidote are not candidates for hemodialysis or hemoperfusion. However, patients who present very late (i.e., 18–24 hours after ingestion) who still have high levels of circulating acetaminophen (i.e., greater then 150 μg/ml) may be considered candidates for dialysis or hemoperfusion. If the procedure is done, it will remove only the acetaminophen that is circulating, which may comprise a fraction of the total dose suggested. It is not clear if removing that amount of drug will improve prognosis; however, because the antidote does not work well when administered very late, extracorporeal techniques to remove the drug may be warranted in very select cases.

9. Does ethanol ingestion alter the prognosis in acetaminophen-poisoned patients?
The role of ethanol in acetaminophen hepatic toxicity is controversial. Chronic ethanol abuse stimulates the P-450 pathway in the liver, which is the pathway responsible for the formation of the toxic metabolite of acetaminophen. However, ethanol itself is partially metabolized by that pathway, and hence competitively inhibits the acetaminophen being metabolized to the toxic metabolite at the same time. It is not clear that chronic alcoholics who ingest a therapeutic dose of acetaminophen (up to 1 gm/dose and the maximum of 4 gm/day) are at increased risk of developing hepatic toxicity. The maximum daily dose for acetaminophen should not be exceeded by either alcoholics or nonalcoholics.

BIBLIOGRAPHY

1. Corcoran GB, Todd EL, Raez WJ, et al: Effects of N-acetylcysteine on the disposition and metabolism of acetaminophen in mice. J Pharmcol Exp Ther 232:857–863, 1985.
2. Hamlyn AN, Douglas AP, James O: The spectrum of paracetamol (acetaminophen) overdose: Clinical and epidemiological studies. Postgrad Med J 54:400–404, 1978.
3. Lin JH, Levy G: Sulfate depletion after acetaminophen administration and replenishment by infusion of sodium sulfate or N-acetylcysteine in rates. Biochem Pharmacol 30:2723–2725, 1981.
4. Linden CH, Rumack BH: Acetaminophen overdose. Emerg Med Clin North Am 2:103–119, 1984.
5. Prescott LF, Illingworth RN, Critchley JA, et al: Intravenous N-acetylcysteine: The treatment of choice for paracetamol poisoning. Br Med J 2:1097–1100, 1979.
6. Prescott LF: Paracetamol overdosage: Pharmacological considerations and clinical management. Drugs 25:290–314, 1983.
7. Rumack BH, Peterson RC, Koch GC, Amara IA: Acetaminophen overdose: 662 cases with evaluation of oral acetylcysteine treatment. Arch Intern Med 141:380–385, 1981.
8. Rumack BH, Matthew H: Acetaminophen poisoning and toxicity. Pediatrics 55:871–876, 1975.
9. Slattery JT, Wilson JM, Kalhorn TF, Nelson SD: Dose-dependent pharmacokinetics of acetaminophen: Evidence of glutathione depletion in humans. Clin Pharmacol Ther 41:413–418, 1987.
10. Smilkstein MJ, Knapp GL, Kulig KW, Rumack BH: Efficacy of oral N-acetylcysteine in the treatment of acetaminophen overdose. N Engl J Med 319:1557–1562, 1988.

117. ANTIDEPRESSANT POISONING

Ken Kulig, M.D.

1. Why are antidepressant overdoses so common?
Antidepressants obviously are prescribed to depressed individuals, who constitute the patient population most likely to overdose in a suicide attempt. It is ironic that some of the most dangerous drugs available, the tricyclic antidepressants, are among those prescribed to depressed individuals. Worldwide, tricyclics probably account for more oral overdose deaths than any other drug class.

2. What are the symptoms and signs after antidepressant overdose?
Very typically, the earliest signs are initial lethargy and perhaps anticholinergic symptoms, including tachycardia and dry mouth. Very rapidly, however, the clinical condition of the patient can deteriorate to include respiratory depression, seizures, myoclonic jerking, hypotension, significant conduction delay, and life-threatening cardiac arrhythmias. This has been termed "catastrophic deterioration," whereby patients can walk into the emergency room with normal vital signs and within 1 hour develop significant life-threatening toxicity.

3. What is the mechanism of death after tricyclic antidepressant overdose?
Up to 80% of fatalities from tricyclic antidepressant overdoses never reach medical attention and victims of overdose are found dead in homes, cars, hotel rooms, etc. Of those who are seen in a hospital, the most common scenario leading to death is a rapid deterioration of vital signs, widening of the QRS on the electrocardiogram, falling blood pressure, and seizures that result in metabolic acidosis, which then makes the cardiac toxicity of the tricyclics worse. Pulseless idioventricular rhythm or asystole then ensues.

4. Are serum levels of tricyclic antidepressants useful?
Serum levels frequently do not correlate well with clinical toxicity, but may be of general academic interest or of forensic interest if the time of the overdose is important. In general, tricyclic antidepressant serum levels greater than 1000 ng/ml usually correspond to life-threatening toxicity. However, levels significantly less than this, even 500 ng/ml, may result in significant CNS and respiratory depression. Many tricyclic antidepressants have active metabolites and the toxicology laboratory will measure these as well. Amitriptyline is metabolized to nortriptyline and imipramine is metabolized to desipramine. Having a higher concentration of the metabolite than the parent compound implies that the overdose occurred many hours previously.

5. Of what value is the electrocardiogram in a patient with normal vital signs after an antidepressant overdose?
Cardiac toxicity can be seen on the electrocardiogram even before significant CNS or respiratory depression occurs. Earliest findings consist of a rightward deflection of the terminal 40 msec portion of the QRS complex, followed by widening of the QRS itself. Widening of the QRS can occur in the absence of other significant toxicity, and means that the patient is more likely subsequently to develop seizures and/or ventricular dysrhythmias. In an unconscious patient in whom the diagnosis is uncertain, seeing a conduction delay on the EKG is useful in diagnosing antidepressant overdose.

6. Which patients need to be admitted after an antidepressant overdose?
Any patient with significant toxicity after tricyclic antidepressant overdose should be admitted to the ICU. It is quite common, however, to see patients with only minimal

disturbances in mental status and with normal EKGs (excluding sinus tachycardia) many hours after an overdose. Persistent resting tachycardia or persistent lethargy should be construed as indicating significant toxicity, and these patients should be admitted to the ICU as well.

7. When can patients safely be discharged from the ICU?

Patients can leave the ICU when all symptoms and signs of major toxicity have resolved, and the EKG, vital signs, and mental status are back to baseline for at least 12 hours. Late dysrhythmias have been reported. These generally occur in patients who have previously had life-threatening toxicity that has not resolved completely.

8. How should GI decontamination be performed in patients after tricyclic antidepressant overdose?

Syrup of ipecac is always contraindicated after tricyclic antidepressant overdose. Patients can become comatose so quickly that they may be unconscious by the time emesis results. Gastric lavage may be of benefit if performed soon after an overdose, but, on the other hand, the lavage fluid may also move tablets through the pylorus and into the small intestines. As a general rule, activated charcoal should always be administered as quickly as possible, either orally down a nasogastric tube, or down the oral gastric hose prior to gastric lavage being performed.

9. Is there a role for multiple-dose charcoal after antidepressant poisoning?

Although some data suggest that the elimination kinetics of the tricyclics can be altered by multiple-dose charcoal, this is not the primary reason to use multiple-dose charcoal. Tricyclic antidepressants have anticholinergic properties, slow gastric emptying, and decreased intestinal peristalsis. After a large overdose of tricyclic antidepressants, it is imperative to give enough charcoal to adsorb all of the drug found in the GI tract. Hence, multiple doses of charcoal, although they may or may not alter elimination kinetics, may be useful to prevent absorption of drug. Multiple-dose charcoal must always be used with care in the unconscious patient and should not be used if bowel sounds are absent. Multiple-dose cathartics should not be used; however, a single dose of a cathartic with the first dose of charcoal may be useful.

10. How should tricyclic antidepressant seizures be treated?

Initial therapy is identical to the treatment of seizures from other causes. IV diazepam may stop the seizure, but IV phenytoin and/or phenobarbital should also be administered to prevent further seizures. Seizures after antidepressant poisoning are particularly dangerous because they cause acidemia, which makes the cardiac toxicity of the tricyclics worse. Therefore, prevention of seizures is crucial. If the patient has already demonstrated life-threatening toxicity, including conduction disturbances on the EKG, seizure prophylaxis may be indicated. If conservative measures (including diazepam, phenytoin, and phenobarbital) do not stop antidepressant-induced seizures within 1–2 minutes, the patient should be paralyzed or given general anesthesia. Continuous, or at least intermittent, EEG monitoring should be done in these cases.

11. How should the cardiovascular toxicity of antidepressants be treated?

Sinus tachycardia by itself does not require treatment. A conduction disturbance on the EKG may respond to intravenous boluses of sodium bicarbonate. Use of phenytoin in this setting is controversial, but there is some evidence that it enhances cardiac conduction and/or prevents seizures in this setting. Slow bicarbonate infusion by putting it in the maintenance IV solution has not been shown to be of benefit. Patients who are intubated should be hyperventilated to keep the arterial pH in the range of 7.45–7.55. Ventricular dysrhythmias can be treated with lidocaine and perhaps bretylium; however, class IA antiarrhythmics (e.g., quinidine) should be avoided.

12. Are the newer antidepressants of different toxicity than the older tricyclics?

Many new antidepressants are on the market and their toxicity does seem to be different. Amoxapine (Asendin) has little or no cardiac toxicity but does seem to cause a higher incidence of seizures and status epilepticus. Trazodone (Desyrel) has little cardiac or CNS toxicity. Fluoxetine (Prozac) likewise appears to have little toxicity after overdose. Large clinical series of overdoses of these agents are currently being collected.

BIBLIOGRAPHY

1. Boehnert MT, Lovejoy FH: Value of the QRS duration versus the serum drug level in predicting seizures and ventricular arrhythmias after an acute overdose of tricyclic antidepressants. N Engl J Med 313:474–479, 1985.
2. Callahan M, Kassel D: Epidemiology of fatal tricyclic antidepressant ingestion: Implications for management. Ann Emerg Med 14:1–9, 1985.
3. Caravati EM, Bossart PJ: Demographic and electrocardiographic factors associated with severe tricyclic antidepressant toxicity. Clin Toxicol 29:31–43, 1991.
4. Foulke GE, Albertson TE: QRS interval in tricyclic antidepressant overdosage: Inaccuracy as a toxicity indicator in emergency settings. Ann Emerg Med 16:160–163, 1987.
5. Foulke GE, Albertson TE, Walby WF: Tricyclic antidepressant overdose: Emergency department findings as predictors of clinical course. Am J Emerg Med 4:496–500, 1986.
6. Frommer DA, Kulig KW, Marx JA, Rumack B: Tricyclic antidepressant overdose: A review. JAMA 257:521–526, 1987.
7. Lavoie FW, Gansert GG, Weiss RE: Value of initial ECG findings and plasma drug levels in cyclic antidepressant overdose. Ann Emerg Med 19:696–700, 1990.
8. Niemann JT, Bessen HA, Rothstein RJ, Laks MM: Electrocardiographic criteria for tricyclic antidepressant cardiotoxicity. Am J Cardiol 57:1154–1159, 1986.
9. Vernon DA, Banner W Jr, Garrett JS, Dean JM: Efficacy of dopamine and norepinephrine for treatment of hemodynamic compromise in amitriptyline intoxication. Crit Care Med 19:544, 1991.
10. Wolfe TR, Caravati EM, Rollins DE: Terminal 40-ms frontal plane QRS axis as a marker for tricyclic antidepressant overdose. Ann Emerg Med 18:348–351, 1989.

INDEX